53.38

2804315175

AF443701

Tumors of the Fetus and Newborn

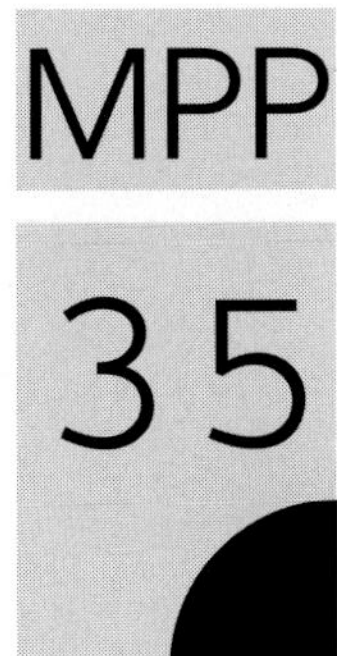

MPP
35

HART ISAACS, JR., M.D.
Attending Pathologist
Children's Hospital San Diego
Associate Clinical Professor of Pathology
University of California, San Diego
San Diego, California

Tumors of the Fetus and Newborn

Volume 35 in the Series
MAJOR PROBLEMS IN PATHOLOGY

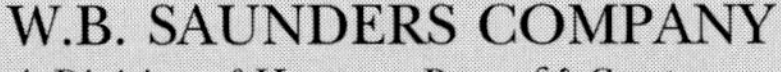

W.B. SAUNDERS COMPANY
A Division of Harcourt Brace & Company
PHILADELPHIA LONDON TORONTO MONTREAL SYDNEY TOKYO

W.B. SAUNDERS COMPANY
A Division of Harcourt Brace & Company

The Curtis Center
Independence Square West
Philadelphia, Pennsylvania 19106

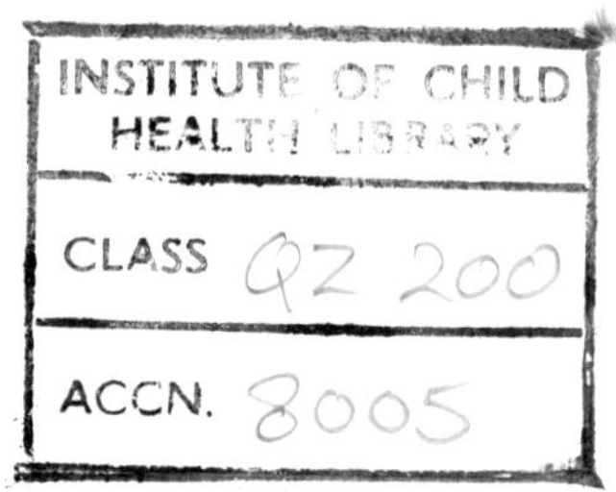

Library of Congress Cataloging-in-Publication Data

Isaacs, Hart.
    Tumors of the fetus and newborn / Hart Isaacs, Jr.
      p.   cm. — (Major problems in pathology ; v. 35)
    Includes index.
    ISBN 0–7216–3813–9
    1. Tumors in children. 2. Infants—Diseases. 3. Infants
(Newborn)—Diseases. I. Title. II. Series.
    [DNLM: 1. Neoplasms—in infancy & childhood. 2. Fetal
Diseases—pathology. 3. Infant, Newborn, Diseases—pathology.
W1 MA492X v.35 1997 / QZ 275 I73t 1997]
RC281.C4I73   1997
618.92′992—dc21
DNLM/DLC
                                              96–38016

NOTICE

Medicine is an ever-changing field. Standard safety precautions must be followed, but as new research and clinical experience broaden our knowledge, changes in treatment and drug therapy become necessary or appropriate. Readers are advised to check the product information currently provided by the manufacturer of each drug to be administered to verify the recommended dose, the method and duration of administration, and contraindications. It is the responsibility of the treating physician relying on the experience and knowledge of the patient to determine dosages and the best treatment for the patient. Neither the publisher nor the editor assumes any responsibility for any injury and/or damage to persons or property.

THE PUBLISHER

TUMORS OF THE FETUS AND NEWBORN   ISBN 0-7216-3813-9

Last digit is the print number: 9   8   7   6   5   4   3   2   1

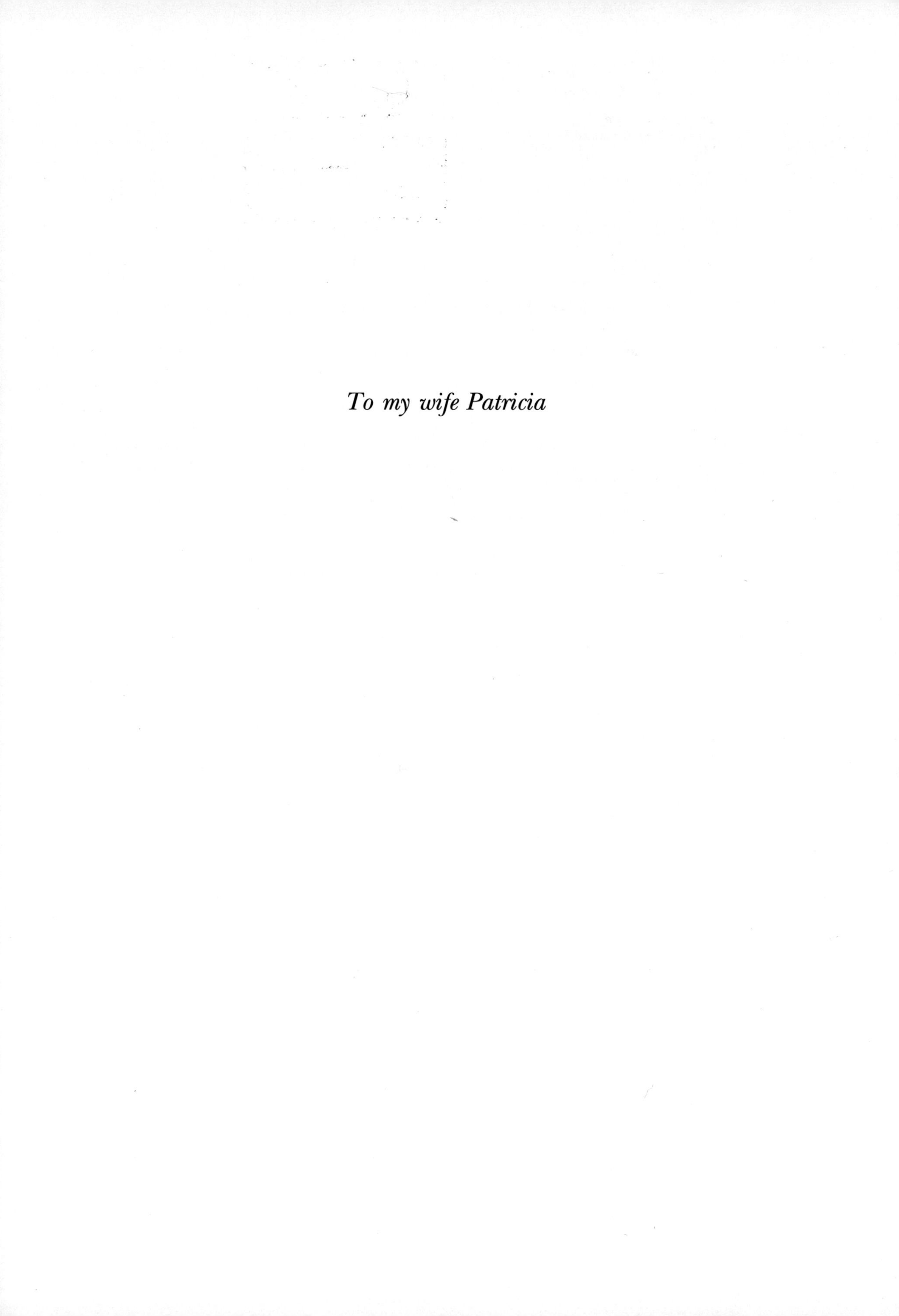

To my wife Patricia

Preface

The purpose of this book is to present an account of the clinical and pathologic features of neoplastic disease and tumor-like conditions in the fetus and newborn. For the past 30 years, I have been intensely interested in this subject. This work is not only a record of my own experience in children's hospitals for more than a quarter of a century but also a comprehensive review of the literature on this subject. Most illustrations have been produced from cases that I have personally studied.

The notable development of neonatology during the past several decades has been accompanied by an awakening interest in perinatal pathology and the recognition of it as a special branch of pathology. Antenatal sonography has enabled the clinician to detect congenital malformations and tumors before birth (see Table 1–2). As a result, a demand has arisen for the services of pathologists who are interested in and familiar with the problems of disease in early life. The neoplasms that affect the fetus and newborn are, in certain respects, different from those encountered at any later age, and they are perhaps the ones most likely to cause difficulty for a pathologist unfamiliar with them. I have attempted to illustrate the various tumors of the young as comprehensively as possible.

The proper handling and processing of tumor specimens, the work-up of the "small cell malignant tumor," and the importance of chromosomal analysis, postmortem examination, and inspection of the placenta have been covered in a previous work* and thus will not be discussed here. Although this book is intended primarily for pathologists, I have endeavored to keep its contents not too far removed from clinical application. It is hoped that it will be of some interest and benefit to obstetricians, pediatricians, pediatric surgeons, and radiologists as well.

Finally, this book is an attempt to provide a basis for the study of neoplasms in the fetus and newborn and to familiarize the pathologist and clinician with these unique tumors and tumor-like conditions. The ultimate goal here is to help the pathologist and clinician achieve an accurate diagnosis and a clear understanding of these lesions so that the proper treatment can be initiated.

Medicine to produce health, has to examine disease . . .
Lives, Demetrius, sec 1.

HART ISAACS, JR., M.D.

---

*Isaacs H Jr: Tumors of the Newborn and Infant. St. Louis, Mosby–Year Book, 1991.

Acknowledgments

I wish to thank my colleagues and friends who have helped me in various ways during the preparation of this book, as well as all who have allowed me to use illustrations from their published work and the publishers of journals and books from which they have been produced. Particular thanks are due Dr. Henry Krous, who gave much time and took much trouble to meet my needs. Dr. Jon Rowland kindly provided me with case material from the Children's Hospital of Los Angeles. The help given me by Darkin Chan and Ann Peters with the electron photomicrographs has been invaluable. I want also to thank the staff at W.B. Saunders, especially Lesley Day, and Joan Saidel for their helpfulness in the preparation and production of this book.

Contents

ETIOLOGY AND INCIDENCE

1

Although tumors of the fetus and newborn are uncommon, they present challenging diagnostic and treatment problems.[1,30,35,38,53,64,101,108] Unfamiliarity with these conditions may lead to an erroneous diagnosis and unnecessarily aggressive treatment.[11,66] Perinatal tumors are not entirely the same as those observed in the adolescent or adult, for the types, incidence, clinical features, behavior, and response to treatment are different (Tables 1–1, 1–2, and 1–3).[4,6,8,9,11,18,22,24,26,30,37,39,50,61–66,87,101,130,148,152,153] Invariably, there is considerable dilemma and terrible parental apprehension when dealing with a tumor in a newborn.

A special problem exists in the histologic distinction between benign and malignant neoplasms occurring before birth. All cell proliferation takes place rapidly in utero, and it may be difficult to determine by examination of tissue immediately after birth whether the cells have been growing independently with complete lack of restraint, which is characteristic of a malignant neoplasm, or whether their growth, although abnormal, has been subject to the same restraining influences as the rest of the body.[106]

No tumor of the adult grows as rapidly as does the normal embryo. Particularly in the early stages of development, normal embryonic cells may have some of the characteristics of neoplastic cells.[106] Generally, pathologists establish a diagnosis of malignant disease based on certain histologic criteria, but these are not always helpful or valid in the young. Several factors must be taken into account. First, normally developing organs and tissues show increased mitotic activity and have immature or embryonic-appearing structures that mimic malignant neoplasms. Because of this, it may be difficult, by microscopic examination of tissue

removed from the fetus or newborn, to determine whether the proliferating cells represent normally differentiating structures or a neoplastic process (see Figs. 4–1, 4–10, and 4–28). Histologic evidence of a malignant tumor is not always a reliable indicator of tumor behavior or prognosis; therefore, any study of perinatal tumors should include both histologically benign and malignant neoplasms.[106] Tumors that are not histologically malignant may cause death because of their location, as in the case of a large lymphangioma, fibromatosis, or mature teratoma involving vital structures in the neck, mediastinum, or brain.[66] Therefore, the pathologist must be familiar with tumors and tumor-like conditions occurring in the young so that the correct diagnosis can be made and the proper treatment begun.

Both benign and malignant neoplasms manifest unique clinical and pathologic findings in the fetus and newborn (see Table 1–3). Establishing a correlation between these findings is necessary not only to diagnose the tumor accurately but also to predict its behavior. It is often only from knowledge of the postnatal course of a tumor that definite proof can be obtained of its malignancy. For example, neuroblastomas are usually considered to be malignant, but some have been observed in which neuroblasts differentiate postnatally into mature ganglion cells or regress and do not behave like a malignant tumor.

Occasionally, it is difficult, if not impossible, to distinguish between certain tumors, congenital malformations, and hamartomas.[11,39,106] Teratoma, melanocytic nevi, nephrogenic rests, and benign soft tissue vascular lesions are examples of this dilemma. The question as to whether the hemangioma, the most common

1

Table 1–1. Comparison of 11 Surveys Consisting of 795 Fetal and Newborn Tumors

Tumor	RWHM	SJCRH	MDA	CHB	CHSD (1983–1994)	CCRG	HSC	CHOP	CHLA (1960–1991)	DCR	RHSC	Total Tumors
Neuroblastoma	6 (13.0)*	19 (55.9)	6 (25)	31 (18)	8 (10.8)	27 (26.7)	48 (47.0)	11 (50)	36 (21.6)	20 (26)	7 (13.7)	219 (27.5)
Teratoma	24 (52.2)	2 (5.9)	—	49 (29)	15 (20.3)	16 (15.8)	—	3 (13.6)	62 (37.1)†	6 (8)	19 (37.2)	196 (24.7)
Leukemia	—	6 (17.6)	3 (12.5)	21 (12)	5 (6.8)	17 (16.8)	8 (7.8)	3 (13.6)	18 (10.8)	12 (16)	—	93 (11.7)
Sarcoma	—	—	8 (33)	17 (10)	5 (6.8)	13 (12.9)	12 (11.8)	3 (13.6)	8 (4.8)	11 (14)	8 (15.7)	82 (10.3)
Brain tumor	5 (10.9)	—	3 (12.5)	14 (8)	11 (14.9)	12 (11.9)	9 (8.8)	—	15 (9.0)	8 (11)	—	74 (9.3)
Renal tumor	2 (4.3)	2 (5.9)	—	8 (5)	1 (1.3)	8 (7.9)	4 (3.9)	1 (4.6)	6 (3.6)	4 (5)	9 (17.6)	45 (5.7)
Liver tumor	1 (2.2)	—	—	8 (5)	5 (6.8)	3 (3.0)	1 (1)	—	18 (10.8)	2 (3)	3 (5.9)	41 (5.1)
Retinoblastoma	—	3 (8.9)	2 (8)	14 (8)	—	—	17 (16.7)	—	4 (2.4)	2 (3)	3 (5.9)	45 (5.7)
Total in Study‡	46	34	24	170	74	101	102	22	167	65	51	795 (100)

Abbreviation key for institutions and references: CCRG, Childhood Cancer Research Group, Oxford;[26] HSC, The Hospital for Sick Children, Toronto, Canada;[30] CHOP, Children's Hospital of Philadelphia;[53] CHLA, Children's Hospital Los Angeles; DCR, Danish Cancer Registry;[24] RWHM, The Royal Women's Hospital and The Mercy Hospital for Women, Melbourne, Victoria, Australia;[145] SJCRH, St. Jude Children's Research Hospital;[35] MDA, M.D. Anderson Hospital;[31] CHB, Children's Hospital, Birmingham, U.K.;[101] RHSC, Royal Hospital for Sick Children, Glasgow, Scotland;[38] CHSD, Children's Hospital San Diego.

*The number in parentheses represents the percent of total cases included in that institution's study.

†2 of 62 were malignant.

‡This figure is the total number of cases recorded for that particular institution's study, not the total number included in the columns in the table.

congenital soft tissue mass, represents a tumor, hamartoma, or congenital malformation has not been settled completely.[43]

Hamartoma is defined as a benign mass lesion composed of cells that are not cytologically abnormal in terms of those ordinarily found at the site of origin. On the basis of this definition, I believe that most hemangiomas represent hamartomas, rather than true neoplasms. *Choristoma* is a term reserved for tissue that is histologically normal for an organ or part other than the one in which it is located. Furthermore, non-neoplastic conditions may mimic tumors. The entities presenting as an abdominal mass in the neonate are a good example of this diagnostic problem (see Table 1–2).

Although the manifestations of some perinatal neoplasms are similar to those of neoplasms observed in the older child, there are notable differences. Correlation of the clinical and pathologic findings is necessary not only to accurately diagnose the tumor in question but also to predict its behavior. A neoplasm of identical histology may have a distinctly different

Table 1–2. Differential Diagnosis and Distribution of Abdominal Masses in the Newborn

Gastrointestinal (15%)	*Urinary* (55%)	*Genital* (15%)
Intestinal atresia	Megacystis	Hydrocolpos
Imperforate anus	Hydronephrosis	Ovarian cyst(s)
Meconium plug	Hydroureter	Granulosa cell tumor
Meconium ileus	Urachal cyst	Ovarian torsion
(Cystic fibrosis)	Urachal diverticulum	
Meconium cyst	Multicystic kidney	
Intestinal duplication	Polycystic kidneys	
Mesenteric cyst	Renomegaly (renal vein thrombosis)	
Lymphangioma	Mesoblastic nephroma	
Intussusception	Wilms' tumor	
Pyloric stenosis	Rhabdoid tumor	
Gastric teratoma		
	Adrenal (5%)	
Liver and Bile Ducts (5%)	Neuroblastoma	
Hemangioma	Hematoma	
Mesenchymal hamartoma	Cyst	
Hepatoblastoma		
Polycystic disease	*Miscellaneous* (5%)	
Choledochal cyst	Sacrococcygeal or retroperitoneal teratoma	
Simple cyst	Anterior meningomyelocele	
Subcapsular hematoma	Splenic hematoma	
Metastatic neuroblastoma, leukemia	Splenic cyst	

Data from Kirks DR, et al.;[70a] Koop CE;[74a] Schwartz MZ, Shaul DB.[121a]

Table 1–3. Unusual Clinical Presentations
of Perinatal Tumors

Maternal Dystocia

Teratoma
Neuroblastoma
Congenital mesoblastic nephroma
Astrocytoma
Ependymoma
Sialoblastoma

Fetal Hydrops

Teratoma
Neuroblastoma
Congenital mesoblastic nephroma
Wilms' tumor
Hepatoblastoma
Cardiac rhabdomyoma
Glioblastoma multiforme
Primitive neuroectodermal tumor
Lymphangioma (cystic hygroma)
Hemangioma
Neurofibroma

Rupture of Tumor during Delivery with Fatal Exsanguination

Teratoma
Neuroblastoma
Hepatoblastoma
Hepatic hemangioma

Congestive Heart Failure Shortly after Birth

Arteriovenous malformation
Cavernous hemangioma
Teratoma
Congenital mesoblastic nephroma
Glioblastoma multiforme
Cardiac rhabdomyoma
Cardiac myxoma
Cardiac fibroma

Polyhydramnios

Teratoma
Hemangioma
Congenital mesoblastic nephroma
Wilms' tumor
Astrocytoma
Bronchopulmonary fibrosarcoma

From Arceci RJ, Weinstein HJ. Neoplasia. *In* Avery GB, Fletcher MA, MacDonald MG (eds): Neonatology: Pathophysiology and Management in the Newborn, 4th ed, p 1211. Philadelphia: JB Lippincott, 1994. Used by permission.

prognosis in a newborn infant as compared to an older child or adolescent. For example, acute lymphocytic leukemia has a much worse prognosis in a newborn.[30,33,47,108,109] The overall survival for the older child with this disease is more than 50%, as compared to practically 0% in the neonate. Conversely, infants with neuroblastoma, particularly those with metastatic stage IV-S disease, generally have a more favorable outcome than do older children.[25,44,45,108]

Perinatal tumors also differ in their present-ing clinical signs and symptoms as compared to those found in older individuals (see Table 1–3).[6,11,66] Maternal dystocia may be the first sign of a large, space-occupying congenital tumor, such as a giant intracranial or retroperitoneal teratoma. The fetal circulation may determine the pattern of metastasis observed at birth.[30,146] Fetal hydrops is another unique manifestation.[68,69,88,95,135,140] Rupture of a large tumor, such as a neuroblastoma or hepatoblastoma, during delivery, with fatal exsanguination of the fetus, is a dramatic illustration of another unusual presentation.

Antenatal diagnosis of tumors is one aspect of fetal care that has recently come to the forefront, allowing insight into the prenatal natural history, pathophysiology, and prognosis of these neoplasms.[54] Advances in imaging techniques, particularly in ultrasonography, have made this possible. Tumors diagnosed most often by antenatal ultrasonography are teratomas, mesoblastic nephroma, liver tumors, and neuroblastoma.[54,79,110–112,140,145,147] The antenatal diagnosis of a neoplasm has important implications for maternal and fetal welfare and for neonatal prognosis.[54] Suspicion of a fetal tumor depends on either sonographic evidence of the fetal abnormality or on maternal effects from the fetal neoplasm.[96] The detection of a tumor alerts the obstetrician to the possible risk for both fetal and maternal disease. Moreover, the discovery of a fetal tumor allows close surveillance by the obstetrician, neonatologist, and pediatric surgeon, as well as anticipation and early recognition of problems during the perinatal period. In utero treatment for the fetus at risk may be considered, but this form of therapy is still in the developmental stages.[54,140]

An Australian perinatal study revealed several important findings: (1) a significant association between malformations and congenital tumors (20%), particularly teratomas; (2) a high frequency of polyhydramnios (33%), which was often the first hint of a congenital tumor; and (3) 17% incidence of a hydrops fetalis, frequently accompanying polyhydramnios.[145] Often, the initial sign of a congenital tumor during pregnancy is polyhydramnios (see Table 1–3).[145] In a study of 46 perinatal tumors conducted by Werb et al., 15 (33%) of the tumors presented with this finding; in two thirds of these cases, the polyhydramnios was attributable to teratomas. These researchers attributed the polyhydramnios to difficulties in the fetal swallowing mechanism, resulting in decreased absorption of amniotic fluid from the gastrointestinal tract. Intracranial teratomas affecting the neural control of swallowing, or epignathi producing mechanical obstruction, were found to be responsible.[145] Hydrops fetalis associated with polyhydramnios was noted in 8 (17%) of the fetuses and newborns in this perinatal study. Hydrops occurred with teratomas, vascular lesions, and cardiac rhabdomyoma. The authors identified the causes of hydrops as circulatory obstruction, leaky tumor vessels, or cardiac dysfunction associated with rhabdomyoma.

Prior to the critical review of congenital tumors by Wells in 1940, it was difficult to determine the accuracy of a large number of reports on this subject.[144] Older published articles were often unsatisfactory and unreliable. Indeed, even now, the varied use of the terms infant and congenital in the literature makes it difficult to conduct an accurate search. Moreover, as Wells pointed out, reporting instances of cancer in adolescents and adults arising from a nevus present at birth as congenital further adds to the nosologic confusion.[144] Therefore, some terms should be defined to ensure accurate communication in this book.

Neoplasms noted at birth and during the first month of life are defined as *congenital* neoplasms, but it is reasonable to assume that any tumor found in the first 3 months of life is congenital.[11] The term *perinatal* pertains to the period shortly before and after birth, and applies to both the fetus and neonate. The *neonatal period* is defined as the first month of life, whereas *infancy* refers to the first year of life. However, in an attempt to include clinically silent tumors that were undoubtedly present at birth and in the neonatal period, this book focuses on patients up to 3 months of age. Clearly, the distinction between a congenital and an acquired tumor identified in the first year of life is difficult. In this text, a *newborn* is defined as a recently born infant, one who is 3 months of age or younger. For the purposes of this discussion, the term *tumor* applies not only to true neoplasms, but also to some tumor-like conditions.

Malignant tumors of the young are sometimes generally referred to as *embryomas* (or embryonic tumors), as initially proposed by Willis[149] and by Bolande,[20,22] Morison,[90] and Wigglesworth.[148] This terminology is based on the microscopic resemblance of these tumors to early phases in the development of the organ or tissue of origin. Embryomas—specifically, Wilms' tumor, retinoblastoma, hepatoblastoma, neuroblastoma, medulloblastoma and rhabdomyosarcoma—are the malignant neoplasms most frequently encountered in early childhood. According to Bolande, some of these neoplasms exhibit a high rate of cytodifferentiation, regression, and benign tendencies.[19,20,22] Furthermore, it should be pointed out that most embryomas are not actually observed at birth or in the first 2 months of life, as initially proposed by Willis, but may be found later in childhood. It is also conceivable that neoplastic transformation could occur during embryogenesis and persist. This might explain the relationship of certain embryonic-appearing lesions, such as Wilms' tumor in situ (nephrogenic rests) or neuroblastoma in situ, to the development of their respective malignant counterparts later on.[22,123]

Blastoma is another term used to denote an embryonic tumor. For example, a pulmonary blastoma is a malignant tumor of the lung composed of primitive-appearing mesenchymal elements and entrapped epithelial elements.[122] (Refer also to Chapter 17, ''Tumors of the Lung'').

The unique physiology of the fetus and still-developing newborn poses unique problems for the clinician in terms of therapy and long-term sequelae. Chemotherapy in the neonate is hindered by poor drug tolerance.[11,26,53,110,127] Complications associated with drug toxicity (e.g., fatal myelosuppression) and increased susceptibility to infections are common.[127] The detrimental effects of radiation therapy on immature, growing tissues have been well documented,[37,108] and mutilating surgery is absolutely contraindicated in newborns and infants. Indeed, the sequelae of therapy, rather than the tumor itself, may cause death. Therefore, the potential long-term effects of surgery, irradiation, and chemotherapy must be fully considered when determining a course of treatment. Moreover, the physician responsible for the patient's care must discuss with the parents the possible risks associated with the selected therapy before it is begun.[11,30,66]

ETIOLOGY

General Aspects

Tumors of the fetus and newborn differ in some respects from those occurring later on in life. They are characterized by unique histologic findings suggestive of an origin linked to abnormal embryogenesis.[20,149] They arise in organs and tissues having an unusually late, ongoing development and varying degrees of imma-

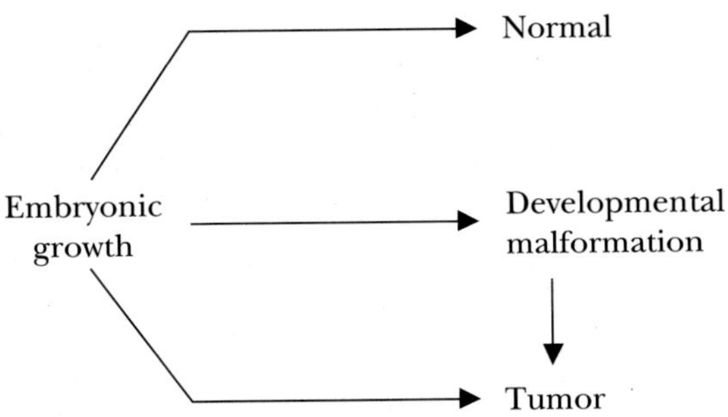

Figure 1–1. Willis'[149] concept of tumorigenesis.

turity in utero, at birth, and during the first few months of life. Willis considered embryonic tumors to be both a neoplasm and a malformation occurring at the same time (Fig. 1–1).[149] According to him, embryomas were not acquired lesions developing from a previously normally formed organ, or even a previously malformed organ, but instead took their origin from some stage of development of that organ (e.g., a Wilms' tumor arising from the renal blastema, or a retinoblastoma arising from developing retinal cells).

Congenital tumors are uncommon, which is surprising in view of the fact that rapid cellular division and growth occur during normal development of the embryo and fetus. Childhood tumors are often composed of persistent embryonal or fetal tissues, suggesting a failure of proper cytodifferentiation or maturation during early life. Wilms' tumor is thought to arise from the metanephric blastema that has lost its propensity for differentiation, but not for growth.[106,149] Similarly, adrenal neuroblastoma develops from neural crest cells that migrate into the gland during embryonic and fetal life. Normally, these cells mature to ganglion cells. Sometimes, however, maturation fails to occur, and proliferation without differentiation results in a neuroblastoma.[21,23,106,149]

Other neoplasms of the fetus and newborn showing morphologic features of embryonic growth include retinoblastoma, medulloblastoma, hepatoblastoma, yolk sac tumor of the testis, and embryonal rhabdomyosarcoma.[106,149] Some teratomas show proliferation of embryonic tissues that fail to mature.[106] On histologic examination, it may be difficult to distinguish between failure of proper maturation of embryonal and fetal tissues and neoplastic growth. Characteristically, a number of tumors in the young are associated with congenital malformations and growth disturbances (Table 1–4).[101,145] Because the histologic features of em-

bryonic tumors appear to recapitulate the developmental stages through which the organ or tissue of origin proceeds to full maturity, knowledge of the embryology of the tissue of origin is helpful in understanding these lesions.[66,149] Therefore, the embryologic development of the organ of origin of the particular tumor being discussed is presented when appropriate.

Some embryonic tumors exhibit an unexpectedly benign behavior despite a malignant microscopic appearance. Examples include stage IV-S neuroblastoma, congenital fibrosarcoma, and nephroblastomatosis.[19,20] For some unexplained reason, these tumors exhibit a tendency to undergo cytodifferentiation and spontaneous regression. These observations have led to the proposal by Bolande that a so-called oncogenic period of grace exists in utero and during the first few months of life, during which time the fetus, newborn, and young infant are "resistant to the full expression or progression" of the malignant tumor.[18] Moreover, according to this concept, the development of a malignant tumor is actively inhibited by some unknown mechanism during embryonic life.[18,42] Consistent with this idea is the fact that malignant neoplasms are seldom seen in the newborn, and only infrequently are responsible for neonatal death or spontaneous abortion. There appear to be certain repressive, protective influences, exerted maximally during intrauterine life (possibly tumor suppressor genes), which prevent the occurrence of neoplasia, particularly malignant neoplasia.[18,42]

These influences could act on the tumor cell by producing cytolysis (e.g., apoptosis-programmed cell death), or by controlling or ar-

Table 1–4. Syndromes and Congenital Malformations Associated with Childhood Tumors

Malformation, Disease, or Syndrome	Neoplasm
Beckwith-Wiedemann syndrome and hemihypertrophy	Wilms' tumor
	Adrenocortical adenoma and carcinoma
	Hepatoblastoma
Aniridia	Wilms' tumor
Genitourinary anomalies	Nephroblastomatosis
	Wilms' tumor
Hirschsprung's disease	Neuroblastoma
Poland's syndrome	Leukemia
Drash syndrome	Wilms' tumor
Perlman syndrome	Nephroblastomatosis
	Wilms' tumor

Data from Berry;[11] Bolande;[18–23] Isaacs;[65,66] Israel;[67] and Mulvihill.[92]

Table 1–5. Chromosomal Abnormalities Associated with Childhood Tumors

Chromosomal Defect	Childhood Tumor
1p deletion	Neuroblastoma
	Melanoma
	Thyroid medullary carcinoma
3p deletion	Wilms' tumor
	Hepatoblastoma
	Embryonal rhabdomyosarcoma
	Adrenal adenoma
11p13 deletion	Wilms' tumor
13q14 deletion	Retinoblastoma
	Osteosarcoma
22q deletion	Neurofibroma
p32p36 deletion	Neuroblastoma
Monosomy 7	Leukemia
t(1;22)	Acute megakaryoblastic leukemia
Trisomy 18	Wilms' tumor
Trisomy 21 (Down syndrome)	Leukemia
Gonadal dysgenesis (45,X/46XY)	Gonadoblastoma
	Germinoma
Klinefelter's syndrome (XXY)	Teratoma
	Breast carcinoma

Data from Isaacs;[65,66] Israel;[67] and Mulvihill.[92]

resting mitotic activity or cytodifferentiation.[18] Other theories have evolved in an attempt to explain the different biological behavior of tumors in the young, but as yet, a full explanation has not been formulated.[21]

Attempts to produce tumors in animal embryos, either by known chemical carcinogens or by irradiation, have proved mainly unsuccessful.[42] Insufficient data are available to implicate environmental factors as the sole cause of congenital tumors. There have been sporadic case reports of certain drugs associated with tumors in early life.[2,56,92,103,126,134] Examples include maternal ethanol ingestion resulting in fetal alcohol syndrome, and hydantoin administration to epileptic mothers associated with neuroblastoma.[2,103,126] No common type of tumor has been described in infants and children affected by fetal alcohol syndrome.[2] Rather, a variety of neoplasms have been associated with this syndrome, ranging from neuroblastoma to Hodgkin's disease.[2] One malignant neoplasm that develops later in life as the result of in utero exposure to diethylstilbestrol (DES) is vaginal clear cell adenocarcinoma.[56] Surprisingly, the administration of chemotherapeutic agents or radiation therapy to pregnant women with cancer has not resulted in significant numbers of offspring with malignant disease.[42,82,89,112] The role of viruses in the etiology of congenital malignant neoplasms remains unclear, although there may be a slight increased risk following in utero exposure to certain viral agents, such as rubella, varicella, influenza, and, possibly, cytomegalovirus, which is responsible for a relatively common congenital infection.[17,46] To date, therefore, no definite causal relationship has been established between environmental factors and congenital tumors, so other etiologies must be sought.

The Etiologic Role of Genetic Factors in the Development of Cancer

Overwhelming experimental evidence suggests that genetic factors play a key role in the etiology of cancer (Tables 1–4, 1–5, and 1–6).[1,7,11,13–16,41,51,67,71–73,84,92,98,105,115,117,129,141–143] Rec-

Table 1–6. Common Features of Hereditary Malignant Tumors

Autosomal dominant inheritance
Onset in early life
Multiple primary tumors
Bilateral involvement of paired organs
Sometimes associated with characteristic syndromes
Increased frequency of identical or related neoplasms
  among family members

From Cancer, Vol 58, 1986, p. 534. Copyright © 1986 American Cancer Society. Reprinted by permission of Wiley-Liss, Inc., a subsidiary of John Wiley & Sons, Inc.

ognition of familial cancer syndromes, the association of impaired DNA repair with increased susceptibility to tumor development, and the various karyotypic abnormalities found in preparations of tumor cells support the premise that DNA is intimately involved with neoplasia.[12,34,36,60,77,78,81,84,91,118] Alterations (mutations) in DNA may be inherited in the germ line chromosomes, or they may occur as a result of the action of environmental agents, such as viruses, chemicals, or irradiation.

Cancer can be regarded as an uncontrolled growth of cells resulting from alterations in their DNA.[14,113] The cell thus altered transforms into a malignant cell, becomes independent of normal regulatory control, and multiplies, producing a clone of cancer cells that subsequently develops into a mass of neoplastic cells. The multistage process by which the normal cell is transformed into a cancer cell is called *carcinogenesis.* The known mechanisms of carcinogenesis are point mutations in the DNA molecule (the replacement of a single correct DNA sequence within a gene by an incorrect one), gene deletions (loss of a large amount of DNA resulting in loss of all or part of the gene), and chromosomal translocations with gene rearrangements (whereby the broken ends of the DNA from two different chromosomes may be joined incorrectly, resulting in parts of each chromosome being exchanged).[34,113]

Growth regulatory genes, called proto-oncogenes, and tumor suppressor genes, which respectively promote and inhibit growth, have a role in normal growth and, when altered, initiate and maintain the formation of tumor cells.[14,48,76,80,117] Moreover, another category of genes has been found to control programmed cell death, or apoptosis, and to play a role in carcinogenesis.[57,75]

Oncogenes

The discovery of cellular oncogenes was the outcome of experimental studies on tumor-producing retroviruses. It was found that normal cells contain genetic sequences similar to those of the retrovirus-transforming genes (viral oncogenes).[14–16,99,131,139,154] Naturally occurring cellular genes, homologous to those of the retrovirus-transforming genes (called proto-oncogenes), were found to occur in non-transformed cells throughout the animal kingdom. Proto-oncogenes are responsible for the normal growth of the cell, and have a role in

the regulation of cell division, differentiation, senescence, and programmed cell death.

Cancer-causing genes (oncogenes) play a pivotal role in tumorigenesis. When the DNA of a proto-oncogene is damaged or altered in some way, an oncogene is formed. Multiple oncogenes act synergistically to produce cancer. Proto-oncogenes may be transformed into oncogenes by one of three mechanisms: chromosomal translocation, point mutation, or gene amplification. Oncoproteins, the protein products of oncogenes (some of which, such as tyrosine kinase, are enzymes), function in several ways: as growth factors, as cell membrane receptors, as intracellular signaling devices (transduction signals), and as nuclear proteins that initiate the cell cycle.[1,97,113,115,119,137] Oncogenes impart to the tumor cell certain properties, such as growth advantage, rapid proliferation, and the ability to metastasize.[14,27,71,139] One example is the N-myc oncogene, which is normally expressed in developing organs and tissues and which is amplified (i.e., copies of the gene are reduplicated) in certain tumor systems, such as neuroblastoma and retinoblastoma.[120,142] Two main cytogenetic changes are associated with gene amplification: (1) homogeneously staining regions on single chromosomes and (2) double minutes, which are paired fragments of chromatin that remain unattached to any chromosome. The product of the N-myc gene is a nuclear protein that is produced in increased amounts in dividing embryonic cells and in some tumor cells. An excessive amount of an oncogene product, as would be found in a neuroblastoma specimen, can serve as an indicator of prognosis, as N-myc amplification is associated with an advanced stage of disease and an unfavorable outcome in patients with neuroblastoma.[27,120]

Malignant cells may arise not only by activation of growth-promoting oncogenes (proto-oncogenes), but also by inactivation of genes that normally suppress cell proliferation (tumor suppressor genes or anti-oncogenes).[14,51,113,117] Tumor suppressor genes operate to restrain the growth of normal cells and to block the formation of tumor cells. Tumor suppressor oncogenes are considered to be recessive because both normal alleles of the tumor suppressor gene must be altered for transformation to occur. On the other hand, mutant proto-oncogenes are regarded as dominant because they transform cells regardless of the presence of normal proto-oncogenes.

Certain pediatric neoplasms are associated

with a loss of growth-inhibiting tumor suppressor genes. The retinoblastoma gene (Rb) is a classic example of a tumor suppressor gene. Individuals experiencing a loss of one or both of these two protective genes have an increased susceptibility to, or actually develop, retinoblastoma (see also Chapter 10, "Tumors of the Eye").[41,84,94,142] There is an important relationship between the integrity (homozygosity) of the 13q14 Rb gene and the development of certain childhood cancers.[52,93,94] Studies indicate that both copies of the 13q14 Rb gene must be altered in some way (e.g., by loss, inactivation, mutation, or deletion) before a tumor can develop. If an individual acquires a defective 13q14 gene from either parent, then that individual is heterozygous for the altered gene and, by definition, is a carrier for the gene. However, before tumorigenesis can occur, a second event (or "second hit") must occur, as originally proposed by Knudson.[74] That is, both retinoblastoma genes must be altered. Furthermore, inheritance of a faulty copy of one allele at the 13q14 locus makes the individual susceptible to various types of cancer. When the second copy becomes altered, deleted, or inactivated at the 13q14 locus, tumorigenesis occurs, with retinoblastoma developing at an early age and secondary malignant neoplasms, such as osteosarcoma, appearing later on.[52,94]

Tumors Associated with Chromosomal Anomalies and Malformation Syndromes

Familial aggregation of specific tumors, such as occurs in the "cancer family syndrome" whereby clustering of more than one type of malignant disease occurs, has been reported.[81,84] An important relationship exists between congenital malformations and inherited syndromes and the development of neoplasms (see Tables 1–4 and 1–6).[10,20,22,23,83,85,86,92,102,125,132,133,136] In this setting, the tumor occurs before or after birth or later on in life in individuals with specific inherited diseases, certain congenital anomalies, or malformation syndromes, many of whom have an underlying chromosomal defect (see Tables 1–4 and 1–5). One such example is the increased incidence of neoplasms associated with gonadal dysgenesis in patients having a Y chromosome (e.g., 45X/46XY), whereby gonadoblastoma and germinoma arise in the dysgenetic gonad(s).[3,22,66,92,132] Aniridia, hemihypertrophy,

and malformations of the genitourinary tract often occur in individuals with Wilms' tumor (see Table 1–4).[20,22,100,102,125,128,132]

The data of Koufos and colleagues indicate that a common chromosomal defect, characterized by the loss of suppressor genes (homozygosity) at loci on chromosome 11p, is responsible for the development of Wilms' tumor, rhabdomyosarcoma, and hepatoblastoma.[77,78] Moreover, children with the autosomal dominant Beckwith-Wiedemann syndrome not only have a high frequency of these three embryonal tumors, but also have the 11p anomaly.[78,136]

Individuals with neurocutaneous syndromes (phakomatoses) have a high incidence of neoplasia. The autosomal dominant conditions of tuberous sclerosis and neurofibromatosis predispose these individuals to the development of astrocytoma, other gliomas, and malignant schwannoma.[8,70,92] Hereditary syndromes and conditions associated with an increased risk of developing tumors are listed in Table 1–4.

Hereditary syndromes characterized by DNA repair defects have been described.[89,113] In the affected individual, the cell is unable to repair a damaged DNA sequence. Such damage may be caused by exposure to ultraviolet light from the sun or by certain chemicals or viruses. The formation of tumors is accelerated in these altered cells. Examples of diseases and associated neoplasms occurring as a result of faulty DNA repair include ataxia telangiectasia (lymphomas), Bloom's syndrome (leukemia), Fanconi's anemia (leukemia), and xeroderma pigmentosa (cutaneous carcinomas).[92,113,132] Except for ataxia telangiectasia, these entities are autosomal recessive conditions. The malignant neoplasms associated with these disorders—namely, carcinoma, leukemia, and lymphoma—rarely, if ever, occur in the perinatal period.

Metastasis of Maternal Malignant Lesions to the Placenta and Fetus

Passage of a maternal malignant tumor across the placenta into the fetus is an unusual event.[5,10,28,29,32,49,58,59,107,114,116,124] This is surprising, as the incidence of cancer in pregnancy is estimated to range from 1 per 1000 to 1 per 5900 cases.[55,107] Maternal-fetal transmission of malignant cells is probably more common than realized.[114] Metastasis of maternal cancer to the placenta and fetus has been reviewed by Benirschke and Kaufmann;[10] Fox;[49] Potter and

Schoeneman;[107] Rushton;[116] Rothman, Cohen, and Astarloa;[114] and by Shanklin.[124] The types of neoplasms transmitted from the mother to the placenta vary. Melanoma is the malignant lesion that has been documented most often (see Chapter 5, ''Tumors and Tumor-Like Conditions of the Skin''). Leukemia, lymphoma, medulloblastoma, and carcinoma of the breast and bronchus are reported infrequently. Potter and Schoenman identified 24 cases of placental metastasis during the period of their review from 1866 to 1966; malignant melanoma was the leading malignant lesion, occurring in 11 of the 24 cases, followed by carcinoma of the breast in 4 of the 24 cases.[107] Horner reported a case of placental metastasis from a cystadenocarcinoma of the ovary,[59] and Brossard et al. reported a case of maternal cerebellar medulloblastoma that metastasized to the placenta (intervillous spaces) but did not spread to the infant, who was well at the time of writing.[29]

Fox published a critical review of the reported cases of placental metastases from maternal neoplasms prior to 1978.[49] He accepted only 29 as valid, compared to the 36 cases reviewed by Rothman and colleagues.[114] Instances of lymphoma and leukemia were excluded by Fox because, in his estimation, there were no well-demonstrated cases of placental involvement by either lymphoma or leukemia. In the reports reviewed, Fox could find no convincing evidence of villous invasion by leukemic cells, although large numbers of maternal blast cells were found to be trapped in the intervillous spaces, particularly in mothers with high leukocyte counts. In a study of 14 fetuses and 34 children born of mothers with leukemia, Diamandopoulos and Hertig found no evidence of transmission of leukemia from these mothers to their offspring.[40]

According to Fox's detailed study, in all 29 cases of placental tumor metastases, tumor cells were situated in the intervillous spaces; in 9, villous invasion was also demonstrated and of these only 2 with proven fetal metastases were attributable to malignant melanoma.[49]

The trophoblast appears to act as an active barrier, both physically and probably immunologically, to prevent tumor cells from being transferred from the mother to the fetus or vice versa.[10,107] This protective mechanism certainly could account for the low incidence and minimal risk of maternal-fetal or fetal-maternal transfer of tumor cells. It is conceivable that, in addition, immunologic factors in the fetus (e.g., allograft rejection of tumor cells) could play a significant role.

When extensive involvement of the placenta occurs, gross examination of the tumor reveals nodular infiltrates that are darkly pigmented, as with malignant melanoma.[10,28,49] Microscopic examination reveals nests or sheets of neoplastic cells in the intervillous space. Villous and fetal vascular invasion are seldom seen, but have been reported in two cases of maternal melanoma. In both instances, there were metastases to the placenta and fetus, resulting in the death of the infant a few months later (see Table 5–3).[28,58]

When there is a maternal history of cancer during pregnancy, the placenta should always be examined carefully and systematically.[114] Unfortunately, many placental specimens are discarded and not examined at all. Some placentas that appear normal on gross inspection will reveal microscopic evidence of tumor, as illustrated in Fox's study in which only 14 of the 29 involved placentas had grossly visible tumor nodules.[49] Careful follow-up evaluation of the infant for signs of metastatic disease is a necessary part of the evaluation.[114]

Development of disseminated choriocarcinoma in the newborn, resulting from a placental primary neoplasm, occurs only rarely. Wells reported five examples in which a choriocarcinoma arising in the placenta was transmitted to the fetus and caused its death. In two of these cases, the mother was found to be free of neoplastic disease.[144] This is not surprising, as choriocarcinoma may be present in the full-term placenta and shed at delivery without affecting the mother. Witzleben and Bruninga[150] summarized five cases from the literature, including one of their own. In these five cases, there was a placental choriocarcinoma noted at the time of delivery or shortly thereafter, or no discoverable primary site in the infants who developed widespread metastases. Recently, Picton et al. described simultaneous choriocarcinoma in a mother and newborn.[104] The infant was born with severe anemia (5.7 g/dL) attributable to fetomaternal hemorrhage. At 3 weeks of age, liver and lung metastases were found in the neonate. The infant died at 5 weeks of age, 5 days after a liver biopsy. The mother, who had lung metastases, was successfully treated with methotrexate.

The diagnosis of choriocarcinoma should be suspected when a newborn presents with hematemesis or hemoptysis, severe anemia, hepatomegaly, lung metastases on chest imaging studies, and/or elevated urinary or plasma levels of chorionic gonadotropin.[150]

INCIDENCE

Estimates of the incidence of perinatal tumors are often imprecise.[101,130] Only a few population-based studies have been published. Most published articles represent the experience of individual health care centers where selection bias seems to reflect referral patterns.[130] In some reported cases, the distinction between classification as a neoplasm or as a congenital malformation has proved difficult, and most reports have excluded lymphangiomas, cutaneous hemangiomas, and melanocytic nevi.[130] Moreover, tumors in both stillborns and neonates may go unrecognized or unreported. With the advent of newer imaging techniques, however, this situation has improved.

The early classic study on the incidence of congenital tumors was published by Wells in 1940.[144] He included in the report all cases reported in the literature as congenital malignant tumors for which he was able to locate the original description.[144] He found that many cases had been copied by one author from another, and that often, there was nothing in the original report to indicate that a particular tumor was malignant or had been present at birth. Of the cases reviewed, only 255 tumors present at birth were considered by Wells to be potentially malignant. Of these, 66 were classified as definitely malignant, 66 as probably malignant, and 123 as possibly malignant. The largest group, representing about half of the total number of cases, were diagnosed as having sarcomas. These neoplasms were primary in bone, muscle, connective tissue, skin, brain, orbit, parotid, vulva, prostate, bladder, pancreas, and intestine. Neuroblastomas comprised the next largest group, followed by Wilms' tumor.

More recent reports indicate that the malignant neoplasms most frequently noted at birth are neuroblastoma and leukemia, followed by sarcomas and brain tumors (see Table 1–1).[8,26,53,62,101] Overall, however, teratoma is the most common neoplasm identified in several perinatal studies, and in only a very small percentage of cases is it found to be malignant on histologic examination.[38,62,101,145] In a review of neonatal neoplasms identified over a 40-year period by the University of Texas M.D. Anderson Cancer Center, sarcoma was found to be the leading malignant solid tumor (13 of 32

[40%] cases).[151] Next, in order of frequency, were brain tumors, neuroblastomas, and retinoblastomas.

Tumors occurring in the fetus and newborn are essentially the same histologically as those found in older individuals, but they differ in terms of order of frequency, localization, distribution, degree of differentiation, and prognosis. Leukemia-lymphoma, brain tumors, neuroblastoma, and soft tissue sarcomas, listed in decreasing order of occurrence, are the most common neoplasms noted in older children and adolescents younger than 15 years of age.[153]

Data derived from the Third National Cancer Survey in the United States from 1969 to 1971 showed an incidence of malignant tumors of 3.65 cases per 100,000 live births.[8] Approximately 653 cancers were recorded annually in infants, and of these, 130 were diagnosed in newborns.[8] By comparison, however, The Childhood Cancer Research Group in Great Britain reported a lower incidence of neonatal malignant disease. From 1970 to 1977, they reported 1.70 cases per 100,000 live births.[9] More recently, the Danish Cancer Registry reported an incidence of 2.38 cases per 100,000 births for the period 1943–1985, a figure that lies between those reported for the United States and Great Britain.[24]

A study of 501 autopsies performed on newborn infants by Valdes-Dapena and Arey during the years 1960 through 1966 revealed only one patient with a neoplasm (frequency of 0.2%), which was identified as a thyroid teratoma.[138] A later survey from the Royal Women's and Woman's Mercy Hospitals, Melbourne, Australia (1939 to 1989) yielded a total of 46 tumors (frequency of 0.26%) collected from an audit of 17,417 perinatal necropsies.[145] Teratoma was the most common neoplasm (n = 24), comprising more than 50% of cases, followed in decreasing order of incidence by vascular tumors (hemangioma and lymphangioma, n = 8); neuroblastoma (n = 6); cardiac rhabdomyoma (n = 3); mesoblastic nephroma (n = 2); and thyroid adenoma, hepatic adenoma, and cerebellar medulloblastoma (n = 1 for each of the three).

In one of the latest reports, probably representing the largest series thus far, a 30-year population-based study from the Children's Hospital of Birmingham, United Kingdom revealed that the incidence of tumors was double that previously reported (7.2 per 100,000 live births per year).[101] According to this study, the age at diagnosis, the almost-equivalent male:female ratio, and the distribution of histologic types remained about the same as reported in previous surveys. The authors of this study noted that the overall incidence increased each year over the 30-year period. Certainly, advances in the accuracy of imaging techniques, particularly sonography and nuclear magnetic resonance imaging, could account for this increase. See Table 1–1 for a comparison of the incidence of fetal and newborn neoplasms from various institutions.

According to Bader and Miller[8] and Campbell and colleagues,[30] less than half of neonatal malignant neoplasms are observed on the day of birth, and two thirds are noted before the end of the first week. These data contrast with the series reported by the Children's Hospital of Philadelphia and Children's Hospital of Los Angeles, in which only one third of neonatal malignant lesions were detected on the first day of life.[53,62] In both the Danish and the Birmingham (United Kingdom) studies, half the cases were diagnosed during the first week of life.[24,101]

Mortality

In the newborn, the incidence of a given tumor is not the same as its mortality. This is because certain malignant lesions may be rapidly fatal, others may lead to death beyond the neonatal period, and still others may respond to therapy or undergo maturation and/or regression.[121] When mortality is used as an indicator of incidence during the first year of life, Bader and Miller[8] have noted that acute leukemia is the most common malignant neoplasm, followed in order of frequency by neuroblastoma, brain tumors, and renal tumors. However, when ranked by incidence, the most frequent cancer was determined to be neuroblastoma, followed by leukemia, Wilms' tumor, sarcoma, retinoblastoma, and brain tumors. To illustrate this point further, leukemia is responsible for more deaths than neuroblastoma in the newborn, although the mortality of the former is one half its incidence, as compared to the mortality of neuroblastoma, which is roughly one tenth its incidence.[8,121] The overall mortality rate for neonatal neoplasms recorded by the Third United States Cancer Survey was approximately one fifth the incidence, which probably reflects the relatively good outcome of several malignant neoplasms in the neonate.

The long-term survival rate associated with neonatal tumors has improved with time. In the Danish Cancer Registry study, it was 25%, which is a rate similar to that reported in other newborn studies.[24,30,53,62] Moreover, individuals with soft tissue sarcoma had the highest 5-year survival rate (55%), followed by those with neuroblastoma (25%), but all patients with leukemia and brain tumors died.[24] The Children's Hospital of Birmingham (United Kingdom) study showed a higher overall survival of 55% at 1 year.[101] Patients with leukemia, as in all other previous reports, had the worst prognosis. The highest survival rate thus far was reported in the St. Jude Children's Hospital study. According to this study, 23 patients (68%) survived (median of 11 years); 4 of 28 with solid tumors died; and 1 of 6 neonates with leukemia, a patient with Down syndrome, lived 5 years.[35]

REFERENCES

1. Aaronson SA. Growth factors and cancer. Science 1991;254:1146.
2. Abel EL. Fetal Alcohol Syndrome, p 78. Oradel, NJ: Medical Economics Books, 1990.
3. Ablin A, Isaacs H Jr. Germ cell tumors. *In* Pizzo PA, Poplack DG (eds): Principles and Practice of Pediatric Oncology, 2nd ed, p 867. Philadelphia: JB Lippincott, 1993.
4. Altman AJ, Schwartz AD. Malignant Diseases of Infancy, Childhood and Adolescence, 2nd ed. Philadelphia: WB Saunders, 1983.
5. Anderson JF, Kent S, Machin GA. Maternal malignant melanoma with placental metastases. A case report with literature review. Pediatr Pathol 1989;9:35.
6. Arceci RJ, Weinstein HJ. Neoplasia. *In* Avery GB, Fletcher MA, MacDonald MG (eds): Neonatology: Pathophysiology and Management in the Newborn, 4th ed, p 1211. Philadelphia: JB Lippincott, 1994.
7. Arthur DC. Genetics and cytogenetics of pediatric cancers. Cancer 1986;58:534.
8. Bader JL, Miller RW. U.S. cancer incidence and mortality in the first year of life. Am J Dis Child 1979;133:157.
9. Barson AJ. Congenital neoplasia: The Society's experience, abstracted. Arch Dis Child 1978;53:436.
10. Benirschke K, Kaufmann P. Pathology of the Human Placenta, 2nd ed, p 426. New York: Springer-Verlag, 1990.
11. Berry PJ. Congenital tumours. *In* Keeling JW (ed): Fetal and Neonatal Pathology, 2nd ed, p 273. Berlin: Springer-Verlag, 1993.
12. Bigner SH, Mark J, Bigner DD. Cytogenetics of human brain tumors. Cancer Genet Cytogenet 1990;47:141.
13. Bishop JM. The molecular genetics of cancer. Science 1987;235:305.
14. Bishop JM. Molecular themes in oncogenesis. Cell 1991;64:235.
15. Bishop JM. Oncogenes and clinical cancer. *In* Weinberg RA (ed): Oncogenes and the Molecular Origins

16. Bishop JM. Viruses, genes and cancer. II. Retroviruses and cancer genes. Cancer 1985;55:2329.

17. Bithell JF, Draper GJ, Gorbach PD. Association between malignant disease in children and maternal virus infections. Br Med J 1973;1:706.

18. Bolande RP. Benignity of neonatal tumors and concept of cancer repression in early life. Am J Dis Child 1971;122:12–14.

19. Bolande RP. Cellular Aspects of Developmental Pathology, p 108. Philadelphia: Lea and Febiger, 1967.

20. Bolande RP. Developmental pathology. Am J Pathol 1979;94:627.

21. Bolande RP. Models and concepts derived from human teratogenesis and oncogenesis in early life. J Histochem Cytochem 1984;32:878.

22. Bolande RP. Neoplasia of early life and its relationships to teratogenesis. *In* Rosenberg HS, Bolande RP (eds): Perspectives in Pediatric Pathology, Vol 3, p 145. Chicago: Year Book Medical Publishers, 1976.

23. Bolande RP. The neurocristopathies. A unifying concept of diseases arising in neural crest mal-development. Human Pathol 1974;5:409–429.

24. Borch K, Jacobsen T, Olsen JH, et al: Neonatal cancer in Denmark 1943–1985. Pediatr Hematol Oncol 1992;9:209.

25. Breslow NE, McCann B. Statistical estimation of prognosis for children with neuroblastoma. Cancer Res 1971;31:2098.

26. Broadbent VA. Malignant disease in the neonate. *In* Roberton NRC (ed): Textbook of Neonatology, 2nd ed, p 879. Edinburgh: Churchill Livingstone, 1992.

27. Brodeur G, Seeger R. Gene amplification in human neuroblastomas: Basic mechanisms and clinical implications. Cancer Genet Cytogenet 1986;19:101.

28. Brodsky I, Baren M, Kahn SB, et al. Metastatic malignant melanoma from mother to fetus. Cancer 1965; 18:1048.

29. Brossard J, Abish S, Bernstein ML, et al. Maternal malignancy involving the products of conception: A report of malignant melanoma and medulloblastoma. Am J Pediatr Hematol Oncol 1994;16:380.

30. Campbell AN, Chan HSL, O'Brien A, et al. Malignant tumours in the neonate. Arch Dis Child 1987;62:19.

31. Cangir A, Shallenberger RC, Choroszy M. Malignant neoplasms in the neonatal period (abstract). Proc Am Soc Clin Oncol 1987;6:215.

32. Cavell B. Transplacental metastasis of malignant melanoma. Acta Paediatr (Suppl) 1963;146:37.

33. Crist W, Pullen J, Boyett J, et al. Clinical and biologic features predict a poor prognosis in acute lymphoid leukemias in infants: Pediatric Oncology Group Study. Blood 1986;67:135.

34. Croce CM. Chromosome translocations and human cancer. Cancer Res 1986;46:6019.

35. Crom DB, Wilimas JA, Green AA, et al. Malignancy in the neonate. Med Pediatr Oncol 1989;17:101.

36. Dal Cin P, Brock P, Casteels-Van Dacle M, et al. Cytogenetic characterization of congenital or infantile fibrosarcoma. Eur J Pediatr 1991;150:579.

37. D'Angio GJ. Oncologic problems in the newborn. Am J Pediat Hematol/Oncol 1981;3:269.

38. Davis CF, Carachi R, Young DG. Neonatal tumors: Glasgow 1966–86. Arch Dis Child 1988;63:1075.

39. Dehner LP. Neoplasms of the fetus and neonate. *In* Naeye RL, Kissane JM, Kaufman N (eds): Perinatal Diseases. International Academy of Pathology, Monograph No. 22, p 286. Baltimore: Williams and Wilkins, 1981.

40. Diamandopoulos GT, Hertig AT. Transmission of leukemia and allied diseases from mother to fetus. Obstet Gynecol 1963;21:150.

41. Dryja TP, Mukai S, Petersen S, et al. Parental origins of the retinoblastoma gene. Nature 1989;339:556.

42. Einhorn L. Are there factors preventing cancer development during embryonic life? Oncodevelopmental Biol Med 1983;4:219.

43. Enzinger FM, Weiss SW. Soft Tissue Tumors, 3rd ed, p 579. St. Louis: CV Mosby, 1995.

44. Evans AE, Baum E, Chard R. Do infants with stage IV-S neuroblastoma need treatment? Arch Dis Child 1981;56:271.

45. Evans AE, Chatten J, D'Angio JG, et al. A review of 17 IV-S neuroblastoma patients at the Children's Hospital of Philadelphia. Cancer 1980;45:833.

46. Fine PEM, Adelstein AM, Snowman J, et al. Long term effects of exposure to viral infections in utero. Br Med J 1985;290:509.

47. Finkelstein JZ, Higgins GR, Rissman E, et al. Acute leukemia during the first year of life. Presentation, chemotherapy and clinical course. Clin Pediatr 1972; 11:236.

48. Finlay CA, Hinds PW, Levine AJ. The p53 proto-oncogene can act as a suppressor of transformation. Cell 1989;57:1083.

49. Fox H. Pathology of the Placenta, p 357. Philadelphia: WB Saunders, 1978.

50. Fraumeni JF Jr, Miller RW. Cancer deaths in the newborn. Am J Dis Child 1969;117:186.

51. Frebourg T, Friend SH. Cancer risks from germline p53 mutations. J Clin Invest 1992;90:1637.

52. Friend SH, Bernards R, Rogel S, et al. A human DNA segment with properties of the gene that predisposes to retinoblastoma and osteosarcoma. Nature 1986; 323:643.

53. Gale GB, D'Angio GJ, Uri A, et al. Cancer in neonates: The experience at the Children's Hospital of Philadelphia. Pediatrics 1982;70:409.

54. Garmel SH, Crombleholme TM, Semple JP, et al. Prenatal diagnosis and management of fetal tumors. Semin Perinatol 1994;18:350.

55. Haas JF. Pregnancy in association with a newly diagnosed cancer: A population-based epidemiologic assessment. Int J Cancer 1984;34:229.

56. Herbst AL, Cole P, Colton T, et al. Age-incidence and risk of diethylstilbestrol-related adenocarcinoma of the vagina and cervix. Am J Obstet Gynecol 1977;128: 43.

57. Hockenberry DM, Nunez G, Schreiber RD, et al. Bcl-2 is an inner mitochondrial membrane protein that blocks programmed cell death. Nature 1990;348:334.

58. Holland E. A case of transplacental metastases of malignant melanoma from mother to fetus. J Obstet Gynaecol Br Emp 1949;56:529.

59. Horner EN. Placental metastases. Obstet Gynecol 1960;15:566.

60. Horsman DE, White VA. Cytogenetic analysis of uveal melanoma. Consistent occurrence of monosomy 3 and trisomy 8q. Cancer 1993;71:811.

61. Isaacs H Jr. Congenital malignant tumors. *In* Reed GB, Claireaux AE, Bain AD (eds): Diseases of the Fetus and Newborn: Pathology, Radiology and Genetics, p 131. London: Chapman Hall, 1989.

62. Isaacs H Jr. Congenital and neonatal malignant tu-

mors: A 28-year experience at Children's Hospital of Los Angeles. Am J Pediatr Hematol/Oncol 1987;9:121.

63. Isaacs H Jr. Neoplasms in infants: A report of 265 cases. Pathol Annu 1983;18(2):165.

64. Isaacs H Jr. Perinatal (congenital and neonatal) neoplasms: a report of 110 cases. Pediatr Pathol 1985;3:165.

65. Isaacs H Jr. Tumors. *In* Gilbert-Barness E (ed): Potter's Pathology of the Fetus and Infant, Vol 2, p 1242. St. Louis: Mosby–Year Book, 1996.

66. Isaacs H Jr. Tumors of the Newborn and Infant. St. Louis: Mosby–Year Book, 1991.

67. Israel MA. Cancer cell biology. *In* Pizzo PA, Poplack DG (eds): Principles and Practice of Pediatric Oncology, 2nd ed, p 57. Philadelphia: JB Lippincott, 1993.

68. Keeling JW. Fetal hydrops. *In* Keeling JW (ed): Fetal and Neonatal Pathology, 2nd ed, p 253. Berlin: Springer-Verlag, 1993.

69. Keeling JW. Hydrops Fetalis and other forms of excess fluid collection in the fetus. *In* Wigglesworth JS, Singer DB (eds): Textbook of Fetal and Perinatal Pathology, Vol 1, p 429. Oxford: Blackwell, 1991.

70. Kinzler KW, Vogelstein B. A gene for neurofibromatosis 2. Nature 1993;363:495.

70a. Kirks DR, Merten DF, Grossman H, et al. Diagnostic imaging of pediatric abdominal masses: An overview. Radiol Clin North Am 1981;19:527.

71. Kirsch IR. Genetics of pediatric tumors: The consequences of chromosomal aberrations. *In* Pizzo PA, Poplack DG (eds): Principles and Practice of Pediatric Oncology, 2nd ed, p 29. Philadelphia: JB Lippincott, 1993.

72. Knudson AG Jr. Genetics of human cancer. Ann Rev Genet 1986;20:231.

73. Knudson AG Jr. Hereditary cancer, oncogenes, and antioncogenes. Cancer Res 1985;45:1437.

74. Knudson AG Jr. Retinoblastoma: A prototypic hereditary neoplasm. Semin Oncol 1978;5:57.

74a. Koop CE. Abdominal mass in the newborn infant. N Engl J Med 1973;289:569.

75. Korsmeyer SJ. Bcl-2: An antidote to programmed cell death. Cancer Surv 1992;12:105.

76. Koskinen PJ, Alitalo K. Role of myc amplification and overexpression in cell growth, differentiation and death. Semin Cancer Biol 1993;4:3.

77. Koufos A, Grundy P, Morgan K, et al. Familial Wiedmann-Beckwith syndrome and a second Wilms' tumor locus both map to 11p15. Am J Genet 1989;44:711.

78. Koufos A, Hansen MF, Copeland NG, et al. Loss of heterozygosity in three embryonal tumours suggests a common pathogenic mechanism. Nature 1985;316:330–334.

79. Kurjak A, Zalud I, Jurkovic Z, et al. Ultrasound diagnosis and evaluation of fetal tumors. J Perinat Med 1989;17:173.

80. Lewin B. Oncogenic conversion by regulatory changes in transcription factors. Cell 1991;64:303.

81. Li FP, Fraumeni JF Jr, Mulvihill JJ, et al. A cancer family syndrome in twenty-four kindreds. Cancer Res 1988;48:5358.

82. MacMahon B. Childhood cancer and prenatal irradiation. *In* Burchenal JH, Oettgen HF (eds): Cancer Achievements, Challenges and Prospects for the 1980s, p 223. New York: Grune and Stratton, 1981.

83. Magee JF, McFadden DE, Pantzar JT. Congenital tumors. *In* Dimmick JE, Kalousek DK (eds): Developmental Pathology of the Embryo and Fetus, p 235. Philadelphia: JB Lippincott, 1992.

84. Malkin D, Friend S. The role of tumour suppressor genes in familial cancer. Semin Cancer Biol 1992;3:121.

85. Miller RW. Neoplasia and Down's syndrome. Ann NY Acad Sci 1970;171:637.

86. Miller RW. Relation between cancer and congenital defects: An epidemiologic evaluation. J Natl Cancer Inst 1968;40:1079.

87. Miller RW, Dalager NA. U.S. childhood cancer deaths by cell type, 1960–1968. J Pediatr 1974;85:664.

88. Moerman P, Fryns J-P, Goddeeris P, et al. Nonimmunologic hydrops fetalis. Arch Pathol Lab Med 1982;106:635–640.

89. Mole RH. Childhood cancer after prenatal exposure diagnostic x-ray examinations in Britain. Br J Cancer 1990;62:152.

90. Morison JE. Foetal and Neonatal Pathology, 3rd ed, p 119. New York: Appleton-Century-Crofts, 1970.

91. Mulligan LM, Gardner E, Smith BA, et al. Genetic events in tumor initiation and progression in multiple endocrine neoplasia type 2. Genes, Chromosomes Cancer 1993;6:166.

92. Mulvihill JJ. Childhood cancer, environment and heredity. *In* Pizzo PA, Poplack DG (eds): Principles and Practice of Pediatric Oncology, 2nd ed, p 11. Philadelphia: JB Lippincott, 1993.

93. Murphree AL, Benedict WF. Retinoblastoma: Clues to human oncogenesis. Science 1984;223:1028.

94. Murphree AL, Munier FL. Retinoblastoma. *In* Ryan S (ed): Retina, 2nd ed, Vol 1, p 571. St. Louis: Mosby–Year Book, 1994.

95. Nakamura Y, Komatsu Y, Yano H, et al. Nonimmunologic hydrops fetalis: A clinicopathological study of 50 autopsy cases. Pediatr Pathol 1987;7:19.

96. Newton ER, Lewis F, Dalton ME, et al. Fetal neuroblastoma and catecholamine-induced maternal hypertension. Obstet Gynecol 65 (Suppl) 1985;49S.

97. Nishizuka Y. The molecular heterogeneity of protein kinase C and its implications for cellular regulation. Nature 1988;334:661.

98. Nowell PC. Cancer, chromosomes and genes. Lab Invest 1992;66:407.

99. Nusse R. The activation of cellular oncogenes by retroviral insertion sites. Trends Genet 1986;2:244.

100. Palmer N, Evans AE. The association of aniridia and Wilms' tumor: Methods of surveillance and diagnosis. Med Pediatr Oncol 1983;11:73.

101. Parkes SE, Muir KR, Southern L, et al. Neonatal tumours: A thirty-year population-based study. Med Pediatr Oncol 1994;22:309.

102. Pendergrass TW. Congenital anomalies in children with Wilms' tumor: A new survey. Cancer 1976;37:403.

103. Pendergrass TW, Hanson JW. Fetal hydantoin syndrome and neuroblastoma. Lancet 1976;2:150.

104. Picton SV, Bose-Haider B, Lendon M, et al. Simultaneous choriocarcinoma in mother and newborn infant. Med Pediatr Oncol 1995;25:475.

105. Ponder BAJ. Inherited predisposition to cancer. Trends Genet 1990;6:213.

106. Potter EL, Craig JM. Pathology of the Fetus and Infant, 3rd ed, p 177. Chicago: Year Book Medical Publishers, 1975.

107. Potter JF, Schoeneman M. Metastasis of maternal cancer to the placenta and fetus. Cancer 1970;25:380.

108. Reaman GH. Special considerations for the infant with cancer. *In* Pizzo PA, Poplack DG (eds): Principles and Practice of Pediatric Oncology. 2nd ed, p 303. Philadelphia: JB Lippincott, 1993.

109. Reaman GH, Zeltzer P, Bleyer WA, et al. Acute lymphoblastic leukemia in infants less than one year of age: A cumulative experience of the Children's Cancer Study Group. J Clin Oncol 1985;3:1513.

110. Reece EA. Fetal neoplasm. *In* Reece EA, Hobbins JC, Mahoney MJ, Petrie RH (eds): Medicine of the Fetus and Mother. Philadelphia: JB Lippincott, 1992.

111. Romero R, Oilu G, Jeanty P, Ghidini A, Hobbins JC. Prenatal Diagnosis of Congenital Anomalies. Norwalk, CT: Appleton & Lange, 1988.

112. Rosenstock JG. Neoplasia: The mother and the neonate. Semin Perinatol 1983;7:226.

113. Ross DW. Introduction to Molecular Medicine, p 121. New York: Springer-Verlag, 1992.

114. Rothman LA, Cohen CJ, Astarloa J. Placental and fetal involvement by maternal malignancy: A report of rectal carcinoma and review of the literature. Am J Obstet Gynecol 1973;116:1023.

115. Rozengurt E. Growth factors and cell proliferation. Curr Opin Cell Biol 1992;4:161.

116. Rushton DI. Pathology of the placenta. *In* Wigglesworth JS, Singer DB (eds): Textbook of Fetal and Perinatal Pathology, Vol 1, p 210. Oxford: Blackwell, 1991.

117. Sager R. Tumor suppressor genes: The puzzle and the promise. Science 1989;246:1406.

118. Sanberg AA, Ture-Carel C, Gemmill RM. Chromosomes in solid tumors and beyond. Cancer Res 1988; 48:1049.

119. Satoh T, Nakafuku M, Kaziro Y. Function of Ras as a molecular switch in signal transduction. J Biol Chem 1992;267:24149.

120. Schwab M. Amplification of N-myc as a prognostic marker for patients with neuroblastoma. Semin Cancer Biol 1993;4:13.

121. Schwartz AD. Congenital malignant disorders. *In* Avery AM, Taeusch HW Jr (eds): Schaffer's Diseases of the Newborn, 5th ed, p 928. Philadelphia: WB Saunders, 1984.

121a. Schwartz MZ, Shaul DB. Abdominal masses in the newborn. Pediatr Rev 1989;11:172.

122. Senac MO, Wood BP, Isaacs H, et al. Pulmonary blastoma—A rare childhood malignancy. Radiology 1991;179:743.

123. Shanklin DR, Sotelo-Avilla C. In situ tumors in fetuses, newborns and young infants. Biol Neonatol 1969;14: 286.

124. Shanklin DR. Tumors of the Placenta and Umbilical Cord. Philadelphia: BC Decker, 1990.

125. Shannon RS, Mann JR, Harper E, et al. Wilms' tumor and aniridia: Clinical and cytogenetic features. Arch Dis Child 1982;57:685.

126. Sherman S, Roizen N. Fetal hydantoin syndrome and neuroblastoma. Lancet 1976;2:517.

127. Siegel SE, Moran RG. Problems in chemotherapy of cancer in the neonate. Am J Pediatr Hematol Oncol 1981;3:287.

128. Sotelo-Avila C, Gooch WM. Neoplasms associated with the Beckwith-Wiedemann syndrome. *In* Rosenberg HS, Bolande RP (eds): Perspectives in Pediatric Pathology, Vol 3, p 255. Chicago: Year Book Medical Publishers, 1976.

129. Stanbridge EJ. Human tumor suppressor genes. Ann Rev Genet 1990;24:615.

130. Stevens MCG. Neonatal tumours. Arch Dis Child 1988;63:1122.

131. Swain A, Coffin JM. Mechanism of transduction by retroviruses. Science 1992;255:841.

132. Swift M, Reitnauer PJ, Rao KW. Hereditary and other antecedent conditions of childhood neoplasia. *In* Finegold M (ed): Pathology of Neoplasia in Children and Adolescents. Major Problems in Pathology, Vol 18, p 1. Philadelphia: WB Saunders, 1986.

133. Tank ES, Kay R. Neoplasms associated with Beckwith's syndrome, hemihypertrophy and aniridia. J Urol 1980;124:266.

134. Tuman KJ, Chilcote RR, Berkow RI, et al. Mesothelioma in a child with prenatal exposure to isoniazid. Lancet 1980;2:362.

135. Turkel SB. Conditions associated with nonimmune hydrops fetalis. Clin Perinatol 1982;9:613.

136. Turleau C, de Grouchy J, Chavin-Colin F, et al. Trisomy 11p15 and Beckwith-Wiedemann syndrome. A report of two cases. Hum Genet 1984;67:219.

137. Ulrich A, Schlessinger J. Signal transduction by receptors with tyrosine kinase activity. Cell 1990;61:203.

138. Valdes-Dapena MA, Arey JB. The causes of neonatal mortality: An analysis of 501 autopsies on newborn infants. J Pediatr 1970;77:366.

139. Varmus HE. An historical overview of oncogenes. *In* Weinberg RA (ed): Oncogenes and the Molecular Origins of Cancer, p 3. New York: Cold Spring Harbor Laboratory Press, 1989.

140. Walton JM, Rubin SZ, Soucy P, et al. Fetal tumors associated with hydrops: The role of the pediatric surgeon. J Pediatr Surg 1993;28:1151.

141. Weinberg RA. Oncogenes, antioncogenes, and the molecular basis of multistep carcinogenesis. Cancer Res 1989;49:3713.

142. Weinberg RA. The retinoblastoma gene and gene product. Cancer Surv 1992;12:43.

143. Weinberg RA. Tumor suppressor genes. Cell 1991; 254:1138.

144. Wells HG. Occurrence and significance of congenital malignant neoplasms. Arch Pathol 1940;30:535.

145. Werb P, Scurry J, Ostor A, et al. Survey of congenital tumors in perinatal necropsies. Pathology 1992;24: 247.

146. Wieberdink J. Metastases in neonatal neuroblastoma. *In* Pochedly C (ed): Neuroblastoma, Clinical and Biological Manifestations, p 13. New York: Elsevier Biomedical, 1982.

147. Wienk MATP, Van Geijn HP, Copray FJA, et al. Prenatal diagnosis of fetal tumors by ultrasonography. Obstet Gynecol Surv 1990;45:639.

148. Wigglesworth JS. Perinatal pathology. *In* Bennington, JL (ed): Major Problems in Pathology, Vol 15. Philadelphia: WB Saunders, 1984.

149. Willis RA. The Borderland of Embryology and Pathology, 2nd ed. London: Butterworths, 1962.

150. Witzleben CL, Bruninga G. Infantile choriocarcinoma: A characteristic syndrome. J Pediatr 1968;73:374.

151. Xue H, Horwitz JR, Smith MB, et al. Malignant solid tumors in neonates: A 40 year review. J Pediatr Surg 1995;30:543.

152. Young JL, Heiss HW, Silverberg E, Myers MH. Cancer Incidence, Survival and Mortality for Children Under 15 Years of Age. American Cancer Society, 1978.

153. Young JL, Miller RW. Incidence of malignant tumors in U.S. children. J Pediatr 1975;86:254.

154. zur Hausen H. Viruses in human cancers. Science 1991;254:1167.

GERM CELL TUMORS

2

Germ cell tumors are an assorted group of benign and malignant neoplasms derived from primordial germ cells.[40,65,92,171] They are found in a variety of sites, both gonadal and extragonadal, with the latter occurring in midline locations, such as the sacrococcygeal area, retroperitoneum, mediastinum, neck, and pineal region (Tables 2–1 and 2–2).

Most germ cell tumors found in the fetus and newborn are histologically benign and are diagnosed as either mature or immature teratomas (see Table 2–1). Occasionally, yolk sac tumors or, rarely, embryonal carcinomas occur in association with a teratoma. The term malignant teratoma is imprecise and is no longer recommended. Yolk sac tumor (endodermal sinus tumor) or embryonal carcinoma with a teratoma is called a mixed germ cell tumor, and each of its components is identified in the diagnosis. Neither choriocarcinoma nor germinoma has been reported to occur in neonatal teratomas.[18,92]

The WHO classification of germ cell tumors is the basis for most contemporary classifications, and is the one that is generally employed (Table 2–3).[150] According to this classification, germ cell neoplasms are divided into eight histologic categories: dysgerminoma, yolk sac tumor, embryonal carcinoma, polyembryoma, choriocarcinoma, teratoma, gonadoblastoma, and germ cell sex cord–stromal tumors.[150] Some pathologists incorporate seminoma and dysgerminoma, as well as pineal germinoma, into an all-inclusive category of "germinoma" because the microscopic appearances of all three are essentially the same. However, the WHO classification uses the term dysgerminoma instead of germinoma in the classification of germ cell tumors. Moreover, gonado-

blastoma, a neoplasm typically observed in dysgenetic gonads, is included in the category of germ cell tumors although Sertoli cell components are found in addition to germ cells (see Fig. 2–21).[40,140] Occasionally, gonadoblastoma involves the gonads of infants without gonadal dysgenesis.[92,140]

EMBRYOLOGY

Knowledge of the embryonic development of the gonads is requisite for understanding the concept and the histopathology of germ cell tumors. Primordial germ cells originate in the yolk sac endoderm and are visible in the developing embryo during the fourth week of gestation.[118] At about the sixth week, they migrate along the dorsal mesentery of the hindgut to the gonadal ridges, where they populate either the developing ovary or testis (Fig. 2–1). Germ cell tumors are thought to arise from these pluripotential primordial germ cells, which evolve into a variety of benign and malignant neoplasms.[40,65,171] Even though they are considered to be primarily gonadal in origin, this diverse group of tumors is also found outside the testis and ovary. One possible explanation for this occurrence is that, when the primordial germ cells migrate from the yolk sac to the genital ridge and eventually to the gonad in the embryo, some migrate away and miss their intended destination, ending up in such extragonadal sites as the pineal area, mediastinum, retroperitoneum, and sacrococcygeal region. For some unexplained reason—perhaps as the result of a DNA mutation—the aberrant cells undergo transformation to a germ cell tumor, the type of which depends on the degree

Table 2–1. Distribution of 128 Perinatal Teratomas, Children's Hospital Medical Center, Boston, 1928–1982

| Location | Histologic Type* | | | Male | Female | Percent of Total |
	Number	*M*	*I*			
Sacrococcygeal	102	82	20	13	89	79.7
Neck	6	1	5	—	—	4.7
Retroperitoneum	4	2	2	—	—	3.1
Mediastinum	4	3	1	—	—	3.1
Head (face)	4	3	1	—	—	3.1
Orbit	2	2	—	—	—	1.6
Pharynx	2	2	—	—	—	1.6
Liver	2	2	—	1	1	1.6
Abdominal wall	1	1	—	1	—	0.8
Spinal canal	1	1	—	—	—	0.8
Totals	128	99	29			100

Data from Tapper D, Lack EE. Teratomas in infancy and childhood: A 54-year experience at the Children's Hospital Medical Center. Ann Surg 1983;198:398. Used by permission.
*M, mature tissue components; I, immature tissue components.

of differentiation. For example, embryonal carcinoma would be on the malignant end of the spectrum, whereas mature teratoma would be on the benign end.[92]

CYTOGENETICS

Nonrandom structural aberrations, most often involving chromosomes 1 and 12, have been described in germ cell tumors.[2] Isochromosome 12p[i(12p)] is found in several different types of germ cell tumors.[2,120,146] Deletions in the long arm of chromosome 12, namely 12q[del(12)(q14)], are proposed as one of the defects associated with malignant transformation of testicular germ cells.[146] Moreover, studies suggest a DNA imbalance, with loss of Y chromosomal DNA and a simultaneous excess of X chromosomal DNA.[131] Investigations of ovarian teratomas show that two thirds of them are derived from a single germ cell after meiosis I and failure of meiosis II or endoreduplication of a mature ovum, and one third arise as a result of failure of meiosis I or mitotic division of premeiotic germ cells.[128,129]

TERATOMAS

A *teratoma* is defined as a true tumor composed of multiple tissues foreign to, and capable of growth in excess of, those characteristic of the part from which it is derived.[133] However, it is sometimes difficult to distinguish between teratomas and structures that result from abor-

Table 2–2. Distribution of 62 Perinatal Teratomas, Children's Hospital, Los Angeles, 1960–1991

| Location | Histologic Type* | | | | Male | Female | Percent of Total |
	Number	*M*	*I*	*YST*			
Sacrococcygeal	45	29	15	1	11	34	72.6
Neck†	5	1	4	—	3	2	8.1
Retroperitoneum	5	3	2	—	3	2	8.1
Epignathus	2	2	—	—	2	—	3.2
Nasopharynx	2	2	—	—	—	2	3.2
Mediastinum	1	—	1	—	1	—	1.6
Pericardium	1	—	1	—	—	1	1.6
Occiput	1	1	—	—	—	1	1.6
Totals	62	38	23	1	20	42	100

*M, mature tissue components; I, immature tissue components; YST, teratoma + yolk sac tumor.
†One newborn had two separate teratomas of the neck and palate.

Table 2–3. WHO Classification
of Germ Cell Tumors

1. **Dysgerminoma ("Germinoma")**
   Variant—with syncytiotrophoblast cells
2. **Yolk Sac Tumor (Endodermal Sinus Tumor)**
   Variants—Polyvesicular vitelline tumor
         —Hepatoid
         —Glandular ("endometrioid")
3. **Embryonal Carcinoma**
4. **Polyembryoma**
5. **Choriocarcinoma**
6. **Teratomas**
   1. Immature
   2. Mature
      Solid
      Cystic (dermoid cyst)
      With secondary tumor (specify type)
      Fetiform (homunculus)
   3. Monodermal
      Stroma ovarii
      Carcinoid
      Mucinous carcinoid
      Neuroectodermal tumors (specify type)
      Sebaceous tumors
      Others
   4. Mixed (specify types*)
7. **Gonadoblastoma**
   Variant—with dysgerminoma or other germ cell
   tumor
8. **Germ Cell Sex Cord–Stromal Tumor**
   Variant—with dysgerminoma or other germ cell
   tumor

From Scully RE, Personal communication, 1995.
*For example, immature teratoma + yolk sac tumor.

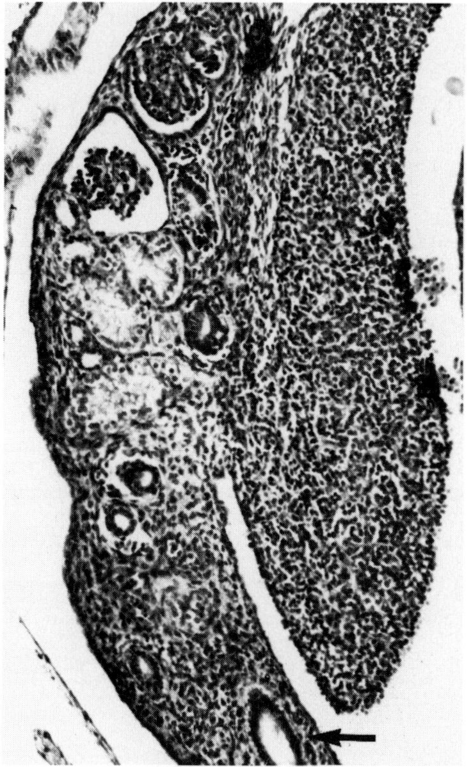

Figure 2–1. Developing gonad in a 12-mm embryo (approximately 6 weeks' gestational age). Photomicrograph of the gonadal ridge with collections of small primordial germ cells that have migrated from the yolk sac. Mesonephric tubules, glomeruli, and the paramesonephric duct (*arrow*) are situated adjacent to the gonad (hematoxylin-eosin, ×150).

tive attempts at twinning. Investigators have tried to explain all teratomas on the basis of modified twinning resulting from isolation of blastomeres, fertilization of a polar body, and parthenogenetic development of an ovum. According to Potter and Craig, an even progression can be traced from normal twins to conjoined twins, parasitic twins, and fetus in fetu.[133] Careful studies reveal a break in the progression from an oriented, longitudinal, partially symmetric structure of a twin to the jumbled, disordered, irregular growth of a teratoma in which one, two, or three tissues predominate.[133] The proper identification of questionable masses requires careful dissection and mapping of the parts, as well as consideration of their interrelationship, the degree to which they are organized, and their growth potential.[133,184] Despite the apparent progression from twins to fetus in fetu to teratomas, Willis and others vehemently deny such a relationship.[184] The distinction is based primarily on the fact that teratomas are capable of independent growth, whereas structures that are classified as malfor-

mations are limited in their potentiality for growth to a rate similar to the part of the body they resemble.[133]

Teratomas are observed in many locations at birth, but particular sites of predilection are the sacrococcygeal area and neck (see Tables 2–1 and 2–2) (Figs. 2–2 to 2–4).[12,17,18,26,40–44,87–92,169] Other locations of teratomas include the brain, pineal body, retroperitoneum, anterior mediastinum, heart and pleura, pharynx, thyroid, base of the skull, spine, pelvis, liver, and subcutaneous tissue (see Tables 2–1 and 2–2).[16,40,42,103–105,169]

Most teratomas and dermoid cysts of the ovary are not discovered until after puberty. Before the age of 12 years, teratomas are the most common ovarian tumor; the youngest individual diagnosed as having teratoma in one series was 4 years of age.[169,175] More than one third of childhood teratomas of the testis are recognized in the first year of life, but they occur only

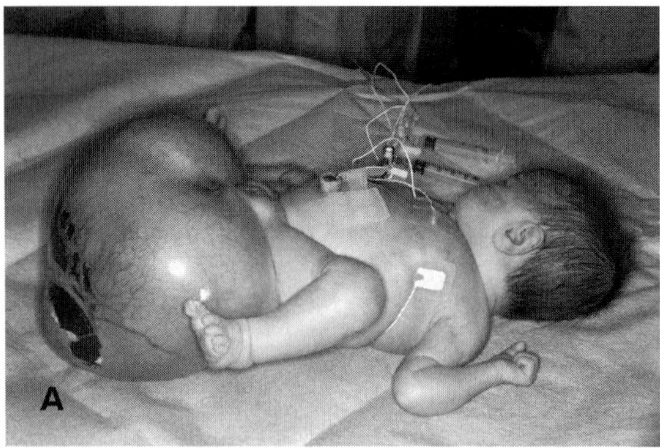
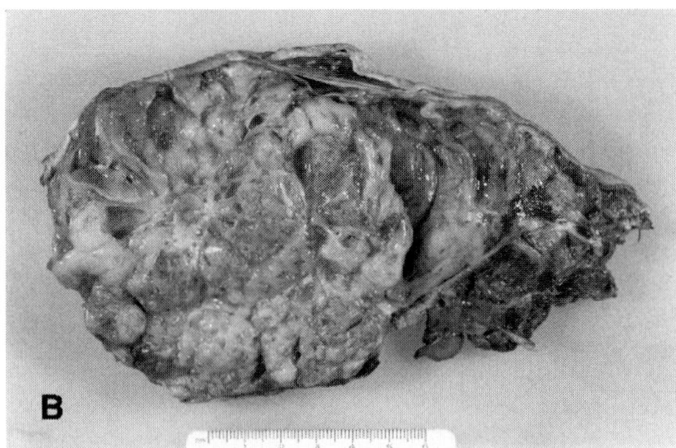

Figure 2–2. Sacrococcygeal teratoma. Sonography at 30 weeks' gestation revealed an abnormality in the sacral region. Shortly before delivery, fetal distress was noted and a cesarean section was performed. *A*, This 4.4-kg female was born at 37 weeks' gestation with a large sacrococcygeal tumor. *B*, The tumor, which was excised at 1 day of age, weighed 1.5 kg (1/3 the birth weight) and measured 15 × 13 × 10 cm. The cut surface of the bissected tumor has a variegated solid and cystic appearance. Skin partially covers the periphery of the specimen. Microscopically, the tumor consists of immature neuroglial elements in addition to a variety of mature tissues characteristically found in these teratomas (see Figs. 2–9, 2–10, 2–11, 2–14, and 2–15). (From Isaacs H Jr. Tumors of the Newborn and Infant. St. Louis: Mosby–Year Book, 1991.)

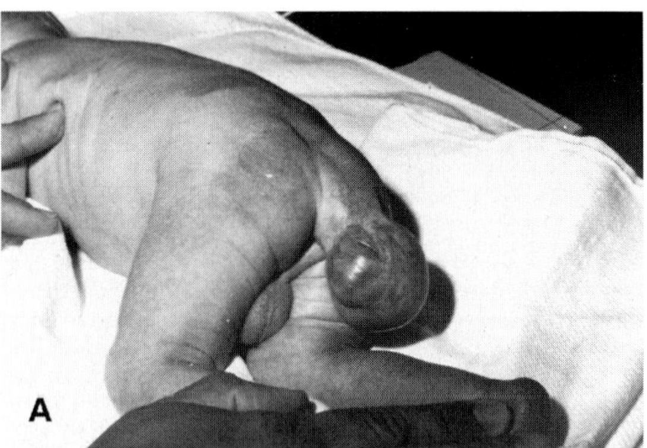
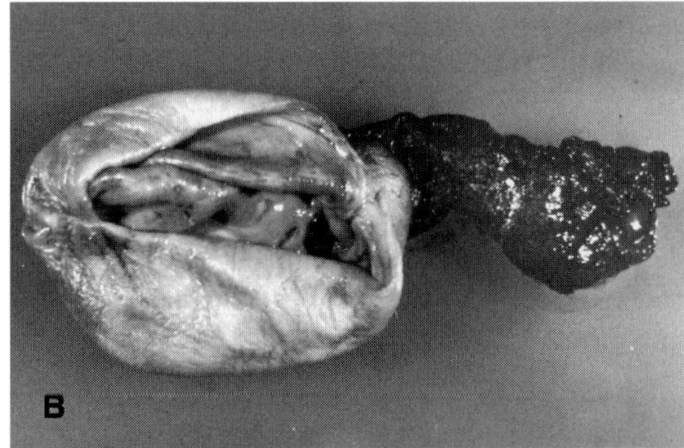

Figure 2–3. Sacrococcygeal teratoma. *A*, A male newborn with a tail-like extension from the sacrococcygeal area. *B*, The tumor is composed of a terminal round cyst measuring 4 × 5 cm, which is connected to the coccyx by solid, fibrofatty tissue. The cyst, which is opened, is composed of skin surrounding respiratory and gastrointestinal components. In addition, choroid plexus, and mature and immature neuroglial tissue are present.

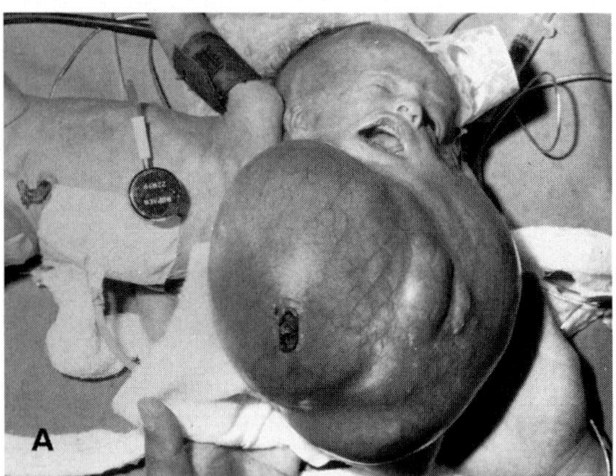
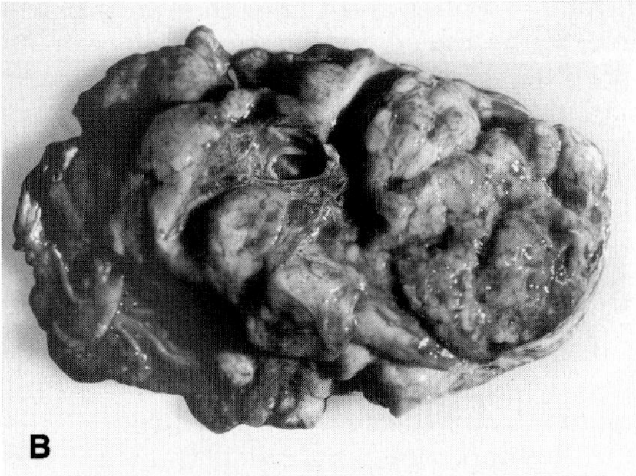

Figure 2–4. Thyrocervical teratoma. *A*, This 2-week-old male infant has a gigantic teratoma arising from the neck that produced maternal dystocia. *B*, The resected specimen weighed 1184 g and measured 24 × 15 × 8 cm. The teratoma was found to consist of both mature and immature neural tissue, in addition to cartilage and respiratory and gastrointestinal epithelium. (From Pediatr Pathol 1985;3:168, Isaacs H Jr., Taylor & Francis, Inc., Washington, DC. Reproduced with permission. All rights reserved.)

rarely in the neonatal period.[96,169] The youngest patient with testicular teratoma in the Boston study was 6 months of age, whereas the youngest in the Los Angeles study was 12 months old.[92,169] Kay listed one newborn with a teratoma in the Prepubertal Testicular Tumor Registry (see Table 3–1).[96]

By definition, teratomas are composed of tissues representing each of the three layers of the embryonic disk. Endodermal components are the least common, but at times, intestinal or gastric mucosa is remarkably well developed and may be surrounded by muscle layers that are complete, even to Auerbach's plexus (see Figs. 2–11 and 2–12). Ectodermal components, especially brain tissue, make up a large portion of most teratomas that are present at birth and are more prominent than in those tumors discovered later in life (see Figs. 2–9, 2–10, 2–14, and 2–15).[92,133] This is particularly true of the sacrococcygeal teratomas. The tissue in these tumors for the most part resembles glia, although ganglion cells and cavities lined by cells resembling ependyma and choroid plexus are not uncommon (see Fig. 2–9). Epidermal and dermal structures, including hairs and sebaceous and sweat glands, are generally present, and there may also be teeth that are fairly well developed. The various types of epithelium include columnar, pseudostratified, stratified, ciliated and nonciliated, and secretory and nonsecretory. Glands, in addition to those derived from the skin, include salivary, mucus, thyroid, pancreas, adrenal, and others. Tissues resembling kidney, liver, and lung are rare (see Figs. 2–12 and 2–13). Mesodermal components, such as fat, cartilage, bone, and muscle, are present in almost all congenital teratomas.[90,92,133]

The immature teratoma consists primarily of embryonic-appearing neuroglial or neuroepithelial components which may coexist along with mature tissues and may display a worrisome histologic appearance because of their hypercellularity, nuclear atypia, and increased mitotic activity (see Figs. 2–14, 2–15, and 2–16). Occasionally, tissues that are other than neural in origin, such as nephrogenic rests, are found in the immature teratoma (see Fig. 2–13).[15,92] In most instances, immature teratomas—high grade or otherwise—occurring in the fetus and newborn are associated with a favorable prognosis.[27,40,90,104] However, their behavior is less predictable in adolescents and adults, in whom they may be associated with a poor outcome. Scully's grading system is a useful guide for predicting prognosis in this age group.[152] The grading system, based on the amount of immature tissue present, is not applicable to either the fetus or newborn because embryonic or immature elements may be appropriate for the stage of fetal growth.[113]

Notable discussions on the classification and biology of teratomas include those by Willis,[184] Teilum,[171] Gonzalez-Crussi,[65] Dehner,[40,42,44] and Fox.[57]

Fetus in Fetu

The relationship between fetus in fetu and teratoma remains controversial and somewhat nebulous, to say the least.[4,54,65,77,109,110,121,184] *Fetus in fetu* is defined as a pedunculated mass with vertebrae or notochord and a structural organization that exceeds that of a teratoma.[65,77] It typically occurs in the retroperitoneum. Federici et al. diligently reviewed the literature on this subject, identifying and listing 41 cases since 1806 and adding 3 of their own.[54]

Both fetus in fetu and teratoma may occur together in the same individual, albeit rarely, and a family history of twinning has been noted in some patients with teratomas.[18,40] Fetus in fetu has been detected by prenatal ultrasonography.[54,77,121] An abdominal retroperitoneal mass is the most common clinical finding.[54] It is reported in association with an undescended testis, which presents as an abdominal mass in neonates.[4] In the author's experience, one newborn with fetus in fetu had a retroperitoneal mass containing vertebra-like bone, gut remnants, and mostly fibrofatty tissue. The oval, amorphous, skin-covered blob with a poorly formed appendage was enclosed within a fibrous membrane attached to the retroperitoneum by a vascular pedicle.

Teratoma and fetus in fetu are probably components of a continuum, with no well-defined distinction between the two.[113,165] Moreover, at the present time, fetus in fetu is regarded as a form of teratoma and is categorized as a mature teratoma according to the WHO classification (Table 2–3). Another term applied to this lesion, particularly when the ovary is involved, is homunculus.[77,150]

Clinical Findings

Teratoma is the foremost germ cell tumor of the fetus and newborn, usually presenting as an obvious mass with signs and symptoms referable to the location of origin. Teratomas are seen more often in the perinatal period than at any other time in childhood.[2,18,40,169,180] Half of childhood teratomas are congenital and, in some perinatal series, they are the most common tumor overall (Table 1–1).[90,127,169,180] Although a mature teratoma is considered to be benign on the basis of histologic findings, it may cause death if vital structures, such as the brain or heart, are involved[65,125,168] or if the airway is compromised.[18,92,113] Teratomas are detected antenatally by ultrasonography. Sonographic findings have been presented by Reece,[138] Kurjak et al.,[102] Wienk et al.,[181] and Chervenak et al.[30,31]

Significant congenital anomalies often occur in association with teratomas.[11,80,127,180] The type of anomaly depends on the site and size of the tumor, and their appearance and extent vary. For example, single or combined malformations of the genitourinary tract, rectum, anus, vertebrae, and caudal spinal cord are found in patients with extensive sacrococcygeal teratomas.[12,106,124,127] Large, disfiguring cleft palate defects are found in newborns with gigantic cranial and nasopharyngeal neoplasms.[65,133]

Unique clinical presentations are associated with large, space-occupying, congenital teratomas. These may present as nonimmune hydrops fetalis (severe generalized edema not attributable to hemolytic disease of the newborn); respiratory distress and/or hemoptysis resulting from compression or extension into the airway; polyhydramnios secondary to the fetus' inability to swallow amniotic fluid; stillbirth; and maternal dystocia.[11,17,18,40,92,141,145,168,180] Gigantic exophthalmos and massive hydrocephalus are associated with orbital and cranial teratomas, respectively.[16,65,125] Failure to establish respirations owing to airway obstruction is the initial finding in a baby with a nasopharyngeal, tonsillar, palatal, cervical, or mediastinal teratoma.[11,18,40,42,90] Some epignathi, thyrocervical, and nasopharyngeal teratomas are so large and extensive that they are unresectable and cause death by asphyxia at the time of birth.[133]

Occasionally, perinatal teratomas are discovered as an unexpected or incidental finding on prenatal or neonatal imaging studies, on a newborn physical examination, or later, during a routine follow-up examination for some other unrelated clinical problem. Internal teratomas arising from the mediastinum, pericardium, and retroperitoneum are prime examples of such neoplasms. The pericardial teratoma listed in Table 2–2 was found incidentally on a chest x-ray film taken for evaluation of an upper respiratory infection.

In a review of 17,417 perinatal postmortem examinations, Werb et al. found 24 teratomas, accounting for 50% of the congenital tumors identified.[180] The teratomas were usually large and, owing to their size and location, were incompatible with extrauterine life. Ten teratomas were associated with hydramnios, 3 with dystocia, 5 with hydrops fetalis, and 4 with malformations at locations distant to the tumor. Twenty teratomas were identified in stillborn fetuses, 50% of whom were macerated.[180] Valdes-Dapena and Arey conducted an analysis of 501 autopsies performed on newborns during the years 1960 through 1966 at St. Christopher's Hospital for Children. They identified one patient with a neoplasm that was identified as a thyroid teratoma. The baby died shortly after birth from respiratory obstruction.[176]

Sites of Origin

Sacrococcygeal Teratoma

Sacrococcygeal teratoma is the leading germ cell tumor and the most common neoplasm of the fetus and newborn in several renowned series (Table 2–3).[7,13,66,67,71,93,116,127,169,177,178,180] The tumor has an estimated incidence of 1:20,000 to 1:40,000 births, with a female predominance ranging from 2:1 to 4:1.[12,40,42,47,113] Although most occur sporadically, familial presacral teratomas and an increased frequency in twins have been reported.[9,60,85,113] In two families investigated by Ashcraft and Holder, teratomas and associated anomalies were found in more than three generations, suggesting a dominant inheritance pattern.[9]

In some studies, as many as 18% of patients with sacrococcygeal teratomas have associated congenital defects, such as tracheoesophageal fistula, imperforate anus, anorectal stenosis, spina bifida, genitourinary malformations, meningomyelocele and anencephaly.[9,12,33,60,85,101,127,180] Some anomalies are related, in part, to the presence of a large, space-occupying mass during development, but others occur elsewhere independently.[113]

Many sacrococcygeal teratomas are small and asymptomatic during pregnancy and so are not discovered until birth.[63,138] However, larger ones may become manifest in utero and may be diagnosed prenatally with imaging studies.[6,21,30,39,55,56,62,63,72,76,79,80,101,119,136,138,148,156,186] Since 1979, increasing numbers of sacrococcygeal teratomas have been diagnosed by antenatal sonography.[62] An enlarged uterus for the expected time of gestation may be the initial finding. Prenatal sonography may reveal an external mass, arising from the sacral area, that is composed of solid and cystic areas, with foci of calcification apparent in about one third of the tumors.[30,55,79,80,82,144] Kuhlman et al. reported one of the earliest prenatal diagnoses at 13 weeks' gestation.[101]

Polyhydramnios, nonimmune hydrops fetalis, placentomegaly, dystocia, stillbirth, and neonatal death have all been attributed to large sacrococcygeal teratomas.[6,30,33,63,80,99,136,138,144,162,180] Hydrops, hepatomegaly, and placentomegaly result from fetal high-output cardiac failure secondary to a vascular shunt created by the tumor. Severe anemia following hemorrhage into the tumor is another contributing factor.

Flake et al. reviewed 22 cases of fetal sacrococcygeal teratoma, including one of theirs, and concluded that most tumors are discovered at 22 to 34 weeks' gestation.[56] In their series, a uterus that was large for gestational dates, with or without hydramnios, was the first sign; detection after 30 weeks' gestation correlated with a fetal survival of 75%, as compared to a 7% survival for tumors presenting before 30 weeks. Fetal hydrops and/or placentomegaly was associated with stillbirth in practically all instances.

Other problems associated with large sacrococcygeal teratomas include rupture or massive hemorrhage into the tumor with fetal exsanguination during delivery.[6,24,33,56,78,86,138,162,180] In the study conducted by Holzgreve et al., three neonatal deaths were attributed to trauma of the tumor mass related to vaginal delivery.[80] Because of this finding, the authors now recommend cesarean section to prevent trauma to the teratoma or dystocia. Hemorrhage into the tumor and complications of prematurity are the main causes of death from sacrococcygeal teratoma in the perinatal period.[62]

Amniotic fluid levels of alpha-fetoprotein (AFP) and acetylcholine esterase are either high normal or increased with this tumor; therefore, these tests are not helpful in distinguishing between a neural tube defect and a sacrococcygeal teratoma in the fetus.[138] Moreover, sacrococcygeal teratoma has been misdiagnosed as a myelomeningocele on the basis of antenatal sonographic findings and an elevated maternal AFP level.[53] Cystic sacrococcygeal teratoma and myelomeningocele show similar findings on sonography, and both are associated with an elevated maternal level of AFP. Physical examination of the affected fetus may reveal the correct diagnosis, but careful histologic evaluation of the cyst wall may be necessary in some instances to distinguish between the two entities.[53]

Sacrococcygeal teratomas may be attached to the inner or outer surface of the sacrum and coccyx (see Figs. 2–2 and 2–3) or may arise from the soft tissues of the pelvis. They are present at the lower end of the trunk, sometimes separating the legs and at other times extending posteriorly from the spine.[133] If they extend into the abdominal cavity, it is usually only for a short distance, and the bulk of the tumor remains exterior. Teratomas can usually be easily shelled out of the lower pelvis, but may be attached to the coccyx more firmly. They are generally large, often measuring 15 to 30 cm or more in diameter at birth, which indicates an origin early in intrauterine life. Immature teratomas tend to be larger and more solid than mature ones.[169] Extension of the teratoma into the spinal canal and attachment to the spinal cord are unusual.[134,170] Earlier, it was mentioned that the tumor may be confused clinically with myelomeningocele, although the latter usually occur at a higher level and are less solid. Most teratomas are composed principally of tissue resembling brain, but elements from all germ layers are usually present. Others may contain, in addition, an immature neuroglial component, sometimes a yolk sac tumor, and rarely, embryonal carcinoma (Tables 2–1 and 2–2) (Figs. 2–2 to 2–16).[5,12,51,63,72,75,79,87]

Teratomas of the Neck

Thyrocervical teratomas are second in frequency to those arising from the sacrococcygeal region (Tables 2–1 and 2–2).[18,40,65,88,169] Six of 128 (5%) newborn teratomas in the Boston Children's Medical Center study, and 8% of 62 newborn teratomas in the Children's Hospital, Los Angeles series occurred in the neck (Tables 2–1 and 2–2).[169] Generally, neonates with thyrocervical teratomas do not have other associated defects, but imperforate anus, congenital heart malformations, chondrodystrophy, pulmonary hypoplasia, anencephalus, hydrocephalus, trisomy 13, and cystic fibrosis are described occasionally.[11,46,69,94,113,144,145] The presence of a cervical mass is the main finding (see Fig. 2–4). The cause of death with extensive teratomas is respiratory distress resulting

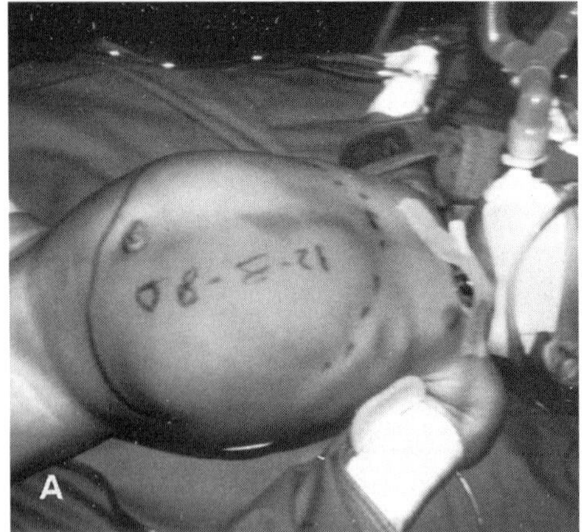

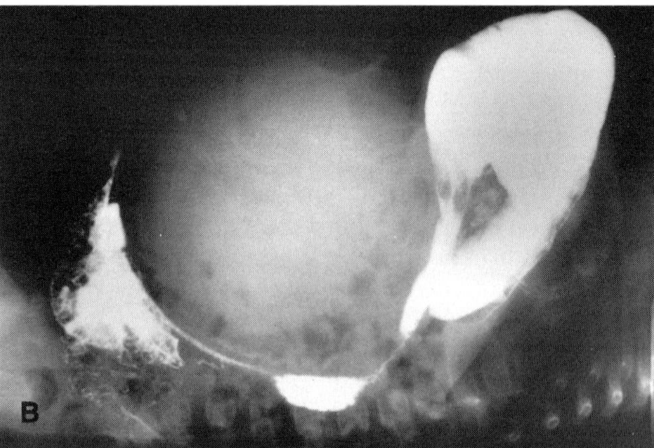

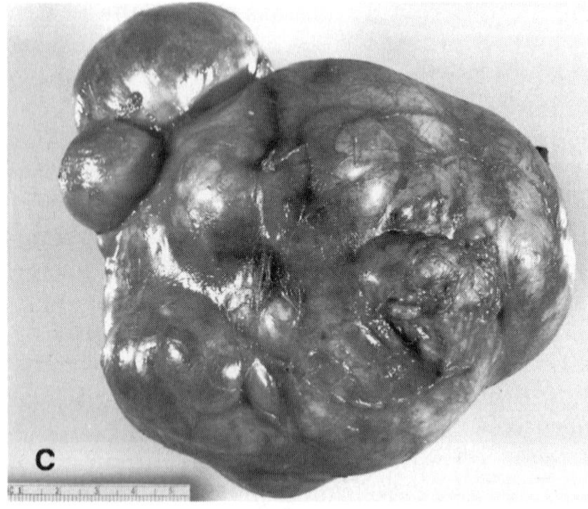

Figure 2–5. Retroperitoneal teratoma. The patient was a 2-month-old male infant with a history of constipation, progressive abdominal distention, and an enlarging abdominal mass since birth. *A,* The infant's protuberant abdomen and tumor are outlined. *B,* The abdominal imaging study reveals compression of the intestine by a large retroperitoneal mass. *C,* The specimen, weighing 799 g and measuring 15 × 15 × 6 cm, consists of solid and cystic areas. (From Isaacs H Jr. Tumors of the Newborn and Infant. St. Louis: Mosby–Year Book, 1991.

from tracheal deviation or compression by the tumor.[23,69,94,145,176] Extension of the teratoma into the mediastinum, which causes pulmonary hypoplasia, further compounds the respiratory problems and increases the mortality.[69]

When large cervical teratomas are detected in utero by sonography,[62] the findings generally reveal a unilateral, asymmetric, well-defined, partially solid and cystic mass, with or without calcifications.[11,14,50,94,113,144,145] Cystic lymphangioma (hygroma) is the main consideration in the differential diagnosis.[62] Polyhydramnios is found in about one third of the cases, particularly when the lesion is large.[62] Gigantic tumors cause dystocia, in which case a cesarean section may be required to deliver the baby.[14,69,94,113,144,145]

Cervical teratomas are often intimately related to the thyroid gland, although evidence that they arise from the thyroid is sometimes lacking. Like the teratomas of the sacrococcy-

geal region, they are overwhelmingly congenital in origin.[133,160] Brain tissue is the most frequent component, and cartilage, bronchial epithelium, and ependyma-lined cysts are not uncommon. Generally, the teratomas are composed of both mature and immature neuroglial tissues.[23,69,91,169] Congenital cervical teratomas with yolk sac tumor are rare.[42,174] Metastasis of immature neuroglial elements from a cervical teratoma to the lungs was described by Baumann and Nerlich, who found a similar case in the German literature.[14] Additionally, cervical lymph node metastases composed of immature neuroglial tissue has been reported by Dunn et al. and Gundry and colleagues.[50,69] Several examples of neonatal malignant cervicofacial teratomas, including some of those just cited, have also been identified by Azizkhan et al.,[11] but their article did not specify the exact head and neck primary sites for each of the malignant lesions, and no histologic details were given.

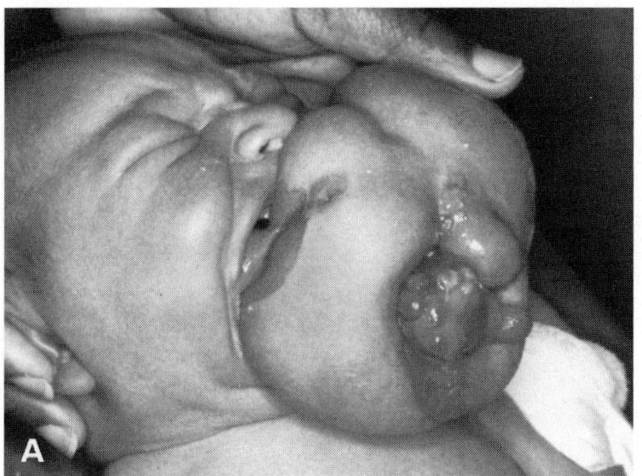 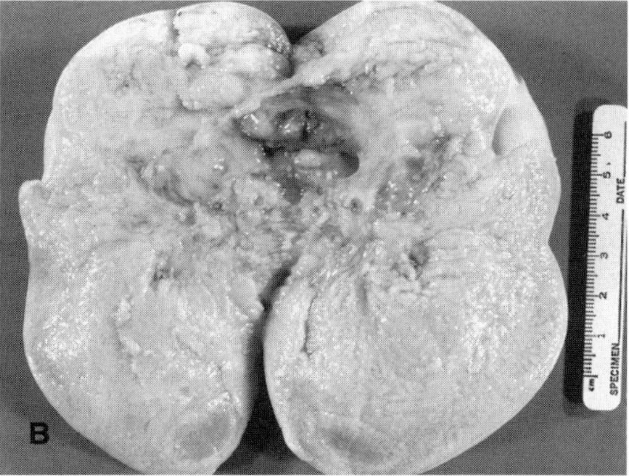

Figure 2–6. Epignathus. *A,* A 4-day-old, full-term male infant with a solid teratoma attached to the right side of the hard palate. *B,* The specimen consists mostly of fat. There is an appendage-like protrusion sticking out on the left side. The central nodular area is composed of mature tissues consisting of brain, gastrointestinal tract, and bone. Although microscopic examination of the tumor suggests fetus in fetu, neither well-defined vertebrae nor structural organization of the tissue components are noted. (From Isaacs H Jr. Neoplasms in infants: A report of 265 cases. Pathol Annu 1983;18(2): 165. Used by permission.)

Immediate surgical intervention in newborns with cervical teratomas has reduced the significant mortality from 80% in nonoperative cases to 10% to 15% in operative cases.[69]

Palatal and Nasopharyngeal Teratoma

Epignathi arise from the soft or hard palate in the region of Rathke's pouch (an upgrowth from the roof of the primitive oral cavity) and vary greatly in size. They generally fill the buccal cavity and extend out through the mouth, although they may arise from the upper surface of the sphenoid bone and extend into the cranial cavity. Occasionally, an isthmus of tissue extends through the sphenoid bone connecting inner and outer masses of tumor tissue.[133,161] Tumors at the base of the skull and hard palate differ only in the direction of their growth. Some extend out of the mouth and contain fairly well-differentiated structures resembling fetal parts (Fig. 2–6). Pharyngeal teratomas

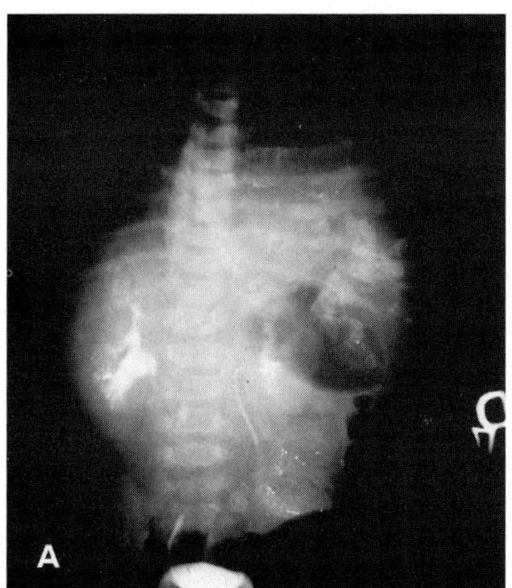 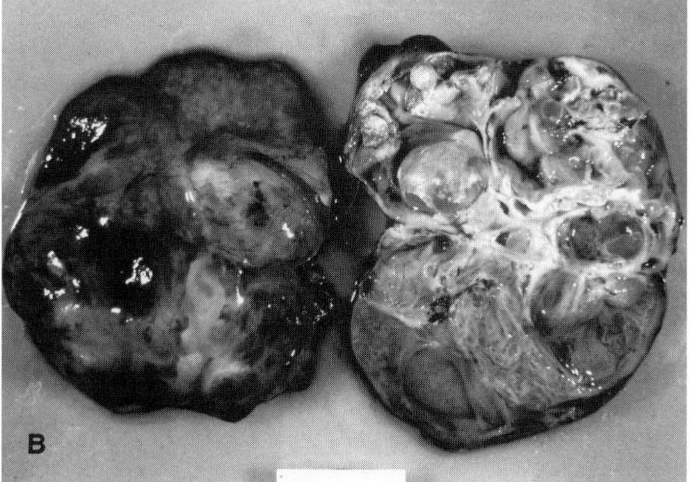

Figure 2–7. Gastric teratoma in a 4-month-old male infant with vomiting, feeding problems, and an abdominal mass. *A,* Intravenous pyelography depicts a tumor arising from the lesser curvature of the body of the stomach. *B,* The cystic and solid tumor measured 16 × 14 cm and contained immature neuroglial tissue, skin, choroid plexus, gastrointestinal and respiratory epithelium, and cartilage.

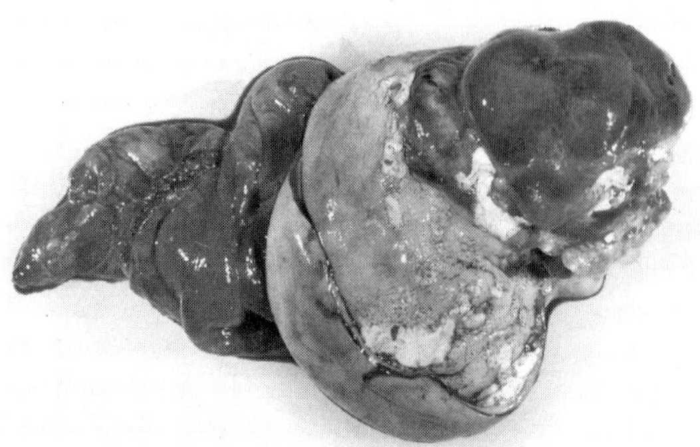

Figure 2–8. Teratoma of the testis. A testicular mass measuring 7.5 × 5 cm was found in an infant during a routine bilateral inguinal hernia repair. The gross photograph shows a tumor composed of skin, white sebaceous material, and a variety of tissues. In addition to skin, bone, and gastrointestinal tract epithelium, immature neuroglial elements were present on histologic examination.

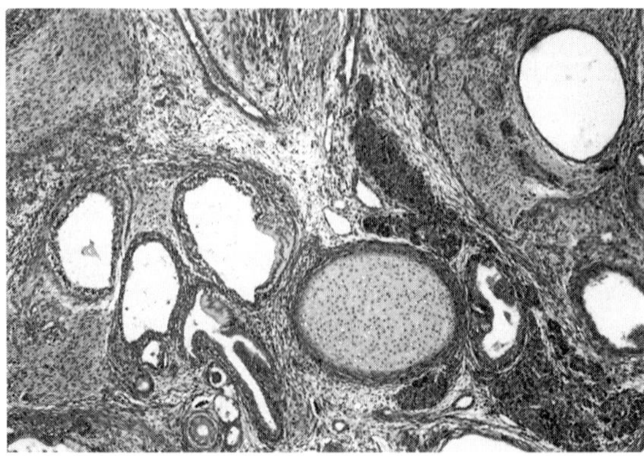

Figure 2–10. Photomicrograph of a mediastinal teratoma composed mainly of mature neuroglial tissue with cysts lined by a variety of epithelia, cartilage, and salivary gland (hematoxylin-eosin, ×50). (From Isaacs H Jr. Tumors of the Newborn and Infant. St. Louis: Mosby–Year Book, 1991.

arise from the posterior nasopharynx and vary considerably in their extent.[5,133]

Large epignathic teratomas are associated with polyhydramnios, which is a poor prognostic sign, and can readily be diagnosed by prenatal sonography.[5,31,35,95,108,113,161] This type of teratoma prevents fetal swallowing, which leads to polyhydramnios.[18] A large, solid and cystic, sometimes calcified mass projecting out from the oral cavity suggests the prenatal diagnosis.[31,35,144]

Less than 10% of newborns with epignathi have associated congenital malformations, which may include cleft palate, hypertelorism,

congenital heart anomalies, umbilical hernia, and facial hemangiomas.[113,144] Facial defects are attributed to the mechanical effects of the teratoma on developing structures.[144] Magee et al. described an inoperable epignathus in a premature female with Aicardi's syndrome (infantile flexor spasms, agenesis of the corpus callosum, and chorioretinal abnormality).[113] Several other examples of palatal and pharyngeal teratomas in neonates and stillborns have been reported in the literature.[5,23,48,112,147]

The differential diagnosis for congenital lesions presenting with an oropharyngeal mass should include epignathus, encephalocele, dermoid cyst, hairy polyp, gastrointestinal cyst, and lingual thyroid.[161]

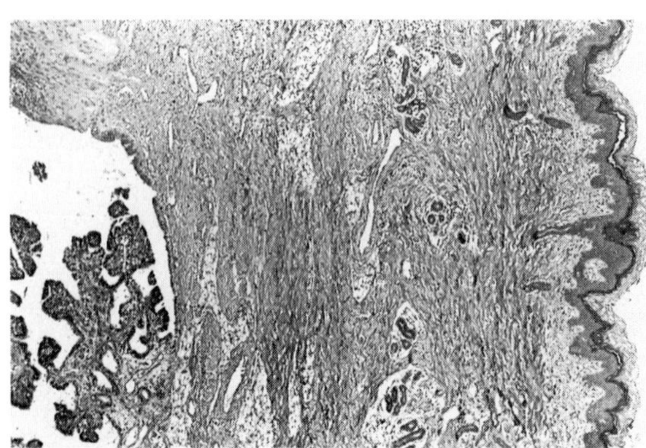

Figure 2–9. Teratoma with skin, neuroglial tissue, and choroid plexus. Most mature teratomas contain these three tissues, as exemplified by the tumors described in Figures 2–2 through 2–8 (hematoxylin-eosin, ×50). (From Isaacs H Jr. Tumors of the Newborn and Infant. St. Louis: Mosby–Year Book, 1991.

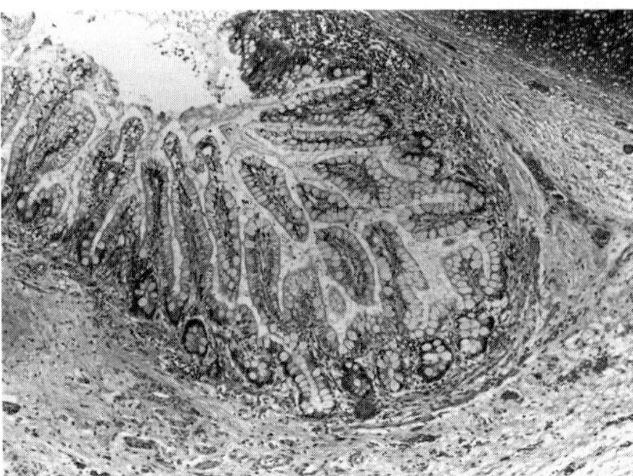

Figure 2–11. Mature sacrococcygeal teratoma with small bowel and cartilaginous components (hematoxylin-eosin, ×50).

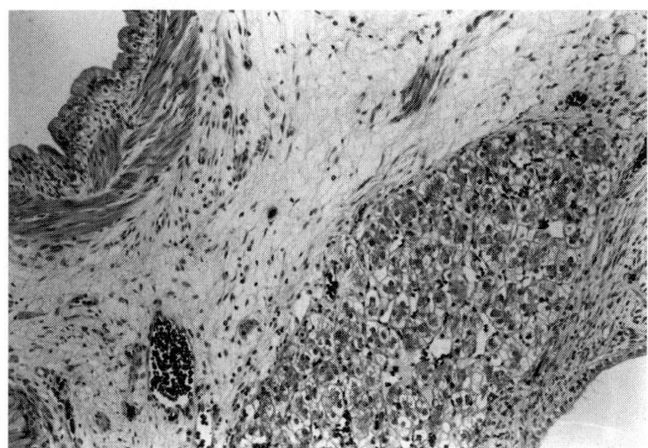

Figure 2–12. Mature sacrococcygeal teratoma with liver and primitive gut (hematoxylin-eosin, ×50). (From Isaacs H Jr. Tumors of the Newborn and Infant. St. Louis: Mosby–Year Book, 1991.)

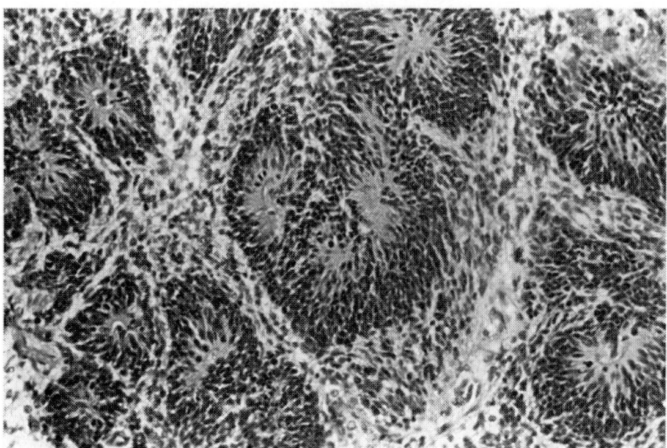

Figure 2–14. Immature, ependymal, rosette-like neuroglial elements are present in this cerebellar teratoma. The main components of immature teratomas, regardless of the primary site of origin, are neuroglial elements, which may be derived from brain germinal matrix, ependyma, choroid plexus, or eye (hematoxylin-eosin, ×150).

Most pharyngeal and epignathic teratomas are histologically benign and are composed of mature tissues, with or without immature neuroglial elements.[23,35,88,161] However, Dehner et al. described three examples of yolk sac tumor, associated with teratomas of the head and neck, that presented as obvious masses at birth.[44] Yolk sac tumor of the nasopharynx was diagnosed in a 3-year-old girl who had a mature teratoma removed from the same site as a newborn.[25] In light of this case, close follow-up examinations and periodic AFP determinations may be indicated for several years. Normal serum AFP values for neonates and infants have been tabulated by Blair and colleagues[20] and Wu et al.[189] (Table 2–4).

The dermoid ("hairy polyp") is one of the main considerations in the differential diagnosis of nasopharyngeal masses in the newborn.[173] The dermoid is related to the teratoma, but it does not contain tissues representative of all three germ layers (Fig. 2–17). Microscopically, it consists only of skin with hair and other appendages, fat, and sometimes, cartilage. The lesion, depending on its size and location, produces intermittent respiratory obstruction and feeding problems that are often related to the infant's position.[112,155,172,173] A lesion that is simi-

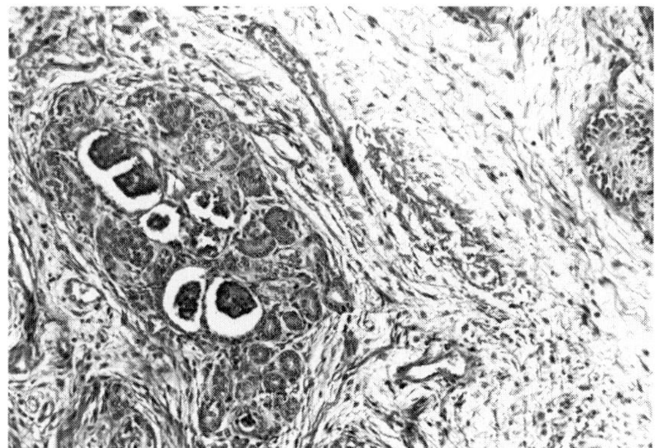

Figure 2–13. Nephrogenic tissue is another example of an uncommon component present in a teratoma, which, in this instance, was from the mediastinum. There is a small cluster of ganglion cells along the right upper margin (hematoxylin-eosin, ×50). (From Isaacs H Jr. Tumors of the Newborn and Infant. St. Louis: Mosby–Year Book, 1991.)

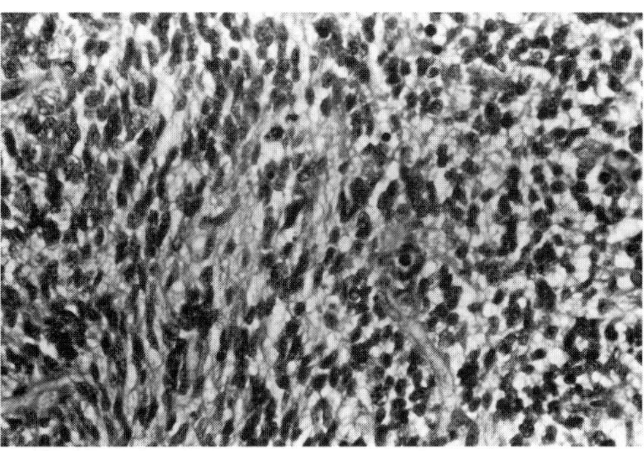

Figure 2–15. Immature cerebellar teratoma with germinal, matrix-like cells having the appearance of a primitive neuroectodermal tumor. Note the numerous, small, dark, round and spindle-shaped cells separated by fibrillar material (neuropil), which are histologic features similar to those observed in both neuroblastoma and medulloblastoma. In most instances, foci of these immature elements blend in with more mature, recognizable neuroglial tissue, which is helpful in establishing the diagnosis (hematoxylin-eosin, ×150).

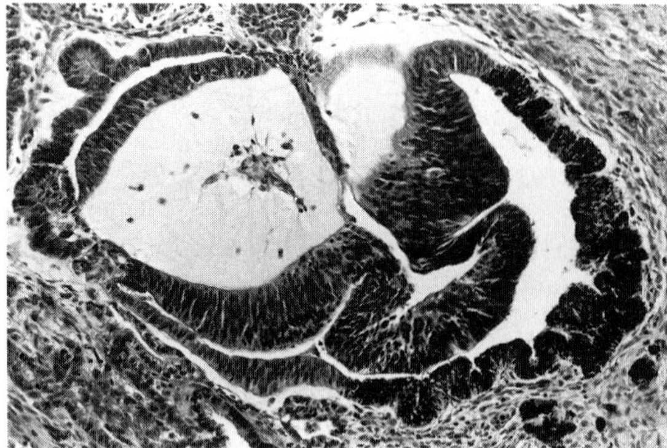

Figure 2–16. Immature cerebellar teratoma with pigmented, optic cup–like structures. Heavily pigmented (possibly retinal) epithelium is present along the right margin of the vesicle (hematoxylin-eosin, ×150).

lar histologically has been known to occur also in the conjunctiva.

Gastric Teratoma

Gastric teratoma is an exceedingly rare form of teratoma.[36,37,40,52,70,92,154] It may present as an abdominal mass in the neonatal period and may be accompanied by vomiting and/or gastrointestinal bleeding (hematemesis or melena), which is noted most often with endophytic lesions (see Fig. 2–7). Respiratory distress occurs when there is displacement of the diaphragm by the tumor.[52] Peritoneal gliomatosis resulting from a congenital gastric teratoma has been reported, and was an incidental finding in hernia sacs removed 10 months after gastrectomy.[36] Histologic examination reveals that gastric teratomas, similar to other tumors found outside the sacrococcygeal area, are composed of mature tissues and, often, immature neuroglial elements. Simple excision of

Table 2–4. Average Normal Serum
α-Fetoprotein Levels in the Perinatal Period

Age	Mean ± SD (ng/mL)
Premature	134,734 ± 41,444
Newborn	48,406 ± 37,718
Newborn to 2 weeks	33,113 ± 32,503
Newborn to 1 month	9,452 ± 12,610
2 weeks to 1 month	2,654 ± 3,080
2 months	323 ± 278
3 months	88 ± 87
4 months	74 ± 56

From Wu JT, Book L, Sudar K. Serum alpha-fetoprotein levels in normal infants. Pediatr Res 1981;15:50. Used by permission.

the teratoma, followed by reconstructive gastric surgery, is the treatment of choice.[52,70] The prognosis for this teratoma is generally favorable.[52,92,154]

Mediastinal Teratoma

Mediastinal teratomas are uncommon in infants and children, constituting only 7% to 10% of all teratomas in this age group.[40,105] Less than 50% of childhood mediastinal teratomas occur in neonates, in whom they are located anteriorly or on either side of the chest, within the pericardium or heart.[27,46,61,92,104,105,130,133,139,169,182] Fourteen cases of teratomas of the heart and pericardium were included in a series by Williams prior to 1962, five of which involved infants younger than 4 months of age.[182] A study by the Boston Children's Medical Center revealed that 4 of 11 children with mediastinal teratomas were 3 months of age or younger.[169] Two newborns had pericardial teratomas with presenting symptoms that mimicked congenital heart disease or idiopathic cardiomegaly. In a study of 15 infants and children with mediastinal teratomas (6 personal cases plus 9 from the literature), Lakhoo et al., of the Hospital for Sick Children, London, found 7 who were younger than 3 months of age.[105] In this study, four tumors were located in the anterior mediastinum, two involved the right chest, and one involved the right cardiac ventricle. A 2-day-old male infant with an encapsulated teratoma attached to the trachea, great vessels, and pericardium was treated successfully with surgical resection performed by Mogilner et al.[117] Magee et al. described a stillborn infant of 26 weeks' gestation with a large mediastinal teratoma and fetal hydrops.[113]

Frequently, patients with mediastinal teratoma have a mass identified on imaging studies, but a definitive diagnosis of teratoma can only be established after microscopic examination of the excised tumor.[105] One such case was diagnosed by prenatal sonography.[179] A multiloculated cystic teratoma located in the anterosuperior mediastinum extended into the neck and was accompanied by polyhydramnios, placental and fetal hydrops, and a fatal outcome. In addition, the neonate had hypoplastic lungs, pleural effusions, and ascites.[179] Froberg et al. documented a similar example of a mature mediastinal teratoma detected by sonography at 25 weeks' gestation.[61] The tumor caused hydrops fetalis and in utero death at 27 weeks' gestation.

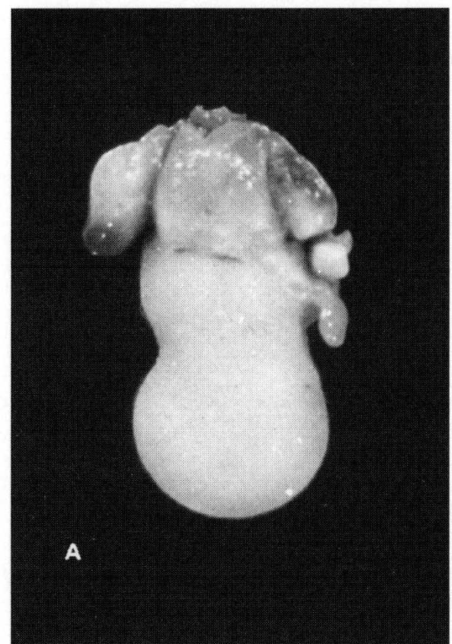 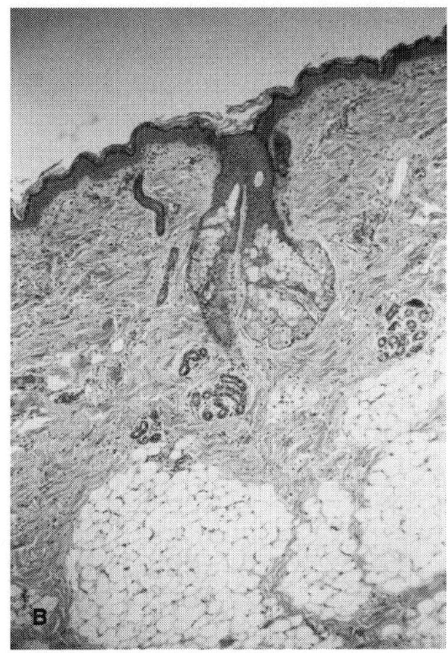

Figure 2–17. Nasopharyngeal hairy polyp. Intermittent respiratory distress related to positioning of the baby was noted shortly after birth. Laryngoscopy revealed a finger-like projection protruding from and obstructing the nasopharynx. *A,* A gross photograph shows a polypoid mass covered by skin with smaller, lateral projections. *B,* On histologic examination, the polyp was found to consist of skin with hair follicles, fat, and cartilage (not shown in this field) (hematoxylin-eosin, ×63).

Fetal hydrops may be the initial manifestation of a pericardial teratoma.[113] Some pericardial teratomas are so large that they practically fill the entire thoracic cavity, preventing respiration at birth.[3,24] The accompanying pericardial effusion also contributes to the respiratory distress, which is one of the main presenting findings in the neonate.[27,105] When present, calcification in an anterior mediastinal mass detected by imaging studies can be an aid in suggesting the diagnosis of teratoma, but calcification is seen in only a small percentage of cases involving the fetus and newborn.[105,117,141,153,179]

Dehner cites a 15% overall malignancy rate for mediastinal teratomas diagnosed in the pediatric age group.[40] However, Carter et al., Lakhoo et al., and Tapper and Lack concluded from their studies that mediastinal teratomas, both mature and immature, occurring in newborns and infants behave in a benign fashion, if resectable, and are associated with a favorable prognosis as compared to those occurring in adolescents and adults.[27,105,169] Of 10 newborns and infants included in the series by Carter et al., only 1 died, as a result of surgical complications.[27] Three of the four patients in the Boston study survived, and one died from compression of the heart and great vessels by an unresectable tumor.[169] Of the 7 patients included in the

London study, one died as a result of a surgical complication.[105] The consensus of opinion is that complete surgical removal is the treatment of choice.

Intrapericardial Teratoma

Intrapericardial teratoma can be detected by prenatal sonography (see Chapter 16, "Cardiac Tumors").[3,137,181] The principal sonographic findings are a mass within the pericardial space that is attached to the base of the great vessels, along with pericardial effusion and, often, polyhydramnios.[3] Older infants may present with respiratory distress and feeding problems.[3,166] The teratoma may be an incidental finding on chest imaging studies performed for evaluation of pneumonia or other condition.

These usually pedunculated masses are attached to the base of the great vessels or the atrioventricular valves (see Fig. 16–3). On histologic examination, mediastinal, pericardial, and intracardiac teratomas are composed of mature tissues, with or without immature neuroglial elements.[3,18,27,92,105,137,141,153,166,169,179]

Retroperitoneal Teratoma

Usually, retroperitoneal teratomas are located in the posterior portion of the abdomen, above the pelvis, presenting as abdominal masses (see Fig. 2–5). They account for about 5% of all childhood teratomas.[114] They are similar to those in the sacrococcygeal region, and are found most often in the first year of life. In Arnheim's study of 44 retroperitoneal teratomas in infants and children prior to 1951, 52% were found in the first year of life and 23% were diagnosed in the first 3 months of life.[8] These tumors may be either unilateral or bilateral. The difficulty of distinguishing between the mature retroperitoneal teratoma and fetus in fetu has already been mentioned. Most teratomas are composed of differentiated (mature) tissues,[8] and less than 15% are associated with yolk sac tumor, which occurs more frequently in older children. Davis et al. described a retroperitoneal teratoma that was resected shortly after birth and was interpreted initially as mature.[39] However, the patient died of a malignant recurrence and metastatic yolk sac carcinoma 3 years after the initial surgery (see Fig. 2–19).[39] Gonzalez-Crussi described an unusual teratoma in a 3-month-old male infant that was composed of both mature tissues and immature nephrogenic tissue (20%) that was indistinguishable from Wilms' tumor.[64] Parenthetically, Dehner also reported an example of an intrarenal teratoma.[41]

Orbital Teratoma

Orbital teratoma is an uncommon neoplasm presenting at birth with unilateral proptosis in an otherwise normal pre-term or full-term infant.[16,107,115] Orbital teratoma can be detected by prenatal sonography.[115] It is characterized by rapid growth, extensive enlargement of the bony orbit, transillumination of part or all of the tumor, and, surprisingly enough, associated normal development of the eye.[16] Occasionally, the tumor extends into the intracranial cavity or is part of an intracranial teratoma with secondary orbital involvement.[16,115] Orbital teratomas contain mature tissues and immature neuroglial elements and, sometimes, embryonic-appearing, optic, cup-like structures, which is unique for teratomas arising in this location (see Fig. 2–16).[115]

Dermoid tumors of the eye arise from the conjunctiva at the margin of the cornea (limbus). They are not true teratomas in that they ordinarily consist only of ectoderm and mesoderm (i.e., skin and fat). Histologically, these lesions resemble pharyngeal hairy polyps and

probably could be assigned to the category of choristoma.

Teratomas in Other Locations

Teratomas characteristically occur in or near the midplane of the body and are usually noted in the face and the eye, but not in the extremities. One example was a massive teratoma measuring 20 cm × 18 cm that was attached to the center of the face, involving the maxillae and orbits, and that extended into the cranial cavity through a patent Rathke's pouch.[185] Another tumor was situated under the scalp near the region of the posterior fontanelle.[133] The tonsil, tongue, intestine, abdominal wall, kidney, liver, and maxillary sinus are uncommon locations for teratomas.[10,17,22,41,44,46] Takehara et al. described a nasal teratoma protruding from an enlarged, distorted, right nostril in a neonate with an acardiac amorphous twin.[167]

Most teratomas in the brain originate from the pineal region or the base of the skull. Recently, a newborn with a midline cerebellar teratoma was operated on at Children's Hospital, San Diego. Intracranial teratomas, the most frequent central nervous system tumors occurring in fetuses and newborns, are discussed in Chapter 9, "Brain Tumors."

Practically all teratomas occurring in unusual sites outside the sacrococcygeal area in the newborn are composed primarily of mature tissues from all three germ layers, with or without immature neuroglial elements. These generally behave, therefore, in a benign fashion.[92]

Testicular teratomas occur in newborns and infants and generally contain mature tissues, with or without immature neuroglial elements (Fig. 2–8).[92] One of 46 (2.2%) teratomas recorded in the Prepubertal Testicular Tumor Registry occurred in a neonate (see Table 3–1).[96] The median age of 46 patients with this tumor who were included in the Registry was 14 months.[96] Intratubular germ cell neoplasia associated with teratoma is very rare in infants and is considered to be a precursor lesion or preinvasive stage of germ cell tumor of the testis. The lesion is found in undescended testes during the first year of life.[164]

Placental teratomas are very uncommon, for only a dozen or so have been reported.[58,113,122,158,183] Most are composed of mature tissues, but the one described by Williams and Williams contained immature elements.[183] Placental teratomas have been discussed in detail by Shanklin[158] and by Magee et al.[113] Parenthetically, persistent omphalomesenteric duct remnants in the umbilical cord, composed of vacuolated cuboidal epithelium, have been mistaken for teratoma.

Prognosis and Treatment

Serial sonographic examinations are indicated for fetuses with teratomas in order to monitor tumor size, amniotic fluid volume, and the status of the fetus.[62] Teratomas, particularly those that are cervical and sacrococcygeal, are associated with an increased frequency of preterm labor and premature delivery related to placentomegaly, polyhydramnios, and the size of the tumor.[62,138,144] Cesarean section may be indicated because of malpresentation and dystocia attributable to the teratoma. In utero fetal surgery is presently being investigated as a treatment option.[62]

Most teratomas diagnosed in infants are classified histologically as mature. The immature teratoma, with or without a mature component, is second in frequency (see Tables 2–1 and 2–2). The sacrococcygeal area is the location associated with the highest incidence of malignancy, usually in the form of either endodermal sinus tumor or, rarely, embryonal carcinoma.[17,41,87,89,124,169] The overall frequency of neonatal sacrococcygeal teratomas with yolk sac tumor is approximately 10%, with values cited in the literature ranging from as low as 2.5% to as high as 25%.[12,17,90,149,169] The presence of immature neuroglial elements in neonatal teratomas, although worrisome, apparently has no bearing on prognosis, as these patients generally have a favorable outcome.[12,90] An important relationship exists between the age at diagnosis of a patient with sacrococcygeal teratoma and outcome. The incidence of malignancy in the neonate is roughly 10%, whereas it approaches almost 100% by 3 years of age.[42,92] According to Bale, there is also a significant relationship between the location of the teratoma and the incidence of malignancy, which varies from 8% for postsacral lesions, to 34% to 42% for dumbbell lesions, to 38% to 75% for presacral lesions.[12]

The recommended treatment for sacrococcygeal teratoma is early diagnosis and complete surgical removal of the tumor, including the coccyx, as soon as possible after birth.[2,34,42,149,169] Often, the infant is cured following surgery. However, in some instances, the patient returns several months or even years after the initial

surgery with a mass in the sacrococcygeal area that is identified on biopsy as a teratoma and/ or yolk sac tumor.[19,169] Recurrences were noted in 3 of 40 patients with sacrococcygeal teratomas in the Birmingham, U.K. series, in 3 of 102 patients in the Childrens' Hospital Medical Center, Boston series, and in 6 of 36 patients included in the Hospital for Sick Children, Toronto study.[19,127,169] The possible explanations for recurrence include an inadequate surgical excision initially, a second primary tumor, sampling error, or an oversight of the subtle yolk sac tumor component by the pathologist.[75,92] According to Hawkins et al., minute, occult yolk sac tumor elements in a sacrococcygeal teratoma can easily be overlooked unless a thorough search is undertaken.[75] These researchers identified six children with mature or immature sacrococcygeal teratomas initially diagnosed during the newborn period who subsequently developed yolk sac tumor recurrences within 7 to 33 months.

The prognosis for an infant with teratoma, whether or not there are immature neuroglial elements, is favorable, particularly if the tumor is situated outside the sacrococcygeal area. Probably the most plausible explanation for this is that teratomas occurring outside the sacrococcygeal region during the first year of life have a considerably lower frequency of association with yolk sac tumor (see Table 2–2).[17,42] Previously, it was noted that the incidence of malignancy in tumors of the sacrococcygeal area is age-related; this does not appear to be true for other sites (except during adolescence and adulthood), although exceptions have been described. Recurrence of yolk sac tumor several years after removal of a congenital nasopharyngeal teratoma has been reported.[25] Moreover, the study by Tapper and Lack revealed that the single most important factor affecting outcome, regardless of site, was whether the teratoma could be resected successfully at the time of initial surgery.[169] Nevertheless, patients should undergo close follow-up, including imaging studies and AFP levels, for at least 3 years after surgical excision of a sacrococcygeal teratoma.[19] Table 2–4 shows the average normal serum AFP values for young infants at various ages.

YOLK SAC TUMOR

Yolk sac tumor (endodermal sinus tumor) is the leading malignant germ cell tumor affecting infants and children.[2,73,74] More arise from the sacrococcygeal area than from any other location during the first year of life. Less common primary sites in this age group include the head and neck, testis, pelvic retroperitoneum, and vagina, and seldom, the ovary.[40,44] Pediatric yolk sac tumor is cytogenetically and biologically distinct from its adult counterpart. Perlman et al. examined six childhood yolk sac tumors and found deletions in chromosomes 1 (1p) and 6 (6q), but no evidence of i(12p) deletion, which is described in adult germ cell tumors.[132]

Yolk sac tumor is the predominant pediatric malignant germ cell tumor involving the testis. Six of 207 (2.9%) such tumors recorded in the Prepubertal Testicular Tumor Registry occurred in newborns.[96] No neonatal examples of yolk sac tumor of the testis were found in the series of either Abell and Holtz (the youngest patient being 6 months of age) or the Children's Hospital, Los Angeles (the youngest patient being 11 months of age).[1,92] The frequencies of yolk sac and juvenile granulosa cell tumors were almost identical in Kay's study;[96] of 20 neonatal testis tumors, 6 were classified as yolk sac tumors and 8 were identified as juvenile granulosa cell or other gonadal stromal tumors (see Table 3–1).

Vaginal yolk sac tumor is a distinctive lesion that is noted in girls younger than 2 years of age.[29,123] Vaginal bleeding or spotting on the diaper and a polypoid mass projecting into the vaginal lumen are the characteristic clinical findings. On gross examination, the mass resembles sarcoma botryoides (embryonal rhabdomyosarcoma) because of its polypoid, grape-like appearance. However, the histologic features are those of a malignant epithelial tumor with a papillary or reticular pattern and positive AFP immunoperoxidase staining (Fig. 2–18), rather than a small cell sarcoma with cytoplasmic cross-striations on hematoxylin-eosin staining, a positive actin and desmin reaction, and thick and thin cytoplasmic filaments observed on electron microscopy. To the author's knowledge, neonatal ovarian yolk sac tumor has not been reported.

On gross examination, yolk sac tumors have a slimy, pale tan-yellow appearance, with greyish-red foci of necrosis and small cyst formations. Generally, they are very soft and mushy, and often fall apart upon removal. When the testis is involved, most of it is replaced by tumor, leaving a barely recognizable, light tan,

thin rim of parenchyma (Fig. 2–18A). Six or more histologic patterns of endodermal sinus tumor are recognized: papillary, reticular, solid, polyvesicular vitelline, hepatoid, and glandular, including the endometrioid-like pattern.[32,40,73,135,150,171] The papillary form consists of papillary projections, with or without the classical perivascular endodermal sinus structures (Schiller-Duval body) (Fig. 2–18B and C). The reticular pattern shows tumor cells arranged in a network situated about spaces containing vacuolated, pink-staining material (Fig. 2–18D). The solid pattern consists mostly of solid nests of cells. The rare polyvesicular vitelline variant displays hourglass-like vesicles with constrictions (the blastocyst yolk sac vesicles described by Teilum[171]) embedded in a cellular mesenchymal background. A distinctive variation of the solid pattern is the hepatoid pattern, which derives its name from the histologic observation that the cells resemble fetal liver cells, suggesting hepatocellular differentiation by the tumor.[73,135] The endometrioid-like variant is found in the ovary of girls older than 11 years of age and is characterized by gland-like formations lined by tall, clear cells similar to early secretory endometrium.[32] There is also a more primitive glandular form described by Chen et al.[29] The papillary and reticular patterns are the ones most frequently observed in the newborn with yolk sac tumor.

Intracellular and extracellular hyaline droplets are present in most yolk sac tumors. The droplets test positive upon periodic acid-Schiff (PAS) staining, are diastase-resistant, and are variably reactive to AFP, which is a useful chemical marker present in the serum of these patients (Fig. 2–18C and E).[40,188]

Prior to the era of improved chemotherapeutic agents, the prognosis of a child with a malignant germ cell tumor was dismal, but now it has improved considerably.[2,74] The Pediatric Oncology Study (1971–1984) showed, however, that neonatal sacrococcygeal teratomas may recur as yolk sac tumors, which are associated with a particularly poor prognosis because of their invasive nature (Fig. 2–19); additionally, the study showed that the polyvesicular vitelline pattern of this tumor was associated with a better prognosis than other histologic forms of sacrococcygeal tumors.[74] In a recent study, 1 of 11 patients with yolk sac tumor and metastatic disease died, having received only one chemotherapeutic agent.[72]

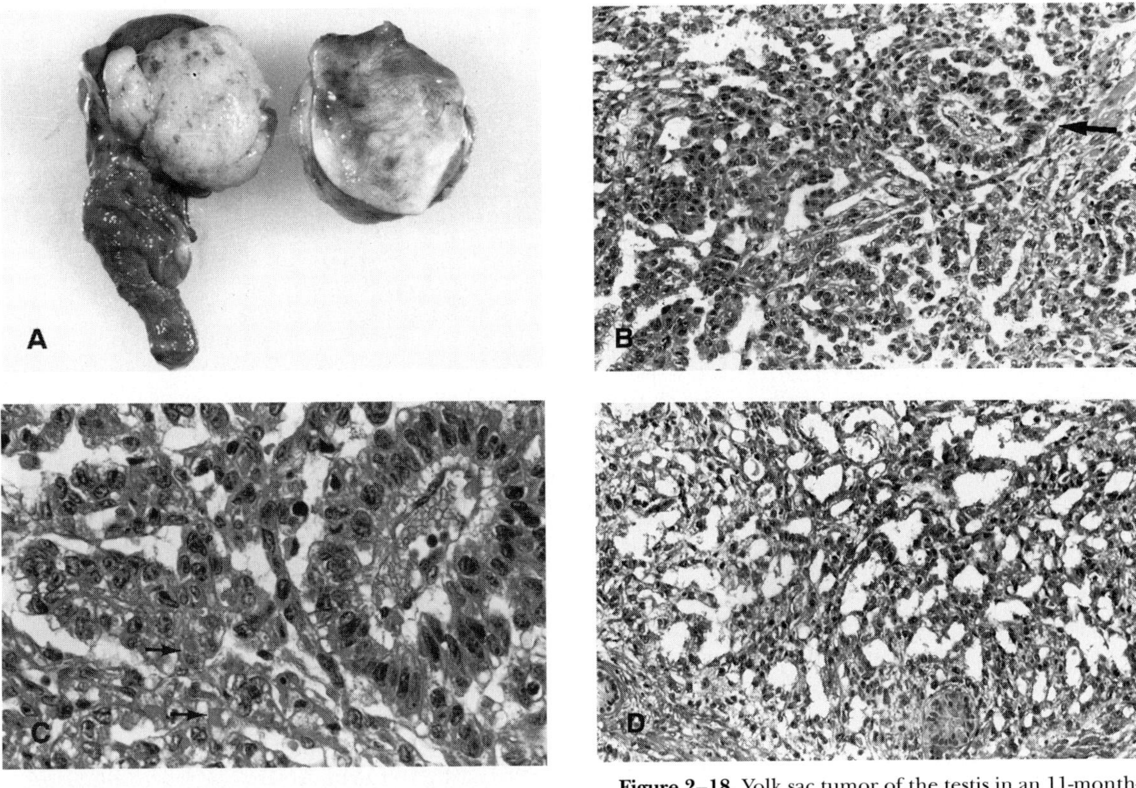

Figure 2–18. Yolk sac tumor of the testis in an 11-month-old male infant with a scrotal mass. *A*, The bisected testicular tumor and attached spermatic cord are shown. *B*, A photomicrograph reveals the papillary pattern of yolk sac tumor and perivascular endodermal sinus structures (Schiller-Duval body) (*arrow*) (hematoxylin-eosin, ×120). *C*, A higher-power view of papillary and endodermal sinus structures. Deposits of hyaline-staining material representing α-fetoprotein are present (*arrows*). *D*, A histologic section shows the reticular (net-like) pattern. Two small immature testicular tubules are present near the lower margin of the photograph (hematoxylin-eosin, ×120). *E*, staining with α-fetoprotein immunoperoxidase reveals a reaction with some of the tumor cells (α-fetoprotein immunoperoxidase, ×300). (From Isaacs H Jr. Tumors of the Newborn and Infant. St. Louis: Mosby–Year Book, 1991.)

EMBRYONAL CARCINOMA

Embryonal carcinoma is the other malignant germ cell tumor that is found in the first year of life.[92,169] It is far less common than yolk sac tumor, occurring alone or in combination with a teratoma. Previously, yolk sac tumors were lumped into the category of embryonal carcinomas (e.g., yolk sac tumor of the testis), which merely added to the confusion with regard to the terminology, classification, and clinical evaluation of these two tumors. On microscopic examination, embryonal carcinoma is a poorly differentiated malignant lesion composed of embryonal-looking epithelial cells with characteristic large nucleoli growing in solid and glandular patterns (Fig. 2–20).[73,152] The results of human chorionic gonadotropin (hCG) and AFP immunoperoxidase staining tests are variable, but cytokeratin is positive. Electron microscopy usually is not helpful in establishing the diagnosis.

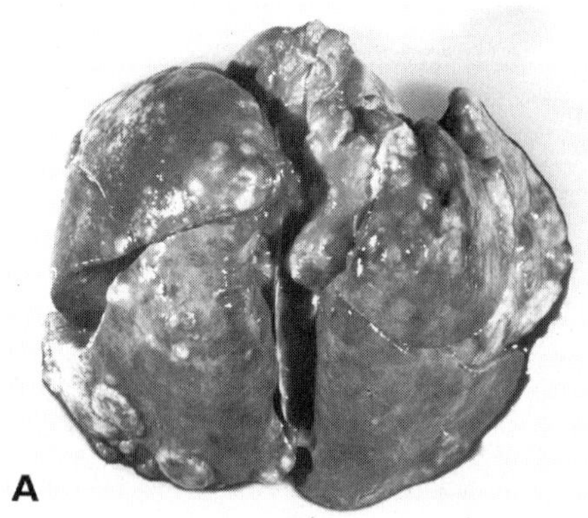

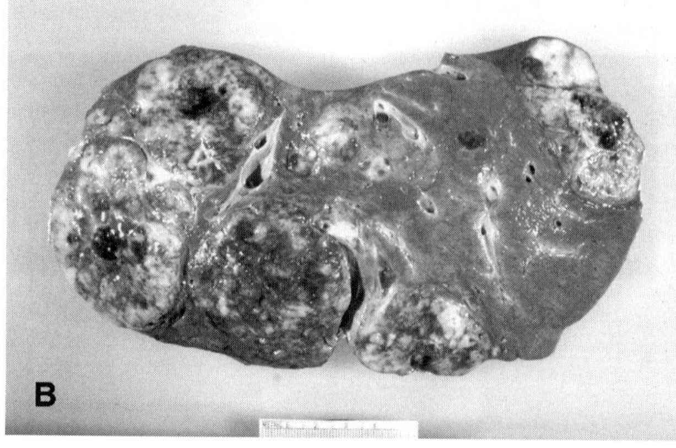

Figure 2–19. Sacrococcygeal teratoma with yolk sac tumor metastases. Yolk sac tumor is the most common malignant component of sacrococcygeal teratomas; it occurs in about 10% of the tumors in this location. *A*, Lung metastases. *B*, Liver metastases. (From Isaacs H Jr. Tumors of the Newborn and Infant. St. Louis: Mosby–Year Book, 1991.)

POLYEMBRYOMA

Polyembryoma is a very infrequent and unusual germ cell tumor of the gonads that is characterized by the presence of embryoid bodies that resemble presomite embryos.[171] Microscopically, the embryoid bodies are similar to tiny embryos, with two vesicles, resembling yolk sac and amniotic cavity, separated by a two- to three-layer embyonic disk. The polyembryoma

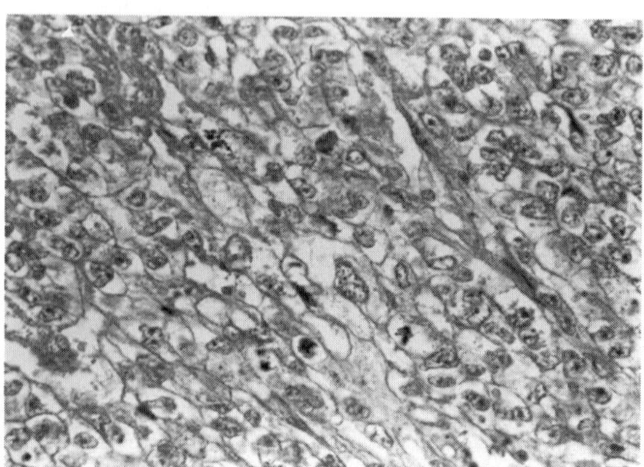

Figure 2–20. Presacral teratoma with embryonal carcinoma and yolk sac tumor. This 1-year-old female patient was found to have a large presacral mass. Histologic sections of the tumor revealed neuroglial tissue, cysts lined by squamous and respiratory epithelium, and nodules of cartilage. In addition, there is a malignant germ cell tumor component composed of both endodermal sinus tumor (predominantly) and embryonal carcinoma. The latter consists of sheets of large, atypical-looking, pleomorphic, epithelial cells with vesicular nuclei and prominent nucleoli, as depicted in the photomicrograph (hematoxylin-eosin, ×300). (From Isaacs H Jr. Tumors of the Newborn and Infant. St. Louis: Mosby–Year Book, 1991.)

stains positively for AFP and β-hCG, suggesting both embryonic and extraembryonic differentiation.[2] In the Children's Hospital, Los Angeles study, two infants had yolk sac tumors of the testis associated with polyembryoma.[92]

DYSGERMINOMA AND CHORIOCARCINOMA

Generally, primary dysgerminoma (germinoma) does not occur in the infant, either alone or in combination with a teratoma.[18,40,92] Choriocarcinoma, on the other hand, is described in the first year of life, occurring either as metastasis secondary to a placental choriocarcinoma[28,38,100,187] or as a primary tumor arising from a variety of locations, such as the liver, lung, brain, kidney, or maxilla.[59,81,97,98,159] The most common site is intracranial, in the pineal region (see Chapter 9, "Brain Tumors").[59,159] As a rule, choriocarcinoma does not occur in association with teratomas in the newborn and infant.[2] In six cases, the malignant neoplasm was found to be congenital, presenting in the first 2 months of life as widespread metastasis accompanied by elevated β-hCG levels resulting from a placental primary neoplasm.[187] It may be impossible to determine whether the choriocarcinoma was primary—for example, originating from the liver, lung, or brain—or metastatic, arising from a small placental lesion that was overlooked.[98] Moreover, if the placenta looks normal on gross examination, it is the practice to discard it, without examining it microscopically. The diagnosis of choriocarcinoma should be considered when a newborn

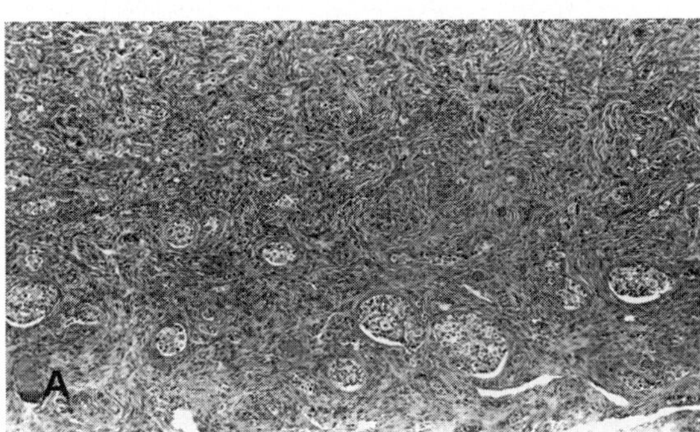 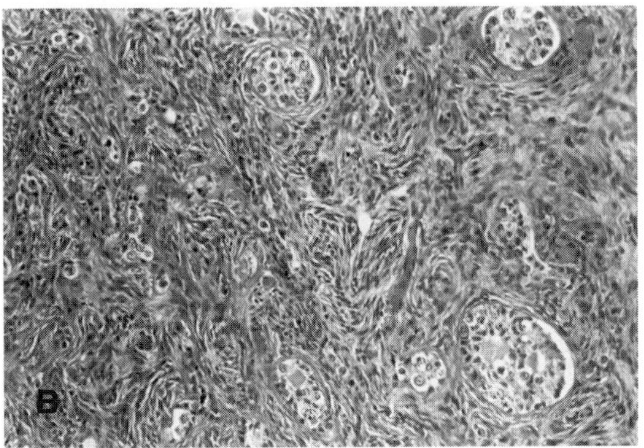

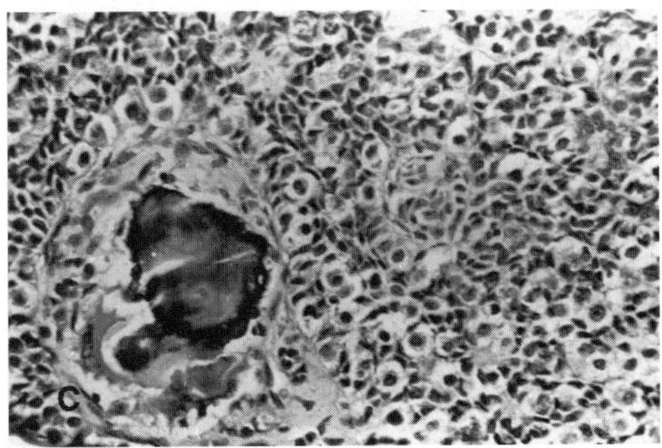

Figure 2–21. Gonadoblastoma arising from a dysgenetic gonad. The patient was a dysmorphic 4-month-old infant with tetralogy of Fallot, ambiguous genitalia, and a karyotype of 45,XO/46,XY. During a bilateral herniorrhaphy, an undescended streak gonad, measuring 2 × 1.3 cm, was found on the right side, and an undescended immature testis measuring 1.5 × 1.5 cm was noted on the left. Tumor was present only in the streak gonad. *A*, A lower-power overall view of the streak gonad shows the cortex in the upper half, along with the ovarian-type stroma and clusters of developing tumor cells in the lower half (hematoxylin-eosin, ×60). *B*, Nests of large germ cells and smaller, dark, round to oval Sertoli cells forming microfollicles are situated in an ovarian-type stroma. Some cell nests contain round spaces filled with hyaline-staining material. According to Teilum, gonadoblastoma recapitulates the structure of the fetal gonad[171] (hematoxylin-eosin, ×150). *C*, In more advanced stages of tumorigenesis, multiple foci of calcification form in the microfollicles, which can be appreciated on gross examination and on imaging studies (hematoxylin-eosin, ×300). (From Isaacs H Jr. Tumors of the Newborn and Infant. St. Louis: Mosby–Year Book, 1991.)

presents with bleeding tendencies, such as hematemesis or hemoptysis, anemia, hepatomegaly, lung metastases, and/or elevated urinary and plasma hCG levels.[187] Histologic examination reveals choriocarcinoma to be composed of two main components—cytotrophoblasts and syncytiotrophoblasts—with cells intermediate between the two. Cytotrophoblasts consist of large, round, cuboidal cells with variable vesicular central nuclei and clear cytoplasm, whereas syncytiotrophoblasts form syncytia or knots and contain much larger cells with abundant pink, vacuolated cytoplasm and large, hyperchromatic, irregular nuclei. Cytotrophoblasts and syncytiotrophoblasts are found adjacent to one another and next to di-lated vascular sinusoids. Extensive necrosis and hemorrhage are characteristic findings on both gross and microscopic examination. Cytoplasmic β-hCG testing is positive by immunoperoxidase staining, whereas AFP test results are negative.

GONADOBLASTOMA

Gonadoblastoma typically arises from an abnormal gonad.[11,151,152] The affected gonad may be of an indeterminate nature, a streak ovary, or a dysgenetic undescended testis.[151] In Scully's study, 61 of 74 (82%) patients with gonadoblastoma were phenotypic females who were obviously virilized, and the remainder were phenotypic males, many of whom had cryptorchidism, hypospadias, or female internal genitalia.[151] Additionally, most patients with this tumor have a 46,XY or a 45,X/46,XY mosaic karyotype.

Perinatal gonadoblastoma is unusual.[33,83,84,151,163] Spear and Martin reported bilateral tumors in a 950-g fetus of 28 weeks' gestation.[163] The patient had multiple congenital anomalies, dysplastic gonads with an ovarian stroma, and a 46,XY karyotype. Occasionally, gonadoblastoma arises from normal testes. Luisiri et al. reported one case of an apparently normal, 46,XY male with descended testes who presented at birth with a cystic mass of the right testis measuring 1.5 cm $\times$ 1.3 cm.[111]

On gross examination, gonadoblastoma consists of one or more small, firm, tan nodules that characteristically contain flecks of calcification which, if sufficiently large, may be visualized on imaging studies. The tumor has a distinctive microscopic appearance consisting of large germ cells surrounded by smaller, round, darker-staining Sertoli cells that form microfollicles and contain hyaline bodies and calcium deposits (Fig. 2–21).[92,151,171]

Gonadoblastoma is regarded as an in situ malignant lesion from which germinoma and other malignant germ cell tumors can develop.[140,151] It is not locally invasive, nor does it metastasize. Gonadectomy is recommended for young patients with mixed gonadal dysgenesis because of the increased frequency of gonadoblastoma and germinoma, as well as the virilizing effects of residual testicular tissue.[140]

REFERENCES

1. Abell MR, Holtz F. Testicular neoplasms in infants and children. I. Tumors of germ cell origin. Cancer 1963;16:965.
2. Ablin A, Isaacs H Jr. Germ cell tumors. *In* Pizzo PA, Poplack DG (eds): Principles and Practice of Pediatric Oncology, 2nd ed, p 867. Philadelphia: JB Lippincott, 1992.
3. Alegre M, Torrents M, Carreras E, et al. Prenatal diagnosis of intrapericardial teratoma. Prenatal Diagn 1990;10:199.
4. Alpers CE, Harrison MR. Fetus in fetu associated with an undescended testis. Pediatr Pathol 1985;4:37.
5. Alter AD, Cove JK. Congenital nasopharyngeal teratoma: Report of a case and review of the literature. J Pediatr Surg 1987;22:179.
6. Alter DN, Reed KL, Marx GR, et al. Prenatal diagnosis of congestive heart failure in a fetus with a sacrococcygeal teratoma. Obstet Gynecol 1988;71:978.
7. Altman RP, Randolph JG, Lilly JR. Sacrococcygeal teratomas. American Academy of Pediatrics Section Survey—1973. J Pediatr Surg 1974;9:389.
8. Arnheim EE. Retroperitoneal teratomas in infancy and childhood. Pediatrics 1951;8:309.
9. Ashcraft KW, Holder TM. Hereditary presacral teratoma. J Pediatr Surg 1974;9:691.
10. Aubert J, Casamayou J, Denis P, et al. Intrarenal teratoma in a newborn child. Eur Urol 1978;4:306.
11. Azizkhan RG, Haase GM, Applebaum H, et al. Diagnosis, management, and outcome of cervicofacial teratomas in neonates: A Children's Cancer Group Study. J Pediatr Surg 1995;30:312.
12. Bale PM. Sacrococcygeal developmental abnormalities and tumors in children. Perspect Pediatr Pathol 1984;1:9–56.
13. Bale PM, Painter DM, Cohen D. Teratomas in childhood. Pathology 1975;7:209.
14. Baumann FR, Nerlich A. Metastasizing cervical teratoma of the fetus. Pediatr Pathol 1993;13:21.
15. Beckwith JB. Pathological aspects of renal tumors in childhood. *In* Broecker BH, Klein FA (eds): Pediatric Tumors of the Genitourinary Tract, p 25. New York: Alan R. Liss, 1988.
16. Berlin AJ, Rich LS, Hahn JF. Congenital orbital teratoma. Child's Brain 1983;10:208.
17. Berry CL, Keeling J, Hilton C. Teratomata in infancy and childhood: A review of 91 cases. J Pathol 1969;98:241.
18. Berry PJ: Congenital tumours. *In* Keeling JW (ed): Fetal and Neonatal Pathology, 2nd ed, p 273. Berlin: Springer-Verlag, 1993.
19. Bilik R, Shandling B, Pope M, et al. Malignant benign neonatal sacrococcygeal teratoma. J Pediatr Surg 1993;28:1158.
20. Blair JL, Carachi R, Gupta R, et al. Plasma α-fetoprotein reference ranges in infancy. Effect of prematurity. Arch Dis Child 1987;62:362.
21. Bond SJ, Harrison MR, Schmidt KG, et al. Death due to high-output cardiac failure in fetal sacrococcygeal teratoma. J Pediatr Surg 1990;25:1287.
22. Bras G, Butts D, Hoyte DA. Gliomatous teratoma of the tongue: Report of a case. Cancer 1969;24: 1045.
23. Byard RW, Jimenez CL, Carpenter BF, et al. Congenital teratomas of the neck and nasopharynx: A clinical and pathological study of 18 cases. J Paediatr Child Health 1990;26:12.
24. Byard RW, Jimenez CL, Moore L. Mechanisms of sudden death in patients with congenital teratoma. Pediatr Surg Int 1992;7:464.
25. Byard RW, Smith CR, Chan HSL. Endodermal sinus tumor of the nasopharynx and previous mature congenital teratoma. Pediatr Pathol 1991;11:297.
26. Carney JA, Thompson DP, Johnson CL, et al. Teratomas in children: Clinical and pathologic aspects. J Pediatr Surg 1972;7:271.
27. Carter D, Bibro MC, Touloukian RJ. Benign clinical behavior of immature mediastinal teratoma in infancy and childhood. Cancer 1982;49:398.
28. Chandra SA, Gilbert EF, Viseskul C, et al. Neonatal intracranial choriocarcinoma. Arch Pathol Lab Med 1990;114:1079.
29. Chen SJ, Li YW, Tsai WY. Endodermal sinus (yolk sac) tumor of vagina and cervix in an infant. Pediatr Radiol 1993;23:57.
30. Chervenak FA, Isaacson G, Touloukian R, et al. Diagnosis and management of fetal teratomas. Obstet Gynecol 1985;66:666.
31. Chervenak FA, Tortora M, Moya FR, et al. Antenatal

sonographic diagnosis of epignathus. J Ultrasound Med 1984;3:235.

32. Clement PB, Young RH, Scully RE. Endometrioid yolk sac tumor. A clinicopathological analysis of eight cases. Am J Surg Pathol 1987;11:767.

33. Coffin CM, Dehner LP. Congenital tumors. *In* Stocker JT, Dehner LP (eds): Pediatric Pathology, Vol I, p 325. Philadelphia: JB Lippincott, 1992.

34. Conklin J, Abell MR. Germ cell neoplasms of sacrococcygeal region. Cancer 1967;20:2105.

35. Conran RM, Kent SG, Wargots ES. Oropharyngeal teratomas: A clinicopathologic study of four cases. Am J Perinatol 1993;10:71.

36. Coulson WF: Peritoneal gliomatosis from a gastric teratoma. Am J Clin Pathol 1990;94:87.

37. Curio MS, Grosfeld JL, Wheetman RM. Gastric teratoma: Unusual case for bleeding of the upper gastrointestinal tract in the newborn. Pediatrics 1981;67:721.

38. Dautenhahn L, Babyn PS, Smith CR. Metastatic choriocarcinoma in an infant: Imaging appearance. Pediatr Radiol 1993;23:597.

39. Davis CF, Carachi R, Young DG. Neonatal tumors: Glasgow 1966–86. Arch Dis Chld 1988;63:1075.

40. Dehner LP. Gonadal and extragonadal germ cell neoplasia in childhood. Human Pathol 1983;14:493–511.

41. Dehner LP. Intrarenal teratoma occurring in infancy: Report of a case with discussion of extragonadal germ cell tumors in infancy. J Pediatr Surg 1973;8:369.

42. Dehner LP. Neoplasms of the fetus and neonate. *In* Naeye RL, Kissane JM, Kaufman, N (eds). Perinatal Diseases, International Academy of Pathology, Monograph No. 22, p 286. Baltimore: Williams and Wilkins, 1981.

43. Dehner LP. Pediatric Surgical Pathology, 2nd ed. St. Louis: CV Mosby, 1987.

44. Dehner LP, Mills A, Talerman A, et al. Germ cell neoplasms of head and neck soft tissues: A pathologic spectrum of teratomatous and endodermal sinus tumors. Hum Pathol 1990;21:309.

45. Dennadayalu RP, Tuuri D, Dewall RA, et al. Intrapericardial teratoma and bronchogenic cyst. J Thorac Cardiovasc Surg 1974;67:945.

46. Dische MR, Gardner HA. Mixed teratoid tumors of the liver and neck in trisomy 13. Am J Clin Pathol 1978;69:631.

47. Donnellan WA, Swenson O. Benign and malignant sacrococcygeal teratomas. Surgery 1968;64:834.

48. Downing GJ, Kilbride HW, Freeman JC, et al. Picture of the month: Nasopharyngeal teratomas. Am J Dis Child 1990;144:795.

49. Dudgeon DL, Isaacs H Jr, Hays DM. Multiple teratomas of the head and neck. J Pediatr 1974;85:139.

50. Dunn CJ, Nguyen DL, Leonard JC. Ultrasound diagnosis of immature cervical teratoma: A case report. Am J Perinatol 1992;9:445.

51. Ein SH, Mancer K, Adeyemi SD. Malignant sacrococcygeal teratoma-endodermal sinus, yolk sac tumor in infants and children: A 32-year review. J Pediatr Surg 1985;20:473.

52. Esposito G, Cigliano B, Paludetto R. Abdominothoracic gastric teratoma in a female newborn infant. J Pediatr Surg 1983;18:304.

53. Evans MJ, Danielian PJ, Gray ES. Sacrococcygeal teratoma: A case of mistaken identity. Pediatr Radiol 1994;24:52.

54. Federici S, Ceccarelli PL, Ferrari M, et al. Fetus in fetu: Report of three cases and review of the literature. Pediatr Surg Int 1991;6:60.

55. Feldman M, Byrne P, Johnson MA, et al. Neonatal sacrococcygeal teratoma: Multi-imaging modality assessment. J Pediatr Surg 1990;25:675.

56. Flake AW, Harrison MR, Adzick NS, et al. Fetal sacrococcygeal teratoma. J Pediatr Surg 1986;21:563.

57. Fox H. Biology of teratomas. *In* Anthony PP, MacSween RNM (eds): Recent Advances in Histopathology, Vol 13, p 33. London: Churchill Livingstone, 1987.

58. Fox H, Butler-Manuel R. A teratoma of the placenta. J Pathol Bacteriol 1964;88:137.

59. Fraser GC, Blair GK, Hemming A, et al. The treatment of simultaneous choriocarcinoma in mother and baby. J Pediatr Surg 1992;27:1318.

60. Fraumeni JF Jr, Li FP, Dalager N. Teratomas in children: Epidemiologic features. J Natl Cancer Inst 1973;51:1425.

61. Froberg MK, Brown RE, Maylock J, et al. In utero development of a mediastinal teratoma: A second-trimester event. Prenatal Diagn 1994;14:884.

62. Garmel SH, Crombleholme TM, Semple JP, et al. Prenatal diagnosis and management of fetal tumors. Semin Perinatol 1994;18:350.

63. Gergely RZ, Eden R, Schifrin BS, et al. Antenatal diagnosis of congenital sacral teratoma. J Reprod Med 1980;24:229.

64. Gonzalez-Crussi F. Case 6: Retroperitoneal teratoma. Pediatr Pathol 1985;4:181.

65. Gonzalez-Crussi F. Extragonadal teratomas. *In* Atlas of Tumor Pathology, second series, fasicle X. Washington, DC: Armed Forces Institute of Pathology, 1982.

66. Gonzalez-Crussi F, Winkler RF, Mirkin DL. Sacrococcygeal teratomas in infants and children. The relationship of histology and prognosis in 40 cases. Arch Pathol Lab Med 1978;102:420.

67. Grosfeld JL, Ballantyne TVN, Lowe D, et al. Benign and malignant teratomas in children: Analysis of 85 patients. Surgery 1976;80:297.

68. Guarisco JL, Butcher RB II. Congenital cystic teratoma of the maxillary sinus. Otolaryngol Head Neck Surg 1990;103:1035.

69. Gundry SR, Wesley JR, Klein MD, et al. Cervical teratomas in the newborn. J Pediatr Surg 1983;18:382.

70. Haley T, Dimler M, Hollier P. Gastric teratoma with gastrointestinal bleeding. J Pediatr Surg 1986;21:949.

71. Harms D, Schmidt D, Leuschner I. Abdominal retroperitoneal and sacrococcygeal tumors of the newborn and the very young infant (report from the Kiel Pediatric Registry). Eur J Pediatr 1989;148:720.

72. Havranek P, Rubenson A, Guth D, et al. Sacrococcygeal teratoma in Sweden: A 10-year national retrospective study. J Pediatr Surg 1992;27:1447.

73. Hawkins EP. Pathology of germ cell tumors in children. Crit Rev Hematol/Oncol 1990;10:165.

74. Hawkins EP, Finegold MJ, Hawkins HK, et al. Nongerminomatous malignant germ cell tumors in children: A review of 89 cases from the pediatric oncology group, 1971–1984. Cancer 1986;58:2579.

75. Hawkins E, Isaacs H, Cushing B, et al. Occult malignancy in neonatal sacrococcygeal teratomas: A report from a combined Pediatric Oncology Group and Children's Cancer Group Study. Am J Pediatr Hematol Oncol 1993;15:406.

76. Hecht F, Hecht B, O'Keefe D. Sacrococcygeal teratoma: Prenatal diagnosis with elevated alpha-fetoprotein and acetylcholinesterase in amniotic fluid. Prenatal Diag 1982;2:229.

77. Heifetz SA, Alrabeeah A, St J Brown B, et al. Fetus in fetu: A fetiform teratoma. Pediatr Pathol 1988;8:215.

78. Heloury Y, Vergnes P, Gauthier F. Prognosis of prenatally diagnosed sacrococcygeal teratomas (abstract). Med Pediatr Oncol 1992;20:418.

79. Holzgreve W, Mahony BS, Glick PL, et al. Sonographic demonstration of fetal sacrococcygeal teratoma. Prenatal Diagn 1985;5:245.

80. Holzgreve W, Miny P, Anderson R, et al. Experience with 8 cases of prenatally diagnosed sacrococcygeal teratomas. Fetal Ther 1987;2:88.

81. Hongo T, Fujii Y, Fukuda T, et al. Long-term treatment in infantile choriocarcinoma. Acta Paediatr Jpn 1992;34:52.

82. Horger EO, McCarter LM. Prenatal diagnosis of sacrococcygeal teratoma. Am J Obstet Gynecol 1979; 134:228.

83. Hughesdon PE, Kumarasamy T. Mixed germ cell tumors (gonadoblastomas) is normal and dysgenetic gonads. Virch Arch [A] 1970;349:258.

84. Hung W, Randolph JG, Chandra R, et al. Gonadoblastoma in dysgenetic testis causing male pseudohermaphroditism in newborn. Urology 1981;17:584.

85. Hunt PT, Davidson KC, Keith W, et al. Radiography of hereditary presacral teratoma. Radiology 1977;122: 187.

86. Ikeda H, Okumura H, Nagashima K, et al. The management of prenatally diagnosed sacrococcygeal teratoma. Pediatr Surg Int 1990;5:192.

87. Isaacs H Jr. Congenital malignant tumors. *In* Reed GB, Claireaux AE, Bain AD (eds): Diseases of the Fetus and Newborn: Pathology, Radiology and Genetics, p 131. London: Chapman Hall, 1989.

88. Isaacs H Jr. Congenital and neonatal malignant tumors: A 28-year experience at Children's Hospital of Los Angeles. Am J Pediatr Hematol/Oncol 1987; 9(2):121.

89. Isaacs H Jr. Neoplasms in infants: A report of 265 cases. Pathol Ann 1983;18(2):165.

90. Isaacs H Jr. Perinatal (congenital and neonatal) neoplasms: A report of 110 cases. Pediatr Pathol 1985;3: 165.

91. Isaacs H Jr. Tumors. *In* Gilbert E (ed): Pathology of the Fetus and Infant, Vol 2, p 1242. St. Louis: Mosby–Year Book, 1996.

92. Isaacs H Jr. Tumors of the Newborn and Infant. St. Louis: Mosby–Year Book, 1991.

93. Izant RJ, Filston HC. Sacrococcygeal teratomas. Analysis of 43 cases. Am J Surg 1975;130:617.

94. Jordan RB, Gauderer MWL. Cervical teratomas: An analysis, literature review and proposed classification. J Pediatr Surg 1988;23:583.

95. Kang KW, Hissong SL, Langer A. Prenatal ultrasonic diagnosis of epignathus. J Clin Ultrasound 1978;6: 330.

96. Kay R. Prepubertal testicular tumor registry. Urol Clin North Am 1993;20(1):1.

97. Kelly DL Jr, Kushner J, McLean WT. Neonatal intracranial choriocarcinoma. J Neurosurg 1971;35:465.

98. Kim SN, Chi JG, Kim YW, et al. Neonatal choriocarcinoma of the liver. Pediatr Pathol 1993;13:723.

99. Kohler HG. Sacrococcygeal teratoma and "nonimmunological" hydrops fetalis. Br Med J 1976;2:422.

100. Kruseman N, van Lent M, Blom AH, et al. Choriocarcinoma in mother and child, identified by immunoenzyme histochemistry. Am Clin Pathol 1977;67: 279.

101. Kuhlmann RS, Warsof SL, Levy DL, et al. Fetal sacrococcygeal teratoma. Fetal Ther 1987;2:95.

102. Kurjak A, Zalud I, Jurkovic Z, et al. Ultrasound diagnosis and evaluation of fetal tumors, J Perinat Med 1989;17:173.

103. Lack EE, Travis WD, Welch KJ. Retroperitoneal germ cell tumors in childhood. A clinical and pathologic study of 21 cases. J Thoracic Cardiovasc Surg 1985;89: 826.

104. Lack EE, Weinstein HJ, Welch KJ. Mediastinal germ cell tumors in childhood: A clinical and pathological study of 21 cases. J Thoracic Cardiovasc Surg 1985;89: 826.

105. Lakhoo K, Boyle M, Drake DP. Mediastinal teratomas: Review of 15 pediatric cases. J Pediatr Surg 1993;28: 1161.

106. Lemire RJ, Beckwith JB. Pathogenesis of congenital tumors and malformations of the sacrococcygeal region. Teratology 1982;25:201.

107. Levin ML, Leone CR, Kincaid MC. Congenital orbital teratomas. Am J Ophthalmol 1986;102:476.

108. Levine AB, Alvarez M, Wedgewood J, et al. Contemporary management of a potentially lethal fetal anomaly: A successful approach to epignathus. Obstet Gynecol 1990;76:962.

109. Lewis RH. Foetus in foetu and the retroperitoneal teratoma. Arch Dis Child 1961;36:220.

110. Lord JM. Intra-abdominal foetus in foetu. J Pathol Bacteriol 1956;72:627.

111. Luisiri A, Vogler C, Steinhardt G, et al. Neonatal cystic testicular gonadoblastoma: Sonographic and pathologic findings. J Ultrasound Med 1991;10:59.

112. Maeda K, Yamamoto T, Yoshimura H, et al. Epignathus: A report of two neonatal cases. J Pediatr Surg 1989;24:395.

113. Magee JF, McFadden DE, Pantzar JT: Congenital tumors. *In* Dimmick JE, Kalousek DK (eds): Developmental Pathology of the Embryo and Fetus, p 235. Philadelphia: JB Lippincott, 1992.

114. Mahour GH, Landing BH, Woolley MM. Teratomas in children: Clinicopathologic studies in 133 patients. Zeitschr Kinderchir 1978;23:365.

115. Mamalis N, Garland PE, Argyle JC, et al. Congenital orbital teratoma: A review and report of two cases. Surv Ophthalmol 1985;30:41.

116. Marsden HB, Birch JM, Swindell R. Germ cell tumours of childhood: A review of 137 cases. J Clin Pathol 1981;34:879.

117. Mogilner JG, Fonseca J, Davies MRQ. Life-threatening respiratory distress caused by a mediastinal teratoma in a newborn. J Pediatr Surg 1992;27:1519.

118. Moore, KL. The Developing Human: Clinically Oriented Embryology, 5th ed. Philadelphia: WB Saunders, 1993.

119. Morrow RJ, Whittle MJ, McNay MB, et al. Prenatal diagnosis of an intra-abdominal sacrococcygeal teratoma. Prenatal Diagn 1990;10:753.

120. Murty VV, Dmitrovsjy E, Basl GJ, et al. Nonrandom chromosome abnormalities in testicular and ovarian germ cell tumor lines. Cancer Genet Cytogenet 1990; 50:67.

121. Naudin Ten Cate L, Vermeij-Keers C, Smit DA, et al. Intracranial teratoma with multiple fetuses: Pre- and post-natal appearance. Human Pathol 1995;26:804.

122. Nickell KA, Stocker JT. Placental teratoma: A case report. Pediatr Pathol 1987;7:645.

123. Norris HJ, Bagley GP, Taylor HB. Carcinoma of the infant vagina: A distinctive tumor. Arch Pathol 1970; 90:473.

124. Noseworthy J, Lack EE, Kozakewich HPW, et al. Sacrococcygeal germ cell tumors in childhood: An updated

experience with 118 patients. J Pediatr Surg 1981;16:358.

125. Odell JM, Allen JK, Badura RJ, et al. Massive congenital intracranial teratoma: A report of two cases. Pediatr Pathol 1987;7:333.

126. Onabanjo SO, Aghadiuno PU, Ogunniyi J, et al. Congenital benign extracranial teeratoma in a Nigerian neonate. Child's Nerv Syst 1987;3:188.

127. Parkes SE, Muir KR, Southern L, et al. Neonatal tumours: A thirty-year population based study. Med Pediatr Oncol 1994;22:309.

128. Parrington JM, West LF, Povey S. Chromosome changes in germ cell tumors. *In* Jones WG, Ward AM, Anderson CK (eds): Germ Cell Tumors, Vol II, p 61. Oxford: Pergamon Press, 1986.

129. Parrington JM, West LF, Povey S. The origin of ovarian teratomas. J Med Genet 1984;21:4.

130. Pate JW, Baker R, Korones SB. Mediastinal teratoma in the newborn. Surgery 1963;5:533.

131. Peltomaki P, Lothe R, Borresen AL, et al. Altered dosage of the sex chromosomes in human testicular cancer: A molecular genetic study. Int J Cancer 1991;47:518.

132. Perlman EJ, Cushing B, Hawkins E, et al. Cytogenetic analysis of childhood endodermal sinus tumors: A Pediatric Oncology Group Study. Pediatr Pathol 1994;14:695.

133. Potter EL, Craig JM. Pathology of the Fetus and Infant, 3rd ed, p 177. Chicago: Year Book Medical Publishers, 1975.

134. Powell RW, Weber ED, Manci EA. Intradural extension of a sacrococcygeal teratoma. J Pediatr Surg 1993;28:770.

135. Prat J, Bhan AK, Dickerson GR, et al. Hepatoid yolk sac tumor of the ovary (endodermal sinus tumor with hepatoid differentiation): A light microscopic, ultrastructural and immunohistochemical study of seven cases. Cancer 1982;50:2355.

136. Pringle KC, Weiner CP, Sopper RT, et al. Sacrococcygeal teratoma. Fetal Ther 1987;2:80.

137. Rasmussen SL, Hwang WS, Harder J, et al. Intrapericardial teratoma. Ultrasonic and pathologic features. J Ultrasound Med 1987;6:159.

138. Reece EA: Fetal neoplasm. *In* Reece EA, Hobbins JC, Mahoney MJ, Petrie RH (eds): Medicine of the Fetus and Mother, p 617. Philadelphia: JB Lippincott, 1992.

139. Reynolds JL, Donahue JK, Pearce CW. Intrapericardial teratoma: A cause of acute pericardial effusion in infancy. Pediatrics 1969;43:71.

140. Robboy SJ, Miller T, Donahoe PK, et al. Dysgenesis of testicular and streak gonads in syndrome of mixed gonadal dysgenesis: Perspective derived from a clinicopathologic analysis of twenty-one cases. Hum Pathol 1982;13:700.

141. Robertson JM, Fee HJ, Mulder DG. Mediastinal teratoma causing life-threatening hemoptysis: Its occurrence in an infant. Am J Dis Child 1981;135:148.

142. Robinson RA, Nelson L. Hepatic teratoma in an anencephalic fetus. Arch Pathol Lab Med 1986;110:655.

143. Rodin AE, Singla P. Teratomas of the tongue at birth. Pediatr Pathol 1985;3:291.

144. Romero R, Oilu G, Jeanty P, Ghidini A, Hobbins JC. Prenatal Diagnosis of Congenital Anomalies, p 34. Norwalk, CT: Appleton & Lange, 1988.

145. Rosenfeld CR, Coln CD, Duenhoelter JH. Fetal cervical teratoma as a cause of polyhydramnios. Pediatrics 1979;64:176.

146. Samaniego F, Rodriquez E, Houldsworth J, et al. Cytogenetic and molecular analysis of human male germ cell tumors: Chromosome 12 abnormalities and gene amplification. Genes Chromosome Cancer 1990;4:239.

147. Sauter ER, Diaz JH, Arensman RM, et al. The preoperative management of neonates with congenital oropharyngeal teratomas. J Pediatr Surg 1990;25:925.

148. Schmidt KG, Silverman NH, Harrison MR, et al. High output cardiac failure in fetuses with large sacrococcygeal teratoma: Diagnosis by echocardiography and Doppler ultrasound. J Pediatr 1989;114:1023.

149. Schropp KP, Lobe TE, Rao B, et al. Sacrococcygeal teratoma: The experience of four decades. J Pediatr Surg 1992;27:1075.

150. Scully RE. Personal communication, 1995.

151. Scully RE. Gonadoblastoma: A review of 74 cases. Cancer 1970;25:1340.

152. Scully RE. Tumors of the Ovary and Maldeveloped Gonads. *In* Atlas of Tumor Pathology, Fascicle 16, 2nd series. Washington, DC: Armed Forces Institute of Pathology, 1978.

153. Seibert JJ, Marvin WJ, Rose EF, et al. Mediastinal teratoma: A rare cause of severe respiratory distress in the newborn. J Pediatr Surg 1976;11:253.

154. Senocak ME, Gulsev K, Buyukpamukcu N, et al. Gastric teratoma in children including the third reported female case. J Pediatr Surg 1990;25:681.

155. Senyuz OF, Rizalar R, Celayir S, et al. Fetus in fetu or giant epignathus protruding from the mouth. J Pediatr Surg 1992;27:1493.

156. Sepulveda WH. Prenatal sonographic diagnosis of congenital sacrococcygeal teratoma and management. J Perinat Med 1989;17:93.

157. Shah BL, Vasan U, Raye JR. Teratoma of the tonsil in a premature infant: Case report and review of the literature. Am J Dis Child 1979;133:79.

158. Shanklin DR. Tumors of the Placenta and Umbilical Cord. Philadelphia: BC Decker, 1990.

159. Shitara T, Oshima Y, Yugami S, et al. Choriocarcinoma in children. Am J Pediatr Hematol/Oncol 1993;15:268.

160. Silberman R, Mendelson IR. Teratoma of the neck. Report of two cases and review of the literature. Arch Dis Child 1960;35:159.

161. Smith NM, Chambers SE, Billson VR, et al. Oral teratoma (epignathus) with intracranial extension: A report of two cases. Prenat Diagn 1993;13:945.

162. Sotelo-Avila C, Gonzalez-Crussi F. Congenital tumours. *In* Wigglesworth JS, Single DB (eds): Textbook of Fetal and Perinatal Pathology, Vol I, p 455. London: Blackwell, 1991.

163. Spear GS, Martin CG. Fetal gonadoblastoid testicular dysplasia. Hum Pathol 1986;17:531.

164. Stamp IM, Barlebo H, Rix M, et al. Intratubular germ cell neoplasia in an infantile testis with immature teratoma. Histopathology 1993;22:69.

165. Stephens TD, Spall R, Urfer AG, et al. Fetus amorphous or placental teratoma? Teratology 1989;40:1.

166. Sumner TE, Crowe JE, Klein A. Intrapericardial teratoma in infancy. Pediatr Radiol 1980;10:51.

167. Takehara H, Komi N, Munoz NA, et al. Nasal teratoma in a neonate associated with an acardiac amorphous twin. Pediatr Surg Int 1994;9:196.

168. Tamura H. Intracranial teratoma in fetal life and infancy. Obstet Gynecol 1966;27:134.

169. Tapper D, Lack EE. Teratomas in infancy and childhood: A 54-year experience at the Children's Hospital Medical Center. Ann Surg 1983;198:398.

170. Teal LN, Angtuaco TL, Jimenez JF, et al. Fetal teratomas: Antenatal diagnosis and clinical management. J Clin Ultrasound 1988;16:329.

171. Teilum G. Special Tumors of Ovary and Testis and Related Extragonadal Lesions: Comparative Pathology and Histological Identification, 2nd ed. Philadelphia: JB Lippincott, 1976.

172. Tharrington CL, Bossen EH. Nasopharyngeal teratomas. Arch Pathol Lab Med 1992;116:165.

173. Thomsen JR, Clayton J, Baker R, et al. Neonatal respiratory distress secondary to an obstructing nasopharyngeal dermoid. Clin Pediatr 1992;31:44.

174. Touran T, Applebaum H, Frost DB, et al. Congenital metastatic cervical teratoma: Diagnostic and management considerations. J Pediatr Surg 1989;24:21.

175. Towne B, Mahour GH, Woolley MM, et al. Ovarian cysts and tumors in infancy and childhood. J Pediatr Surg 1975;10:311.

176. Valdes-Dapena MA, Arey JB. The causes of neonatal mortality: An analysis of 501 autopsies on newborn infants. J Pediatr 1970;77:366.

177. Valdiserri RO, Yunis EJ. Sacrococcygeal teratomas: A review of 68 cases. Cancer 1981;48:217.

178. Waldhausen JA, Kilman JW, Vellios F, et al. Sacrococcygeal teratoma. Surgery 1963;54:933.

179. Weinraub Z, Gembruch U, Fodisch HJ, et al. Intrauterine mediastinal teratoma associated with non-immune hydrops fetalis. Prenatal Diagn 1989;9:369.

180. Werb P, Scurry J, Ostor A, et al. Survey of congenital tumors in perinatal necropsies. Pathology 1992;24:247.

181. Wienk MATP, Van Geijn HP, Copray FJA, et al. Prenatal diagnosis of fetal tumors by ultrasonography. Obstet Gynecol Surv 1990;45:639.

182. Williams GEG. Teratoma of the heart. J Pathol Bacteriol 1961;82:281.

183. Williams R, Williams V. Immature placental teratoma—A placental neoplasm (abstract). Pediatr Pathol 1994;14:539.

184. Willis RA. The Borderland of Embryology and Pathology, 2nd ed. London: Butterworths, 1962.

185. Wilson JW, Gehweiler JA. Teratoma of the face associated with a patent canal extending into the cranial cavity (Rathke's pouch) in a three-week-old child. J Pediatr Surg 1970;5:349.

186. Witte DP, Kissane JM, Askin FB. Hepatic teratomas in children. Pediatr Pathol 1983;1:81.

187. Witzleben CL, Bruninga G. Infantile choriocarcinoma: A characteristic syndrome. J Pediatr 1968;73:374.

188. Wold LE, Kramer SA, Farrow GM. Testicular yolk sac and embryonal carcinomas in pediatric patients: Comparative immunohistochemical and clinicopathologic study. Am J Clin Pathol 1984;81:427.

189. Wu JT, Book L, Sudar K. Serum alpha-fetoprotein levels in normal infants. Pediatr Res 1981;15:50.

3

NON–GERM CELL GONADAL TUMORS

Neoplasms of the testis and ovary seldom occur in the perinatal period.[1,4,8,11,25–27] Most primary tumors of the testis in older infants and children are of germ cell origin—namely, teratoma and yolk sac tumor, and occasionally, gonadoblastoma.[7,11–13,16] However, according to the review by Kay, the frequency of testicular germ cell tumors and sex cord–stromal tumors is about equal in the newborn (Table 3–1).[13] Ovarian cysts are more prevalent than ovarian tumors in the perinatal period (Fig. 3–1).

Over the years, terminology relating to non–germ cell gonadal tumors has been somewhat nebulous and controversial, to say the least. The use of identical names for histologically different tumors has led to endless nosologic confusion. As a result of this dilemma, the World Health Organization (WHO) chose the term "sex cord–stromal tumors" to include all ovarian and testicular tumors that are composed of elements of sex cord derivation—namely, granulosa and Sertoli cells—and those of stromal origin—namely, theca and Leydig cells—either alone or in combination.[15]

In the differential diagnosis of a scrotal mass in a neonate, hydrocele should be the first consideration. Other entities in the differential diagnosis should include testicular torsion (Fig. 3–2), juvenile granulosa tumor, gonadoblastoma, and leukemic involvement of the testis (see Fig. 7–4B).[4,12] Pigmented neuroectodermal tumor of infancy and meconium periorchitis are examples of peritesticular masses occurring in the newborn.[4]

Large ovarian follicular and theca-lutein cysts may present as cystic abdominal masses in the fetus and newborn, creating diagnostic and treatment problems.[21,26] The cysts may be large and single, but usually are small and multiple (see Fig. 3–1). The diagnosis of ovarian cyst is suggested by antenatal or postnatal sonography.[14,21,22,26] Perinatal juvenile granulosa cell tumor of the ovary is the subject of a few case reports.[15,19,23,29,30] To the author's knowledge, ovarian teratoma has not been documented in the newborn.

JUVENILE GRANULOSA CELL TUMOR

The gonadal stromal tumors—i.e., juvenile granulosa cell, Sertoli cell, and theca and Leydig cell tumors—occur more often in adults than in infants and children. Juvenile granulosa cell tumor is not only the most common stromal tumor, but is also the leading ovarian tumor, overall, occurring in the perinatal period.[9,15,18] Of the 25 or so Sertoli cell tumors reported in children, 3 were found in neonates.[7,10,18] The author's research indicates that pure Leydig cell tumor has not been described in the newborn.

The juvenile granulosa cell tumor of the testis is histologically analogous to its ovarian counterpart and its clinical manifestation is likewise benign. A favorable outcome for the infant can be anticipated with orchiectomy as the sole treatment.[15] Over 50% of the cases are diagnosed in neonates, 90% by 6 months of age.[13,15] The findings in 14 cases of infantile granulosa cell tumor of the testis have been reviewed by Lawrence et al.; 11 were younger than 3 months of age.[15] In a later series of 25

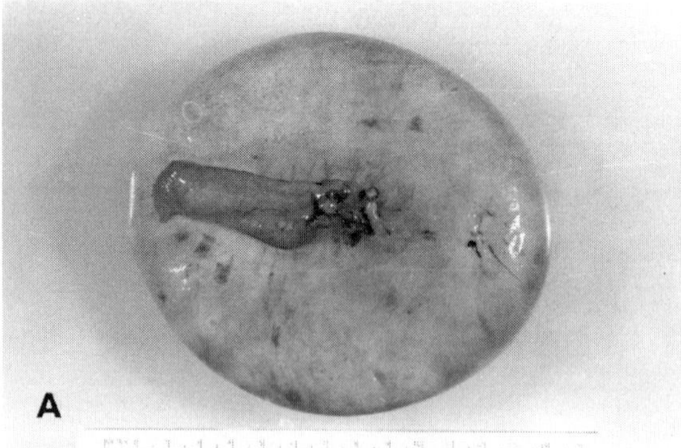
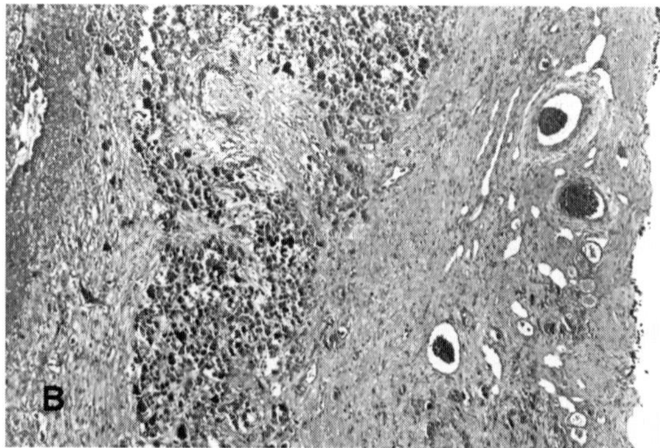

Figure 3–1. Follicular cyst of the ovary in a 3-week-old female infant with an abdominal mass. *A*, The left ovary was replaced by a 40-g cystic mass measuring 6 × 4.5 cm and containing brown, cloudy fluid and old blood clot. *B*, A histologic section reveals atrophic ovary and cyst wall elements containing foci of necrosis, calcification, old hemorrhage, and fibrosis. The histologic findings are consistent with an old torsion, probably occurring in utero, of a large follicular cyst followed by infarction (hematoxylin-eosin, ×60).

patients studied by Groisman et al., 23 were younger than 3 months of age.[9] Chromosomal anomalies and ambiguous genitalia are associated with this tumor.[9,20,24,28] For example, the Wilms' tumor suppressor gene WT1, located at chromosome 11p13, is observed in children with the Denys-Drash syndrome and Wilms' tumor and in those with juvenile granulosa tumor.[5]

Testicular enlargement (the most frequent sign), abdominal swelling, or torsion of the testis, an incidental finding in a hernia sac or at necropsy, are the various presenting findings in the neonate with this tumor.[2,9,10,15,17,25] Crump found an intra-abdominal testicular juvenile granulosa cell tumor measuring 11 cm × 7 cm in a 1000-g male fetus who died of pulmonary hyaline membrane disease.[6]

Granulosa cell tumors of the ovary occur in the newborn as well.[28,29] Bilateral tumors have been reported in this age group and may be associated with endocrinologic manifestations.[19,23,30] Sexual precocity has been described in stillborn infants and neonates with this neoplasm.[29] Pigmented external genitalia, endome-

Table 3–1. Histopathologic Diagnoses of 20 Testicular Tumors of Newborns

Tumor	Number	(%)*
Germ cell tumors	9	(45)
Yolk sac tumor	6	(30)
Gonadoblastoma	2	(10)
Teratoma	1	(5)
Sex cord–stromal tumors	8	(40)
Gonadal stromal tumor	6	(30)
Juvenile granulosa cell tumor	2	(10)
Other	3	(15)
Granular cell tumor	2	(10)
Hamartoma	1	(5)

Data from Kay R. Prepubertal Testicular Tumor Registry. Urol Clin North Am 1993;20(1):2. Used by permission.

*Percent of 20 (total) cases.

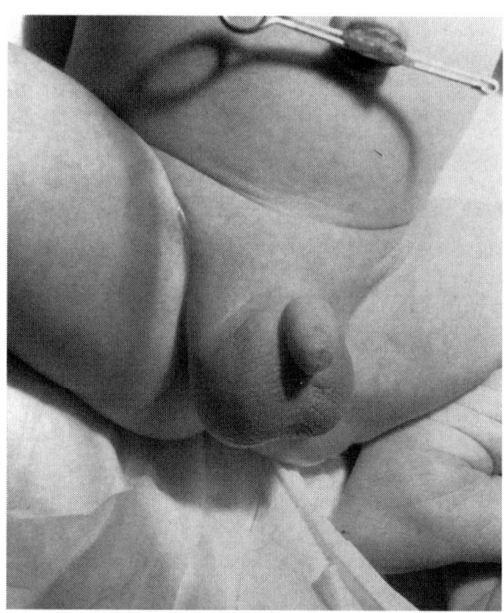

Figure 3–2. Testicular torsion in a newborn. A 3-day-old male presented with edematous enlargement of the right testis. Surgical exploration of the scrotum revealed torsion with hemorrhagic infarction, which was confirmed by histologic studies. Hydrocele and torsion are more common than a neoplasm, and thus should be given prime consideration in the differential diagnosis of testicular enlargement in the newborn. (From Isaacs H Jr. Tumors of the Newborn and Infant. St. Louis: Mosby–Year Book, 1991.)

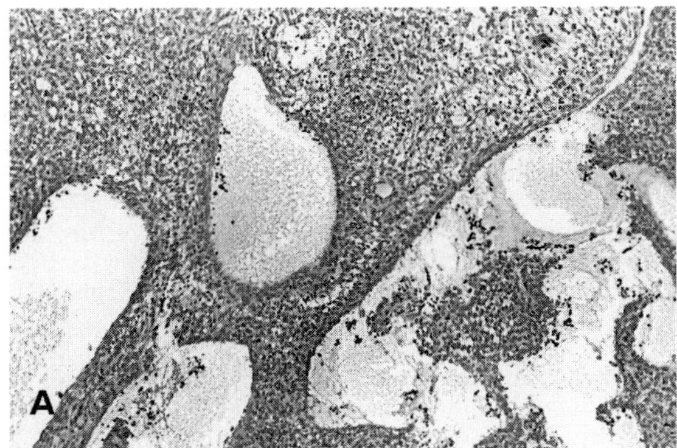 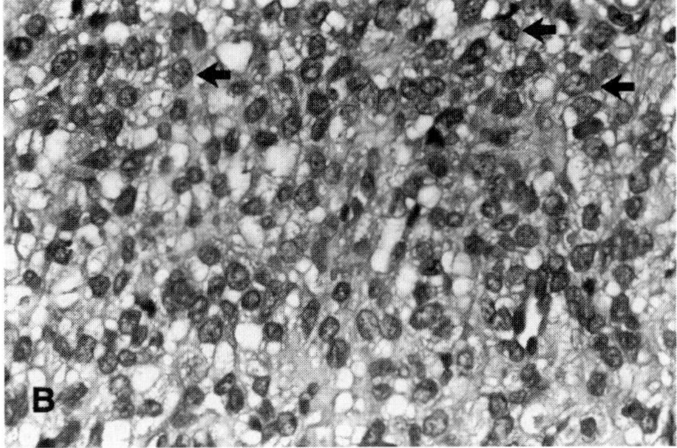

Figure 3–3. Juvenile granulosa cell tumor of the testis removed from a 5-month-old male infant. *A*, Diffuse infiltrates of granulosa cells containing large cystic follicles are filled with pale-staining secretion, giving the tumor a Swiss cheese–like appearance (hematoxylin-eosin, ×60). *B*, A higher-power view shows a bubbly, microcystic appearance and tumor cells with mild nuclear atypia and nuclear grooving (*arrows*). Two mitotic figures are present (hematoxylin-eosin, ×400).

trial hemorrhage, and bilateral granulosa cell tumors of the ovary were found at necropsy in a 2-day-old premature female infant with pulmonary hyaline membrane disease (Case no. A-89-179, Children's Hospital, Los Angeles). The tumor has also been described in association with leprechaunism, a fatal disorder characterized by gnome-like facies, hirsutism, breast enlargement, cliteromegaly, decreased adipose tissue, abdominal distention, cystic ovaries, and growth retardation.[3]

On gross examination, juvenile granulosa cell tumor has both solid areas and multiple cysts, some of which are very large. Occasionally, the ovaries are replaced by numerous multilocular cysts filled with clear fluid.[3] Histologically, the neoplasm shows diffuse sheets of granulosa cells and contains cystic follicles of various sizes accompanied by pale-staining secretion. The large cystic areas in some fields resemble Swiss cheese under low magnification (see Fig. 3–3A). The septae contain spindle cells resembling ovarian stroma and the cysts are lined by granulosa cells with clear cytoplasm. The nuclei are round and slightly hyperchromatic, but may or may not have the grooved appearance characteristic of the adult granulosa cell tumor (see Fig. 3–3B). Marked nuclear atypia is seen in some tumors with 5 to 7 mitoses per 10 high-power fields.[9,15,18,20,28] The immunohistochemical findings of congenital granulosa cell tumors of the testis are described by Groisman et al. and by Tanaka et al.[9,24] The polyhedral tumor cells and normal Sertoli and granulosa cells stain positive for cytokeratin and vimentin. The spindle cells and normal peritubular myoid and theca externa cells react with vimentin, actin, and, focally, with desmin. Leydig cells and theca interna cells from normal infant ovaries and testes express only vimentin.[9] These studies confirm the premise that granulosa tumor cells are related to ovarian and testicular stromal cells.[9]

Electron microscopic findings corroborate the immunohistochemical features just described. Ultrastructurally, the granulosa cell tumor consists of three main cellular components: nonluteinized granulosa cells, immature Sertoli cells, and theca cells.[18,19]

Most newborn juvenile granulosa tumors are usually classified as stage la; that is, they are confined to the ovary. Therefore, the recommended treatment is unilateral salpingo-oophorectomy. Generally, these patients have a good prognosis.[29]

REFERENCES

1. Abell MR, Holtz F. Testicular neoplasms in infants and children. I. Tumors of germ cell origin. Cancer 1963; 16:965.
2. Batsakis JG. Tumors of the testis in infancy and childhood. Arch Pathol 1961;72:27.
3. Brisigotti M, Fabbretti G, Pesce F, et al. Congenital bilateral juvenile granulosa cell tumor of the ovary in leprechaunism: A case report. Pediatr Pathol 1993;13:549.
4. Coffin CM, Dehner LP. Congenital tumors. *In* Stocker JT, Dehner LP (eds): Pediatric Pathology, Vol I, p 325. Philadelphia: JB Lippincott, 1992.
5. Coppes MJ, Rackley R, Kay R. Primary testicular and paratesticular tumors of childhood. Med Pediatr Oncol 1994;22:329.
6. Crump WD. Juvenile granulosa cell (sex cord-stromal) tumor of the fetal testis. J Urol 1983;129:1057.

7. Culp DA, Frazier RG, Butler JJ. Sertoli cell tumor in an infant. J Urol 1956;76:162.

8. Dehner LP. Neoplasms of the fetus and neonate. *In* Naeye RL, Kissane JM, Kaufman, N (eds): Perinatal Diseases. International Academy of Pathology, Monograph No. 22, p 286. Baltimore: Williams and Wilkins, 1981.

9. Groisman GM, Dische MR, Fine EM, et al. Juvenile granulosa cell tumor of the testis: A comparative immunohistochemical study with normal infantile gonads. Pediatr Pathol 1993;13:389.

10. Holtz F, Abell MR. Testicular neoplasms in infants and children. II. Tumors of non-germ cell origin. Cancer 1963;16:982.

11. Isaacs H Jr. Perinatal (congenital and neonatal) neoplasms: A report of 110 cases. Pediatr Pathol 1985;3:165.

12. Isaacs H Jr. Tumors of the Newborn and Infant. St. Louis: Mosby–Year Book, 1991.

13. Kay R. Prepubertal Testicular Tumor Registry. Urol Clin North Am 1993;20(1):1.

14. Kurjak A, Zalud I, Jurkovic Z, et al. Ultrasound diagnosis and evaluation of fetal tumors. J Perinat Med 1989;17:173.

15. Lawrence WD, Young RH, Scully RE. Juvenile granulosa cell tumor of the infantile testis: A report of 14 cases. Am J Surg Pathol 1985;9:87.

16. Mostofi FK, Price EB. Tumors of the Male Genital System. *In* Atlas of Tumor Pathology, 2nd series, fascicle 8. Washington, DC: Armed Forces Institute of Pathology, 1973.

17. Mostofi FK, Theiss EA, Ashley DJB. Tumors of specialized gonadal stroma in human male patients. Cancer 1959;12:944.

18. Pinto MM. Juvenile granulosa cell tumor of the infant testis: Case report with ultrastructural observations. Pediatr Pathol 1985;4:277.

19. Pysher TJ, Hitch DC, Krous HF. Bilateral juvenile granulosa cell tumors in a 4-month-old dysmorphic infant: A clinical, histologic and ultrastructural study. Am J Surg Pathol 1981;5:789.

20. Raju U, Fine G, Warrier R, et al. Congenital testicular juvenile granulosa cell tumor in a neonate with X/XT mosaicism. Am J Surg Pathol 1986;10:577.

21. Reece EA: Fetal neoplasm. *In* Reece EA, Hobbins JC, Mahoney MJ, Petrie RH (eds): Medicine of the Fetus and Mother, p 617. Philadelphia: JB Lippincott, 1992.

22. Romero R, Oilu G, Jeanty P, Ghidini A, Hobbins JC. Prenatal Diagnosis of Congenital Anomalies. Norwalk, CT: Appleton & Lange, 1988.

23. Roth LM, Nicholas TR, Ehrlich CE. Juvenile granulosa cell tumor. A clinicopathologic study of three cases with ultrastructural observations. Cancer 1979;44:2194.

24. Tanaka Y, Sasaki Y, Tachibana K, et al. Testicular juvenile granulosa cell tumor in an infant with X/XY mosaicism clinically diagnosed as true hermaphroditism. Am J Surg Pathol 1994;18:36.

25. White JM, McCarthy MP. Testicular gonadal stromal tumors in newborns. Urology 20:121, 1982.

26. Widdowson DJ, Pilling DW, Cook RCM. Neonatal ovarian cysts: Therapeutic dilemma. Arch Dis Child 1988;63:737.

27. Woodside JR, Borden TA. Sertoli cell tumor (gonadal stromal tumor) in an infant. J Pediatr Surg 1979;14:138.

28. Young RH, Lawrence WD, Scully RE. Juvenile granulosa cell tumor—Another neoplasm associated with abnormal chromosomes and ambiguous genitalia: A report of 3 cases. Am J Surg Pathol 1985;9:737.

29. Zaloudek C, Norris HJ. Granulosa tumors of the ovary in children: A clinical and pathologic study of 32 cases. Am J Surg Pathol 1982;6:503.

30. Zemke EE, Herrel WE. Bilateral granulosa cell tumors. Successful removal from a child of fourteen weeks of age. Am J Obstet Gynecol 1941;41:704.

4

SOFT TISSUE TUMORS

The soft tissues give rise to a wide variety of neoplasms and tumor-like conditions, often presenting in the newborn as palpable masses. Soft tissue tumors of the fetus and newborn are different in many respects from those of adults insofar as their incidence, anatomic location, histopathologic characteristics, and prognosis are concerned.[23,79,104,185,187,284,381]

This group of tumors is relatively common in the fetus and newborn as compared to other neoplasms occurring in this age group.[7,8,74,79,80,82,102,109,185,187,203,292] Excluding vascular hamartomas and malformations, they are second only to teratomas in frequency in some studies.[100,187] For example, soft tissue tumors comprised 22% of the total 110 perinatal neoplasms in the Children's Hospital Los Angeles review and were exceeded in number only by teratomas (36%) (see Table 1–1).[185] The series from the Hospital for Sick Children, Toronto, consisted of 102 neonatal tumors, and soft tissue tumors ranked third (12%) following neuroblastoma and retinoblastoma.[60]

The fibrous connective tissue tumors—fibromatosis, myofibromatosis, and fibrosarcoma—comprise most of the perinatal soft tissue neoplasms, both benign and malignant (Tables 4–1 and 4–2).[79,80,104,187] More than half involve the extremities, and approximately one third are malignant (Table 4–2).[74,79,104,185,284,336] Fibrosarcoma is the leading malignant soft tissue tumor in most newborn series, followed by (in decreasing order) rhabdomyosarcoma, primitive neuroectodermal tumor, and rhabdoid tumor.[79,104,184,185,187,203,284] However, 8 of 12 mesenchymal malignant lesions reported by Campbell et al. were rhabdomyosarcomas and 3 were undifferentiated sarcomas.[60]

When a soft tissue tumor (e.g., a fibrosarcoma or rhabdomyosarcoma) occurs in a fetus or neonate, sometimes it is difficult to determine whether it formed early in development from tissues that were still in embryonic stages or later on, from those that were already mature.[376] Willis was one of the first to draw attention to the similarity between the histologic appearance of developing tissues and of tumors in the young (see Fig. 4–1).[376]

In the normal developing fetus and newborn, cells appear to be immature, making the distinction between some benign and malignant tumors difficult or impossible. This is particularly problematic in the interpretation of soft tissue tumors in the young, in whom the diagnosis of sarcoma must be made with caution.[30,72,182,266,317] Kaufman and Stout were the first to suggest that congenital mesenchymal tumors are seldom malignant despite their large size or microscopic resemblance to soft tissue sarcomas in adults.[79,203] Although soft tissue lesions are considered to be benign microscopically, lesions such as hemangioma or fibromatosis may cause death if they involve a vital structure, such as in the neck or thorax. Nevertheless, most soft tissue neoplasms diagnosed in the first year of life, including some of the sarcomas, deserve a conservative therapeutic approach and generally have a favorable outcome.[49,72,75,79,80,109,183,184,186,187,317,345]

FIBROUS CONNECTIVE TISSUE (MYOFIBROBLASTIC) TUMORS

The so-called fibrous connective tissue tumors comprise the largest category of soft tissue neoplasms found in the newborn. They include the fibromatoses (desmoid type), digital fi-

Table 4–1. Soft Tissue Tumors During the First 3 Months of Life, University of Minnesota Hospital and Clinic, 1960–1984

Diagnosis*	Number (% of total)
Myofibromatosis	15 (26.3)
Torticollis (fibromatosis colli)	9 (15.8)
Fibrous histiocytoma	6 (10.5)
Lipoblastoma	4 (7.0)
Congenital-infantile fibrosarcoma	11 (19.3)
Peripheral primitive neuroectodermal tumor	6 (10.5)
Embryonal rhabdomyosarcoma	5 (8.8)
Sarcoma, NOS†	1 (1.8)
Total	57 (100)

*The study included 11 capillary hemangiomas and 17 lymphangiomas that are not listed here.

†NOS = not otherwise specified.

Data abstracted from Pediatr Pathol 1990, 10:514, Coffin CM, Dehner LP, Taylor & Francis, Inc., Washington, DC. Reproduced with permission. All rights reserved.

bromatosis, myofibromatosis, infantile fibrosarcoma, and fibrous hamartoma (Table 4–3; refer to Figs. 4–2 to Fig. 4–12).[72,78,80,128,169,184,185,187] According to Enzinger, fibrous proliferations in the young can be divided into two main groups: (1) those corresponding in terms of location, histology, and behavior to identical tumors found in adults, such as the desmoid fibromatoses; and (2) those having neither clinical nor morphologic counterparts in adults (e.g., myofibromatosis and fibrous hamartoma of infancy).[126] The latter are relatively uncommon, are found primarily in newborns and infants, and, because of their unusual features, often present specific diagnostic problems.[126] In the fibrous connective tissue group of tumors, the histologic appearance frequently does not correspond precisely with clinical behavior. Histologic findings, such as hypercellularity, an immature appearance, and rapid growth, may be mistaken for evidence of malignancy, resulting in needless and excessive therapy.[126]

Electron microscopic and immunohistochemical studies show that the fibrous connective tissue tumors—namely, fibromatosis, myofibromatosis, fibrous hamartoma, and infantile fibrosarcoma—are composed primarily of myofibroblasts and fibroblasts.[38,128,134,234,257] Although these tumors share a common clinical presentation—a palpable mass—and, possibly, a similar histogenesis, they show a variety of distinct gross and microscopic appearances. Generally, tumors included in this classification are associated with a favorable outcome.[187]

In a study conducted by Coffin and Dehner, myofibromatosis was the most common connective tissue tumor in 57 infants younger than 3 months of age, followed in frequency by fibrosarcoma and then torticollis (see Table 4–1).[80] In a similar review by the author, torticollis was the leading lesion, followed by fibrosarcoma and myofibromatosis (see Table 4–2).

Fibromatosis

Fibromatosis (juvenile or infantile desmoid fibromatosis) is a benign, fibrous, connective tissue tumor presenting as a palpable mass in the fascia, skeletal muscle, or periosteum (Figs. 4–2 to 4–4).[7,8,21,49,109,128,180,187,346] In the newborn, the most frequent locations affected are the extremities and the head and neck region.[184,185,319] The lesion also occurs in unusual sites (e.g., subglottic fibromatosis manifesting as congenital laryngeal airway obstruction and severe respiratory distress).[359] The tumor is found more often in male than in female children.[128,319,346] Occasionally, it is difficult to distinguish between a cellular fibromatosis and a low-grade fibrosarcoma on the basis of histologic findings, and the nebulous, confusing term of "aggressive fibromatosis" has sometimes been applied.[128,185] Both fibromatosis and fibrosarcoma are aggressive locally and often recur; the latter occasionally metastasizes, but the former does not.[8,49,128,184,185,313,319]

One of the largest pediatric studies, which included 59 cases, was conducted by Schmidt and Harms.[319] Five of 14 fibromatoses (desmoid type) were found in newborns, all of whom were male. The so-called abdominal and extra-abdominal fibromatoses did not occur in the perinatal period.

On gross examination, a fibromatosis consists of a firm, light gray or white mass with a rubbery, whorled, cut surface (Fig. 4–3*B*). It appears to be encapsulated, but the tumor often is found to have invaded insidiously or to have blended into the adjacent soft tissues. Fibrosarcoma shows similar gross features, but tends to be considerably softer, more friable, and more myxoid or gelatinous in appearance than a fibromatosis (see Figs. 4–10*A* and 4–11*A*).[184,185] Fibromatoses tend to be smaller than fibrosarcomas, averaging 2 cm in greatest dimension and 15 cm in diameter or more, respectively.

Table 4–2. Newborn* Soft Tissue Tumors, Children's Hospital, Los Angeles, 1958–1991

Patient No.	Sex	Diagnosis	Site
Benign Tumors			
1	M	Fibromatosis	Scalp
2	M	Digital fibromatosis	Thumb
3	M	Digital fibromatosis	Multiple, fingers
4	M	Myofibromatosis	Neck
5	M	Myofibromatosis	Back
6	M	Myofibromatosis	Back
7	M	Myofibromatosis	Multiple: arms, face, bones
8	M	Torticollis	Neck
9	F	Torticollis	Neck
10	F	Torticollis	Neck
11	F	Torticollis	Neck
12	M	Torticollis	Neck
13	M	Torticollis	Neck
14	M	Torticollis	Neck
15	F	Hemangiopericytoma†	Neck and mediastinum
16	M	Hemangiopericytoma	Forearm
17	F	Hemangiopericytoma	Chest wall
18	M	Hemangiopericytoma	Thigh
19	M	Hemangiopericytoma	Thigh
20	M	Hemangiopericytoma	Thigh
21	F	Fibrous histiocytoma	Foot
22	M	Schwannoma	Palate
23	F	Granular cell tumor	Gingiva and tongue
24	F	Granular cell tumor	Gingiva
25	F	Granular cell tumor	Gingiva
26	F	Granular cell tumor	Gingiva
27	M	Lipoma	Buttock
28	M	Lipoma	Thigh
29	M	Xanthogranuloma	Foot

Patient No.	Sex	Diagnosis	Site	Status
Malignant Tumors				
1	F	Fibrosarcoma	Face and maxillary sinus	L
2	M	Fibrosarcoma	Neck	LTF
3	M	Fibrosarcoma	Flank	LTF
4	M	Fibrosarcoma	Thigh	L
5	M	Fibrosarcoma	Thigh	D
6	M	Rhabdomyosarcoma	Eyelid	L
7	M	Angiomatoid malignant fibrous histiocytoma	Thigh	L
8	M	Polyphenotypic small cell tumor	Forearm	L
9	M	Sarcoma, NOS	Epidural	D
10	M	Sarcoma, NOS	Chest wall	L
11	M	Sarcoma, NOS	Paraspinal	D

*Patients younger than 3 months of age.
†Patient died.
NOS = not otherwise specified; L = living; LTF = lost to follow-up; D = dead.

However, size is not a reliable indicator of malignancy.[184,185]

Fibromatoses are basically spindle cell neoplasms with moderate variations in cellularity and the amount of intercellular collagen present (see Figs. 4–3 and 4–4). Some are hypocellular with abundant collagen resembling scar tissue, whereas others are more cellular with an occasional mitosis and a prominent, pale-staining, myxoid background.[109,184,185] Occasionally, these histologic differences can be appreciated in the same tumor, especially if it is large. Sampling error plays a critical role in the diagnosis. The tumors stain positively with vimentin immunoperoxidase, but do not react with desmin, S-100 protein, actin, or cytokeratin.[186,319,322] Ul-

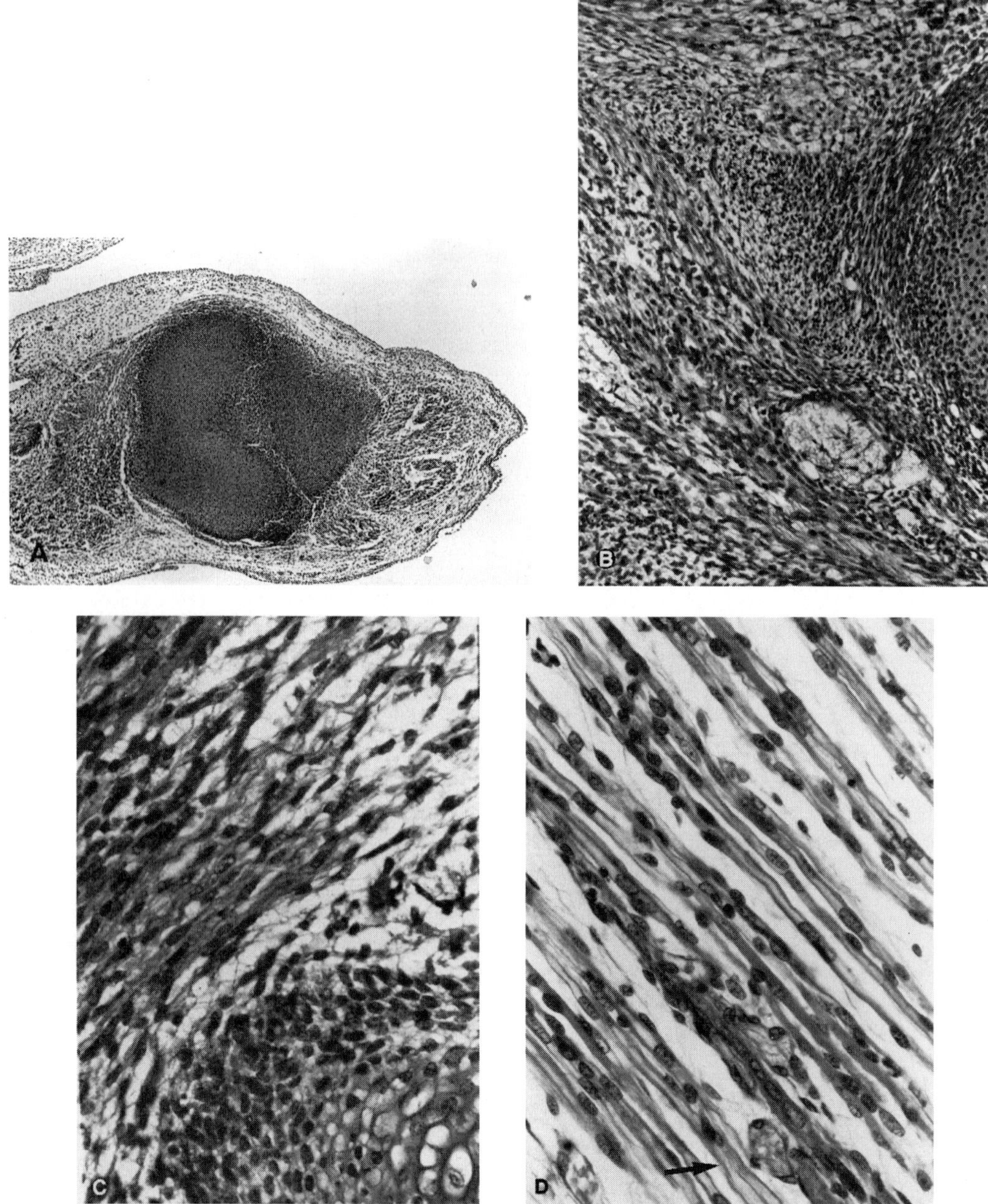

Figure 4–1. Developing limb bud from a 12-mm embryo. _A,_ A low-power view reveals the cartilage plate and early digit formation (hematoxylin-eosin, ×48). _B,_ Cartilage, connective tissue, skeletal muscle, and adipose tissue elements are evident (hematoxylin-eosin, ×150). _C,_ A high-power view depicts hypercellularity, hyperchromatism, and nuclear atypia observed in developing mesenchyme (hematoxylin-eosin, ×380). _D,_ Skeletal muscle from the same embryo shows fusion of myoblasts, forming elongated myotubes. Some myoblasts contain cytoplasmic cross-striations (_arrow_) (hematoxylin-eosin, ×380).

Table 4–3. Classification of Perinatal Myofibroblastic Tumors

---

Congenital (infantile) myofibromatosis
  Solitary
  Multiple
  Generalized
Infantile (desmoid-type) fibromatosis
Infantile digital fibromatosis
Fibrous hamartoma of infancy
Torticollis (fibromatosis colli)
Congenital (infantile) fibrosarcoma

---

trastructural studies show that the tumor cells are both fibroblasts and myofibroblasts (see Fig. 4–4D).

Early, wide excision with adequate surgical margins is the treatment of choice. However, just shelling out a fibromatosis, leaving tumor at the lines of resection, will not result in cure. The lesion recurs if not completely excised, and will cause fatal complications particularly if a vital structure is involved.[187] For recurrent or unresectable fibromatoses, chemotherapy or radiation therapy may be an option.[180]

Digital Fibromatosis (Recurring Digital Fibroma)

Infantile digital fibromatosis is considered to be a form of fibromatosis (myofibromatosis) that characteristically involves the dorsolateral aspects of the distal phalanges of the fingers and toes (see Fig. 4–4).[32,33,57,129,305,305a,346] Stout's 1954 classification of "fibromatoses of the hands and feet" included four infants and children, ranging in age from birth to 5 years, with fibrous tumors exclusively affecting the digits, recurring frequently after excision, and showing no evidence of metastases.[346] Eleven years later, Reye described six similar cases, demonstrated the pathognomonic intracytoplasmic inclusion bodies, and termed the lesion recurring digital fibrous tumor of childhood.[305a] Almost 50% of such tumors are discovered within the first month of life, most are diagnosed by 1 year of age, and most recur after simple excision.[128,187,267,305a,313] Some have been described in association with the Beckwith-Wiedemann syndrome.[90] The tumors are single or multiple and are composed of white, firm nodules with a broad base and shiny surfaces (see Fig. 4–4).[128,187,313]

Digital fibromatoses have a firm, white, whorled cut surface. Histologic examination reveals the usual characteristics of a fibromatosis in this age group: small, regular, spindle-shaped cells arranged in an interlacing bundle or herringbone growth pattern, exhibiting little or no mitotic activity, and embedded in a collagenous matrix invading the dermis and subcutaneous tissue (see Fig. 4–4).[305a] The presence of cytoplasmic inclusion bodies distinguishes the digital fibromatosis from all other fibrous tumors.[305a] Sometimes, the inclusions can be seen with hematoxylin-eosin staining (see Fig. 4–4C). The trichrome stain variably displays round or oval, red, paranuclear, intracytoplasmic inclusions which, by electron microscopy, are seen to consist of packets of actin filaments[188] (see Fig. 4–4D). This finding is confirmed by immunohistochemical and cy-

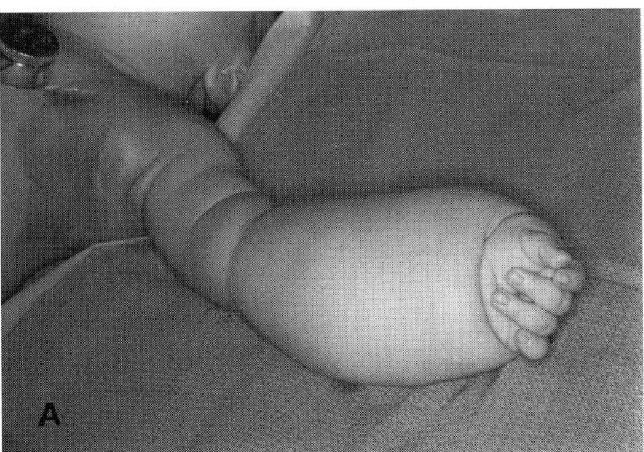
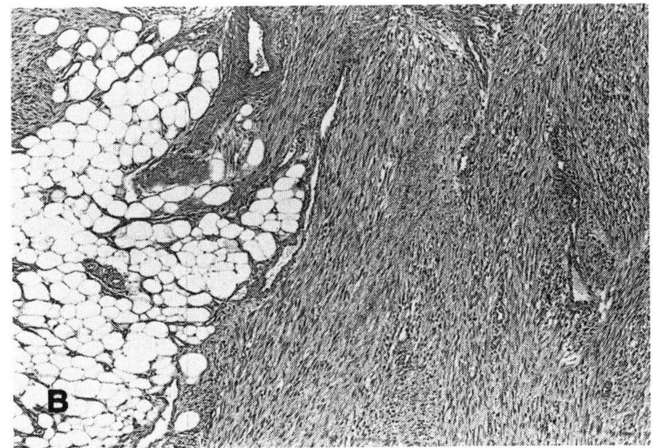

Figure 4–2. Congenital fibromatosis involving the forearm of a 3-month-old male child. *A,* The left forearm is diffusely enlarged by a firm mass. Note the cafe-au-lait spots on the patient's chest and axilla. *B,* A photomicrograph reveals uniform, spindle-shaped cells invading the subcutaneous fat and surrounding blood vessels (hematoxylin-eosin, ×120). (From Isaacs H Jr. Tumors of the Newborn and Infant. St. Louis: Mosby–Year Book, 1991.)

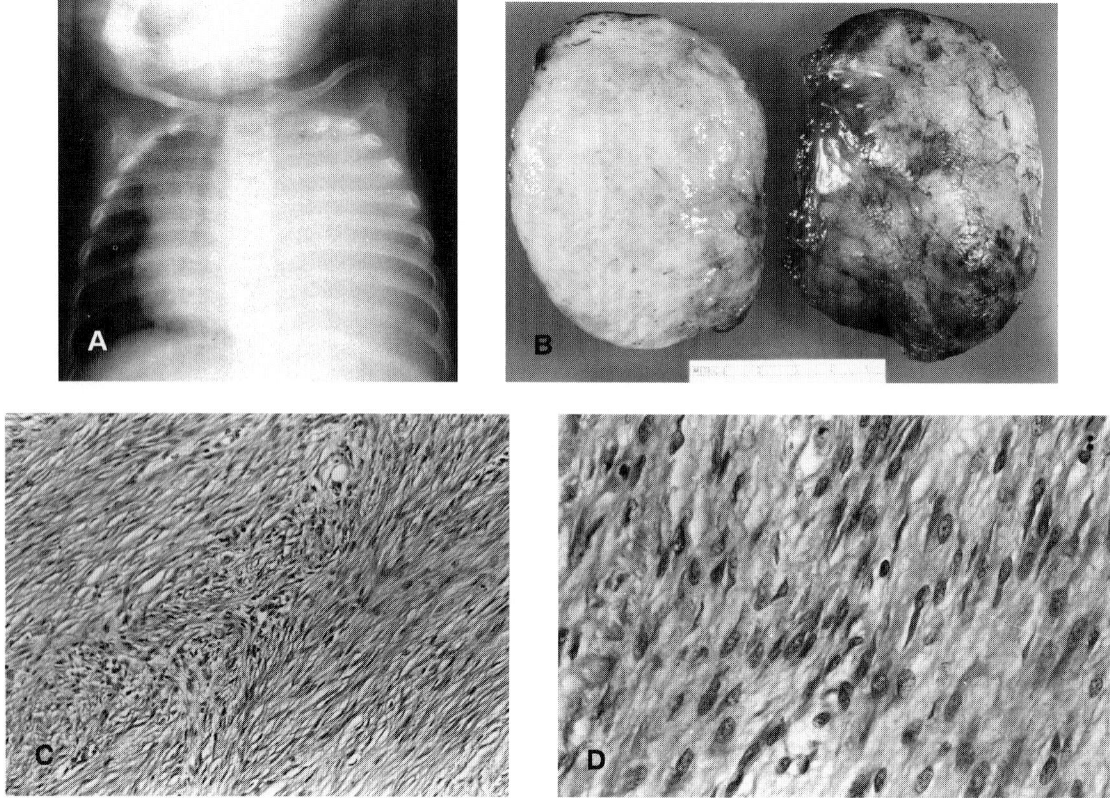

Figure 4–3. Fibromatosis of the mediastinum and left supraclavicular area in a 7-month-old female child who presented with a mass in the shoulder and chest. *A,* A chest radiograph shows a large left mediastinal mass occupying much of the left thorax and displacing the mediastinal structures to the right. *B,* The excised gross specimen, which measures 10.5 × 8 cm, was divided in half; the cut surface is shown on the left of the picture, whereas the external surface is pictured on the right. The cut surface has a pale, gelatinous appearance. *C,* The interdigitating (herringbone) and fan-like storiform (middle of field) patterns of growth are typical for this group of tumors (hematoxylin-eosin, ×300). *D,* A higher-power view depicts the tumor cells in greater detail. The cells resemble tissue culture–like fibroblasts (hematoxylin-eosin, ×480). (From Isaacs H Jr. Neoplasms in infants: A report of 265 cases. *In* Sommers SC, Rosen PP (eds): Pathol Annu 1983;18: 165. Used by permission.)

tochemical studies.[133,267] The tumor cell cytoplasms react positively with vimentin and actin and negatively with desmin and keratin.[133,267,383] Like the other fibromatoses of infancy, ultrastructurally, the cell of origin is considered to be the myofibroblast and fibroblast.[38,78,188,267,313,383] Digital fibromatoses invade locally (including bone) and frequently recur, and many eventually regress spontaneously and disappear.[72] Conservative surgical excision is the recommended form of therapy.

Torticollis

Torticollis (fibromatosis colli, sternocleidomastoid tumor) is a tumor-like condition that produces a neck mass in a young child. It presents as a firm, palpable nodule in the sternocleidomastoid muscle, usually appearing within the first 2 weeks of life and causing a deformity called "wry neck." Torticollis is observed in less than 1% of newborn infants.[89] It is usually unilateral, but in some instances, bilateral neck masses may occur.[180] The condition has also been called fibromatosis colli and sternocleidomastoid tumor, implying that the lesion is a neoplasm. Controversy still exists as to whether the lesion represents a true neoplasm or a reparative process.[7,8,128,187] Currently, it is regarded as the latter.[187]

One classic review of torticollis was done by MacDonald, who described 50 newborns presenting with masses in the sternocleidomastoid muscle.[242] Although reported almost 30 years ago, the study portrays the course and natural history of the disease. The average age at the time of diagnosis was 3 weeks. There was a slight male predominance (60%). More than 50% of the affected neonates were the product

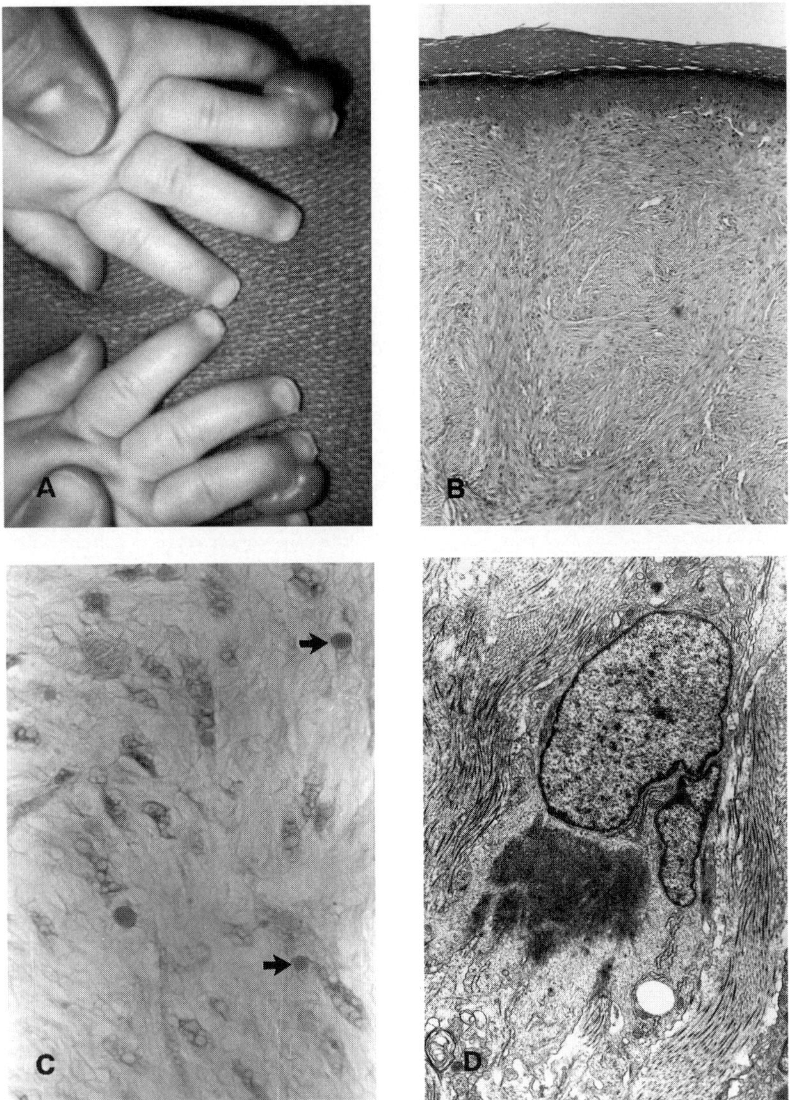

Figure 4–4. Digital fibromatosis. A 1-year-old boy presented with a history of nodules on the lateral aspects of the distal phalanges of the fourth fingers since birth. The nodules were excised but recurred each time; eventually, they disappeared. *A,* Note the mirror image distribution of the lesions. *B,* The tumor is moderately cellular and composed of small, regular, spindle-shaped cells involving the dermis and subcutaneous tissue. The tumor displays an interdigiting or herringbone growth pattern. The epidermis is not involved (trichrome, ×120). *C,* Intracytoplasmic hyaline inclusions (*arrows*) are evident (hematoxylin-eosin, ×615). *D,* The intracytoplasmic inclusions are composed of actin-like filaments, which are noted beneath the nucleus (×13,200). (*A* and *B:* From Isaacs H Jr. Neoplasms in infants: A report of 265 cases. *In* Sommers SC, Rosen PP (eds): Pathol Annu 1983;18:165. Used by permission. *D:* Courtesy of Ann Peters, Children's Hospital, San Diego, CA.)

of a breech or forceps delivery, and more than 50% were firstborn children. Most of the lesions were located on the right side of the neck, and many were associated with breech birth. The patients were either not treated or were treated with stretching exercises. The results of a 6-year follow-up study revealed that 22 of 50 of the lesions completely resolved, with the affected patients returning to normal; slight tightness or a band with minimal asymmetry was noted in 7 cases; and torticollis resulted in

another 7 cases.[242] A review of 23 patients with torticollis, published by Enzinger 4 years before MacDonald's study, revealed similar findings except that the lesions occurred with almost equal frequency on either side, and two patients had bilateral disease.[125a]

The histologic features of torticollis are time-dependent. During the first few months of life, the histologic picture is similar to that of desmoid fibromatosis. However, a few years later, bland, acellular-appearing fibrosis, accompa-

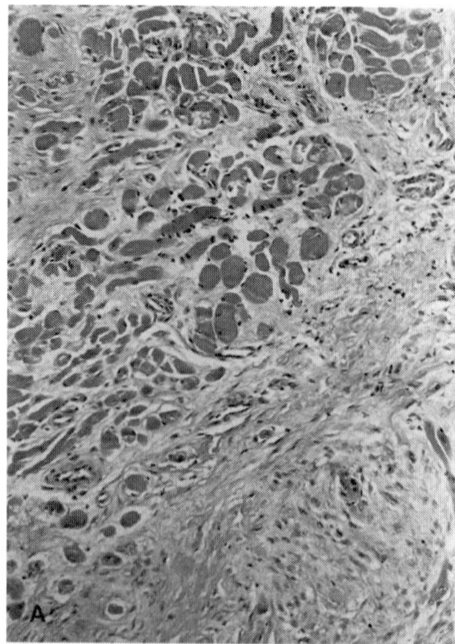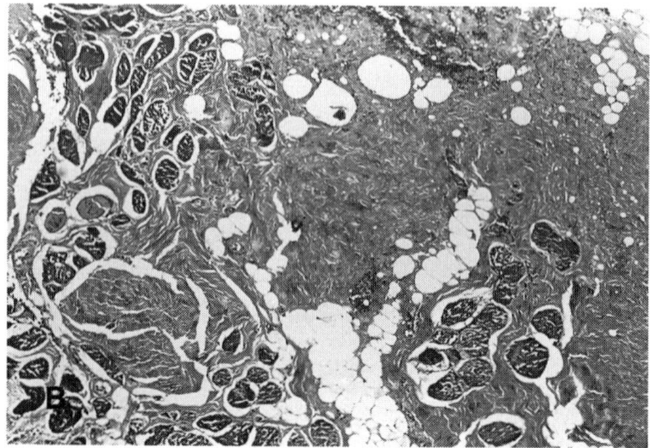

Figure 4–5. Torticollis (fibromatosis colli). The appearance of the lesion is age-dependent. *A,* A photomicrograph of a portion of the sternocleidomastoid muscle removed from a 6-week-old male with torticollis. There is extensive skeletal muscle fibrosis and atrophy. At this early stage of the disease, the histologic appearance of interstitial fibrosis in some areas is indistinguishable from fibromatosis (hematoxylin-eosin, ×240). *B,* A section taken from the sternocleidomastoid muscle of a 7-year-old boy with torticollis. In comparison to Figure 4–5*A,* Figure 4–5*B* shows much greater loss of skeletal muscle fiber in a background of hypocellular, bland, interstitial fibrosis (trichrome, ×240). (From Isaacs H Jr. Tumors of the Newborn and Infant. St. Louis: Mosby–Year Book, 1991.)

nied by atrophy and loss of skeletal muscle fiber, is observed on biopsy study, and the process becomes stationary (Fig. 4–5).

Myofibromatosis

Myofibromatosis is an unusual neoplasm found primarily in the first year of life. It generally presents as one or more nodular lesions involving the skin, soft tissues, and, sometimes, the bones and viscera. In the medical literature, it appears under a variety of names, including congenital multiple fibromatosis, congenital generalized fibromatosis, multiple vascular leiomyomas, and mesenchymal hamartoma. Many examples have been reported.[4,25,34,35,48,54,62,75,83,84,185,187,194,262,269,313,332,333,351,367,377]

Myofibromatosis occurs in solitary, multiple, or generalized forms having the same histologic findings but with different prognoses. In 1965, Kauffman and Stout suggested the term multiple myofibromatosis when the lesions were confined to bone, muscle, and subcutaneous tissues, and generalized myofibromatosis when the viscera were involved.[203] The congenital generalized form is characterized by a poor prognosis. Death occurs in the first few months of life owing to the involvement of vital struc-

tures during the active phase of rapid growth, and regression which can cause, for example, cardiac and respiratory failure and intestinal obstruction.[84,258] Ts'o and Teoh described a myofibromatosis involving the left side of the larynx that was responsible for airway obstruction in a 2-day-old male infant; in addition, at necropsy, solitary tumors were found in the tongue, myocardium, and lungs.[354] The suggested origin of the tumors was vascular subintimal mesenchymal or smooth muscle myofibroblasts.[84]

Rosenberg et al. classified congenital generalized fibromatosis (myofibromatosis) into two main types.[313] Type I included patients with involvement of the skin, subcutaneous tissue, muscle, and bone, whereas type II included patients with visceral involvement in addition to skin and skeletal muscle tumors.[313] This classification is similar to the one proposed by Kauffman and Stout, alluded to earlier.[203] Of the 33 cases investigated by Rosenberg et al., which included 2 of their own, the distribution was 16 patients with type I disease and 17 with type II. These researchers showed that their classification had important prognostic implications. Except for one patient, all those with type I lesions survived. Of the 17 patients with type II disease, 13 died before 4 months of age. Moreover, the four survivors with type II disease did not have pulmonary involvement.[313] One notable conclusion derived from this study was that the presence or absence of lung lesions was a significant factor in determining the course of disease in patients with type II lesions.

Chung and Enzinger subsequently presented the clinicopathologic findings in 61 patients with infantile myofibromatosis: 45 had solitary tumors, whereas 16 had multicentric tumors.[75] Solitary myofibromatoses were more common than multiple ones, and a male predominance was noted.[75] Multiple tumors usually were discovered by 1 month of age, whereas about 50% of solitary tumors were found at birth. Solitary myofibromatosis involved primarily the soft tissues of the head, neck, and trunk. By contrast, the multicentric tumors arose not only from the skin and subcutaneous tissues situated over various parts of the body, but also from the muscles, bones, and viscera, and a female predominance was noted.[75] This renowned study showed that myofibromatosis was a distinct entity that differed from fibromatosis.[75]

Additional reviews on this subject have been published by Brill et al., who described 63 patients with congenital generalized myofibromatoses;[48] Wiswell and colleagues, whose study included 166 infantile myofibromatoses (125 neonates);[377] Bracko et al., who reported 25 familial cases (including 20 newborns);[47] Roggli and associates, who cited 16 congenital examples with visceral involvement;[310] and Soper and DeSilva, who reported 9 infantile cases (7 neonates).[333] Myofibromatoses rarely occur in the brain and spinal cord of patients with multicentric tumors; indeed, less than 10 such cases have been documented.[25,75,112,316,333,351,377] Usually, the lesions are situated within the arachnoid or spinal dura. An unusual case of a fatal solitary myofibromatosis occurring in a 48-day-old female was reported; the tumor originated from the epidural space of the posterior fossa and resulted in brain compression, ventricular obstruction, and hydrocephalus.[62]

The typical clinical manifestation of myofibromatosis is one or more firm, rubbery nodules located within the skin, subcutaneous tissue, or muscle. The superficially situated nodules tend to be freely movable, whereas the deep-seated ones are fixed.[75] Sometimes, the overlying skin is ulcerated. Large, disfiguring facial masses have been described in newborns.[54,328] Facial tumors are often extensive, involve the adjacent sinuses and craniofacial bones, and may extend into the cranial cavity.

Compression of the spinal cord by tumor in the dura may cause hypotonia and flaccid paralysis of the extremities.[10] The 48-day-old female infant with a large, solitary, epidural, posterior fossa tumor (described earlier) presented with macrocrania, a semicomatose state, generalized hypotonia, and bilateral papilloedema.[62] Solitary or multiple congenital myofibromatosis of the small and large intestine may produce signs of neonatal bowel obstruction with vomiting and abdominal distention or an abdominal mass. Signs of an acute abdomen are noted following intestinal perforation.[75,151,340,367]

Infantile myofibromatosis may occur as either a solitary lesion or as multicentric lesions in bone.[67,181] According to the Mayo Clinic study, most solitary tumors (13 of 14) were found in the craniofacial bones.[181] Multiple, radiolucent, lytic lesions involving the metaphysis of the long bones of the upper and lower extremities and the skull were found in a newborn male described by Chan et al.[67]

Major malformations (e.g., porencephaly with hemiparesis, hemiatrophy, esophageal atresia, and hypoplastic kidney) have been reported in newborns with multiple myofibromatosis.[256,339] However, these associations may be merely coincidental.[339]

A familial occurrence has been documented in several reports, but it is not certain whether infantile myofibromatosis is a recessive or an autosomal dominant disorder.[25,47,75,83,194,316] Salamah et al. described three siblings who had multiple myofibromatoses and whose parents were first cousins.[316] Bracko et al. reported two brothers with multicentric tumors, and listed 23 additional cases with familial disease.[47] Jennings et al. described a father and daughter with congenital tumors.[194] Two male siblings with fatal congenital generalized myofibromatosis were reported by Coffin et al.; pulmonary involvement was determined to be the cause of the siblings' death.[83]

Both the solitary and generalized forms of myofibromatosis display essentially identical gross and microscopic findings. They are characterized by rather well-circumscribed, light tan-gray, rubbery nodules with foci of central necrosis and calcification ranging in size from 0.5 to 5 cm in diameter.[187] Histologic examination reveals the nodules to be composed of spindle-shaped, smooth muscle cells and fibroblasts, a central vascular pattern, and foci of necrosis and calcification. The tumor cells are arranged in short bundles or interdigitating fascicles that closely resemble a leiomyoma in

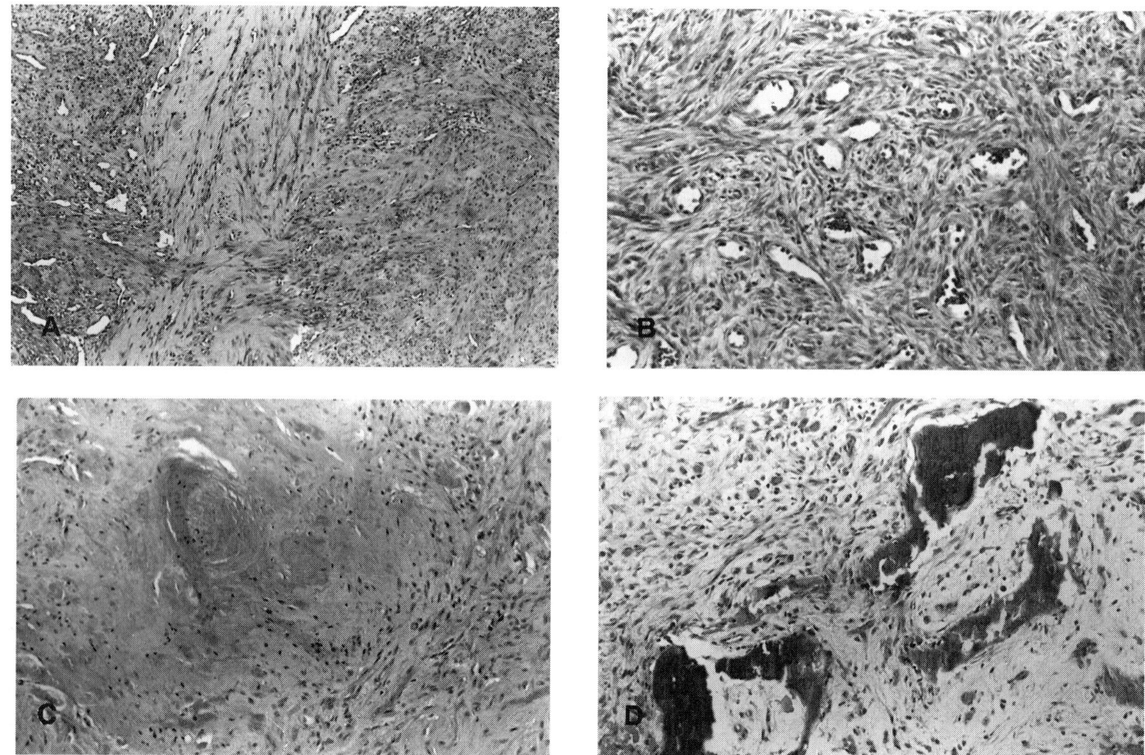

Figure 4–6. Infantile myofibromatosis. The lesions may be single or multiple and may involve the subcutaneous tissue, viscera, or bones. *A,* A photomicrograph of a solitary, tannish-pink, subcutaneous nodule, measuring 2 × 1.8 cm, which was removed from a 2-month-old boy. This benign-appearing, spindle-cell tumor displays spindle-shaped myofibroblastic cells with a fibrous background and a focal vascular pattern (trichrome, ×120). (From Isaacs H Jr. Tumors of the Newborn and Infant. St. Louis: Mosby–Year Book, 1991.) *B,* The vascular pattern resembles a hemangioma or hemangiopericytoma (trichrome, ×120). *C,* An area of necrosis is evident (trichrome, ×120). *D,* An area of calcification is noted (hematoxylin-eosin, ×150).

some areas (Fig. 4–6). The superficially located lesions tend to be well-circumscribed compared to the deep-seated tumors, which are infiltrative.[132] Vascular invasion by the tumor is seen occasionally, but it does not have prognostic significance. Older lesions exhibit mostly fibrosis, eventually form a fibrous scar, and, if small enough, disappear with time (personal observation).

Myofibromatosis of the gastrointestinal tract has been described under various names, including fibromatosis, spindle cell tumors, leiomyosarcoma, and other sarcomas.[68,243,340] Solitary lesions of the small intestine were first documented in two newborns by Kauffman and Stout in 1965,[203] and later by Gonzales-Crussi and Noronha.[151] The tumor is a rare cause of neonatal bowel obstruction. Srigley and Mancer reviewed 12 cases of congenital spindle cell tumors of the intestinal tract and concluded that many represent myofibromatoses rather than sarcomas or other tumors.[340] If completely

excised, solitary intestinal myofibromatoses have a good prognosis.[68,340,367]

Ultrastructural observations confirm the light microscopic findings. Fibroblasts, smooth muscle cells, and cells that are intermediate between the two (myofibroblasts) are observed. The tumors are immunoreactive with actin and estrogen receptor.[83] They react negatively with cytokeratin, S-100 protein, or myoglobin, and are focally positive with desmin.[132] The myofibroblastic nature of the tumor has been confirmed by several investigators.[62,332,340]

Fibromatosis and myofibromatosis share certain features, such as the distribution of solitary lesions and the presence of fibroblasts and myofibroblasts on light and electron microscopy.[4] Central necrosis and a prominent vascular pattern in myofibromatosis are diagnostic criteria that help to distinguish the two (Fig. 4–6*C* and *D*).[75,128] However, sometimes, the microscopic distinction between the two is not well defined, particularly in extremely small biopsy samples, as both lesions are composed of spindle cells with interdigitating growth patterns and fibrosis.[184,187] Infantile hemangiopericytoma is another consideration in the differential diagnosis. In this condition, the vascular spaces are slit-like and tend to be located peripherally, whereas in myofibromatosis, the spaces are situated centrally. The reticulin stain shows reticulin fibers surrounding individual cells (hemangiopericytoma pattern) and groups of cells (hemangioma pattern).

Variend et al. suggest that myofibromatosis, congenital fibrosarcoma, and hemangiopericytoma are histogenetically related, as they share overlapping histopathologic and clinical features.[364] These researchers contend that these entities actually represent a "histological continuum."[364]

Nodular fasciitis, although rare in the newborn, should also be mentioned.[75] Giant fibroblasts resembling ganglion cells are pathognomonic of this reactive process (see Fig. 4–39).[128,187] The clinical setting of generalized myofibromatosis suggests the diagnosis once the entity has been thought of, but the solitary form may be more difficult to distinguish from other soft tissue lesions.

Myofibromatosis has a much greater tendency to regress and resolve spontaneously than does fibromatosis, which is more aggressive locally and is characterized by a greater recurrence rate.[75] Spontaneous regression of the former has been documented on several occasions, including pulmonary nodules.[34,35,258,269,313,332,377] The end result in lesions that have regressed is fibrosis or disappearance of the tumor. When there is extensive involvement of multiple viscera, particularly the lungs, patients with multicentric myofibromatosis have a poor prognosis.[4,48,75,83,310,377] It is the location and the extent of the lesions that determine the ultimate outcome.[333] More extensive imaging studies—namely, computerized tomography and magnetic resonance imaging—at the time of diagnosis, may uncover silent visceral lesions in patients who were thought to have only skin and soft tissue tumors.[262,333] Therefore, these studies are recommended as part of the patient's initial evaluation, as the findings of these studies will definitely affect the prognosis.

The recurrence rate of single lesions is about 7% after primary excision, but the recurrence can be cured, usually after re-excision.[75] According to Wiswell et al.,[377] the mortality rate for the multicentric form with visceral involve-

ment is 73%. Death ensues in cases of cardiopulmonary or intestinal complications. Typically, the natural history is distinguished by spontaneous regression; therefore, aggressive treatment should be delayed unless a vital structure is involved.[25,333]

Fibrous Hamartoma of Infancy

Fibrous hamartoma is a relatively uncommon soft tissue neoplasm that is usually observed within the first year of life, with 10% to 20% of cases presenting at birth.[72,126,132a,334] The entity was first described by Reye in 1956 as one of the "subdermal fibromatous tumours of infancy."[305] Subsequently, Enzinger collected and reviewed 30 case examples, clearly defined the clinical and histopathologic features, and suggested the term "fibrous hamartoma of infancy."[126] Most of his cases were diagnosed during the first year of life, and five were diagnosed at birth. The tumor presents as a slowly growing, painless, palpable mass most often involving the axilla and shoulder and, less frequently, the chest wall, upper arm, neck, and inguinal region arising from the lower dermis or subcutaneous tissue (Figs. 4–7 and 4–8).[126,158,132a,313] The lesion is usually freely movable, but occasionally, the underlying skeletal muscle and nerves may be involved, in which case it becomes fixed. Only rarely is more than one lesion found in the same patient. Male patients are affected more often than female patients.[126,313,334] Although most lesions arise from the subcutaneous tissues, unusual locations, such as the lung, have been described in the neonate.[197]

The tumor consists of a round, bulging mass, arising from the lower dermis and subcutaneous tissue, which is composed of firm, glistening, gray-white fibrous tissue and yellow nodules of fat. On gross examination, it resembles a lipoma with grayish fibrous bands coursing through it. Fibrous hamartomas rarely exceed 8 cm at their greatest diameter. Some appear to be well circumscribed, whereas others blend imperceptively with the surrounding subcutaneous fat (see Figs. 4–7 and 4–8).[313]

Histologic examination reveals that fibrous hamartoma displays three main components:[126] nests of immature-looking, spindle-shaped cells embedded in a myxoid background; interlacing, dense, fibrous trabeculae or cords resembling tendon; and lobules of mature adipose tissue situated between the other two compo-

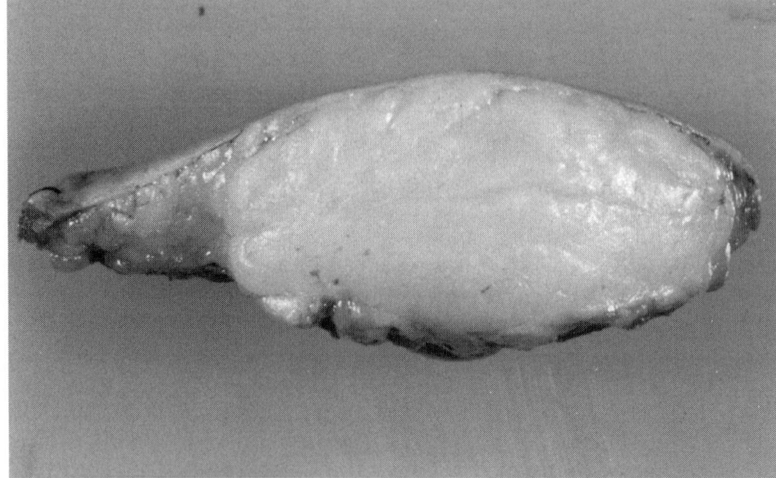

Figure 4–7. Fibrous hamartoma of infancy. Gross appearance of a subcutaneous mass, weighing 30 g and measuring 7.4 × 3.6 cm, which was removed from the lateral aspect of the upper right arm of a 4-month-old girl. The tumor had been present since birth. It consists mostly of adipose tissue, which blends imperceptively with the adjacent subcutaneous fat. The overlying skin is essentially normal. (From Isaacs H Jr. Tumors of the Newborn and Infant. St. Louis: Mosby–Year Book, 1991.)

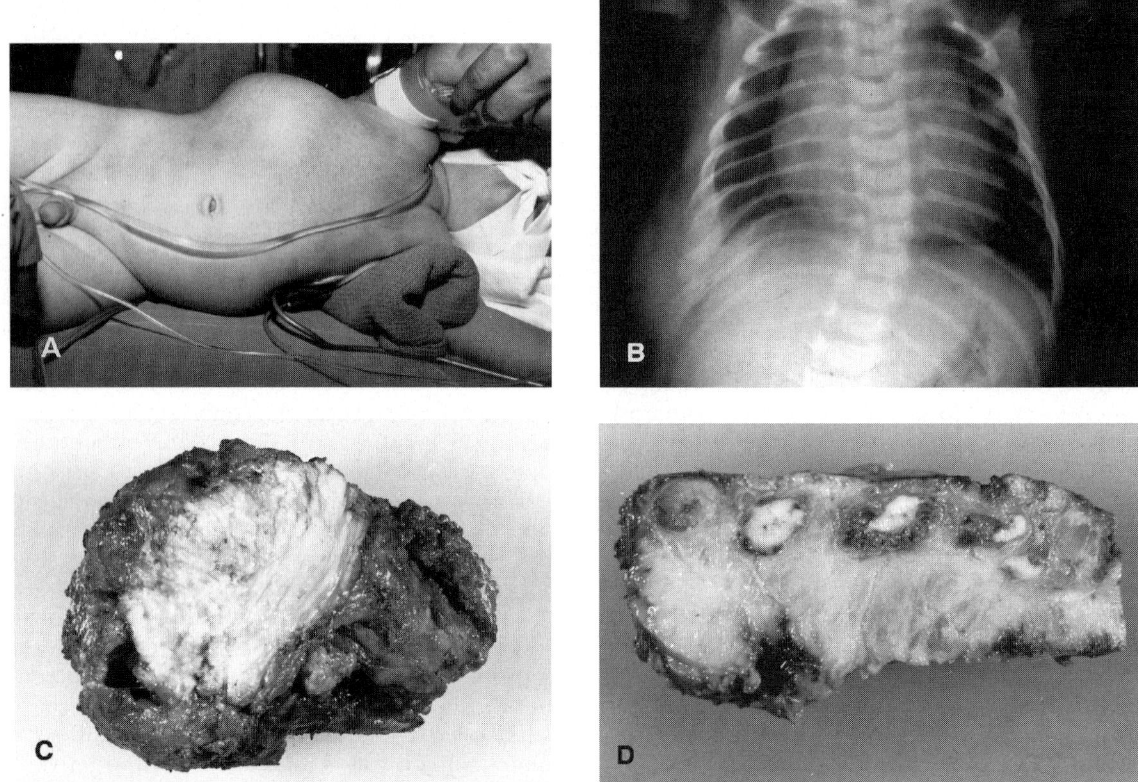

Figure 4–8. Fibrous hamartoma of infancy. *A,* A 2-month-old boy with a mass in the right chest wall. *B,* A chest x-ray film reveals a soft tissue lesion with rib involvement. Scoliosis is present. *C,* The cut surface of the soft tissue component. *D,* The tumor appears to surround the ribs, rather than arising from them, as is the case with chest wall hamartoma of osseous origin (compare with Fig. 18–1).

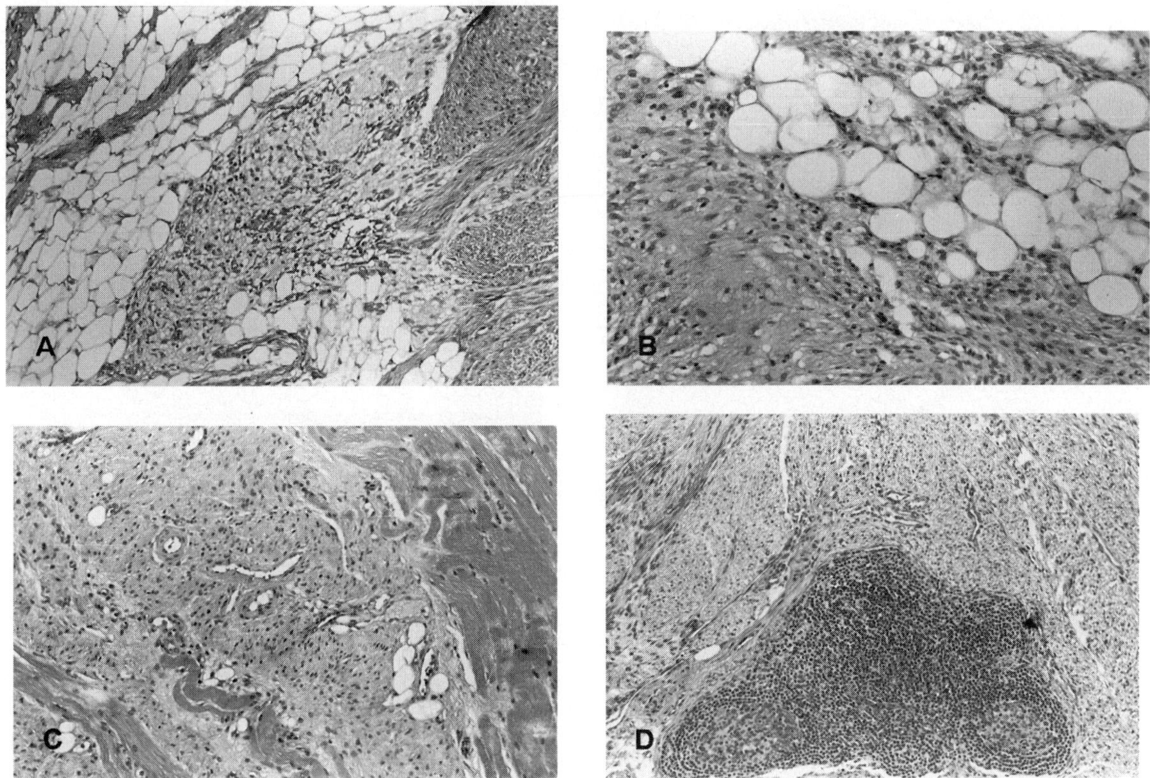

Figure 4–9. Fibrous hamartoma of infancy. *A,* The tumor consists of the three components, other than fat, that are required to establish the diagnosis: fibroblastic areas on the right of the photograph, myxoid areas in the center, and cord-like fibrous bands traversing the upper left hand corner (hematoxylin-eosin, ×80). (From Isaacs H Jr. Tumors of the Newborn and Infant. St. Louis: Mosby–Year Book, 1991.) *B,* A higher-power view demonstrates the immature spindle cells (hematoxylin-eosin, ×150). *C,* Tumor is seen to have invaded the skeletal muscle (hematoxylin-eosin, ×120). *D,* Lymph node surrounded by tumor (hematoxylin-eosin, ×120).

nents (Fig. 4–9).[126] Blood vessels are prominent in the myxoid areas. Tumor cells in the myxoid and fascicular fibroblastic areas are positive for vimentin.[132a] On electron microscopy, the tumor is composed of both fibroblasts and myofibroblasts, the latter consisting of intracytoplasmic myofibrils with dense bodies, pinocytotic vesicles, and basement membranes.[158,257,313] Greco and associates suggest that the cellular myxoid areas resemble the developing blood vessels and fat observed in fetal tissues (see Fig. 4–1).[158] The dense fibrous cords conceivably represent the end stage of fibrous proliferation.[158]

Usually, the tumors do not recur if excision is complete.[187,313] Enzinger has stated that 4 of 30 (13%) patients in his series developed a recurrent tumor.[126] No recurrences were reported in nine patients with this tumor who underwent follow-up study at Children's Hospital, Los Angeles.[187] The histogenesis and biological behavior of this benign fibrous lesion remain enigmatic. Judging from cases personally examined, the tumors tend to regress spontaneously by fibrosis or disappear into the surrounding fat, which would explain the low rate of recurrence. It is conceivable that some fibrolipomas removed from older individuals actually represent a matured fibrous hamartoma of infancy.

Giant Cell Fibroelastoma

Giant cell fibroelastoma is a very uncommon fibroblastic neoplasm found predominantly in male patients younger than 10 years of age.[118] Less than 40 cases have been reported, with the youngest on record involving a 4-month-old child. Characteristically, the tumor is superficial and occurs mostly on the trunk, but also in the inguinal region, scrotum, thigh, or neck.[118] The microscopic findings include moderately cellular solid areas, angiectoid (sinusoidal) spaces resembling lymphatics, and foci of dense

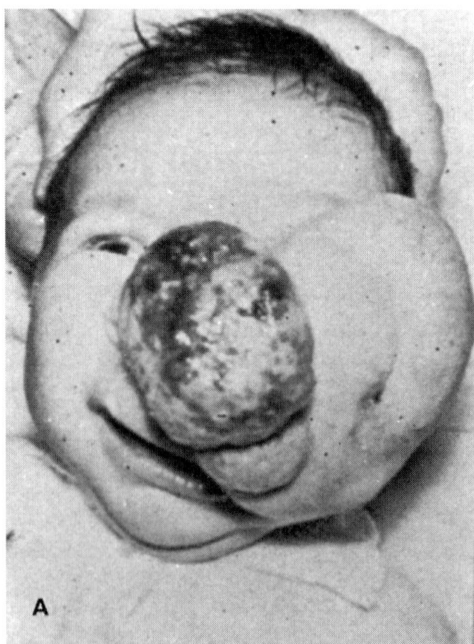
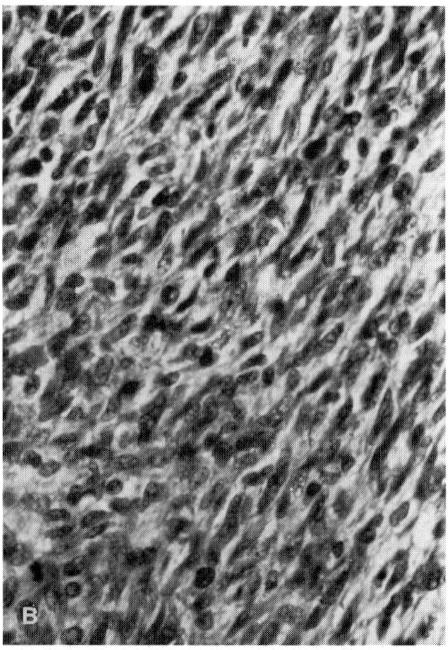

Figure 4–10. Congenital fibrosarcoma. *A,* A 3-day-old girl with a massive lesion involving the face, nose, and maxillary sinus. The lesion, which measured 16 × 16 × 10 cm, was cured by wide local excision. *B,* The hypercellular tumor is composed of spindle-shaped, fibroblast-like cells with a fascicular pattern (hematoxylin-eosin, ×380). (From Hays DM, Mirabal VQ, Karlan MS, et al. Fibrosarcomas in infants and children. J Pediatr Surg 1970;5:176. Used by permission.)

collagen having a myxoid background containing entrapped fat. Fibroblasts and floret-type giant cells are requisite features for definitive diagnosis. Not unlike the other benign fibroblastic tumors of infancy, fibroelastoma is associated with a good prognosis, but will recur if not completely excised.

Congenital Fibrosarcoma

Although congenital (infantile) fibrosarcoma is relatively uncommon, it is the foremost sarcoma of the newborn.[3,16,17,28,40,74,80,146,153,159,170,171,182,183,185,187,190,239,244,247,309,312,313,325,336,345,368] Some controversy exists over the terminology for this lesion, and whether or not it behaves in a malignant fashion.[82,187] Most congenital fibrosarcomas originate in the extremities, whereas others occur in axial locations—namely, the back, head, neck, and retroperitoneum (see Table 4–2; Figs. 4–10 and 4–11).[28,74,336] The tumor has been described in stillborn infants.[239] Although the rate of local recurrence is significant—as high as 50% in some series—metastases seldom occur.[74,102,109,128,170,185,313,336,345]

The first detailed review on this subject that showed a much improved prognosis in young children was presented by Stout in 1962.[345] This classic article, published before the era of effective chemotherapy, serves as a historical control. Of 14 infants and children with fibrosarcoma, 3 (21%) had congenital tumors.[345] Two of these involved the lower extremities (gastrocnemius muscle and foot), and one involved the triceps muscle. The lower leg and trapezius tumors recurred following excision. Patients with the extremity lesions were cured after amputation, but the baby with the triceps tumor died from metastatic disease. The University of Texas M.D. Anderson Hospital group described five newborns with fibrosarcoma.[28] All but one had lesions involving an extremity, two experienced recurrent disease, but all survived. Soule and Pritchard reviewed 110 cases of children with fibrosarcoma, including 70 cases from the literature plus 40 of their own.[336] Slightly more than one third of those affected (40 of 70) were younger than 3 months of age at the time of diagnosis. Most tumors originated in the extremities (11 of 13), followed, in order of frequency, by tumors involving the legs, feet, and hands. The recurrence rate for newborns in the study was 2 of 13 (15%), and the frequency of metastasis ending in death was 1 of 13 (7.7%).

Chung and Enzinger reported their findings for the period of 1948 to 1975 in 53 patients

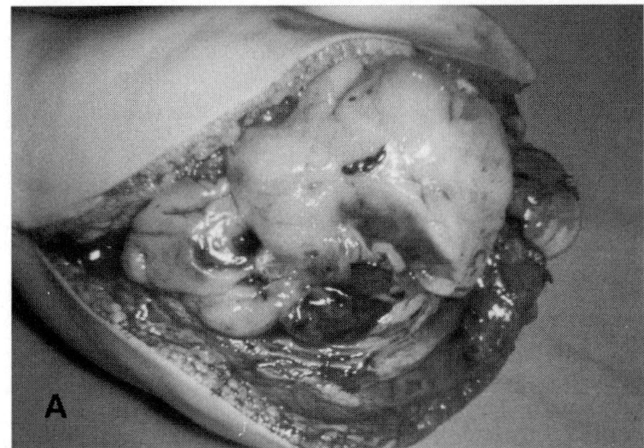

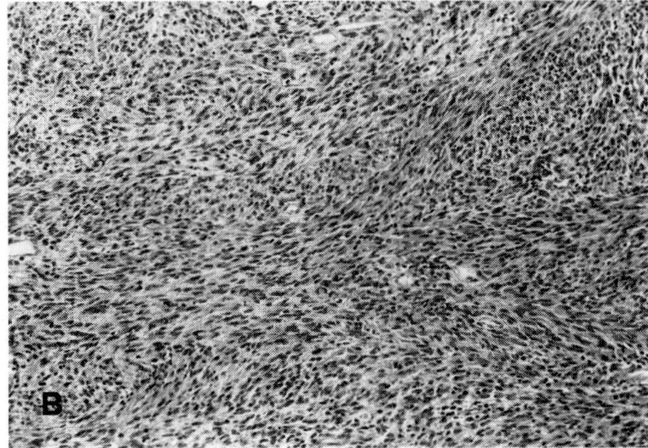

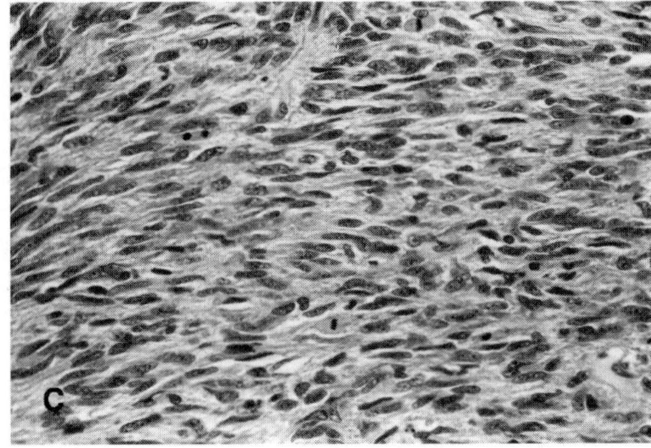

Figure 4–11. Congenital fibrosarcoma. A 5-month-old boy had a rapidly growing tumor in the right thigh discovered at 1 week of age. *A,* The amputation specimen consists of a large, soft, gelatinous tumor occupying most of the thigh. The head of the femur is visible on the medial aspect. *B,* A photomicrograph shows the interdigitating, fascicular growth pattern of the tumor (hematoxylin-eosin, ×120). *C,* The cellular, spindle-cell neoplasm displays moderate nuclear atypia, three or four mitoses, and the presence of interstitial collagen (hematoxylin-eosin, ×600). (From Isaacs H Jr. Neoplasms in infants: A report of 265 cases. *In* Sommers SC, Rosen PP (eds): Pathol Annu 1983;18:165. Used by permission.)

with infantile fibrosarcoma who ranged in age from birth to 5 years.[74] Forty-one patients were diagnosed in the first year of life, 20 (38%) were diagnosed at birth, and 27 (50.9%) were diagnosed before 3 months of age. There was a male predominance (60%). Most of the perinatal fibrosarcomas arose in the extremities, with the remainder occurring in the back, head and neck, and retroperitoneum. Data, including age, sex, primary site, treatment, and outcome, were not tabulated specifically for each patient, but the overall recurrence rate was 15% and the frequency of metastases was 8.3%, which is in agreement with the Mayo Clinic findings reported by Soule and Pritchard.[336]

Table 4–2 includes data from a Children's Hospital, Los Angeles study, which includes five patients from the previous reports of Hays et al.[170] (see Fig. 4–10) and Isaacs,[184] plus a more recent fatal case. There is a male:female ratio of 5:1 and a predominance of extremity lesions. Three tumors of the thigh recurred, necessitating amputation in two patients, and the third patient died of metastatic disease. The latter underwent an inadequate biopsy study shortly after birth at another hospital, resulting

in an erroneous diagnosis. The child's parents were told that the lesion would eventually "go away." Several years later, the fibrosarcoma rapidly increased in size and local and distant metastases appeared.

Blocker et al. described five patients with congenital fibrosarcoma and reviewed 47 additional cases from the literature.[40] Three of their patients had axial tumors, two of which were located in the thoracolumbar region and one in the anterior neck. One neonate with a thoracolumbar tumor survived without recurrence following a wide local resection and the other experienced a recurrence with chest wall and pleural metastases. The infant with the cervical fibrosarcoma died from residual tumor and airway obstruction. Two with extremity lesions, situated in the lower leg and foot, respectively, survived after amputation as the main treatment.[40] Blocker and colleagues concluded from their study that: (1) congenital fibrosarcoma occurs more often in the extremities (71%) than in axial locations (29%); (2) the local recurrence rate for axial tumors is the same as that for tumors involving an extremity (namely, 33%); (3) the metastatic and mortality rates are much greater for axial (26% and 26%, respectively) than for extremity tumors (8% and 5%, respectively); and (4) the overall mortality rate is 11.5% and the metastatic rate is 13.5%, which, according to the authors, is similar to that for older children.[40] Blocker et al. concluded from their findings that infants with either axial or extremity congenital fibrosarcomas should be treated the same as older children, and that young patients should receive adjuvant therapy if necessary.[40]

Kynaston et al. reported six cases of neonatal fibrosarcoma treated with chemotherapy, five of which involved an extremity and one of which involved the lumbosacral area.[220] The one patient that died had an axial lesion. Schofield et al. analyzed 17 cases of infants and children with fibrosarcoma (8 of whom were younger than 3 months of age) and compared the results in this group with the results achieved in 3 of their patients with fibromatosis (2 neonates). Except for one with a back lesion, neonates with fibrosarcomas of the extremity (3 examples), neck, chest wall, buttock, and retroperitoneum survived after various forms of therapy.[322]

Coffin et al. published the clinicopathologic findings in 26 cases of congenital-infantile fibrosarcoma, 19 of which were personal cases and 7 of which were referrals from other institutions.[82] Twenty-one patients were younger than 3 months of age. The anatomic distribution of tumors was as follows: extremities, 9; truncal, 7; and head and neck, 5. All of the patients with extremity lesions survived, whereas 2 of 7 patients with truncal and 3 of 5 patients with head and neck fibrosarcomas died.

Cytogenetic studies performed on congenital fibrosarcomas have revealed a trisomy of chromosomes 8, 11, and 20 (48,XY, +11, +20).[3,16,220,322,338] Trisomy 11 appears to be the most consistent chromosomal anomaly associated with congenital fibrosarcoma, and it is also found in association with cellular mesoblastic nephroma[37] (Fig. 4–12D). James et al. have also described an example of a scapular lesion with a diploid cell population and a favorable outcome.[190]

Clinical Findings

Recognition of an obvious tumor mass at birth or later on in infancy by the parents or pediatrician is the usual clinical presentation. The newborn with a fibrosarcoma may have an impressive soft tissue mass measuring 10 to 20 cm or more that involves an extremity, the trunk, head, or neck (see Figs. 4–10 and 4–11).[3,7,8,39,102,128,153,159,170,184,185,247] Giant congenital tumors may produce a grotesque appearance, as with a fibrosarcoma of the face that involves the paranasal sinuses, as reported by Hays et al. (see Table 4–2; Fig. 4–10).[170] The tumors generally grow rapidly, reaching a large size within a few weeks or months. However, spontaneous regression of an unresectable congenital fibrosarcoma of the forearm has been documented.[244] There are no definite hereditary diseases or congenital malformations associated with this malignant tumor.

The tumor is composed of firm, light gray, occasionally gelatinous tissue that is partially surrounded by a fibrous capsule (see Fig. 4–11A). The larger tumors show areas of hemorrhage, necrosis, and small cystic formations. The gross appearance may be deceptive because extensions of tumor blend subtly with the adjacent soft tissues of the affected part so that just "shelling it out" leaves residual tumor behind. Therefore, wide local excision is required, preferably at the initial surgery, if this is technically feasible. Extremity lesions may involve the underlying bone, producing a pathologic fracture.[28]

Histologic findings reveal small, spindle-shaped cells arranged in fascicles that are separated by variable amounts of myxoid stroma that stains pale gray (see Figs. 4–10 and 4–11). Differing amounts of eosinophilic-staining collagen are present, depending on the degree of differentiation. The microscopic features are essentially the same as those seen in the older child and adult, but the tumor cells tend to be smaller and less mature in appearance (see Figs. 4–10 to 4–12).[102,123,128,153,159,336] Some congenital fibrosarcomas have slightly different features consisting mostly of small, round cells, rather than the customary fibroblastic spindle cells, embedded in an abundant, pale-staining myxoid stroma resembling fetal mesenchyme. This form of the tumor displays only moderate cellular atypia and a low mitotic rate.

Fibrosarcoma may show a similar histologic picture as fibromatosis except that the former displays more cellularity, nuclear atypia, increased mitotic activity and areas of necrosis. The herring bone and storiform (whorled) growth patterns are present in both tumors.[28,82,196,336,345]

Prominent, cleft-like, vascular spaces mimicking those of hemangiopericytoma are noted

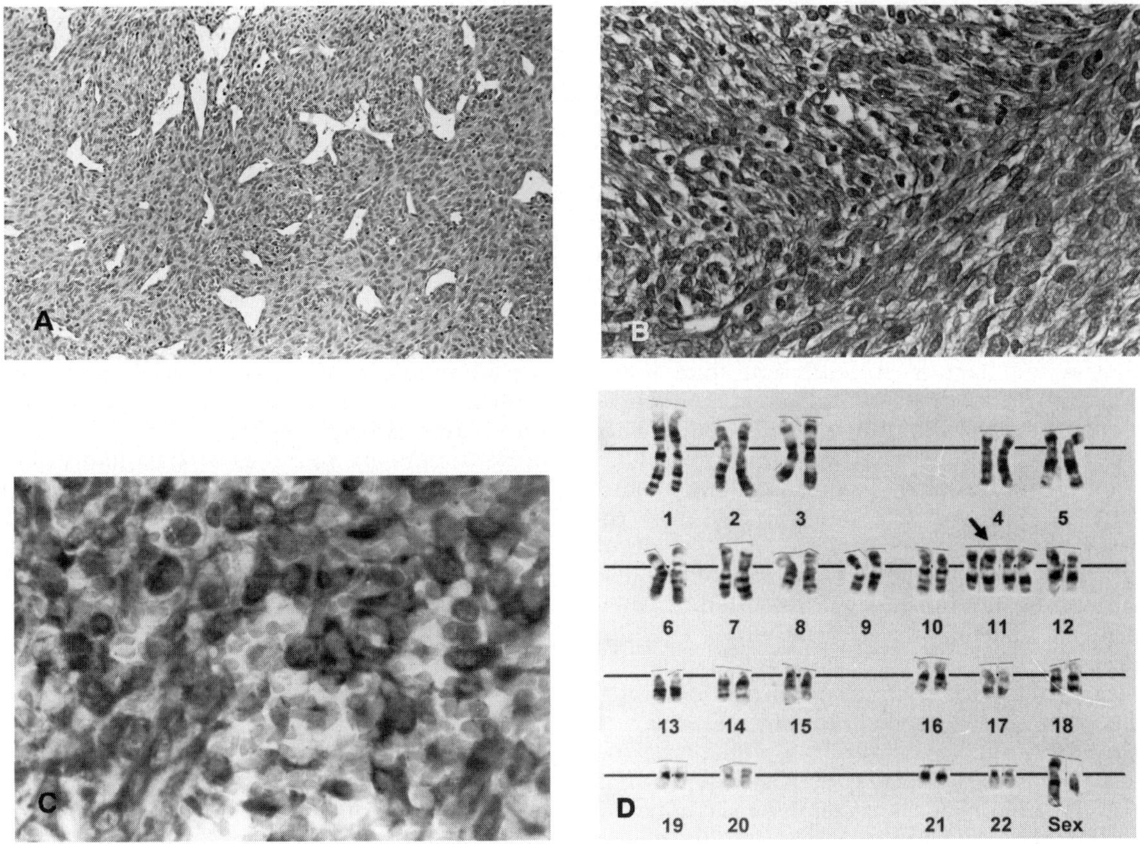

Figure 4–12. Congenital fibrosarcoma. *A,* A hemangiopericytoma-type pattern which may be confused with this tumor (hematoxylin-eosin, ×120). *B,* A reticulin stain reveals reticulin fibers separating the tumor cells (reticulin, ×400). *C,* The tumor cells are reactive with vimentin, but not with actin, desmin, or neuron-specific enolase (vimentin immunoperoxidase, ×600). *D,* The karyotype of a fibrosarcoma from the shoulder of a 2-day-old boy shows a trisomy 11. (Courtesy of James Mascarello, PhD, Children's Hospital, San Diego, CA.)

in some tumors, and may present a diagnostic problem (Fig. 4–12*A*). Moreover, the abnormal karyotype (48,XY, +11, +20) appears to be specific for congenital fibrosarcoma (Fig. 4–12*D*).[3,220]

Prior to the availability of immunoperoxidase methods, a silver reticulin stain was used to demonstrate silver-positive reticulin fibers surrounding individual tumor cells, a feature that was considered helpful in establishing the diagnosis (Fig. 4–12*B*).[74,345] The Masson trichrome stain outlines the cells nicely and demonstrates small deposits of interstitial collagen. Fibrosarcomas generally react positively with vimentin and type IV collagen, but negatively for cytokeratin, epithelial membrane antigen, neurofilament, S-100 protein, actin, and desmin (Fig. 4–12*C*).[16,82,322]

Ultrastructural studies support the view that the tumor is primarily of fibroblastic ori-

gin.[16,153,312] Tumor cells are spindle-shaped and lack basement membranes and well-developed cell junctions. Deposits of electron-dense material are noted, both within dilated rough endoplasmic reticulum and within the extracellular matrix. Cytoplasmic fibrils attached to the dense deposits and extracellular collagen fibers are additional features.[312] Some congenital fibrosarcomas have a prominent histiocytic component in addition to the fibroblastic elements.[153] In one of their recent reviews, Coffin et al. described immature mesenchymal cells with fibroblastic, myofibroblastic, and histiocytic features.[82]

Lundgren et al. describe a form of infantile fibrosarcoma they term rhabdomyofibrosarcoma, which has a desmoplastic fibrosarcomatous microscopic appearance but which, in addition, shows rhabdomyoblastic differentiation by electron microscopy and immunohistochemical study.[239] They described three patients with infantile rhabdomyofibrosarcoma, the youngest of whom was 13 months of age, and five patients with "conventional" congenital fibrosarcomas, the ages of whom ranged from birth to 3 months. According to the authors, this tumor does not behave clinically like the usual infantile fibrosarcoma because it is more rapidly progressive and has a greater tendency to metastasize. They suggest that cases of infantile fibrosarcoma that metastasize could represent this variant. However, their data show that several factors are different than those observed in cases of typical congenital fibrosarcoma, including the age of the patients (greater than 1 year of age), the cytogenetic findings (monosomy for chromosomes 19 and 22), the immunohistochemical findings (reactive myoglobin and desmin), and the ultrastructure (actin filaments and sarcomere-like structures). On the basis of these findings, they propose that this tumor represents a separate entity.[239]

Several reports from various institutions indicate that the incidence of distant metastases in patients with congenital fibrosarcoma is 8% or less overall and appears to be site-dependent (8% for tumors of the extremities as compared to 26% for axial tumors).[39,74,336,345] The tumor spreads to the lungs and lymph nodes, and may metastasize to unusual sites such as the choroid of the eye.[312] No relationship has been established between the histologic findings in newborns with fibrosarcoma, including the grade of malignancy, and either recurrence or metastases.[74,82,185]

Management of congenital fibrosarcoma is of particular concern because of its aggressive behavior and the functional impairment which may result from local treatment. Wide excision is the treatment of choice if it can be done without mutilation. Amputation is the last resort if the tumor has caused a dysfunctional extremity.[17,74,170,247,336] Adjuvant chemotherapy is recommended for those patients with unresectable lesions of the axial and proximal extremities.[3,40,159,220,273,309] Ninane et al. reported three neonates with fibrosarcoma involving the forearm, gluteal region, and chest wall who were treated with preoperative chemotherapy and conservative surgery; all three are alive without evidence of disease.[273] Kynaston et al. described nine additional perinatal cases treated in this manner with similar results.[220] Chemotherapy has been used following limb salvage surgery in the newborn with some success.[309] The prognosis of fibrosarcoma in the infant is much better

than in the older child and adult. The estimated overall survival is greater than 90%, and the rate of recurrence is 32%.[74,82,159,336]

FIBROUS HISTIOCYTOMA

Fibrohistiocytic tumors are composed of histiocytes and fibroblasts and comprise a wide variety of both benign and malignant conditions involving the skin and the soft tissues. Although fibrous histiocytomas have traditionally been considered to be of histiocytic origin, recently, a mesenchymal progenitor cell or immature fibroblast has been implicated.[123,205,388] Most of these tumors are found as subcutaneous nodules or soft tissue masses. Both benign and malignant forms of fibrous histiocytoma occur in newborns and infants, but most are benign.[123,125,128,187,205,370,388] One of the largest series of fibrous histiocytoma reported in children was published by Kauffman and Stout in 1961.[205] Of 39 cases, 5 (12.8%) occurred in infants younger than 3 months of age. The tumors, all of which were benign histologically, were found in various sites, including the scalp, lip, back, abdominal wall, and groin. Four of the 5 patients for whom follow-up information was available were living and well, without evidence of recurrence.[205] Nasopharyngeal fibrous histiocytoma has been responsible for neonatal respiratory distress.[326]

The principal fibrohistiocytic lesions found in the perinatal period are juvenile xanthogranuloma, which is probably an inflammatory or reactive process rather than a neoplastic one, benign fibrous histiocytoma, and the rare malignant fibrous histiocytoma.[125,128,185,187,205,375]

Typically, the benign fibrous histiocytoma is a firm, well-circumscribed, or encapsulated, tan-gray to yellow, 2- to 3-cm nodule (Fig. 4–13). The malignant angiomatoid fibrous histiocytoma, on the other hand, has a much different gross appearance, as it resembles a soft tissue hematoma or a hemorrhagic hemangioma (Figs. 4–14 and 4–15).

The fibrous histiocytoma is a moderately cellular tumor composed of spindle-shaped fibroblastic cells, smaller numbers of round or oval vacuolated histiocytes ("foam cells"), and multinucleated giant cells (see Fig. 4–13). Interdigitating (herringbone) and storiform (cartwheel-like) growth patterns are usually present.[205] It should be kept in mind that these histologic patterns are observed also in the fibromatoses and congenital fibrosarcoma. Early, deep-seated juvenile xanthogranulomas

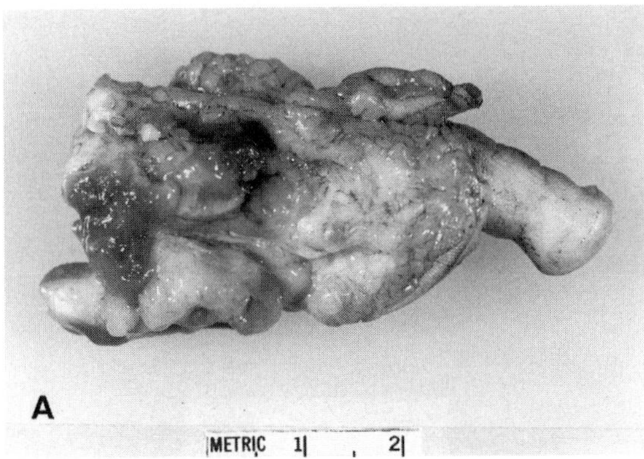
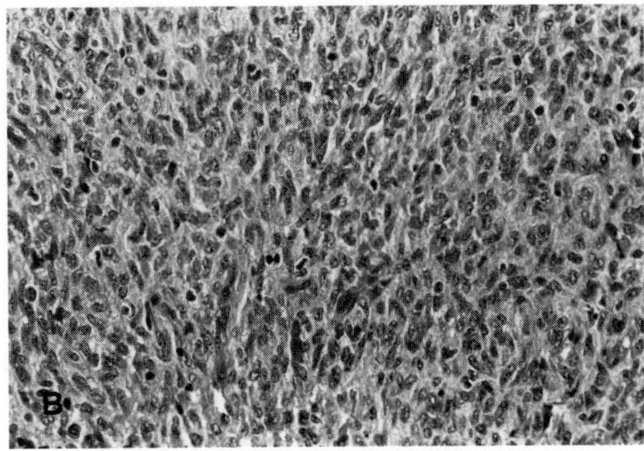

Figure 4–13. Fibrous histiocytoma. A 6-month-old girl underwent an excisional biopsy of a mass on the dorsum of the left foot at 1 month of age. *A,* A recurrent, brownish yellow mass was situated in the interosseous muscles and fat. *B,* The tumor consists of histiocytes and fibroblasts with noticeable mitotic activity and mild to moderate nuclear atypia (hematoxylin-eosin, ×600). (From Isaacs H Jr. Tumors of the Newborn and Infant. St. Louis: Mosby–Year Book, 1991.)

have been mistaken for fibrous histiocytoma. The mitotic rate observed in the benign fibrous histiocytomas usually does not exceed 1 or 2 mitoses per high-power field. Nuclear atypia and anaplasia are absent. The low mitotic rate and lack of anaplasia are important diagnostic findings for distinguishing the benign tumors.

The vimentin immunoperoxidase stain is positive, but the histiocytic markers—namely, alpha$_1$-antitrypsin and alpha$_1$-antichymotryp-

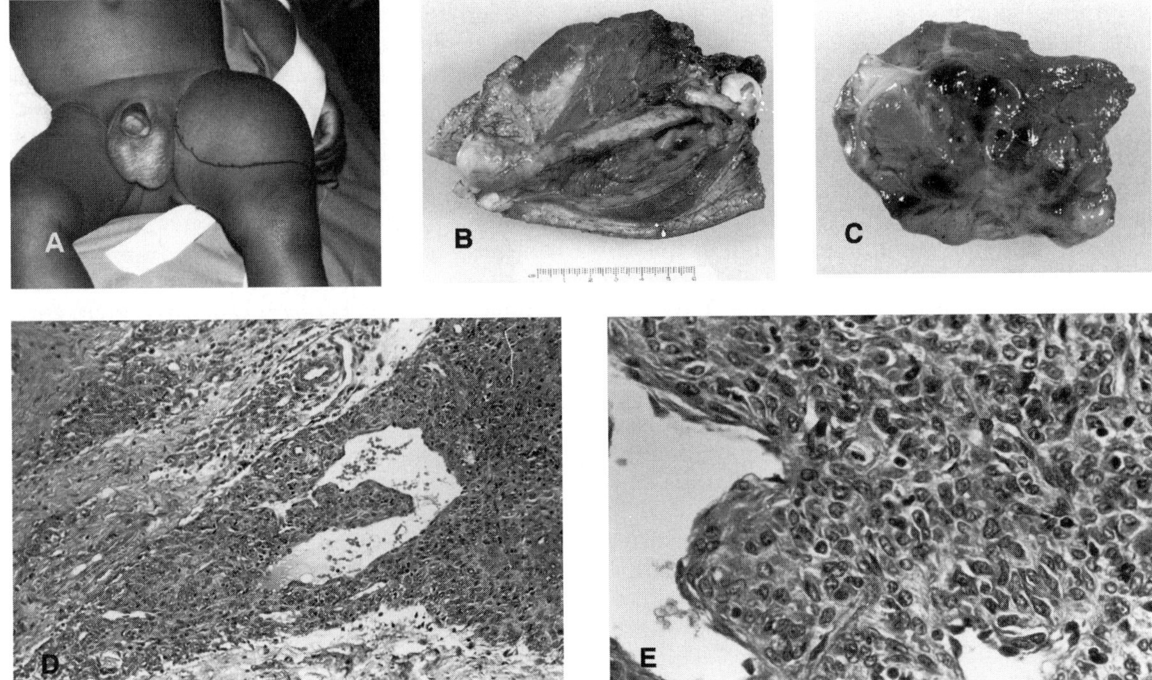

Figure 4–14. Angiomatoid fibrous histiocytoma. *A,* A 3-month-old boy with a left thigh mass that had gradually increased in size since birth. *B,* The amputation specimen demonstrates the tumor (*dark area*) situated beneath the proximal femur in the bed of the vastus medialis muscle. The head of the femur is situated on the right side of the photograph, and the femoral condyles are on the left. *C,* A close-up view of the involved muscle; the tumor is composed of several dark, cyst-like cavities. *D,* Vascular-like channels are bordered by atypical histiocytes and fibroblastic cells (trichrome, ×240). *E,* Tumor cells, rather than endothelial cells, line the channels (trichrome, ×750). (From Isaacs H Jr. Tumors of the Newborn and Infant. St. Louis: Mosby–Year Book, 1991.)

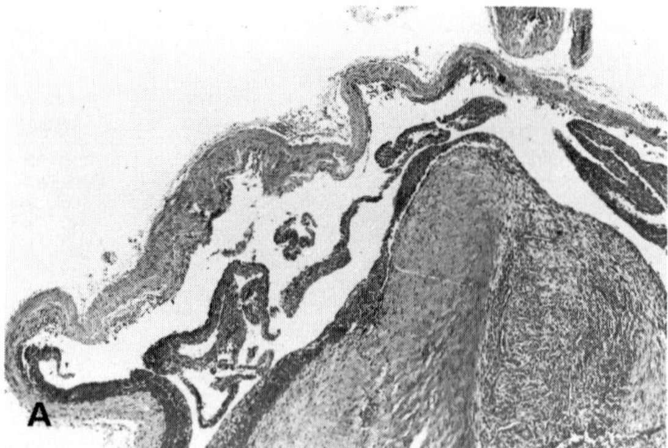 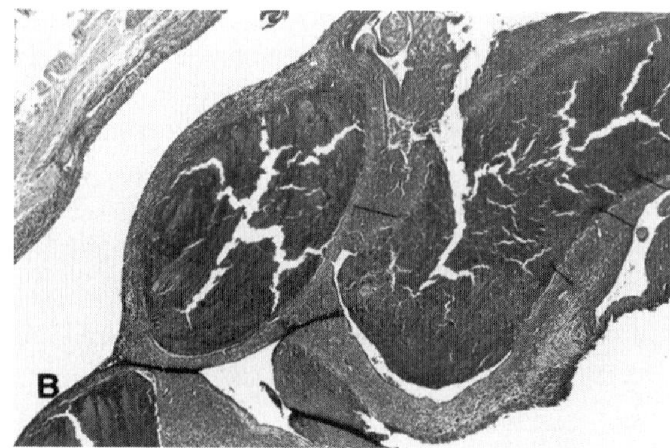

Figure 4–15. Angiomatoid fibrous histiocytoma from the neck of a 3-month-old boy. *A,* The partially cystic tumor mass is surrounded by a dense, fibrous pseudocapsule (trichrome, ×30). *B,* The prominent vascular component is evident (trichrome, ×30).

sin—are variable in their degree of staining, and may be only weakly reactive.[187] Sometimes, the ultrastructural findings are more helpful than immunohistochemical methods in establishing the diagnosis of fibrous histiocytoma. Electron microscopy reveals spindle-shaped fibroblasts, macrophage-histiocytes, and fibrohistiocytic cells that are intermediate between the two.[301,375,388] The fibroblasts are spindle-shaped, composed of a moderate amount of cytoplasm, and surrounded by a cell membrane that lacks a basement lamina. The oval nuclei contain a prominent nucleolus. Variable amounts of rough endoplasmic reticulum, free ribosomes, and mitochondria are present. The histiocytes are larger and rounder than fibroblasts and have round, notched, or reniform nuclei with coarse chromatin clumping adjacent to the nuclear membrane. The cytoplasm contains Golgi apparatus, numerous vacuoles, lysosomal dense bodies, few profiles of rough endoplasmic reticulum, and multiple, pseudopod-like extensions that impart a ruffled appearance to the cell membrane. Both the fibrous and histiocytic components are less mature than their adult counterparts, showing less phagocytosis and production of typical collagen fibers.[375]

Wigger and Mitsudo described the unusual occurrence of a fibrous histiocytoma of the soft tissues, cranial, pelvic, and long bones in a 2-day-old female infant with symptoms of respiratory distress and upper hemiparesis.[375] The clinical and radiologic findings were interpreted as consistent with congenital fibromatosis (myofibromatosis), but light and electron microscopic findings revealed a malignant tumor composed of both histiocytes and fibroblasts.

The malignant angiomatoid fibrous histiocytoma has a distinctive gross and light microscopic appearance (see Figs. 4–14 and 4–15). On gross examination, the lesion may resemble a hemorrhagic cavernous hemangioma. Microscopic examination reveals central, cystically dilated, vascular-like spaces lined by atypical-appearing fibroblasts and histiocytes with pleomorphic and hyperchromatic nuclei displaying moderate numbers of mitoses (Fig. 4–14D and E). Anastomosing vascular channels, lined by endothelial-like cells, resemble angiosarcoma. About the periphery, lymphoid follicles surround the central hemorrhagic zone, giving the tumor the appearance of a lymph node with a hemorrhagic center under low-power magnification.[15,125] Because of these vascular and inflammatory changes and the extensive hemorrhage, the tumor is sometimes misdiagnosed (see Fig. 4–15). Ultrastructural studies by Argenyi et al. reveal three main types of cells: fibroblasts, myofibroblasts, and histiocytes.[15] In addition, intermediate cells with features of both fibroblasts and histiocytes are often found.

One of the largest series of angiomatoid fibrous histiocytoma, published by Costa and Weiss, consisted of 108 patients with tumors, the youngest of whom was 2 months old.[88] Given the frequency of recurrence and metastases, which was 12% and 5%, respectively, the authors concluded that angiomatoid malignant fibrous histiocytoma is a tumor of intermediate malignancy.[88] Two congenital tumors that were successfully surgically resected have been described, one involving the upper arm of an 8-month-old girl[15] and another consisting of a thigh mass in a 3-month-old male infant.[187]

Plexiform fibrohistiocytic tumor is an uncommon, potentially malignant, fibrohistiocytic tumor that occurs in both children and young adults and has a female predominance.[129] Of 65 cases described by Enzinger and Zhang, 23 were diagnosed in children younger than 9 years of age, the youngest of whom was 2 months old.[129] The subcutaneous tissues of the upper extremity and shoulder region are the most common sites of origin. The tumor is a multinodular or plexiform lesion composed of histiocytes, fibroblasts, and distinctive, multinucleated, giant cells. Under low-power magnification, the lesion resembles fibrous hamartoma of infancy or plexiform neurofibroma. In one third of the patients, the tumor recurred, and in 2, the tumor metastasized to regional lymph nodes.[129]

One of the main difficulties in establishing the diagnosis of fibrous histiocytoma is determining whether the tumor in question is benign or malignant.[205] The criteria used to determine malignancy are the location of the tumor (deep-seated versus superficial), the mitotic rate (greater than 3 mitotic figures per high-power field), and the degree of nuclear atypia (significant nuclear pleomorphism and bizarre giant cells).[128,388] Most fibrous histiocytomas of infants are benign, but will recur if not completely removed. Childhood malignant fibrous histiocytoma of soft tissue appears to be similar to rhabdomyosarcoma in terms of the manner in which its spreads and its response to therapy.[299] The youngest of seven patients in a Children's Hospital of Philadelphia study was a 6-month-old male infant with a primary tumor of the chest wall who survived following surgery and chemotherapy.[299]

JUVENILE XANTHOGRANULOMA

Juvenile xanthogranuloma is a fibrohistiocytic proliferation that occurs most often in newborns and infants and is characterized by one or more cutaneous nodules or, less frequently, by lesions in the deep soft tissues or organs.[104,128,191,217,232,331] About 20% of such lesions are present at birth.[191] Cutaneous xanthogranulomas occur as red to yellow-brown papules distributed on the head, neck, and extremities; these usually regress within 2 years of diagnosis.[104,128,232,331] Less than 5% of these lesions are found in other sites, such as the eye, heart, lung, retroperitoneum, and deep soft tissues, and they may or may not be associated with cutaneous lesions.[101,104,128,191,217,232,331,385]

Deep-seated, extracutaneous xanthogranulomas can occur in the newborn (Figs. 4–16 and 5–12).[101,373,385] For example, de Graaf et al. describe a 3-month-old female infant with an abdominal mass, a history of weight loss, and hypercalcemia.[101] The xanthogranuloma involved the omentum, peritoneum, intestinal wall, and hilus of the liver. A diagnostic omentectomy was performed, after which the remaining tumors disappeared within 1 year. A 1-month-old female infant had multiple lesions involving the neck, trunk, limbs, and retroperitoneum.[385] White and Garen described two paravertebral tumors in the midthoracic region of the back that involved the subcutaneous tissues and skeletal muscle and were attached to several vertebral spinous processes.[373]

Xanthogranulomas consist of firm nodules averaging 2 cm to 5 cm in size that vary in color from tan-gray to tan-yellow on cross section.[104,191,373] Soft tissue xanthogranulomas have the same histologic appearance as cutaneous lesions (see Chapter 5, "Tumors and Tumor-Like Conditions of the Skin") (see Fig. 5–12). Moreover, the morphologic and immunohistochemical features of juvenile (patients younger than 2 years of age) and adult xanthogranulomas, as well as of solitary and multiple xanthogranulomas, are essentially the same.[385] Sheets of well-differentiated histiocytes with eosinophilic or foamy cytoplasms and vesicular nuclei are noted. Variable numbers of multinucleated Touton giant cells, which are helpful in establishing the diagnosis, are present, in addition to small numbers of eosinophils, lymphocytes, and plasma cells (Figs. 4–16 and 5–12). Oil red-O–positive lipid droplets are noted in the histiocyte cytoplasm.[191] Touton giant cells may be difficult to find in some instances, particularly in early juvenile xanthogranulomas with monotonous histiocytic infiltrates (Fig. 4–16). In older lesions, prominent foam cells, foci of fibrosis, and the storiform growth pattern of fibrous histiocytoma and the fibromatoses may be present.[128,385]

Immunoperoxidase studies performed on xanthogranuloma cells show variable results. Judging from light microscopy studies, one would anticipate that the histiocytic markers lysozyme, alpha$_1$-antitrypsin, and alpha$_1$-antichymotrypsin would be unequivocally positive; instead, they are either nonreactive or focally or faintly positive.[191] However, the macrophage or monocyte antigens CD68 (KP-1) and HAM56 stain positively, as does the mesenchymal cell marker vimentin.[101,191,385] The cortical thymo-

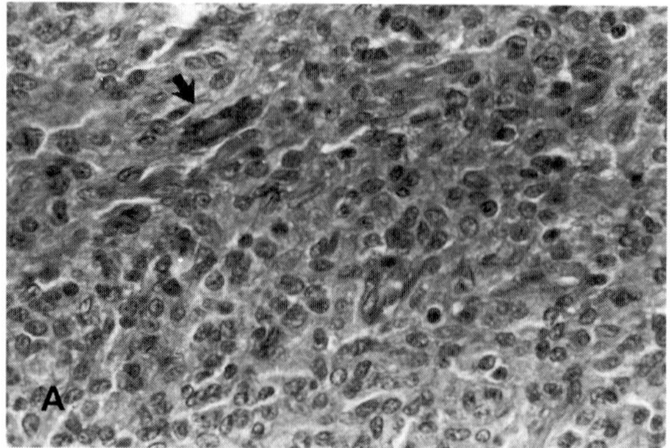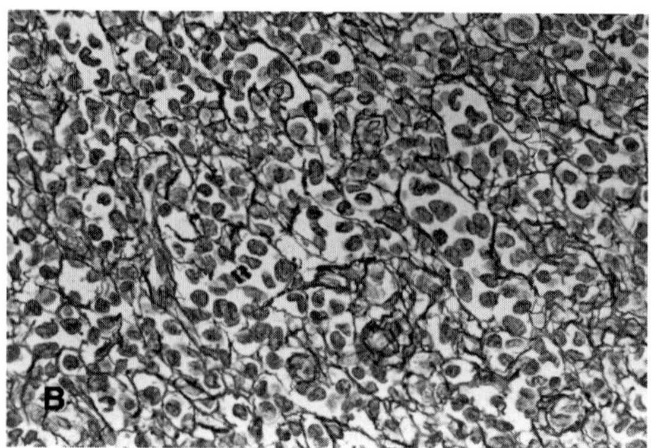

Figure 4–16. Congenital juvenile xanthogranuloma. _A,_ The tumor consists of histiocytes with vacuolated and amphophy-lic-staining cytoplasms. A Touton giant cell is present (_arrow_). Early, deep-seated lesions are hypercellular and have few or no Touton giant cells, which sometimes makes the distinction from fibrous histiocytoma difficult. Langerhans histiocytes have characteristic infolded nuclei, react with S-100 protein, and contain Birbeck granules on electron microscopy (see Fig. 8–1) (periodic acid–Schiff, ×400). _B,_ Histiocytes are surrounded by a prominent reticulin network (reticulin, ×400).

cyte antigen CD1a is positive as well, suggesting a dermal "indeterminate" or possibly dermal dendritic cell lineage for the xanthogranuloma cell, which migrates from the skin to other sites.[101] The negative reactivity to S-100 protein and peanut agglutinin distinguishes the xanthogranuloma cell from the Langerhans cell, an important factor to remember in considering the differential diagnosis.

The histiocytic nature of the xanthogranuloma cells is confirmed also by electron microscopy. The tumor histiocytes are composed of pseudopodia, lysosomes, and lipid droplets.[101,128,148,191] However, the racquet-shaped Birbeck granules that are diagnostic of Langerhans cells are characteristically absent.[101,148,191]

Chromosomal studies of xanthogranulomas show normal 46,XX or 46,XY karyotypes, and DNA flow cytometry reveals diploid stem lines.[101] The prognosis is excellent for xanthogranulomas in both cutaneous and extracutaneous sites.[101,128,191]

Immunohistochemical studies suggest that the xanthogranuloma histiocyte may be related to the dermal dendritic cell.[101] de Graaf et al. have proposed that juvenile xanthogranuloma represents a defect in processing antigens in the cutaneous histiocytes that migrate from the skin to other sites.[101] Possibly, this situation is analogous to that of the Langerhans cell histiocyte and disseminated Langerhans cell histiocytosis.

Patients with juvenile xanthogranuloma are expected to have an excellent outcome follow-ing surgical excision. The tumors usually do not recur. Spontaneous regression has been described in infants, even in those with unresect-able, deep-seated visceral lesions.[101]

VASCULAR TUMORS AND TUMOR-LIKE CONDITIONS

Most vascular lesions occurring in the fetus and newborn are hamartomas and vascular anomalies—namely, hemangioma, lymphangioma, and arteriovenous malformation—rather than neoplasms. Vascular lesions constitute more than two thirds of all soft tissue tumors and tumor-like conditions in the perinatal period.[81,184,185,187] Of these, hemangioma, lymphangioma, and hemangiopericytoma occur most frequently, in that order.[185,187] Hemangioma is the cause of a soft tissue mass more often than any other neoplastic-like condition or tumor, and the head and neck are the most frequent sites. Clinically, this entire group of tumors is characterized by a favorable outcome, provided vital structures are not involved. The vascular malignant conditions of angiosarcoma and Kaposi's sarcoma are extremely rare in the perinatal period.[81,161,187]

Hemangioma

Hemangioma is the most common soft tissue mass found in the newborn.[102,128,184,292] It occurs in nearly 2% of neonates and 10% of infants, and roughly 10% are multiple.[189,314] During a 28-year period at Children's Hospital, Los Angeles, there were 102 soft tissue tumors diagnosed; at the same time, 133 hemangiomas were recorded.[187] Hemangiomas may be single or multiple and are extremely variable in extent. After birth, they may remain their original size, grow with the body, or exhibit a more rapid growth. Cutaneous hemangiomas may not be noticed until the child is a few weeks old. Most of these masses regress after a limited period of growth and disappear by the end of the second year. Although at times they are very cellular (particularly, the solid capillary hemangioma) and show little elaboration into recognizable vascular structures, those present at birth rarely, if at all, prove to be malignant. The skin is the most common site of hemangiomas, although they may be found in the mucous membranes, deep connective tissue, or internal organs, such as the liver, heart, and brain.[292] Of 108 consecutive hemangiomas diagnosed in infants at Children's Hospital, Los Angeles, from 1958 to 1983, the most frequent sites were the skin of the neck (21 cases), the face (18 cases), scalp (12 cases), skin of the extremities (10 cases), back (8 cases), chest (7 cases), and shoulder (6 cases).[187]

Clinical complications arising from hemangiomas are the result of their size, location, and physiology. They may impair vision by encroaching upon the eye, produce respiratory distress by tracheal compression, cause high-output congestive cardiac failure associated with nonimmune hydrops fetalis and polyhydramnios, produce central nervous system or gastrointestinal hemorrhage, or cause a consumptive coagulopathy from platelet and fibrinogen trapping within the lesion, as in the Kasabach-Merritt syndrome.[13,94,115,154,163,201,208]

Simultaneous occurrence of thrombocytopenia with giant hemangiomas in the newborn is responsible for a syndrome characterized by hemorrhagic tendency and bleeding into the hemangioma.[154] Hemorrhagic manifestations are often severe and sometimes prove fatal. Purpuric lesions may be extensive; some, for example, may involve an entire extremity. This syndrome was first described by Kasabach and Merritt in 1940.[201] Since then, several other examples have been reported.[94,225] Good and associates reviewed 10 infants and children with this syndrome, including 3 cases of their own.[154] One third were younger than 3 months of age at the time of diagnosis.[154] Six additional infants and children, including two newborns, were

reported by Larsen et al.[225] In three patients, the hemangiomas remained small for many months and then suddenly enlarged, and hemorrhagic diathesis appeared. Consumptive coagulopathy of antenatal onset, associated with multiple capillary hemangiomata, has been documented by Pierce et al.[289] The affected patient, a postmature male infant, was delivered by cesarean section performed for bradycardia. No spontaneous respirations occurred after birth. At necropsy, the lungs showed diffuse hemorrhage. Hemangiomata with fibrin thrombi were found in the lungs, heart, soft tissues, and several other organs.

Large facial hemangiomas occur in association with the Dandy-Walker syndrome (cystic dilatation of the fourth ventricle and absence of the cerebellar vermis) and other posterior fossa developmental anomalies.[303] Most of these patients have hydrocephalus, and one third have unusual ophthalmologic findings, such as palpebral occlusion, microphthalmos, and optic nerve hypoplasia.[303]

Diffuse neonatal hemangiomatosis is an uncommon disease of the perinatal period that is characterized by multiple hemangiomata of the skin and viscera involving at least three organ systems.[58,145,176,342,343] Several cases have been reported (see Fig. 12–3).[55,56,58,145,176,342,343] The risk of visceral involvement increases with the number of cutaneous hemangiomas.[342] Although the hemangiomas are benign histologically, most infants and newborns with this disease die during the first few months of life. Death occurs as the result of high-output cardiac failure secondary to arteriovenous shunting through the hemangioma, massive hemorrhage from fragile vessels complicated by thrombocytopenia, or involvement of the central nervous system.[58,176] The organs most often affected by the hemangiomata, excluding the skin (100%), are the liver (64%), brain (52%), gastrointestinal tract (52%), lungs (52%), oral cavity (44%), and eyes (32%).[145,342] The hemangiomata vary in size from 0.2 to 2 cm and range in number from 50 to 500.[145,342] The female:male ratio is 2:1. Thus far, no genetic factor has been implicated.[145,342] Benign neonatal hemangiomatosis, on the other hand, is a condition characterized by multiple small hemangiomas involving primarily the skin; it is characterized by a good prognosis.[314,342] Rothe and colleagues outlined the clinical characteristics and management of 10 patients with this disease, including 1 of their own.[314]

Holden and Alexander describe two newborns with diffuse neonatal hemangiomatosis: one with thrombocytopenia and hemorrhaging at birth and the other with progressive neurologic signs and hydrocephalus.[176] They reviewed six additional cases from the literature. Byard et al. reported five fatal cases diagnosed before 10 weeks of age.[58] All of these patients had skin and liver lesions. Other organs involved with hemangiomas included the adrenal, skeletal muscle, leptomeninges, choroid plexus, lungs, spleen, pancreas, bone, bowel, trachea, thymus, and pituitary.[58] Stillman et al. described a neonate with extensive hemangiomatous involvement of the small bowel and mesentery, as well as facial, ocular, and palatal hemangiomas.[343] The baby experienced recurrent and severe gastrointestinal blood loss; melena and anemia were the presenting clinical findings. The presence of hepatomegaly, cardiac failure, unexplained anemia, or thrombocytopenia in a newborn with cutaneous hemangiomas should suggest the diagnosis of diffuse hemangiomatosis.[58,342]

Facial cutaneous hemangiomas are sometimes associated with similar lesions in the eye and central nervous system.[176,292] Hemangiomas in the region of the distribution of the trigeminal nerve may occur with vascular anomalies of the choroid of the eye, the pia, and the brain adjacent to the involved skin. Known as the Sturge-Kalischer-Weber syndrome, this disease is accompanied by other findings, such as congenital glaucoma and buphthalmos, local thickening of the skull, atrophy of the body on the side opposite the cutaneous hemangioma, paralysis, aphasia, epilepsy, and mental retardation. As early as the latter part of the first year of life, slowing of the circulation may cause calcification near the cerebral surface; imaging studies reveal characteristic double-contoured opacities from calcific deposits about small blood vessels in two adjacent gyri (and not from calcification of individual vessels) (see Fig. 9–13).[292]

The hemangiomas of von Hippel-Lindau disease (cerebellar-retinal hemangiomatosis) may be present in early life, but symptoms are rarely recognizable until the second decade.[292] The vascular lesions may be single or multiple, cavernous, or composed of masses of solid capillary hemangiomata. They may involve the skin, cerebellum, retina, spinal cord, and liver. Adenomas or cystic disease of the pancreas, liver, and kidney may be present also. The disease is familial in approximately 20% of cases.

Patients with the Maffucci syndrome have enchondromas at birth. Capillary, cavernous, or solid hemangiomas in the skin and subcutaneous tissue develop before puberty.[292]

Hemangiomas are classified into several histologic types on the basis of the caliber and type of vessels comprising the lesion.[128,224,292] Generally, they are divided into three main types: capillary, cavernous, and arteriovenous (Figs. 4–17 to 4–19). The last entity is most likely a vascular malformation, whereas the first two are probably hamartomas—that is, local overgrowths of blood vessels normally present in the involved area.[187]

Clinically, the capillary hemangioma produces a pink to purple, noncompressible area on the skin surface, but forms no tumor mass. An example is the nevus flammeus or port-wine stain (nevus venosus). Other manifestations are bluish elevated nodules of various sizes within the skin and subcutaneous tissue.[292]

On microscopic examination, the capillary hemangioma has a multilobular configuration consisting of lobules of anastomosing capillaries lined by endothelium supplied by prominent "feeding" vessels. The cells and constituent vessels are closely distributed among normal muscle, subcutaneous tissue, or parenchymal elements of the part involved. Occasionally, the lesions are solid and very cellular, with increased mitotic activity that gives the hemangioma a worrisome appearance (see Fig. 4–17). The ominous, confusing, and nebulous name sometimes applied to this form of capillary hemangioma is "hemangioendothelioma." Rarely, it may be necessary to resort to an elastic stain, immunocytochemical analysis, or electron microscopy to prove its vascular origin.[187] Tumor cells react negatively to antidesmin antibody and positively to vimentin and actin.[152] According to Gonzalez-Crussi and Reyes-Mugica, five cell types are consistently found by electron microscopy: endothelial cells, pericytes, fibroblasts, mast cells, and so-called interstitial cells.[152]

Cavernous Hemangioma

The cavernous hemangioma is less common than the capillary type. Frequently, it involves the head and neck area, but occasionally it affects the brain and viscera. These hemangiomas have larger vascular spaces than the capillary hemangiomas and are compressible because of the large amounts of blood they con-

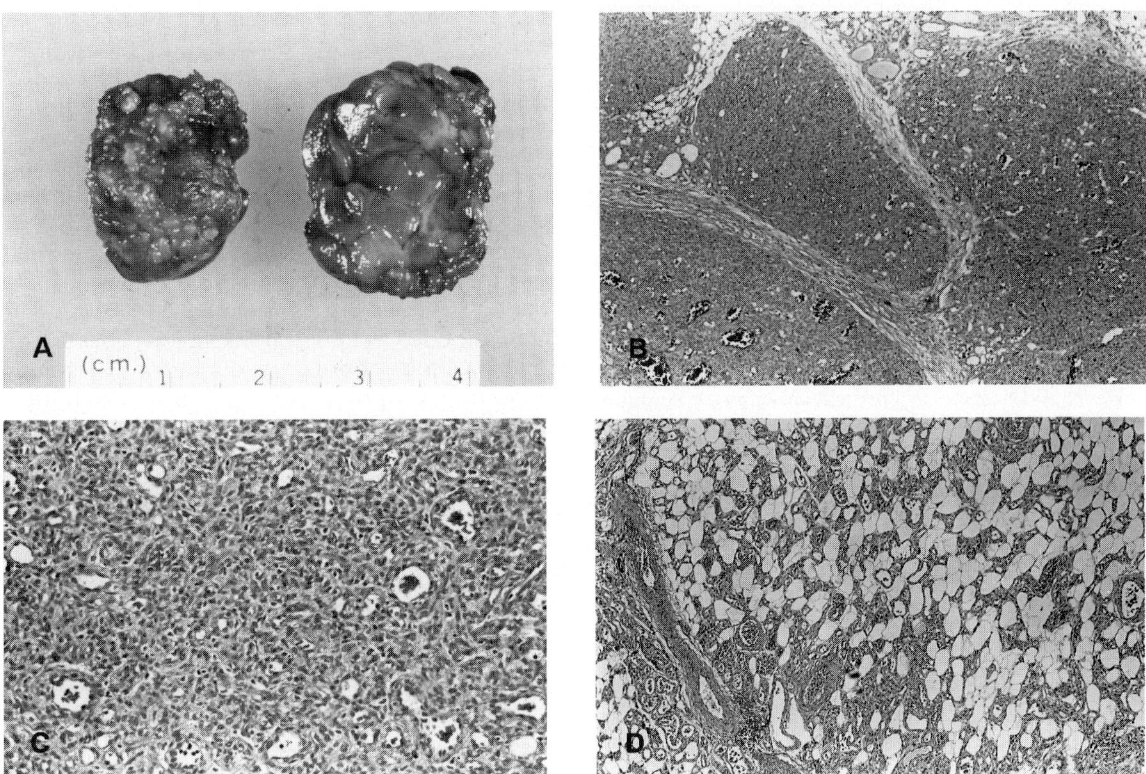

Figure 4–17. Capillary hemangioma. *A,* A nodule measuring 2.5 × 1.5 cm was removed from the neck of a 3-month-old boy. The lesion was brownish-red and nodular, resembling a mat of lymph nodes. *B,* A low-power view displays the lobular architecture just described (hematoxylin-eosin, ×32). *C,* The "open and closed hemangioma pattern" consists mostly of dense clusters of endothelial cells with a few capillary lumina (hematoxylin-eosin, ×150). *D,* An involuting capillary hemangioma taken from a 6-month-old girl shows abundant fat in the lobule separating residual nests of hemangioma. Large "feeding" vessels situated along the left side of the picture are frequently noted in the periphery of the lobules of most capillary hemangiomas (hematoxylin-eosin, ×32). (From Isaacs H Jr. Tumors of the Newborn and Infant. St. Louis: Mosby–Year Book, 1991.)

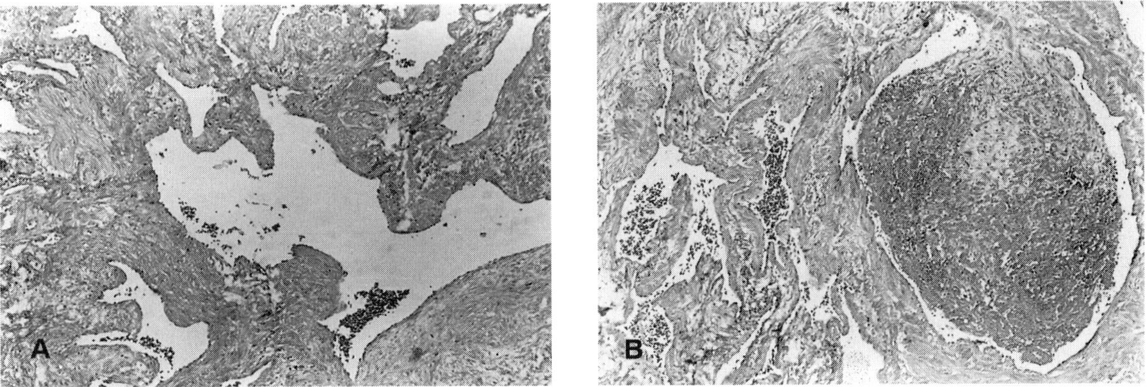

Figure 4–18. Cavernous hemangioma. A red-brown, nodular mass measuring 6 × 4 cm and consisting of many dilated blood vessels was removed from the forearm of a male infant. *A,* Large, irregular, vascular channels are lined by endothelium containing erythrocytes (hematoxylin-eosin, ×40). *B,* An organizing thrombus is also present (hematoxylin-eosin, ×40). (From Isaacs H Jr. Tumors of the Newborn and Infant. St. Louis: Mosby–Year Book, 1991.)

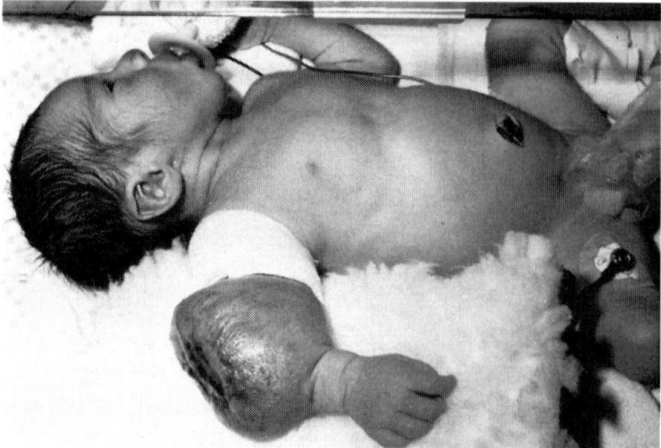

Figure 4–19. Arteriovenous malformation. A newborn had a large arteriovenous malformation of the right forearm which functioned as an arteriovenous fistula, producing a high-output congestive heart failure shortly after birth. Ligation of the artery leading into the malformation was required to control the life-threatening effect of the fistula. (From Isaacs H Jr. Tumors of the Newborn and Infant. St. Louis: Mosby–Year Book, 1991.)

tain. Those involving the skin are raised above the general skin level and often have a reddish-purple, warty, granular surface. The raised vascular nevi, such as strawberry nevi (see Fig. 5–1), contain mixtures of cavernous and capillary nets. The vascular channels vary greatly in size and extent and, on rare occasions, may involve extensive portions of the body.[292]

The liver is the internal organ that is most often the site of a cavernous hemangioma. The extent of involvement may vary from an area measuring a few millimeters to one of several centimeters. When extensive, a consumptive coagulopathy with secondary thrombocytopenia may result (Kasabach-Merritt syndrome) (see Chapter 12, "Liver Tumors"). If superficial, trauma may cause rupture of some of the outermost channels, and fatal intra-abdominal hemorrhage may result (e.g., during delivery). If it is deep in the liver, the tumor may remain silent and remain undiscovered. The larynx and intestines are other locations for cavernous hemangioma. When the larynx is affected, there may be a life-threatening problem with the airway (see Fig. 5–1). There is one case report of cavernous hemangioma of the lung.[137]

Microscopic examination reveals the cavernous hemangioma to consist of anastomosing, thin-walled, vascular channels lined by endothelial cells larger than those in the capillary hemangioma (see Fig. 4–18). Vascular thrombi are common in these lesions.

Arteriovenous Malformation

The arteriovenous malformation (arteriovenous hemangioma, arteriovenous angioma) are developmental anomalies, rather than true tumors.[292] Some are congenital, some massive in size, causing focal gigantism of the affected part; occasionally, they are life-threatening in the neonatal period (see Fig. 4–19). The malformations are composed of thin- and thick-walled vascular channels filled and distended with blood. Certain lesions behave like large arteriovenous shunts, producing a potentially fatal high-output cardiac failure, which may already be present at birth (see Fig. 4–19). Extensive lesions involving the brain, most often the cerebral hemispheres, are usually fatal in the newborn.[185,292,319] Two congenital arteriovenous angiomas involving the cerebral arteries and the venous sinuses of the brain were associated with cardiac failure.[292] Drut et al. reported a stillborn male infant of 31 weeks' gestation with hydrops fetalis, polyhydramnios, and microcephaly who was found to have an arteriovenous angioma of the tentorium and venous sinus confluens at necropsy.[117]

Microscopic examination reveals thick- and thin-walled vessels that are adjacent to one another. Frequently, it is impossible to determine whether the affected vessels are arteries or veins. In some instances, tying off or embolization of the feeding vessels, or even amputation, are required to control the effects of the malformation.

Venous Angioma

Venous angiomas consist of large, endothelium-lined channels that may have smooth muscle in their walls. They may involve a large body area, such as an extremity. They are considered to be malformations, rather than neoplasms.[292]

Malignant vascular tumors, although rare in infancy, do occur in the liver, skin, and soft tissues. Here, the cells have large and variable nuclei and less cytoplasm. Some cellular capillary hemangiomas of the liver and soft tissues have been mistakenly classified as malignant. Kaposi's sarcoma, a malignant lesion involving the skin and soft tissues that is composed of both capillary and spindle-cell connective tissue elements, is unusual in the newborn. However, in this era of acquired immunodeficiency syndrome (AIDS), the number of pediatric cases

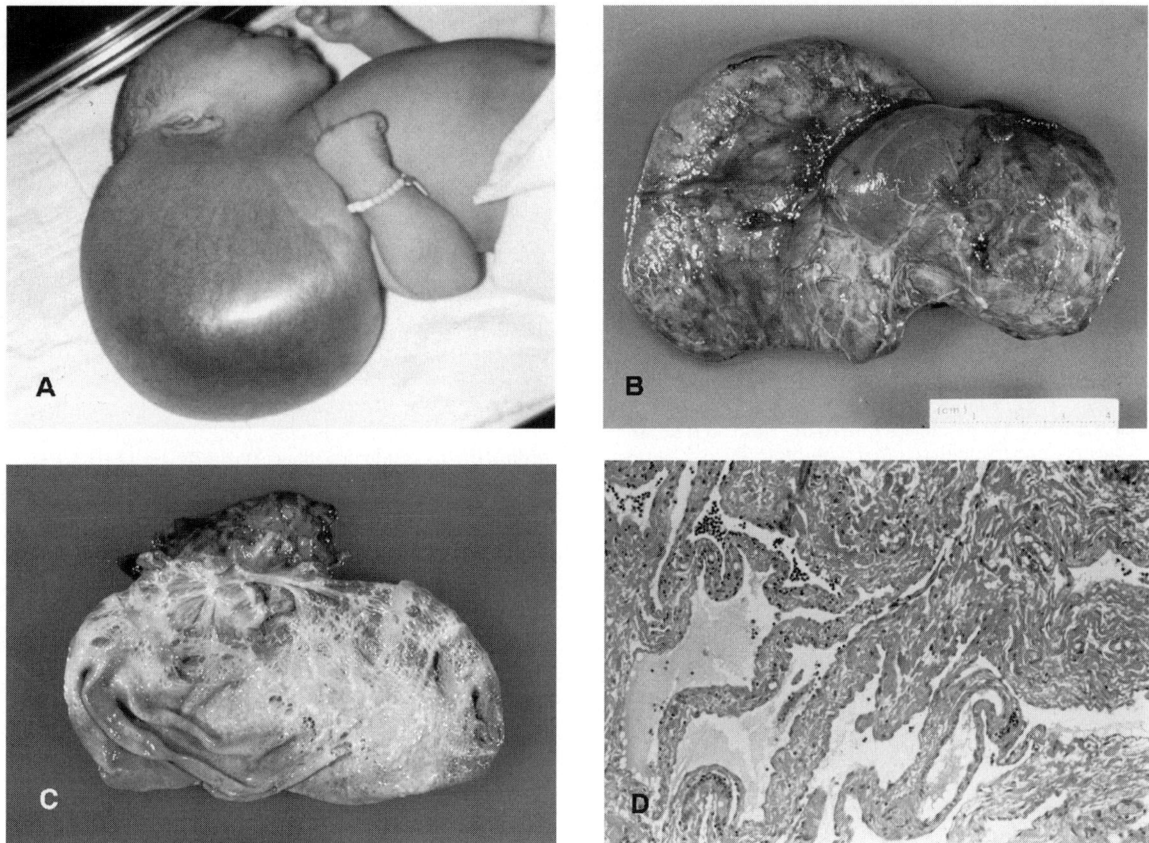

Figure 4–20. Cystic lymphangioma (hygroma) of the neck. *A,* A newborn with a large cystic lesion arising from the back of the neck and shoulder. *B,* An unopened specimen taken from another infant with an identical, but smaller, hygroma measuring 10 × 7 cm. *C,* The opened specimen shows one large cyst with a smaller, solid, microcystic component (top of the photograph). The cyst was filled with clear lymph fluid. *D,* Several large vascular channels are lined by a single row of endothelial cells and are filled with lymph (hematoxylin-eosin, ×240). (From Isaacs H Jr. Tumors of the Newborn and Infant. St. Louis: Mosby–Year Book, 1991.)

is steadily increasing. One such example is a 6-day-old male infant with placentally transmitted human immunodeficiency virus (HIV) and Kaposi's sarcoma.[161]

Lymphangioma

Lymphangioma is a benign vascular malformation composed of cystically dilated lymphatics. Many cystic lymphangiomas (hygromas) and diffuse lymphangiomas are present at birth (Figs. 4–20, 4–21, and 4–23).[187,292] They are second to hemangioma as a cause of a soft tissue mass in the newborn.[184] The incidence of cystic hygroma is estimated to be 1 in 6000 pregnancies.[70,384] The lesions range in size from small, barely visible subepidermal skin blebs (lymphangioma circumscriptum) to massively di-

lated cystic masses (hygroma), and they can occur in almost any location, including the viscera and bones. However, the soft tissues of the neck, axilla, thorax and lower extremities are the major sites (Figs. 4–20 to 4–23). Of 97 consecutive lymphangiomas diagnosed in infants at Children's Hospital, Los Angeles, 45 occurred in the neck, 22 in the chest wall, 12 in the extremities, and 4 in the abdominal wall. In this study, the less common locations were the omentum (n = 3), mesentery (n = 2), larynx (n = 2), tongue (n = 2), and one each in the bowel, retroperitoneum, mediastinum, conjunctiva, and mouth.[187]

Embryology

The lymphatic system begins to develop at the end of the fifth week, approximately 2

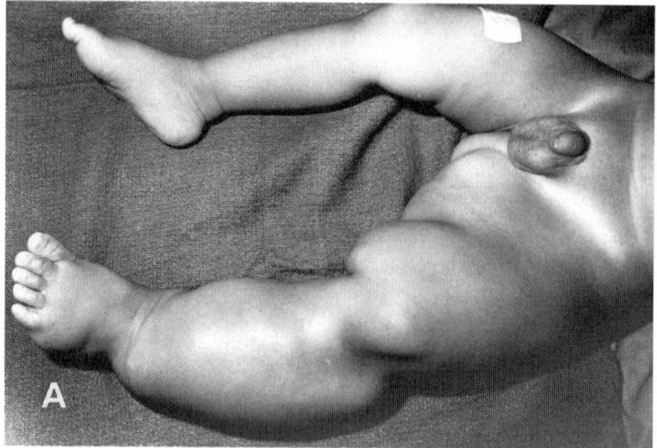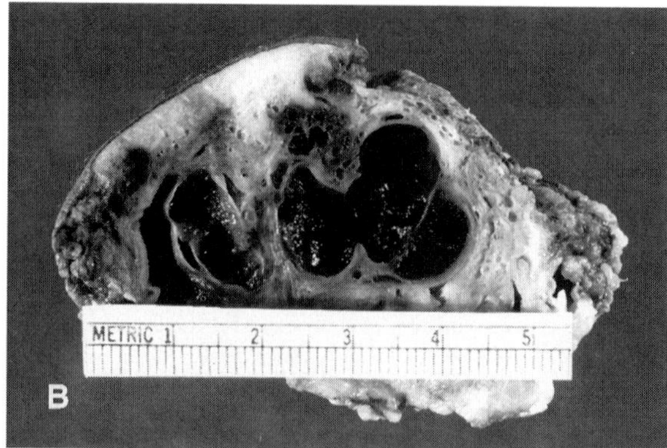

Figure 4–21. Lymphangioma producing focal gigantism of an extremity. *A,* A 1-year-old boy was born with a left lower extremity that was much larger than the right. *B,* The subcutaneous tissue has been replaced by cystically dilated lymphatics of various sizes. Some are filled with blood, which is probably attributable to surgical artifact. (From Isaacs H Jr. Tumors of the Newborn and Infant. St. Louis: Mosby–Year Book, 1991.)

weeks later than the cardiovascular system.[263] Lymphatic vessels sprout from the six primary lymph sacs situated in the neck, iliac, and retroperitoneal regions, and grow along the major veins and supply various parts of the body. Goetsch concluded from her studies that lymphangiomas are developmental defects secondary to a sequestration of lymphatic tissue in early embryonic life.[142] Those in the cervical region are thought to be derived from primitive jugular lymph sacs that fail to join the lymphatic system in a normal way. Dilatation of the jugular lymph sac leads to the formation of cystic hygroma. Peripheral extension occurs as a result of the development of fibrillar sprouts from the margins of existing cystic spaces. These spaces secrete lymph-like fluid that causes local distention and formation of additional, gradually enlarging cysts. As the walls of older cysts become thick and fibrotic, the lesions are composed of endothelium-lined spaces separated by connective tissue. Variable numbers of lymphocytes are present.[70,292]

Lymphangiomas are discovered in utero by ultrasonography. Fetal cystic hygromas are associated with Turner's syndrome, hydrops fetalis, and a high mortality rate.[52,59,64,70,71,202,219,268,290,302,311,371,384]

The use of the terms cystic lymphangioma and cavernous lymphangioma varies, with little reason to distinguish between the two conditions, as they both result from failure of communication and obstructive dilatation of lymphatics. Traditionally, lymphangiomas have

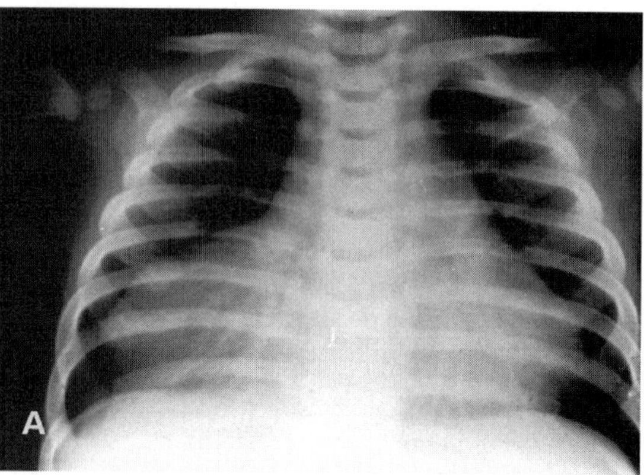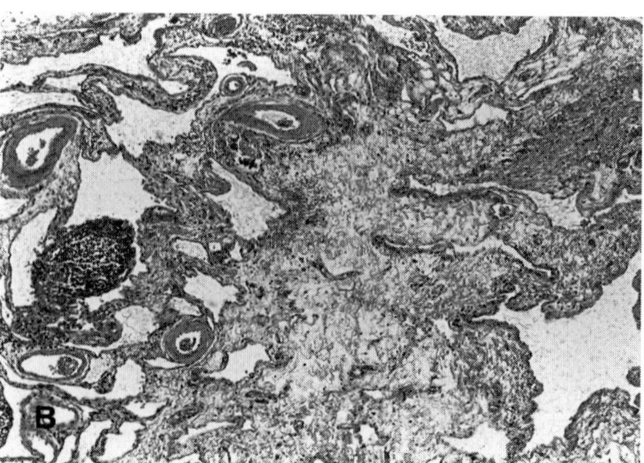

Figure 4–22. Lymphangioma of the mediastinum. *A,* A chest x-ray film of a 5-month-old boy with a history of increasing respiratory distress demonstrated a large mediastinal mass with radiating vessels. *B,* A biopsy reveals numerous, cystically dilated lymphatics and a few blood vessels. Lymphoid nodules characteristically are noted in lymphangiomas (hematoxylin-eosin, ×120). (From Isaacs H Jr. Tumors of the Newborn and Infant. St. Louis: Mosby–Year Book, 1991.)

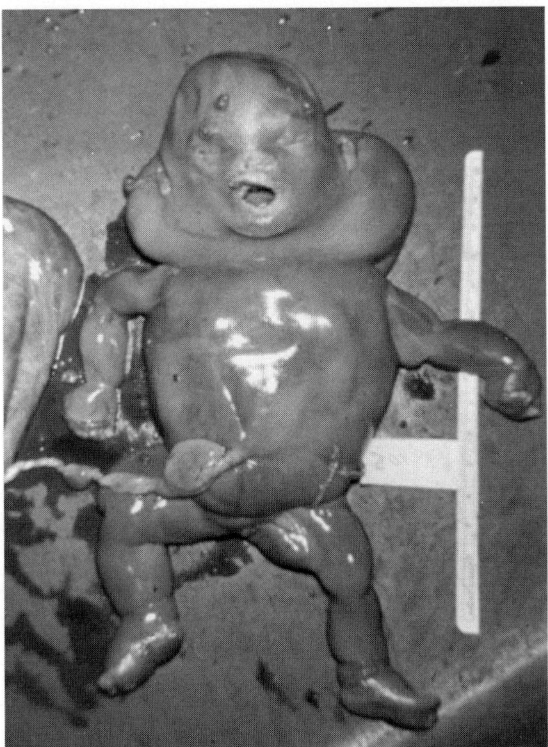

Figure 4–23. Bilateral cervical cystic lymphangiomas (hygromas) occurring in a macerated, stillborn, female fetus (weight, 390 g; length, 21 cm crown-heel; age, 24 weeks' gestation). No other malformations were found at necropsy. There is a high incidence of Turner's syndrome associated with bilateral cervical hygromas. (From Isaacs H Jr. Tumors of the Newborn and Infant. St. Louis: Mosby–Year Book, 1991.)

been classified histologically into three main categories—capillary, cavernous, and cystic (hygroma)—on the basis of the thickness of the lymphatic vessel walls and the size of the cysts.[224] This classification has no significant clinicopathologic correlation, however, as all the lesions essentially appear the same under the microscope. They are essentially composed of cystically dilated lymphatics. Moreover, all lymphangiomas are treated in the same way—namely, by surgical excision if this is feasible.

The term cystic lymphangioma, or hygroma, is applied particularly to large, single, or slightly multilocular, fluid-filled cavities that most often are located on one side of the neck (see Fig. 4–20). Occasionally, they are multiple and may be found in other locations, such as the extremities and mediastinum (see Figs. 4–21 and 4–22).[268] Bilateral hygromas of the neck occurring with widespread lymphangiectasis are not uncommon in aborted fetuses (see Fig. 4–23).

Lymphangiomas discovered in utero by sonography are found in fetuses with Turner's syndrome, hydrops, oligohydramnios, single-vessel umbilical cord, Noonan's syndrome, fetal alcohol syndrome, diaphragmatic hernia (with Fryns syndrome [diaphragmatic defects, acral anomalies, pulmonary hypoplasia, coarse facies, and short, webbed neck]), and trisomy 18 and trisomy 21.[52,70,71,144,290,371] The lesion occurs also in normal individuals.

Chromosomal anomalies are found in more than 60% of fetuses with cystic hygromas, and most of these are female patients with a 45,X karyotype.[87,311,371] Moreover, the association of cystic hygroma with trisomy 21 is probably more frequent than is actually reported.[371] On the other hand, fetuses with hygromas may have normal karyotypes, and these individuals usually have a more favorable prognosis.[352]

In one study, 11 of 15 fetuses with cervical cystic hygroma had 45,X karyotypes, and 13 were hydropic.[70] Seven autolyzed, aborted fetuses had similar findings (Fig. 4–23).[59] The overall prognosis of a fetus with cystic hygroma of the neck is poor.[2] The incidence of this lesion in 405 fetuses with malformations was 5.4%, and the frequency of fetal chromosomal anomaly was 65%. Approximately 60% of these had Turner's syndrome. In one prenatal study, more than 50% of the cystic hygromas were associated with other anomalies, such as fetal hydrops and a two-vessel umbilical cord.[290]

Additional chromosomal defects have been noted in fetuses with cystic hygroma, including trisomy 13,18,21,22,13q-, 18q-, and partial 11q-.[2,59,87,290,311] Welborn and Timm described six fetuses, having an average gestational age of 14 weeks, with cystic hygroma and trisomy 21.[371] According to these authors, many cases of cystic hygroma with this chromosomal anomaly go undetected, as approximately 24% of fetuses with trisomy 21 spontaneously abort prior to the 16th week. They suggest that hygromas occurring before 16 weeks are probably clinically different than those discovered later in gestation.[371]

Lymphangiomas in fetuses with chromosomal anomalies and major malformations are associated with a high mortality rate. Studies show that there is only a 27% chance for the fetus with a cystic hygroma to have a normal karyotype, a 24% chance for survival, and 10% chance for a completely normal anatomy; no survivors with abnormal karyotypes have been reported, and the probability of having a completely normal infant is only 2% to 3%.[2,290]

The lesions associated with Turner's syndrome are single cavities, whereas isolated cystic hygromas tend to be multiloculated.[292] Venous aneurysms have been described in association with giant cystic hygromas.[155] Preoperative knowledge of this associated venous anomaly is a requisite for a successful outcome.

On microscopic examination, hygromas are thin-walled, filled with pink proteinaceous fluid, lined by a single layer of flat endothelial cells, and surrounded by varying amounts of connective tissue and smooth muscle (see Figs. 4–20D and 4–22B). The endothelium-lined, dilated lymphatic channels react positively with factor VIII antibody.[64] Frequently, the endothelial lining is absent.

Lymphangiomas are not compressible and are not visibly connected to lymphatic channels. They may grow in size after birth because of increased secretion of fluid. Evacuation of the fluid gives only temporary relief, and unless the wall is completely removed, the fluid will reappear.[268]

At birth, these lymphatic defects usually appear to have destroyed or prevented the development of muscles and other structures in the involved areas. They are almost never encapsulated, and surgical removal is usually difficult and sometimes impossible.[292]

Hemangiopericytoma

Hemangiopericytoma is an uncommon vascular neoplasm that was initially defined and named by Stout and Murray in 1942.[348] The neoplasm consists primarily of pericytes (pericapillary mesenchymal cells), which are intimately related to capillaries and which share some ultrastructural and immunohistochemical features in common with fibroblasts and smooth muscle cells.[97,193,255,279,306,348] Most lesions present as soft tissue masses in a variety of sites, but they may occur also in other locations, such as the tongue, nasopharynx, stomach, and central nervous system.[9,24,127,204,287,295,324] Hemangiopericytoma is primarily a tumor that affects adults. It is seldom seen in the first decade of life, and less than 10% of the total number of cases have been found in children.[127] Nevertheless, it has been detected prenatally by ultrasonography and has been noted in stillborns.[24,204,363] Perinatal hemangiopericytomas may mimic the clinical manifestations of hemangiomas, presenting as life-threatening hemorrhage and hypovolemic shock from an ul-

cerated subcutaneous hemangiopericytoma; bleeding diathesis (anemia and hypofibrinogenemia) associated with a retroperitoneal primary tumor; hematemesis from a gastric tumor; or high-output congestive heart failure.[24,295,304]

When the tumor occurs in young children, it may have a gross and histologic appearance and biological behavior that differ from those manifested in older children or adults. Because of these distinguishing features, some have been called congenital (infantile) hemangiopericytoma.[127] The prognosis for patients diagnosed with this neoplasm in the first 3 months of life is generally favorable.[20,24,128,184,185,187,190,193,295,362,363] After a comprehensive literature review, Chen and colleagues concluded that congenital hemangiopericytomas behave in a benign fashion, whereas later on in infancy, they are potentially malignant.[69] Metastases have been observed in newborns with hemangiopericytoma.[24,265] One infant had a primary lesion involving the face, which spread to the lungs soon after resection.[265] The other had a neck mass removed at 4 days of age, only to return 28 months later with intrathoracic and brain metastases.[24] The latter case emphasizes the importance of close follow-up examination for an extended period of time, as metastases may occur 1 year or more after the initial surgery.

Of 120 congenital mesenchymal tumors described by Kauffman and Stout, 11 (9%) were classified as hemangiopericytoma.[204] About 50% of these involved the extremities. Except for the two infants with intracranial tumors, the other nine survived without recurrence or metastases. Enzinger and Smith[127] reviewed 106 cases of hemangiopericytoma, including 8 (7.5%) that occurred in infants ranging in age from 1 day to 7 months. All the lesions presented as soft tissue masses located in a variety of sites. The 8 patients in their series, as well as most others diagnosed in the first year of life who were reported subsequently had a favorable outcome.[9,20,113,184,185,279,324,363,365]

van Baarlen and Bax culled 39 examples of infantile hemangiopericytoma from the literature, adding 1 case of their own.[363] Of the 40 patients, 32 were diagnosed before 3 months of age. The subcutaneous tissue of the extremities (34%) and the head and neck (34%) were the most frequent sites. Most patients were treated with radical excision. Follow-up data were available for 25 patients, 19 (76%) of whom survived. Ordonez et al. described a 3-day-old male with a cervical tumor having a similar histologic appearance to the "classic" or "adult" form;

this patient also had a favorable outcome.[279] Multiple congenital hemangiopericytomas are rarely documented. Seibert et al. described a neonate with tumors arising from the occipital region of the scalp and nasopharynx who was successfully treated.[324] It is conceivable that some newborns who are diagnosed with multiple hemangiopericytomas actually have myofibromatoses, which are more common in this age group and behave differently.[255]

Bailey et al. reported five cases of congenital hemangiopericytoma, all occurring in female patients.[24] The sites of origin were the neck, parotid, axilla, and the retroperitoneum. Four had an uneventful recovery and long-term survival after surgical resection, including the infant with the retroperitoneal tumor. However, the one patient with the primary tumor of the neck developed intrathoracic metastases 2 years after the initial surgery.[24] In one Anglo-American study, 5 of 11 patients were younger than 3 months of age at the time of diagnosis, and all 5 survived without recurrence or metastases after surgical resection.[255]

In a recent review of perinatal soft tissue tumors (see Table 4–2), six hemangiopericytomas, comprising 15% of the total soft tissue tumors in that study, were recorded. Two thirds occurred in the extremities, and one each in the neck and mediastinum and chest wall, respectively. Except for the neonate with a mediastinal tumor, all survived.

Two forms of hemangiopericytoma with different gross and microscopic findings are recognized in the newborn and infant. One is the congenital (infantile) type, as described initially by Enzinger and Smith,[127] and the other is the "classic" type or "adult" form, which is observed in older children and adults. To add to the nosologic confusion, examples of the classic type reported in the perinatal period have been termed congenital.[69,193,279] Nevertheless, the prognosis appears to be almost the same, regardless of the type, and immunohistochemical and ultrastructural evidence suggests that both probably represent the same tumor.[279] Moreover, Mentzel et al. disagree that there are two forms of hemangiopericytoma in the young.[255] They believe that the congenital form shares some histologic features in common with myofibromatosis (see the earlier discussion of myofibromatosis).

On gross examination, hemangiopericytomas vary in size from 1 cm to as much as 15 cm in diameter and display a variable appearance. They are firm, tan-yellow to dark red-brown, and nodular, with bulging cut surfaces containing areas of necrosis and calcification (Figs. 4–24B and 4–25B). The classic tumors are friable and tan-gray, with foci of hemorrhage, necrosis, and blood-filled cystic spaces similar to those observed in older patients (Fig. 4–25A).[279]

On histologic examination, the tumor shows a nodular vascular pattern composed of plump or spindle-shaped pericytes with round or oval glassy nuclei situated outside the capillary basement membranes demonstrated on reticulin stain. Those tumors that are found in neonates typically display slit-like, crescent-shaped, endothelium-lined spaces (stag horn-like structures) situated about the periphery of the tumor nodules, as well as a mixed histologic appearance characterized by both hemangiopericytoma and capillary hemangioma components (see Fig. 4–24).[127] The hemangioma component consists of lobules of capillaries and endothelial cells situated inside the capillary basement membrane (Fig. 4–24F). Blend zones are noted between the pericytoma and hemangioma components, which can be appreciated by electron microscopy as cells that are intermediate between the two. Extensive necrosis and fibrosis and foci of calcification are present in most specimens (Fig. 4–24D).[127,183,190] Vascular invasion or the protrusion of tumor cells into vascular lumina is noted in about 50% of the specimens (Fig. 4–24E).

Myofibromatoses are characterized by spindle-shaped cells, necrosis, calcification, and a central vascular zone, which should be kept in mind when considering the differential diagnosis. Both congenital hemangiopericytoma and myofibromatosis are usually associated with a favorable outcome, provided a vital anatomic structure is not involved.

The classic or adult form of hemangiopericytoma, observed in older children and adults, has been noted to occur in the newborn.[193,279] Compared with congenital tumors, this tumor has a much more uniform, densely cellular microscopic appearance, with numerous, anastomosing, dilated, thin-walled, vascular structures that vary in size, increased nuclear atypia, and increased mitotic activity (Fig. 4–25B). Usually, a single neoplastic cell type is recognizable by light microscopy.[279] It may be difficult, in some instances, to distinguish the classic hemangiopericytoma from congenital fibrosarcoma with a prominent vascular pattern (Fig. 4–12A).[107]

The immunohistochemical and electron microscopic findings in hemangiopericytoma

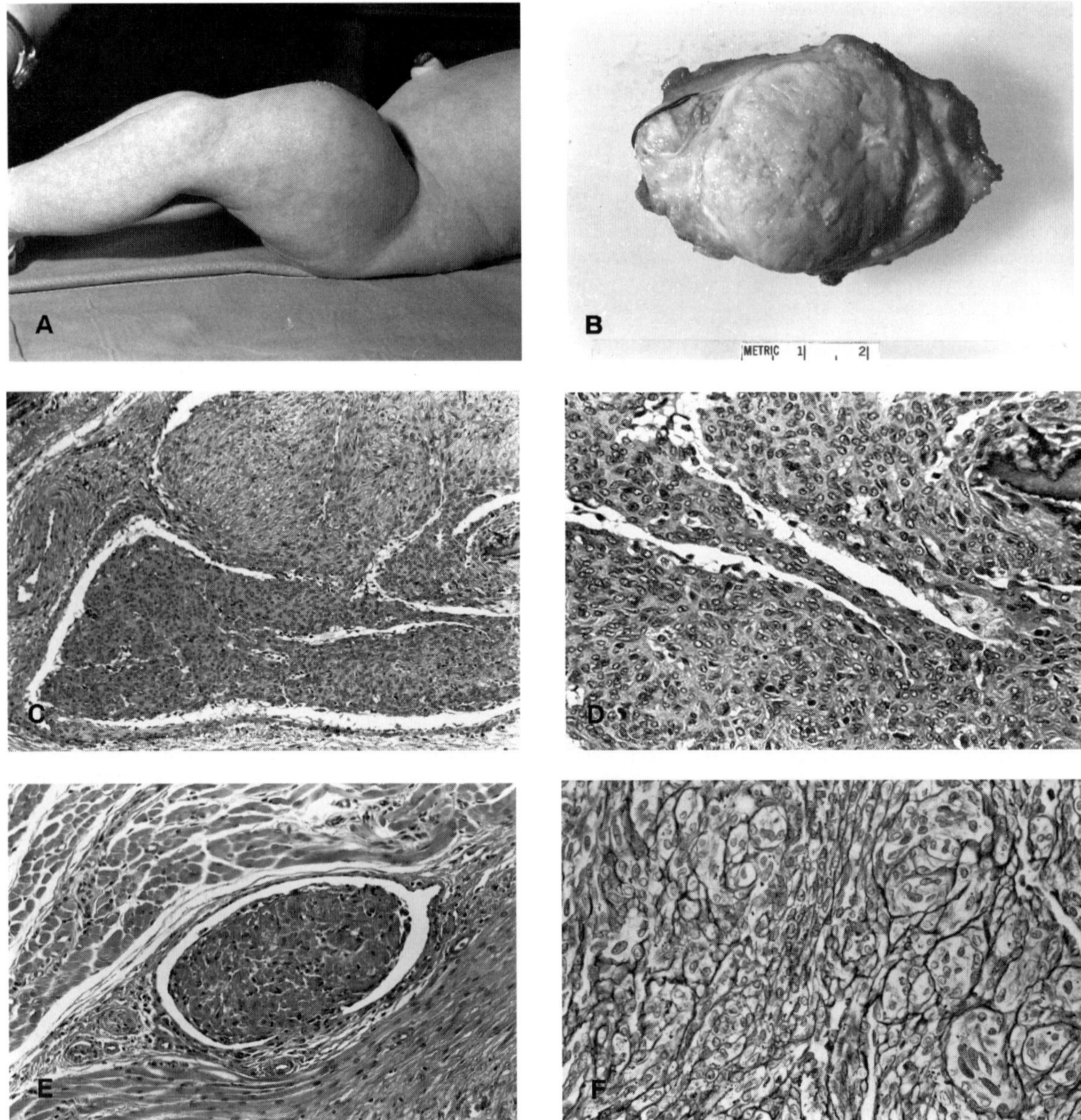

Figure 4–24. Infantile hemangiopericytoma. *A,* A 1-month-old female infant had a left thigh mass discovered at birth. *B,* The tumor weighed 43.6 g and measured 5.5 × 4.5 cm. The cut surface is lobular, bulging, and tan-gray to yellow-brown (owing to extensive necrosis). *C,* A low-power view displays the lobular architecture of the tumor. The lobules are rimmed peripherally by slit-like vascular spaces, which are helpful diagnostic features (hematoxylin-eosin, ×120). *D,* The tumor consists of cells with regular, round to oval, vesicular nuclei and inconspicuous nucleoli. A focus of calcification is seen at the lower left side of the picture (hematoxylin-eosin, ×200). *E,* An intravascular tumor thrombus within skeletal muscle (hematoxylin-eosin, ×150). *F,* A reticulin stain reveals reticulin fibers surrounding nests of cells (hemangioma pattern), as well as individual cells (hemangiopericytoma pattern), with transition zones between the two (Verhoeff's elastic stain, ×300). (From Isaacs H Jr. Neoplasms in infants: A report of 265 cases. *In* Sommers SC, Rosen PP (eds): Pathol Annu 1983; 18:165. Used by permission.)

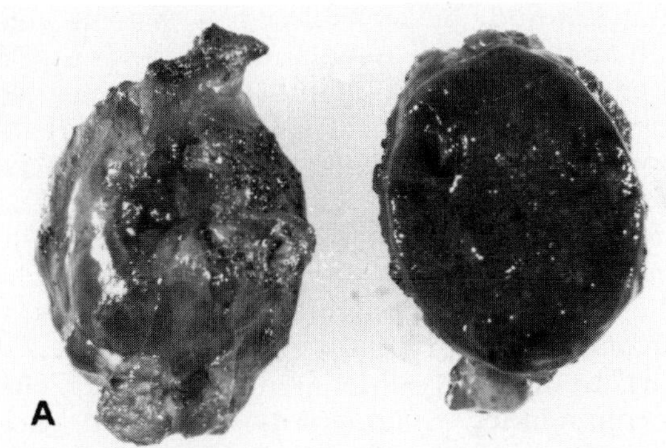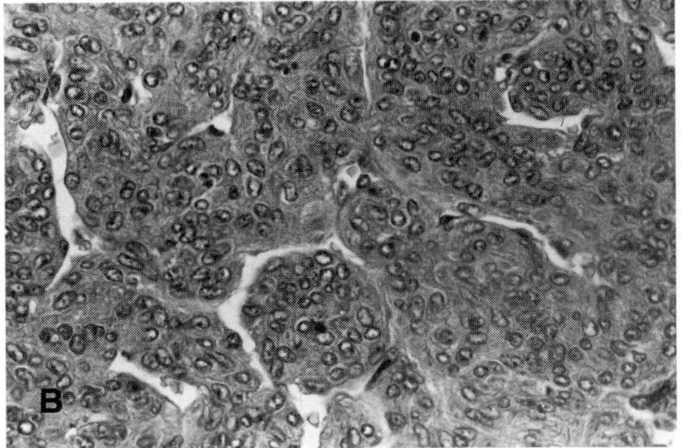

Figure 4–25. Infantile hemangiopericytoma. *A,* A hemorrhagic nodule measuring 2 × 1.5 cm was removed from the posterior thigh of a 5-day-old male infant. *B,* The tumor displays a lobular growth pattern observed in the "adult" form and consists of cells with round to oval, "glassy," vesicular nuclei (hematoxylin-eosin, ×400).

have been described by various investigators.[31,97,193, 255,279,363] Factor VIII antigen staining of endothelial cells and a positive reaction of tumor cells to vimentin have been noted.[279] The tumor cells are nonreactive to desmin, S-100 protein, and keratin, and muscle actin (HHF35) stains focally positive.[97] Ultrastructural features that are supportive of the diagnosis include interdigitating cytoplasmic processes, pinocytotic vesicles and cytoplasmic filaments (sometimes of the smooth muscle type), and poorly formed, intercellular, desmosomal-type attachments.[9,31,97,120,276] Basement membrane–like material partially surrounds individual cells. Tumor cells with features intermediate between hemangiopericytoma and hemangioma are also found, suggesting that the two neoplasms share a common histogenesis.[31,120] DNA ploidy analysis reveals a predominantly diploid cell population.[190]

In the perinatal study shown in Table 4–2, all patients except for one were cured by surgical excision alone. The newborn with the cervical-mediastinal tumor died at the age of 1½ months as a result of pulmonary hemorrhage secondary to tracheal involvement. This case is another tragic example of a histologically benign tumor causing death as the result of involvement of a vital structure. In contrast to the Children's Hospital, Los Angeles study alluded to earlier, all eight infants with hemangiopericytoma reported by Enzinger and Smith survived.[127] Other reports describe a generally favorable outcome for the newborn with hemangiopericytoma.[9,20,24,69,193,255,304,324,362, 363,365] Spontaneous regression after partial resection has also been reported.[9,69,324,363] A conservative surgical approach with careful follow-up is the treatment of choice.[20,24]

SKELETAL MUSCLE TUMORS

Tumors of skeletal muscle are separated into two main groups: rhabdomyoma and rhabdomyosarcoma. The former is an infrequent, benign, skeletal muscle lesion comprising less than 2% of all striated muscle tumors, whereas the latter is the most common soft tissue sarcoma in childhood.[26,27,79,110,114,128,178,211] Rhabdomyosarcoma follows fibrosarcoma in terms of its frequency in the newborn (see Tables 4–1 and 4–2).[100,185,238]

Rhabdomyoma

Rhabdomyoma is classified into fetal, juvenile, and adult forms.[92] Generally, fetal rhabdomyomas are found in infants, and they more closely resemble developing skeletal muscle than the adult form, which is found in later life.[92,374] Juvenile rhabdomyoma is considered to be an intermediate form, occurring in both infants and children.[92] Sites of predilection include the head and neck.[92,110,199] Rhabdomyomas of the female genital tract usually do not occur in infants, and are regarded as a special form of fetal rhabdomyoma.[114] Cardiac rhabdomyoma is a distinct lesion found in cardiac muscle that is probably hamartomatous in nature (see Chapter 16, "Cardiac Tumors").

Of nine cases of extracardiac fetal rhabdomyomas reported by the Armed Forces Institute of Pathology (AFIP) in 1972, three occurred in newborns, all but one of whom were male.[110] All three involved the subcutaneous tissue of the posterior auricular region. A more recent AFIP study included 24 fetal rhabdomyomas. In this series, 10 patients were younger than 1 year of age (42%), and 4 (17%) were younger than 4 months of age.[199] The rhabdomyomas presented as slowly growing, solitary masses within the soft tissue or submucosa, most often arising in the posterior auricular area. This site of origin was followed in frequency by the neck, nasopharynx, and tongue.[199] Only 1 of the 10 infants had a local recurrence. Two additional examples of congenital fetal rhabdomyoma in locations other than the head and neck region have been described, one arising from the abdominal wall and the other from the retroperitoneal area.[215,374] The youngest patient diagnosed as having juvenile (intermediate) rhabdomyoma in the study of Crotty et al. was a 5-month-old female infant with a foot lesion.[92] A clinical manifestation attributed to fetal rhabdomyomas, other than the most common one (a mass), is airway obstruction.[199]

On macroscopic examination, fetal rhabdomyomas are circumscribed (but not encapsulated), light gray to tan-pink nodules that, on average, measure 1.5 to 8 cm in size.[110] Microscopically, they display haphazardly arranged, fetal-appearing, slender, skeletal muscle cells with cross-striations separated by a pale-staining myxoid stroma containing small, oval to spindle-shaped, undifferentiated, mesenchymal cells.[92,110,199,374] Muscle fibers are seen in various stages of differentiation. The juvenile rhabdomyoma has a similar histologic appearance as the fetal type, except that the small mesenchymal cell component is absent.[92] Distinguishing this tumor from the well-differentiated embryonal rhabdomyosarcoma, including the spindle-cell variant, is the chief concern in the differential diagnosis.[110,199,215] Foci of necrosis, cells with large nucleoli, nuclear atypia, and brisk mitotic activity are findings typical of sarcoma but absent in rhabdomyoma.

The skeletal muscle markers actin, desmin, myosin, and myoglobin test positive.[46,199] Adenosine triphosphatase (ATPase) is strongly reactive. Ultrastructural studies reveal bundles of myofibrils, situated in parallel rows, that consist of cytoplasmic filaments with cross-banding. Only a few cells contain rod-like, Z-band material. Skeletal myocytes are found in different stages of development.[46,92,199,215,374]

A debate persists as to whether rhabdomy-

oma should be considered a hamartoma, rather than a true neoplasm. Progression of a fetal rhabdomyoma of the tongue in an 18-month-old child to an alveolar-embryonal rhabdomyosarcoma has been described,[211] indicating that the diagnosis of rhabdomyoma of the soft tissues in a young child should be made with caution because the tumor is so rare. On the other hand, recognition of fetal rhabdomyoma is important in preventing unnecessary therapy and subsequent morbidity.[199] The recommended treatment is wide local excision. Recurrence of a fetal rhabdomyoma is rare.[110,199]

Congenital Cardiac Rhabdomyoma

Cardiac rhabdomyomas are probably hamartomas, rather than true neoplasms, and are the most common mass lesion of the heart in the fetus and newborn (see Chapter 16, "Cardiac Tumors" and Table 16–8). They may exist as single, subendocardial nodules that distend the wall of the chamber in which they are located (see Figs. 16–1 and 16–2), or they may consist of multiple small lesions, in which case, they are often associated with other disturbances in development. In many individuals, rhabdomyomas of the heart are part of a general syndrome of tuberous sclerosis, with involvement of the brain and other organs.[292] Renal cysts and adenomas, as well as malformations of the meninges, pancreas, palate, and other anatomic sites, may also be noted. The tumors are 1 to 2 cm in diameter and usually extend into the cavity of the heart. On histologic examination, they are characterized by large, vacuolated, "spider" cells that contain abundant glycogen and often show radial extensions with transverse striations of their peripheral cytoplasm (Fig. 16–2A and B, heart). Often, they are multiple and consist of numerous small areas, some of which are visible only microscopically. Less often, the myocardium is diffusely affected, with no discrete lesions (see Fig. 16–2C).[292]

Rhabdomyosarcoma

Rhabdomyosarcoma is a neoplasm that primarily affects children and adolescents, comprising more than 50% of all sarcomas in this age group.[104,128,300] Traditionally, it is considered to be a sarcoma derived from the embryonic skeletal muscle cell, the rhabdomyoblast.[123,178] Rhabdomyosarcoma is a highly malignant neo-

Table 4–4. Neonatal Rhabdomyosarcoma (Intergroup Rhabdomyosarcoma Study)

Patient No.	Sex	Primary Site	Group	Histology	Grade	Treatment	Survival Status
1	M	Bladder	III	Embryonal	F	S, XRT, CT	Alive
2	F	Buttock (S-C)	III	Embryonal	U	S, CT	Alive
3	M	Thigh	IIA	Embryonal	U	S, CT, XRT	Dead
4	M	Paraspinal	IIA	Undifferentiated	U	S, CT	Alive
5	F	Vagina	III	Botryoid	U	S, CT	Dead
6	M	Perirectal	IB	Botryoid	F	S, CT	Alive
7	M	Perirectal	IA	Undifferentiated	U	S, CT	Alive
8	F	Paraspinal	III	Embryonal	F	S, XRT, CT	Dead
9	F	Neck	III	Embryonal	F	S, XRT, CT	Dead
10	M	Neck	IV	Undifferentiated	U	S, CT	Dead
11	F	Chest wall	III	Undifferentiated	–	S, CT	Dead
12	M	Oropharynx	IV	Embryonal	U	S, CT	Dead
13	M	Buttock (S-C)	III	Embryonal	F	S, CT	Alive

F = favorable histology; U = unfavorable histology; S-C = sacrococcygeal area; S = surgery; CT = chemotherapy; XRT = radiation therapy.

Modified from Lobe TE, Weiner ES, Hays DM, et al. Neonatal rhabdomyosarcoma: The IRS experience. J Pediatr Surg 1994;29:1167. Used by permission.

plasm that accounts for the majority of soft tissue sarcomas in infants, and it is second or third in frequency in the newborn (following fibrosarcoma), depending on the study (see Tables 4–1 and 4–2).[102,104] Although neonatal rhabdomyosarcoma is uncommon, it was the dominant soft tissue sarcoma identified (in 8 of 12 cases) in the study by Campbell et al.[60]

Associations between rhabdomyosarcoma and hereditary diseases and congenital malformations have been reported.[249,300] An increased frequency of breast carcinoma and brain tumors in families of patients with this sarcoma has been documented as part of the so-called family cancer syndrome.[233,249,285] Rhabdomyosarcoma is one of the malignant tumors found in patients with neurofibromatosis.[250] Postmortem studies performed on 43 children enrolled in the Intergroup Rhabdomyosarcoma Study disclosed that 7 (16%) of the children had congenital malformations, more than 50% of which involved the central nervous system.[315]

Cytogenetic analyses performed on rhabdomyosarcomas show karyotypic differences between embryonal and alveolar rhabdomyosarcoma. The former exhibits a loss of heterozygosity on the short arm of chromosome 11, whereas the latter displays a translocation between chromosomes 2 and 3, t(2; 3).[281,281a] Mutations of p53 cancer suppressor gene are found in a variety of soft tissue tumors, both benign and malignant, including rhabdomyosarcoma. Therefore, the detection of this gene mutation is not diagnostically useful in distinguishing rhabdomyosarcoma from other mesenchymal neoplasms.[281] On the other hand, the detection of the p-glycoprotein transmembrane protein, the product of the multiple drug resistance (MDR) gene, appears to be more specific and has diagnostic and prognostic significance.[281] The presence of p-glycoprotein immunoreactivity is associated with a decreased survival rate in children with rhabdomyosarcoma.

Rhabdomyosarcoma is seldom noted at birth. Less than 1% of the pediatric patients with this neoplasm are diagnosed in the first month of life. A recent Intergroup Rhabdomyosarcoma Study of 3217 infants and children revealed that 13 (0.4%) were younger than 30 days old at the time of diagnosis.[238] Half of the neonatal tumors arose caudally: buttock/sacrococcygeal (2 cases), perirectal (2 cases), bladder (1 case), and vagina (1 case). The remaining tumors occurred in various other locations: neck (2 cases), thorax (2 cases), oropharynx (1 case), chest wall (1 case), and thigh (1 case) (see Table 4–4). One of the largest collections of neonatal rhabdomyosarcoma was described by the Hospital for Sick Children, Toronto group.[60] The tumor accounted for 8% of a total of 102 malignant lesions, and 8 of 12 soft tissue sarcomas. The locations cited for the alveolar rhabdomyosarcomas were the neck, arm, and foot; the sites of the botryoid, embryonal, and unspecified rhabdomyosarcoma types included the vagina, axilla, tongue, and paraspinal area, respectively.[60]

In the newborn, the head and neck region and the genitourinary tract are the most com-

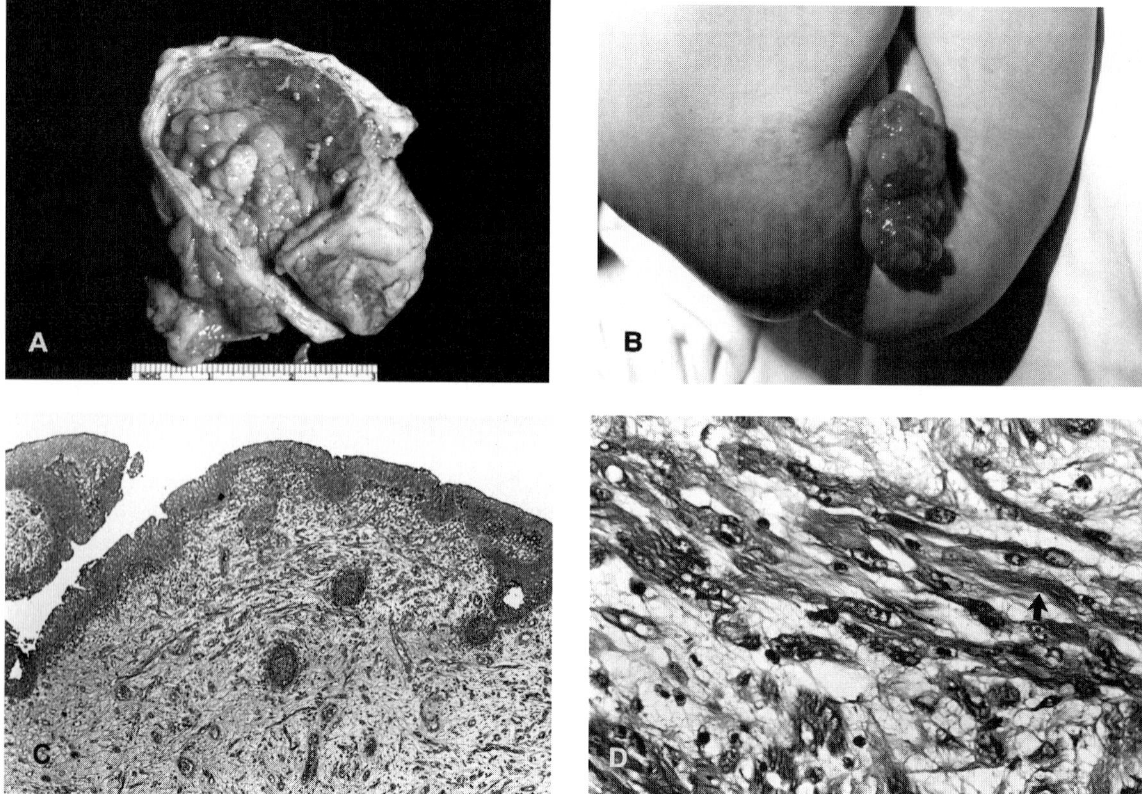

Figure 4–26. Botryoid embryonal rhabdomyosarcoma. *A,* A 1-year-old boy with a grape-like tumor mass invading the trigone and posterior wall of the urinary bladder. *B,* A 7-month-old girl with a similar lesion protruding from the vagina. *C,* A low-power view of two tumor nodules. Directly beneath the vaginal mucosa, there is a cellular rind or mantle composed of rhabdomyoblasts (hematoxylin-eosin, ×120). *D,* The rhabdomyoblasts are shown in greater detail. Some contain cytoplasmic cross-striations (*arrow*) (hematoxylin-eosin, ×480). (*B, C,* and *D:* From Isaacs H Jr. Tumors of the Newborn and Infant. St. Louis: Mosby–Year Book, 1991.)

mon sites for primary rhabdomyosarcoma, followed by the extremities (see Table 4–4 and Fig. 4–26).[60,100,166,203] Of 120 congenital mesenchymal tumors reviewed by Kaufman and Stout, rhabdomyosarcoma was third in order of frequency, following fibromatoses and mesenchymoma, and it was the leading soft tissue malignant tumor.[203] In this series, there were 15 rhabdomyosarcomas with the following distribution: head and neck, 6 cases; urogenital tract, 3 cases; upper extremity and perineal area, 2 cases each; and lower extremity and trunk, 1 case each.

Perinatal rhabdomyosarcoma occurs in various locations and presents clinically in a variety of ways, depending on the site of origin. When the tumor arises from the tongue, it may fill the oral cavity and protrude out of the mouth, causing airway obstruction and feeding problems.[14,211,260] The sarcoma may be responsible for a suprapubic abdominal mass when arising from the urinary bladder.[209] Ober and col-

leagues described two patients with vaginal botryoid rhabdomyosarcomas that were diagnosed at birth as vaginal polyps; both patients survived after hysterectomy.[277] Lower extremity tumors have been detected prenatally by ultrasonography.[61,163a] Zuniga and co-workers described a pedunculated embryonal rhabdomyosarcoma arising from a giant pigmented nevus of the neck and shoulder of a neonate with neurocutaneous melanosis.[387] Gormley et al. collected six cases of congenital orbital rhabdomyosarcoma from the literature and added one of their own; all but one proved fatal before 1 year of age despite various forms of treatment.[156,175,211,337,372] Kauffman and Stout reported another similar case.[203] Embryonal rhabdomyosarcoma can also occur as a mass lesion in the eyelid.[168,183] Hayashi et al. reported a neonate who presented with multiple skin metastases secondary to an alveolar rhabdomyosarcoma of the neck and who died of brain involvement.[167]

Gonzalez-Crussi and Black-Schaffer de-

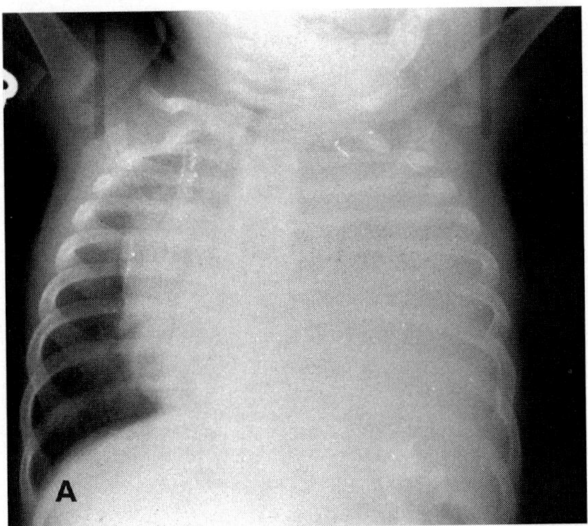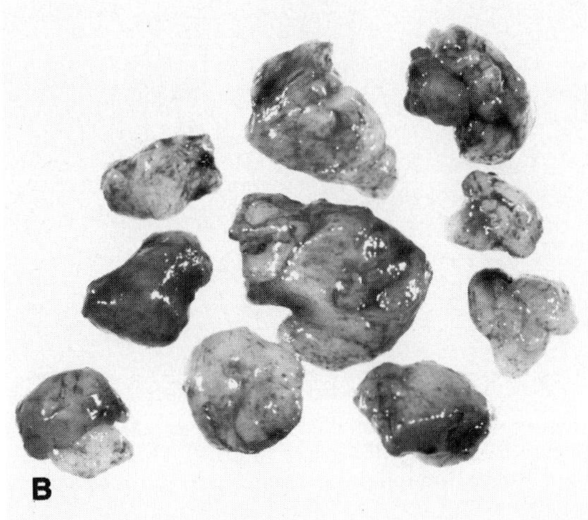

Figure 4–27. Embryonal rhabdomyosarcoma of the mediastinum. *A,* A chest x-ray film was obtained in an 8-month-old boy with a 1-week history of a cough and progressive respiratory distress beginning 3 days prior to hospital admission. The radiograph revealed consolidation of the left thorax with displacement of the mediastinum to the right. *B,* Biopsy material obtained from the mediastinal mass. The tumor has a soft, gray, gelatinous appearance. (From Isaacs H Jr. Tumors of the Newborn and Infant. St. Louis: Mosby–Year Book, 1991.)

scribed 25 infants and children with rhabdomyosarcoma, 3 of whom were younger than 3 months of age.[147] The three patients with embryonal rhabdomyosarcomas had lesions in the neck, upper extremity, and perianal region, respectively, and all survived.[147] A later series from the Texas Children's Hospital, 1954–1984, consisted of 47 patients, 5 (10.6%) of whom were younger than 3 months of age.[166] The distribution of the tumors was as follows: orbit, nasopharynx, pelvis, vagina, and buttock. All but the orbital tumor, which had an alveolar pattern, were classified as embryonal. The survival rate was low (20%); only the newborn with the pelvic embryonal rhabdomyosarcoma survived.[166]

Traditionally, rhabdomyosarcomas have been divided into five main histologic types: embryonal, botryoid, alveolar, pleomorphic, and mixed.[178] As in the older child and adolescent, most rhabdomyosarcomas diagnosed in the first year of life are classified histologically as either embryonal or botryoid type.[128,147,187] The alveolar form, which is associated with the worst prognosis, ranks third in terms of frequency, but pleomorphic rhabdomyosarcoma rarely occurs, if at all, in the young.[60,147,187,203] The newborn Intergroup Rhabdomyosarcoma Study mentioned earlier classified rhabdomyosarcoma into three histologic types: embryonal, botryoid/embryonal, and undifferentiated.[238] The distribution of cases was as follows: embryonal, 7; undifferentiated, 4; and botryoid, 2. The term alveolar rhabdomyosarcoma was not

mentioned, although it is assumed that the alveolar-type tumors would be assigned to the undifferentiated group.

The botryoid form of embryonal rhabdomyosarcoma, which arises from mucosal-lined body cavities (e.g., the vagina, urinary bladder, middle ear, and biliary system), has a distinctive appearance (see Fig. 4–26). Typically, lobulated, grape-like, polypoid projections with pale gray gelatinous cut surfaces are seen (Fig. 4–26*A* and *B*). Microscopic examination shows tiny, round, or spindle-shaped rhabdomyoblasts situated directly beneath the epithelium located in a submucosal cellular rind or mantle (Fig. 4–26*C* and *D*). Well-defined cytoplasmic cross-striations are often very difficult to identify. The desmin and actin immunoperoxidase stains are helpful in identifying the small cells as rhabdomyoblasts. The remainder of the polyp consists of pale-staining, myxoid-appearing, connective tissue and blood vessels. The botryoid rhabdomyosarcoma is associated with the most favorable prognosis of all the histologic types.

Embryonal and alveolar rhabdomyosarcomas form grey-white, myxoid-appearing, infiltrative masses that are seldom encapsulated and that have more extensive necrosis and hemorrhage than that observed in the botryoid type (Fig. 4–27). Embryonal rhabdomyosarcoma displays considerable and characteristic variation in its histologic pattern, with cellular areas alternating with myxoid areas (Fig. 4–28).[128] The more differentiated tumors show

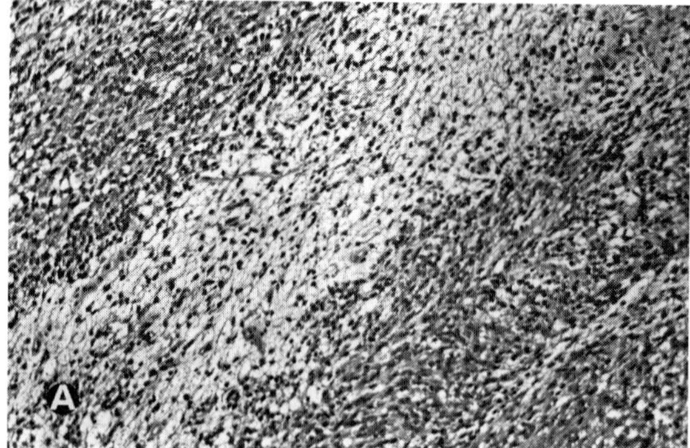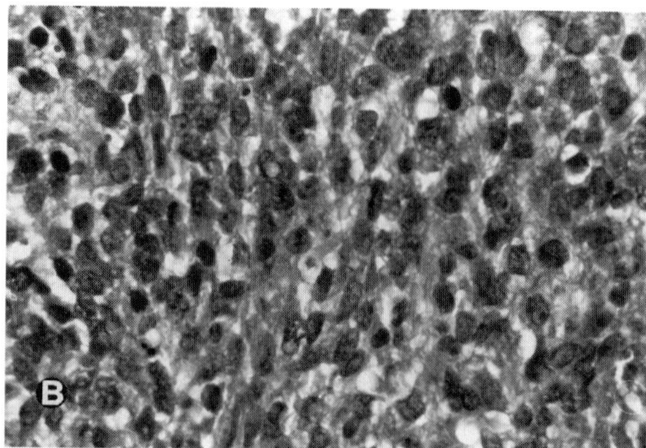

Figure 4–28. Embryonal rhabdomyosarcoma. *A,* Myxoid areas alternating with hypercellular areas are characteristic of this tumor (hematoxylin-eosin, ×150). *B,* This cellular area is composed of small, poorly differentiated cells (hematoxylin-eosin, ×480). Immunohistochemical analysis revealed cells that were reactive with desmin, actin, and vimentin.

round to oval, or sometimes tadpole- or racket-shaped, cells with irregular nuclei and an eosinophilic-staining cytoplasm; occasionally, cytoplasmic cross-striations are present (Fig. 4–29). The poorly differentiated embryonal rhabdomyosarcoma has a histologic appearance that resembles other small cell malignant tumors of infancy and childhood (Fig. 4–28). Ultrastructural and immunocytochemical studies are required to establish the diagnosis. Table 4–5 lists the histologic differential diagnoses of the small blue cell malignant tumors.

One form of embryonal rhabdomyosarcoma that has a better prognosis is termed spindle-cell rhabdomyosarcoma.[65,187,231] The paratesticular area is the most common primary site for this type of tumor. The youngest patient reported was 7 months of age. Microscopic examination reveals a tumor with uniform, spindle-shaped rhabdomyoblasts and an interdigitating (herringbone) growth pattern similar to that of the fibromatoses and fibrosarcoma (Fig. 4–30).

Alveolar rhabdomyosarcoma has a characteristic microscopic appearance consisting of small, round to spindle-shaped cells forming irregular cyst-like spaces that mimic pulmonary alveoli (Fig. 4–31).[124,178] With adequate preservation, the rhabdomyoblasts attached to the lining of the fibrovascular septae appear to "spin off" into the lumen. Eosinophilic giant cell forms are present in the alveoli.[178] Even though well-defined cross-striations are difficult or sometimes impossible to find, positive reactions to vimentin and desmin immunoperoxidase staining, as well as the Z-band material and/or thick and thin filaments observed in the tumor cells by electron microscopy, establish the diagnosis (Fig. 4–31*D*) (see Table 4–5).

To compound the diagnostic difficulties presented by the small cell malignant tumor, there is even a less well-differentiated form of rhabdomyosarcoma called solid alveolar rhabdomyosarcoma, which consists of monotonous sheets of primitive-appearing small cells without fibrous septae.[281] Cytogenetic analysis reveals a t(2:13) translocation. This form of alveolar rhabdomyosarcoma is associated with an agressive clinical behavior and a poor outcome.[281] The National Cancer Institute has proposed a classification whereby the histologic subtypes are reduced to three: namely, embryonal rhabdomyosarcoma ("favorable histology"); alveolar, open and solid round cell ("unfavorable histology"); and pleomorphic, which, as stated earlier, is very rare in young children.[358]

More recently, another classification system —called the universal classification scheme— has been devised for rhabdomyosarcoma and related sarcomas.[355] It is based on the histologic presentation and prognosis of the tumors. The classification consists of three main groups: tumors with favorable prognosis, those with intermediate prognosis, and those with unfavorable prognosis. According to this scheme, the botryoid and spindle-cell rhabdomyosarcomas are assigned the favorable prognosis group, embryonal rhabdomyosarcoma and extraosseous Ewing's sarcoma are assigned to the intermediate prognosis group, and alveolar rhabdomyosarcoma and undifferentiated sarcoma are assigned to the unfavorable prognosis category.[355] For a detailed discussion of this classification and the problems in diagnosing the various subtypes of rhabdomyosarcoma and related sarcomas, the reader is referred to the review article by Tsokos.[355]

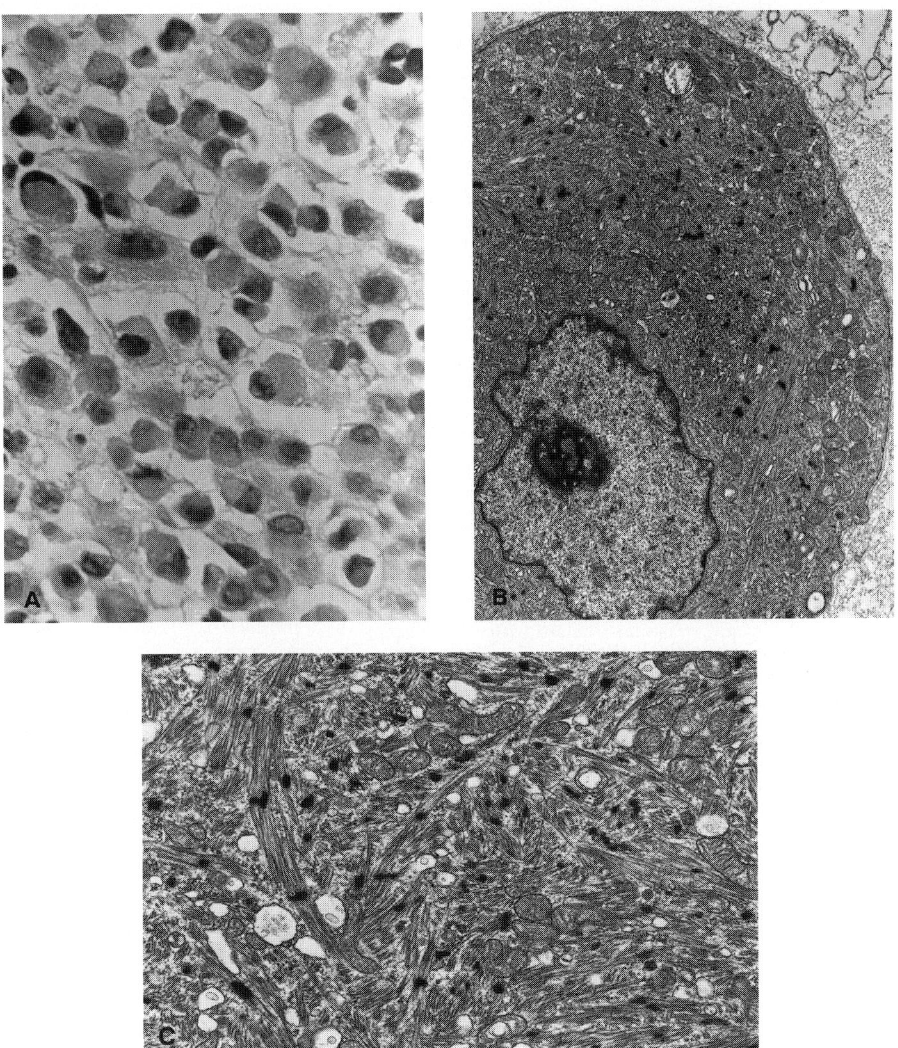

Figure 4–29. Embryonal rhabdomyosarcoma involving the neck of a 2-year-old girl. *A,* The tumor consists mainly of well-differentiated rhabdomyoblasts (hematoxylin-eosin, ×380). *B,* Ultrastructural studies reveal thick and thin filaments and a prominent basement membrane (×5200). *C,* A higher-power view of the thick and thin filaments with Z-bands (×17,800). (Electron photomicrographs courtesy of Ann Peters, Children's Hospital, San Diego, CA.)

The prognosis of adults and children with rhabdomyosarcoma depends on three main factors: the tumor's location, stage (group), and histologic features.[119,138,160,210,227,249,300] The Intergroup Rhabdomyosarcoma Study staging system is the one currently used in many pediatric centers in this country (see Table 4–6).[231,300] Most newborns and infants in the Intergroup Study were classified as having group III tumors (54% and 47%, respectively).[238]

Eight of the 15 patients with congenital tumors in Kauffman and Stout's series survived without known recurrence; 6 died as a result of their tumor, and 1 was lost to follow-up evaluation.[203] All underwent surgical excision, but none were treated with chemotherapy, as the study was done prior to the availability of effective agents; two received radiotherapy. This early study in 1965 serves as an important historical control. The event-free survival rate for infants with rhabdomyosarcoma in the German Soft Tissue Sarcoma Study Group reported in 1989 was 70%, compared to 47% for older children.[216] One Intergroup Rhabdomyosarcoma Study focusing primarily on infants (1986) revealed that the overall 5-year survival rate was almost the same as for older children and adolescents—namely, 63% for infants, compared

Table 4–5. Histopathologic Differential Diagnosis of the Small
Blue Cell Malignant Tumors of the Newborn

Tumor	Light Microscopy	Immunohistochemistry	Ultrastructure
Neuroblastoma	Small, round cells; rosettes; neurofilaments; nuclei with a peppery chromatin pattern	NSE+, NFP+, VIM+, DES−, MSA−, LCA−, CK−, HBA71−, β_2MG−, M1C2−	Neurosecretory granules, microtubules, neurofilaments
Rhabdomyosarcoma	Spindle cells, eosinophilic cytoplasms, cross-striations, embryonal and alveolar patterns	DES+, MSA+, VIM+, NSE±, NFP−, HBA71−, CK−, LCA−	Spindle cells, primitive attachments, Z-bands, thick and thin filaments, basement membranes, glycogen±
Leukemia	Diffuse infiltrates of small, round cells; granules±	LCA+, VIM±, MSA−, NFP−, CK−, HBA71−	Round cells, no attachments, no matrix, granules±
Primitive neuroectodermal tumor (PNET)*	Small, round cells; rosettes; lobular pattern	NSE+, VIM+, NFP±, HBA71+, β_2MG+, LCA−, DES−, MSA−, CK−, M1C2+	Primitive cells, few organelles, rare neurosecretory granules, few intermediate filaments, primitive attachments±
Rhabdoid tumor	Polygonal cells with eosinophilic cytoplasms; intermediate filament inclusions; round, vesicular nucleus with one large nucleolus	VIM+, CK+, DES−, MSA−, NFP−, LCA−	Bundles of cytoplasmic intermediate filaments

*Includes the Askin thoracopulmonary tumor, Ewing's sarcoma, and peripheral neuroepithelioma.
− = negative; + = positive; ± = variable; NSE = neuron-specific enolase; NFP = neurofibrillary protein; VIM = vimentin; DES = desmin; LCA = leukocyte common antigen; MSA = muscle-specific actin; CK = cytokeratin; β_2MG = anti-β_2-microglobulin.
Modified from Isaacs H Jr. Tumors of the Newborn and Infant, p 19. St. Louis: Mosby–Year Book, 1991.

to 67% for the older patients.[296] Eight years later, the Intergroup Rhabdomyosarcoma Study presented the clinicopathological findings in 13 neonatal cases.[238] Patients with so-called caudal rhabdomyosarcomas (involving the buttock/sacrococcygeal area, perirectal region, bladder, or vagina) had the most favorable outcome. The 3-year survival rate for neonates with caudal tumors was 86%, as compared to 14% for those with tumors arising from noncaudal sites (see Table 4–4). The overall survival rate was low: 49% at 3 years. Although 50% survived, the tumor group (stage), tumor size, histologic type (embryonal, botryoid, or undifferentiated), or form of surgery apparently had no bearing on prognosis. However, certain microscopic findings did correlate with outcome. The presence of necrosis and the small round cell pattern, regardless of the type of rhabdomyosarcoma, was associated with a poor prognosis.[238] None of 8 neonates with rhabdomyosarcomas described by Campbell et al. survived with surgery, with or without chemotherapy and/or radiation therapy,[60] and only 1 of 3 neonates with extremity lesions who were included in the Royal Hospital for Sick Children, Glasgow study survived.[100]

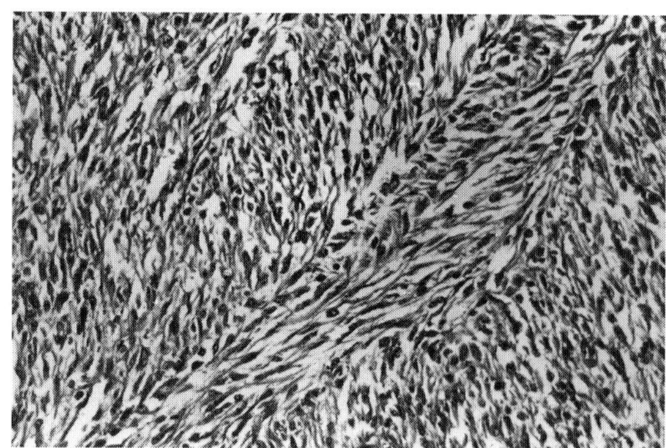

Figure 4–30. Embryonal rhabdomyosarcoma, spindle-cell variant. Biopsy examination of a large, unresectable, pelvic mass arising from the prostate and urinary bladder in a 6-month-old boy revealed a tumor that consisted of spindle-shaped rhabdomyoblasts displaying an interdigitating (herringbone) growth pattern (hematoxylin-eosin, ×300). (From Isaacs H Jr. Tumors of the Newborn and Infant. St. Louis: Mosby–Year Book, 1991.)

RHABDOID TUMOR

Rhabdoid tumor of the kidney was identified as a neoplasm distinct from Wilms' tumor in

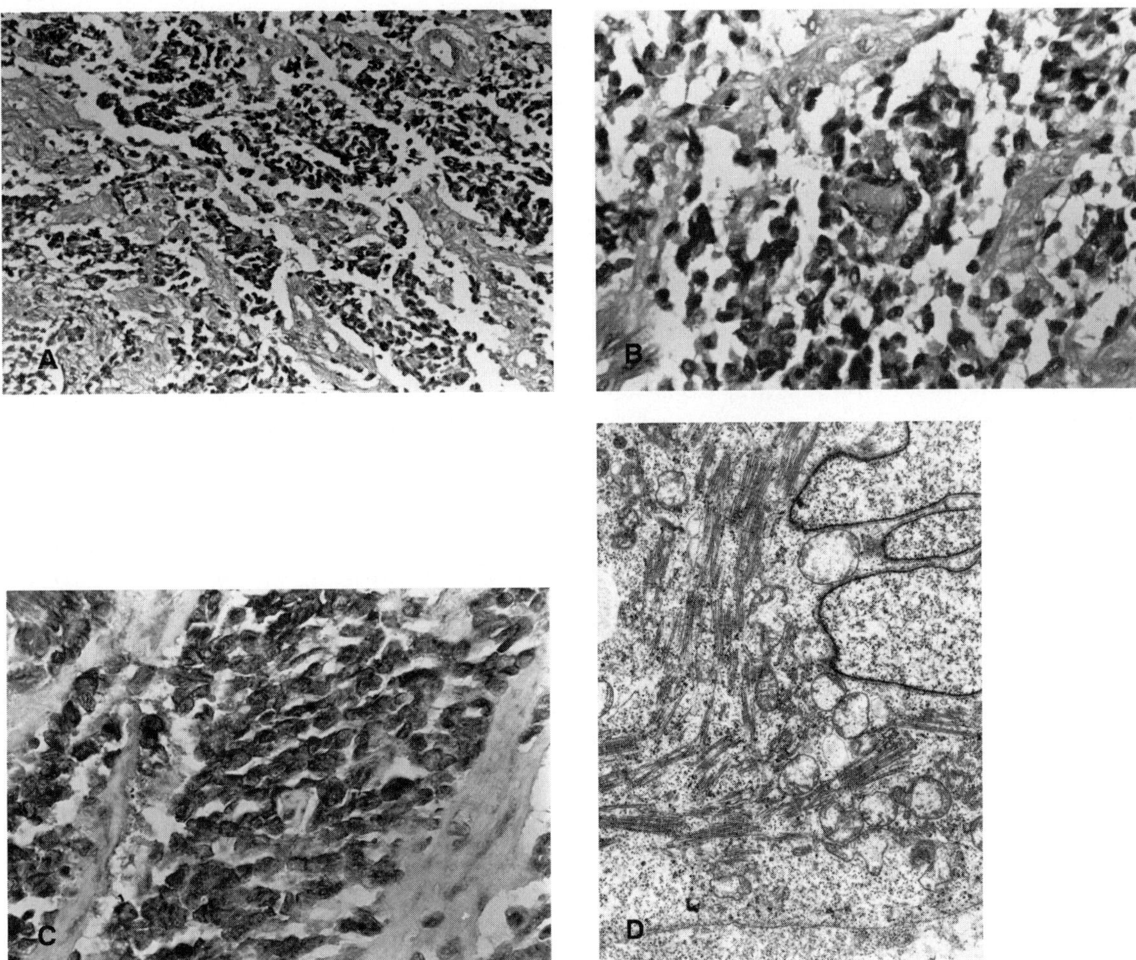

Figure 4–31. Alveolar rhabdomyosarcoma in a 7-month-old boy with a thigh mass and metastases to the lip and cervical lymph nodes. *A,* Small, darkly staining, tumor cells are situated in alveolar-like spaces separated by slightly vascular fibrous septa (hematoxylin-eosin, ×300). *B,* At higher magnification, the variable morphology of the tumor cells is revealed. There is a tumor giant cell in the center of the field (hematoxylin-eosin, ×750). *C,* The tumor cells stain positively for skeletal muscle markers (desmin immunoperoxidase, ×750). *D,* An ultrastructural study shows diagnostic cytoplasmic myofilaments (×18,000). (Photomicrograph courtesy of Darkin Chan, Children's Hospital, Los Angeles, CA.) (From Isaacs H Jr. Tumors of the Newborn and Infant. St. Louis: Mosby–Year Book, 1991.)

Table 4–6. Intergroup Rhabdomyosarcoma Study Clinical Grouping (Staging) System

Clinical Group	Definition
I	A: Localized, completely resected, confined to the site of origin
	B: Localized, completely resected, infiltrated beyond the site of origin
II	A: Localized, grossly resected, microscopic residual
	B: Regional disease, involved lymph nodes, grossly resected
	C: Regional disease, involved lymph nodes, grossly resected with microscopic residual
III	A: Local or regional grossly visible disease after biopsy only
	B: Grossly visible disease after ≥50% resection of primary tumor
IV	Distant metastases present at the time of diagnosis

From Raney RB Jr, Hays DM, Tefft M, et al. Rhabdomyosarcoma and the undifferentiated sarcomas. *In* Pizzo PA, Poplack DG (eds): Principles and Practice of Pediatric Oncology, 2nd ed, p 769. Philadelphia: JB Lippincott, 1993. Used by permission.

the 1970s.[369] The tumor was given the name "rhabdoid" because microscopically, it resembles a rhabdomyosarcoma although it does not exhibit skeletal muscle components either by immunohistochemical analysis or by electron microscopy (see Table 4–5). This highly malignant neoplasm, characterized clinically by early metastases and a high mortality rate, occurs in the newborn and during the first year of life, and only rarely in older age groups (see Chapter 11, "Renal Tumors"). Rhabdoid tumor is found in the soft tissues, skin, central nervous system, heart, genitourinary tract, and other extrarenal sites.[99,240,330,335,360] Familial cases have been reported to occur in siblings.[240]

Diagnosis of the extrarenal rhabdoid tumor depends on its morphologic resemblance to the classic rhabdoid tumor of the kidney, namely, the presence of cells with abundant cytoplasm, a large round nucleolus, and filamentous cytoplasmic inclusions.[282] However, it should be mentioned that Parham and co-workers found that rhabdoid cells occur in a variety of tumors of known origin, raising a question as to the validity of the diagnosis of some extrarenal rhabdoid tumors.[282] Nevertheless, tumors exhibiting the histologic features of rhabdoid tumors are associated with perhaps the worst prognoses of all pediatric neoplasms, regardless of the age at diagnosis.

The frequency of rhabdoid tumor is very low compared to other soft tissue malignant lesions in childhood. Only 26 examples of this tumor (0.9%) were found among 3000 childhood sarcomas entered in the Intergroup Rhabdomyosarcoma Studies I–III;[213] 11 of the 26 (42%) occurred in infants. Only one such tumor was diagnosed in the 0- to 3-month-old age group, in a 2-month-old male infant with a thigh lesion (clinical group III) (see Table 4–6). These studies showed that the tumor most frequently involved the soft tissues of the proximal extremities, trunk, and retroperitoneal area.[213] A later series by Parham et al., which included 42 children and adults, identified 6 infants whose tumors were either congenital or diagnosed before 3 months of age.[281] The tumors occurred in a variety of locations, including ankle soft tissue, scalp, lip, forehead, neck, and skin of the shoulder.

Other patients who were diagnosed with soft tissue rhabdoid tumors at 3 months of age or younger have been described. The primary sites affected are the upper arm, foot, chest wall (2 examples), forehead, and thymus.[99,150,213,230,]

[240,335,360] One soft tissue tumor of the chest wall described by Gonzalez-Crussi et al. occurred in a stillborn infant with disseminated metastases; the other patient in their study was a newborn with a tumor on the dorsum of the foot who died of multiple metastases.[150]

On histologic examination, rhabdoid tumors of the soft tissues are similar to those involving the kidney.[213,335,360] However, the histogenesis of both the renal and extrarenal tumors remains unknown. The tumors consist of polygonal cells with large, vesicular nuclei that characteristically have one large, round nucleolus and an eosinophilic-staining cytoplasm containing inclusions composed of intermediate filaments, which can be demonstrated by electron microscopy and by immunohistochemical analysis (see Fig. 11–17).[213,360] The tumor cells are reactive to vimentin, keratin, and epithelial membrane antigen, but nonreactive to the muscle antibodies desmin and actin. Tsokos et al., however, reported neural and muscle markers, in addition to vimentin, keratin, and epithelial membrane antigen positivity, in some of their renal and extrarenal rhabdoid tumors, and proposed that the tumors "express a diverse morphological and immunocytochemical phenotype."[357] Perhaps it is findings like these that concerned Parham and associates regarding the validity of the separate diagnosis of extrarenal rhabdoid tumor.[282]

Patients with renal and extrarenal rhabdoid tumors experience a similarly discouraging clinical course characterized by early metastases and a poor response to therapy.[335] The survival time for patients with rhabdoid tumor is short, usually less than 6 months. It is significant that many infants with this malignant tumor are at an advanced stage of disease (i.e., clinical group III or IV) at the time of diagnosis. The main sites of metastases in patients with extrarenal rhabdoid tumors are the lungs, liver, and lymph nodes.[335]

Only 1 of 10 infants with rhabdoid tumors in the Intergroup Rhabdomyosarcoma Study survived, and 1 was lost to follow-up evaluation. The tumor in the infant who lived was staged as clinical group I, whereas the others were classified as either stage III or IV.[213] It is impossible to determine accurately the survival rate for the six patients reported by Parham et al. because follow-up data on three of these patients were not available; there was one death and two others survived. The infants with the soft tissue tumors of the scalp and shoulder had widespread metastases at the time of diagnosis.[282]

SMOOTH MUSCLE TUMORS

Smooth muscle tumors are unusual in the pediatric age group.[45,221,350] In perusing the literature, one finds only isolated case reports and very few series. Botting and co-workers described two infants with congenital leiomyomas of the skin and subcutaneous tissue.[45] Cutaneous smooth muscle lesions are described occasionally in the neonate, but these are probably best regarded as hamartomas (i.e., overgrowths of smooth muscle bundles in the lower dermis associated with arrector pili muscles, rather than true leiomyomas)[128] (see Chapter 5, "Tumors and Tumor-Like Conditions of the Skin"). The gastrointestinal tract is the most common site for smooth muscle tumors in the perinatal period, followed by the skin and soft tissues.[11,39,143,270,350] It is likely that some smooth muscle tumors reported in newborns are actually myofibromatoses, which are far more prevalent in this age group.

The distal ileum and transverse colon are the most frequent locations for neonatal smooth muscle tumors of the gastrointestinal tract.[11,39,270] Clinical findings are variable, and may include an abdominal mass, intestinal obstruction, and perforation. Neonatal intestinal obstruction following an intrauterine perforation, and the development of a meconium cyst has been described.[11,270] Angel et al. described a 4-month-old male infant who presented with an ileocecal intussusception secondary to a leiomyosarcoma that had metastasized to the liver.[11]

Leiomyosarcoma of the soft tissues is a very uncommon tumor in infants and children.[11,350] Although leiomyosarcomas in this age group have clinicopathologic features that are similar to those occurring in adults, they may be mistaken for neoplasms of myofibroblastic or fibroblastic origin. Because of this, the diagnosis of leiomyosarcoma in the young is established with some difficulty.[350] Moreover, some cases that have been described as leiomyosarcomas in the newborn, particularly those whose primary site is in the intestine, are most likely myofibromatoses, which are associated with a favorable outcome. To compound the problem, the histologic criteria for distinguishing leiomyoma from leiomyosarcoma are unclear. A large tumor and increased mitotic activity are features that are considered to suggest malignancy.[221] If a prominent vascular pattern and necrosis with calcification are present, then the diagnosis would be myofibromatosis, rather than a true smooth muscle tumor.

Swanson and colleagues reviewed 34 cases of childhood leiomyosarcoma, including 6 cases of their own.[350] Of the 34 patients, 3 were younger than 3 months of age. The scalp was the most common site, followed by the thigh; all three of these patients survived. Electron microscopy, considered in conjunction with immunohistochemical findings (namely, positive reactivity to vimentin, desmin, and actin), is helpful in establishing the diagnosis. The light microscopic findings are essentially the same as those for leiomyosarcomas found in adults; that is, small, pleomorphic, spindle-shaped cells arranged in interwoven bundles (herringbone pattern).[221,350]

ADIPOSE TISSUE TUMORS

Tumors of fatty tissue origin are not as common in infants and children as they are in adults, in whom they are the most common soft tissue neoplasms.[104,128] Benign adipose tissue tumors are classified into several categories:[128] lipoma (single, multiple, superficial, and deep); variants of lipoma, such as lipoblastoma and angiomyolipoma; heterotopic lipoma (e.g., intramuscular and intermuscular lipoma and neural fibrolipoma); infiltrating proliferations of mature fat cells (lipomatosis); and hibernoma, a benign neoplasm of brown fat.[128] Neural fibrolipomas frequently occur in young patients as a component of spinal dysraphic malformation (myelomeningocele).[187]

Lipoblastoma occurs in infancy and during the first 3 years of life, and sometimes is diagnosed at birth.[275] It is a benign tumor composed of immature adipose tissue that may be confused with myxoid liposarcoma.[73,128] Moreover, morphologically, both neoplasms resemble developing adipose tissue.[42] Associations with syndromes, malformations or other tumors have not been described.[85] Liposarcoma occurring in the first year of life was the subject of an isolated case report; the youngest patient in the AFIP's series of 17 children was 8 months of age.[321]

Of a total of 102 soft tissue tumors occurring in infants, 23 were diagnosed as lipomas and 2 were classified as lipoblastomas. The extremities were involved in 7 cases and the spermatic cord was involved in 14 cases. These were the main locations of the lipomas, whereas the shoulder and back were the primary sites of the lipoblastomas.[187] Lipomas of the buttock and thigh were the only perinatal adipose tissue

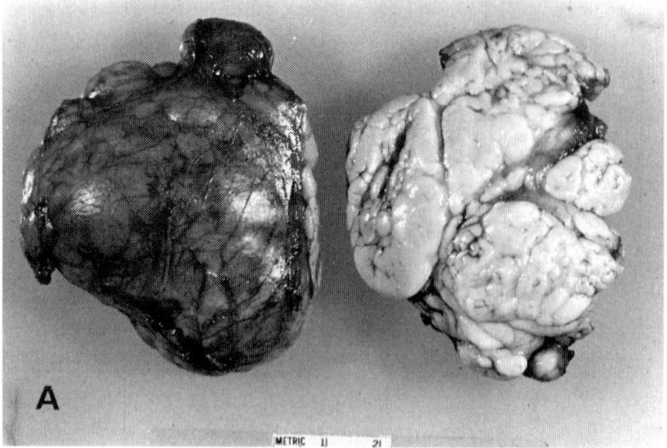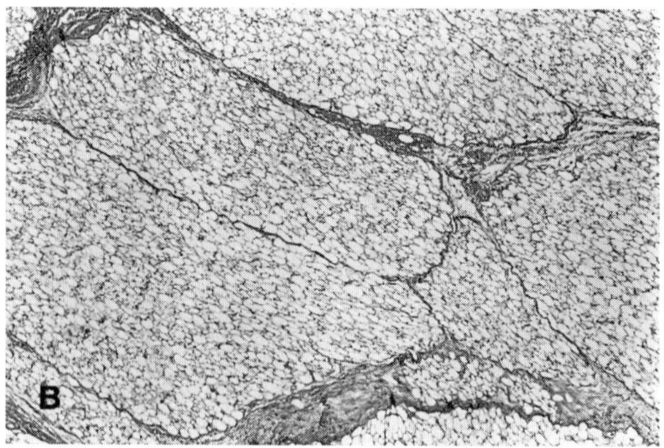

Figure 4–32. Lipoma. A mass measuring 6 × 5.5 cm was present for several months before being removed from the right side of the neck of a 6-month-old boy. *A,* The cut surface demonstrates the typical lobular pattern seen in lipomas. *B,* A low-power view displays the lobular pattern and the uniform, mature fat cells comprising the lesion (hematoxylin-eosin, ×48). (From Isaacs H Jr. Tumors of the Newborn and Infant. St. Louis: Mosby–Year Book, 1991.)

tumors noted (see Table 4–2). In a Minneapolis study, 4 of 57 (7%) soft tissue tumors in infants younger than 3 months of age were lipoblastomas, and all occurred on the trunk.[80] The largest series of lipoblastomas, consisting of 35 cases, was reported by the AFIP; 3 of these cases were diagnosed at birth.[73] The tumor most often involved the soft tissues of the lower and upper extremities. Lipoblastoma was defined as a circumscribed form, whereas the term lipoblastomatosis referred to the diffuse type of this tumor.[73] The diffuse type usually arises in deep soft tissue, has an infiltrative growth pattern, and has an increased tendency for recurrence. The neoplasm may compress or impair function of adjacent structures because of its size and location. Congenital lipoblastoma involving the eyelid, face, hand, and finger has been described.[122,254]

Lipoma

Both the clinical features and the pathologic appearance of a lipoma is essentially the same in infants as in older children and adults.[73,187] Most lipomas present as slowly growing, painless, soft, subcutaneous masses (Fig. 4–32). Less than one third are noted at birth.

Lipoblastoma

Lipoblastomas tend to grow slightly more rapidly than lipomas, have a much firmer consistency, and are paler and more myxoid or greyish in appearance than a typical lipoma on cross section (Fig. 4–33*A*). The tumors range in diameter from 2 cm to more than 14 cm.[73,187]

Microscopic examination reveals immature fat cells with varying degrees of differentiation that are separated by connective tissue septa and loose, greyish, myxoid areas. The presence of lipoblasts with a bubbly, vacuolated cytoplasm is a requisite for the diagnosis. Mitoses are not seen. In some instances, the underlying skeletal muscle is involved. More than half of the tumors consist of mature fat cells, and thus have the appearance of a lipoma (Fig. 4–33*B* and *C*). The absence of mitoses and nuclear atypia help to distinguish lipoblastoma from liposarcoma, which has not been documented in the newborn. Immunoperoxidase studies performed on lipoblastoma show that the tumor cells react positively to S-100 protein but are nonreactive to antibodies to vimentin, actin, Leu-7, and factor VIII.[85] The ultrastructural features of lipoblastoma are those of developing fat cells, as discussed by Greco and associates,[157] Gaffney and colleagues,[136] and Bolen and Thorning[42] (see Fig. 4–1*B*).

Lipoblastomas and lipoma are cured by complete excision of the mass, and generally are associated with a favorable outcome.[141,245] Chung and Enzinger quoted a low recurrence rate (14%), which they attributed to incomplete removal.[73] Sequential biopsies demonstrate that some lipoblastomas spontaneously mature to lipomas, which probably accounts for their good prognosis despite an inadequate excision.[42,73,85,245]

PERIPHERAL NERVOUS SYSTEM TUMORS

The peripheral nervous system tumors are considered to originate from the neural crest

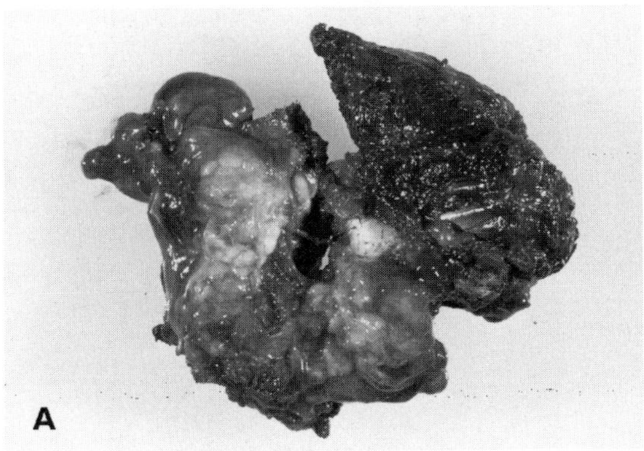

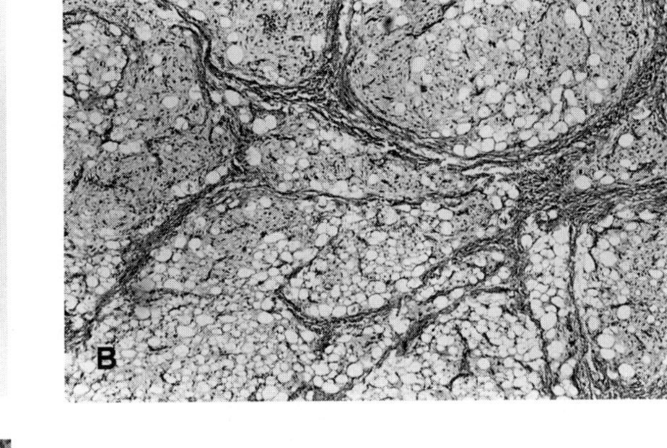

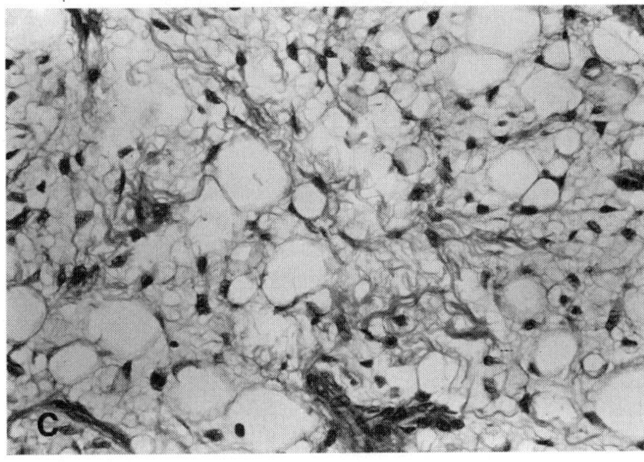

Figure 4–33. Lipoblastoma. *A,* A mass measuring 4×2 cm was removed from the back of a 1-year-old girl. The tumor had a tan to yellow, nodular cut surface. *B,* The tumor has a lobular pattern consisting mostly of immature fat cells and myxoid areas separated by fibrous septa (hematoxylin-eosin, $\times 120$). *C,* Vacuolated lipoblasts are situated in myxoid areas (hematoxylin-eosin, $\times 600$). (From Isaacs H Jr. Tumors of the Newborn and Infant. St. Louis: Mosby–Year Book, 1991.)

and include a wide variety of both benign and malignant conditions.[1,43,79,91,104,128,140,164,165,173,200,218,294,323,341,379] Not all tumors assigned to this group occur in the newborn. However, neurofibroma and the primitive neuroectodermal tumor (PNET), melanotic PNET, ectomesenchymoma, and malignant "triton" tumors are the ones that have been described.[50,200,212] Schwannoma (neurilemoma) and malignant peripheral nerve sheath tumors (malignant schwannoma, neurofibrosarcoma) are uncommon before adolescence.[103,128] Nevertheless, a few examples of congenital malignant peripheral nerve sheath tumors are reported.[248,252,253] Of the malignant soft tissue tumors in infants younger than 3 months of age included in the University of Minnesota series, peripheral PNET ranked second in frequency, following congenital fibrosarcoma (see Table 4–1).[80]

Although melanotic neuroectodermal tumor of infancy, intra-abdominal desmoplastic small cell tumor, and polyphenotypic small cell tumors share some histologic, immunohistochemical, and ultrastructural features with PNET and Ewing's sarcoma, their relationship otherwise has not been clearly defined.[108]

Neurofibroma

Neurofibroma occurs either as a single dermal or soft tissue mass, or as multiple tumors in association with cafe-au-lait spots and neurofibromatosis type 1, an autosomal dominant disorder (von Recklinghausen's disease).[307] Some neurofibromas are evident at birth, whereas others are not observed until later on in childhood, adolescence, or adulthood (Fig. 4–34). Essentially, they occur in any area in the body where nerve fibers are found. About 50% of individuals with neurofibromatosis have evidence of the disease at birth, with the most common sign being the cafe-au-lait spot.[12,93] Occasionally, in the newborn, neurofibromas may present clinically in extraordinary ways, such as congenital stridor resulting from a laryngeal tumor or an airway obstruction secondary to tracheal compression;[100,291] such cases represent part of a "congenital neurocristopathy," occurring together with neuroblastoma and Schwannoma and manifesting as episodes of apnea and cyanosis or bilateral proptosis secondary to orbital tumors,[294] progressive respiratory obstruction secondary to rapidly growing

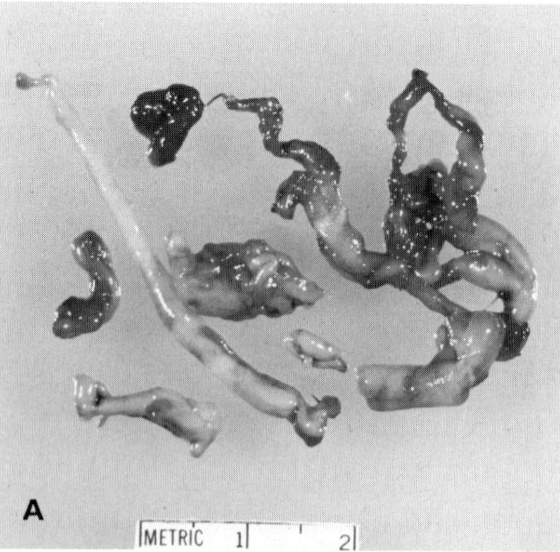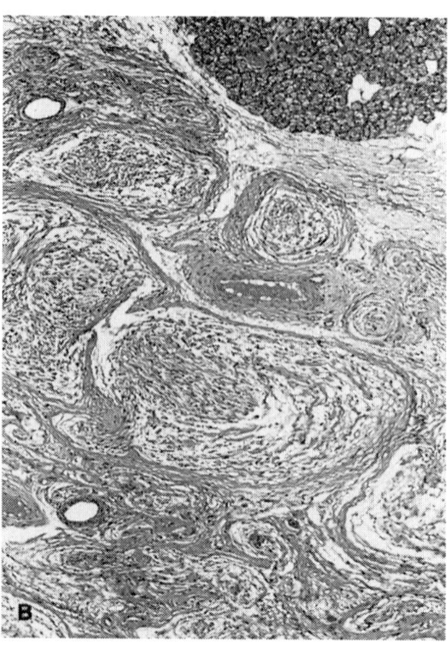

Figure 4–34. Plexiform neurofibroma. A 1-year-old boy with neurofibromatosis had a disfiguring mass involving the face and forehead that had been present since birth. *A,* The excised specimen consists of several elongated, white, shiny, wormlike pieces of tissue. *B,* The tumor consists of enlarged, myxoid-appearing nerve trunks with proliferations of neurites and Schwann cells. A portion of the parotid gland is seen in the upper righthand corner (hematoxylin-eosin, ×120). The face and parotid gland are common sites for this lesion in young children. (From Isaacs H Jr. Tumors of the Newborn and Infant. St. Louis: Mosby–Year Book, 1991.)

neurofibromas of the tongue, oval cavity, neck, and mediastinum,[12] and fetal hydrops with compression of the neck vessels by tumor leading to intractable generalized edema.[382]

According to the study of Matsui et al., the risk for glioma and malignant schwannoma is significantly increased in children with neurofibromatosis type 1, as is the risk for rhabdomyosarcoma, neuroblastoma, and acute myelogenous leukemia.[248] In the Japan Children's Cancer Registry review, 56 children with cancer had neurofibromatosis type 1, a frequency rate of 0.21%. The incidence of optic nerve glioma in patients with neurofibromatosis type 1 was 12.5%, whereas the incidence for other tumors was as follows: central nervous system gliomas, 0.9%; malignant schwannoma, 31.4%; rhabdomyosarcoma, 1.36%; and acute myelocytic leukemia, 0.27%.[248] That study included two neonates, one with an abdominal neuroblastoma and another with a retroperitoneal malignant schwannoma.

Cases have been described that suggest a clinically recognizable neurocristophy linking neuroblastoma and neurofibromatosis.[293,294,382] Qualman et al. documented two examples of neonatal neurofibromatosis with biopsy-proven neurofibromas and cafe-au-lait spots noted at birth.[294] In addition, at postmortem examination, multiple Schwann cell tumors and neuroblastomas involving the orbit, neck, posterior mediastinum, and retroperitoneum were found in a midline or bilaterally symmetric pattern in one 3-month-old female infant. Composite tumors were noted also in the genitourinary tract (prostate) in their other patient. Similar examples of peripheral nerve tumors and neuroblastoma-ganglioneuroblastoma occurring in a midline and symmetric distribution within the adrenals and sympathetic ganglia have been reported in aborted fetuses and stillborn infants.[293,294] Moreover, according to Bolande and Towler, a neurofibroma early in its development may histologically resemble a differentiating neuroblastoma.[41]

Neurofibromas are classified into several histologic types: solitary, plexiform, and diffuse.[128] On microscopic examination, the solitary type is seen to consist of neurites, Schwann cells, and collagen bundles surrounded by a pale-staining myxoid stroma. The plexiform neurofibroma—the hallmark of von Recklinghausen's disease—resembles a bunch of pale white worms on gross inspection, and microscopic examination reveals expansion of nerve fibers by irregular, tortuous, haphazardly arranged proliferations of Schwann cells, neurites, and collagen fibers with a pale-staining stroma (see

Fig. 4–34). The diffuse form occurs in children with or without neurofibromatosis, as well as in association with congenital melanocytic nevi with neural differentiation. The diffuse neurofibroma subtly infiltrates the lower dermis and subcutaneous tissue as a firm, homogeneous, white mass and, on histologic examination, is found to consist of small, round to oval Schwann cells, wavy neurites, and a pale-staining connective tissue stroma. Because of their infiltrative nature, large tumors cannot be excised completely and recurrences are common.

Skeletal malformations are noted in less than 50% of the patients with neurofibromatosis.[91,128] Spinal deformities, including vertebral dysplasia and kyphoscoliosis, are the most frequent bone abnormalities, followed in frequency by congenital tibial pseudoarthrosis.[91] Congenital tibial pseudoarthrosis is a relatively common related skeletal condition. Essentially, the lesion consists of nonunion of the tibia secondary to an in utero fracture. There is extensive fibrosis between the bones in the fracture site, resulting in a false joint (pseudarthrosis). Occasionally, synovia-lined spaces are noted in the area of fibrosis. However, neurofibroma is not identified in the fracture site per se. En bloc resection or, rarely, amputation may be required to treat the pseudarthrosis because the fractured ends generally fail to heal properly.[187]

Several other neoplasms have been described in association with neurofibromatosis, including ganglioneuroma, pheochromocytoma, benign and malignant schwannoma (neurofibrosarcoma), rhabdomyosarcoma, Wilms' tumor, and leukemia.[22,79,128,165,294,341] Although primarily a condition of adults, malignant peripheral nerve sheath tumors have been described in infants and children as well.[252,253] The AFIP reported nine cases of a peripheral nerve sheath tumor variant called plexiform malignant peripheral nerve sheath tumor, two of which were congenital. Both tumors occurred in boys. One, which was located in the orbital region, proved fatal within 6 months; the other newborn with a lesion in the right leg survived. On microscopic examination, the tumor is seen to be well circumscribed, with expanding margins and nodules having a nodular and plexiform appearance with fibrous septa. The tumor has a hypercellular appearance consisting of spindle-shaped cells with a low to medium mitotic rate. The cellular areas resemble fibrosarcoma. Nuclear pallisading and a storiform pattern are also observed in some tumors. According to the authors, this neoplasm should be considered to be a low-grade, locally aggressive malignant tumor with a tendency to recur.[253] The clinical behavior of the plexiform malignant peripheral nerve sheath tumor appears to be somewhat less aggressive than other malignant peripheral nerve sheath tumors in children. A wide local excision and close follow-up monitoring for recurrence constitute the recommended therapeutic approach.[253]

Granular Cell Tumor

Granular cell tumor (congenital epulis) is a neoplasm of controversial histogenesis that is found primarily in the gingiva of newborns and infants.[104,128,222,223,235,283] Two forms of granular cell tumor have been defined: (1) the classical congenital epulis that involves the gums and (2) another form that involves the skin; the mucosa of the respiratory, gastrointestinal, and genitourinary tracts; and various sites throughout the body, usually in older children and adults.[128,222,283] A neural origin has been proposed for the granular cell tumor found in older individuals because of its close relationship to nerves and its immunohistochemical and ultrastructural properties.[128] However, granular cell tumor of the newborn may have a different histogenesis.[283,361]

In their review of congenital granular cell tumor, Lack et al. culled 60 cases reported since 1910 and added 21 cases of their own.[223] The granular cell tumor arises as one or more mucosal-covered nodules from the gingiva of the anterior alveolar ridge and gum line of either the mandible or the maxilla; it occurs predominantly in female patients. Occasionally, the tongue is involved. In rarer instances, the tumor may grow in utero to such an extent that it presents as a large mass attached to the gingiva of the upper jaw, causing airway obstruction and feeding problems, thereby mimicking an epignathic teratoma (Fig. 4–35).[66,130,187,223,297] Nasal flattening and asymmetry are associated with nasal obstruction by large tumors.[297] Congenital granular cell tumor with systemic involvement occurred in a male fetus of 29-weeks' gestational age.[283] The pregnancy was terminated after fetal hydrops was discovered on ultrasonography. In addition to the gingival lesions, multinodular tumors were found within the kidney and in the heart, lungs, esophagus, intestines, thyroid, adre-

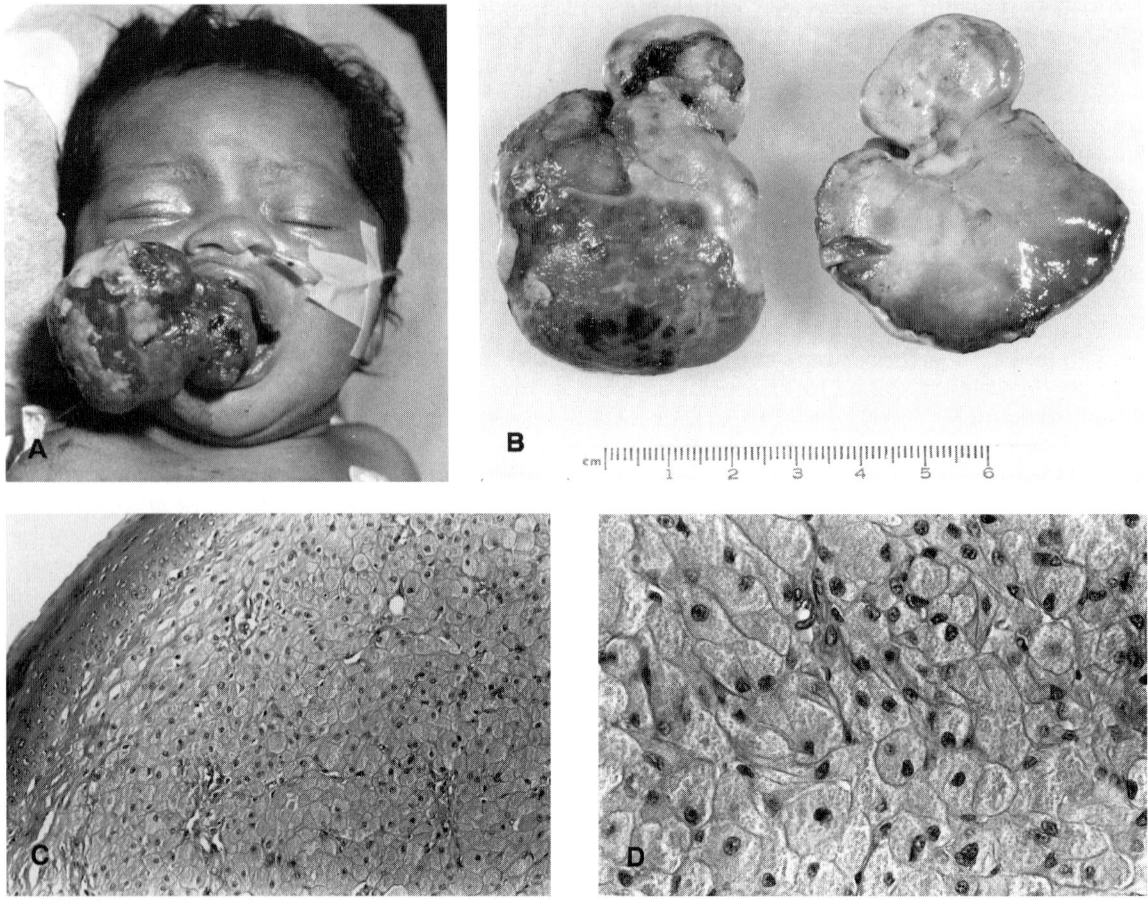

Figure 4–35. Congenital epulis (gingival granular cell tumor). A 5-day-old, full-term female infant delivered by cesarean section was born with a mass arising from the upper midline gingiva and alveolar ridge. *A,* The mass is seen to obstruct the oral cavity. *B,* The tumor, measuring 6 × 5.5 cm and weighing 39 g, has a uniform, gelatinous, and gray-tan to yellow cut surface. *C,* Closely packed, polygonal granular cells with prominent cell membranes are situated beneath the mucosa (hematoxylin-eosin, ×120). *D,* The tumor cells have characteristic cytoplasmic granules and regular, round nuclei with inconspicuous nucleoli. The granules stain positive with periodic acid–Schiff (hematoxylin-eosin, ×480). (From Isaacs H Jr. Tumors of the Newborn and Infant. St. Louis: Mosby–Year Book, 1991.)

nals, spleen, urinary bladder, testis, pituitary, and leptomeninges.[283] This case is unique in the English medical literature.

Granular cell tumors are composed of polygonal cells with pink, granular cytoplasms and regular, round, dark, basophilic-staining nuclei (Fig. 4–35 *C* and *D*). The granules are periodic acid–Schiff (PAS)–positive and diastase-resistant. Acid phosphatase is strongly positive within the tumor cells.[222] Immunostaining is reactive with vimentin and nonreactive with S-100 protein, smooth and skeletal muscle, and histiocytic markers. The ultrastructural features of the congenital granular cell tumor include membrane-bound, pleomorphic, cytoplasmic granules, cell membranes, and intermediate filaments with fusiform electron densities that are consistent with myofibroblasts.[283,361]

Granular cell tumors are cured by simple excision. Spontaneous regression has also been documented following incomplete removal or no surgical treatment at all.[192,223] Therefore, conservative management is recommended, provided there are no feeding or airway problems in the neonate or reason to doubt the diagnosis.[192]

Primitive Neuroectodermal Tumor

The PNET is a small cell malignant neoplasm that occurs in the central and peripheral nervous systems and soft tissues.[106,179,320,355] The category of PNET comprises a wide variety of neoplasms, including entities such as medulloblastoma, retinoblastoma, neuroblastoma, Askin thoracopulmonary tumor, melanotic PNET of the jaws, and peripheral neuroepithelioma of the soft tissues.[106,179]

Previously, peripheral small cell malignant tumors with neuronal differentiation were considered to be the same as neuroblastomas, but recent studies have revealed that the former are indeed biologically distinct neoplasms, although both are thought to be of neural crest origin. Moreover, PNET and neuroblastoma exhibit similar histologic, immunohistochemical, and ultrastructural findings. Because their clinical behavior and treatment differ considerably from the other small blue tumors of childhood, accurate diagnosis is essential.[280] Table 4–5 lists the histopathologic differential diagnoses.

Advances in histopathology and genetics reveal that entities, such as Ewing's sarcoma (both osseous and extraosseous), PNET of bone, small cell malignant tumor of the thoracopulmonary region (Askin tumor), and neuroepithelioma, are probably histogenetically related and, therefore, would fall into the category of the primitive neuroectodermal tumor.[103,135,355] Moreover, neuronal differentiation is observed on electron microscopy and immunohistochemical analysis. The former shows the presence of neurosecretory granules and neurofilaments, whereas the latter reveals reactivity to S-100 protein and neuron-specific enolase (NSE), in addition to vimentin. In addition, cytogenetic findings are practically the same: a t(11;22) (q24;q11–12) chromosomal translocation.[135,179,320,356] Both PNET and Ewing's sarcoma express P-glycoprotein, a transmembrane protein, which functions in the transport of substances (e.g., drugs) across cell membranes.[174] Multidrug resistance is thought to be mediated by P-glycoprotein. Rhabdomyosarcoma and other malignant lesions are immunoreactive with this protein also.[174] According to Pappo et al., peripheral neuroepithelioma (PNET) can be differentiated immunohistochemically from neuroblastoma on the basis of HBA71 and anti-β_2-microglobulin antibodies, which are reactive in the former tumor and unreactive in neuroblastoma (Table 4–5).[280]

PNETs are sometimes the cause of death in fetuses and infants.[18,98,102,162,320] The chest wall, extremities, and face are the primary sites.[98,320,366] It is conceivable that some chest wall and pulmonary PNETs are actually the same entity as Askin tumor (see Chapter 17, "Tumors of the Lung").

Voss et al. described a 3-month-old female infant who presented with an enlarging mass in the left arm (biceps muscle) and liver metastases at the time of diagnosis.[366] Despite chemotherapy, the patient developed brain metastases 11 months later. The urinary vanillylmandelic (VMA) levels were moderately elevated, but the homovanillic acid (HVA) levels were not. Microscopically, the tumor consisted of small cells with scant cytoplasms, vesicular nuclei, and inconspicuous nucleoli. Abundant pink fibrillary material and numerous irregular pseudorosettes were present. Rare dense-core granules, microfilaments, and macula adherens–type junctions were found ultrastructurally. This case illustrates the biologically aggressive nature of the PNET, which is generally refractive to therapy and is responsible for a rapidly progressive, downhill course. PNET and rhabdoid tumor are probably the two most highly malignant tumors of childhood.

Melanotic Neuroectodermal Tumor of Infancy

Difficulty in deciding the cellular origin (histogenesis) of the unique pigmented neoplasm called melanotic neuroectodermal tumor of infancy has led to a multitude of interesting names, including melanotic progonoma, retinal anlage tumor, melanotic adamantinoma, pigmented neuroectodermal tumor, and pigmented congenital epulis.[6,76,95,111,128,229,349] Odontogenic, neural tube, pineal, and retinal origins have been postulated but have not been documented. However, studies suggest that the melanotic neuroectodermal tumor shares certain biochemical, immunohistochemical, and morphologic features with other neoplasms of neural crest origin.[44,63,95,102,111,229,237,288]

Typically, the melanotic neuroectodermal tumor is seen at birth or during the first year of life as a rapidly growing mass, usually arising from the anterior maxilla and less often from the brain, skull, and mandible (Fig. 4–36).[19,63,95,111] Within the cranium, the anterior fontanelle is the most common site.[19] In addition, it occurs in the oropharynx or outside the head in the soft tissues and epididymis.[63,229,288,308,344] It is reported in association with the fetal hydantoin syndrome.[195] Serum alphafetoprotein and urinary VMA levels are in-

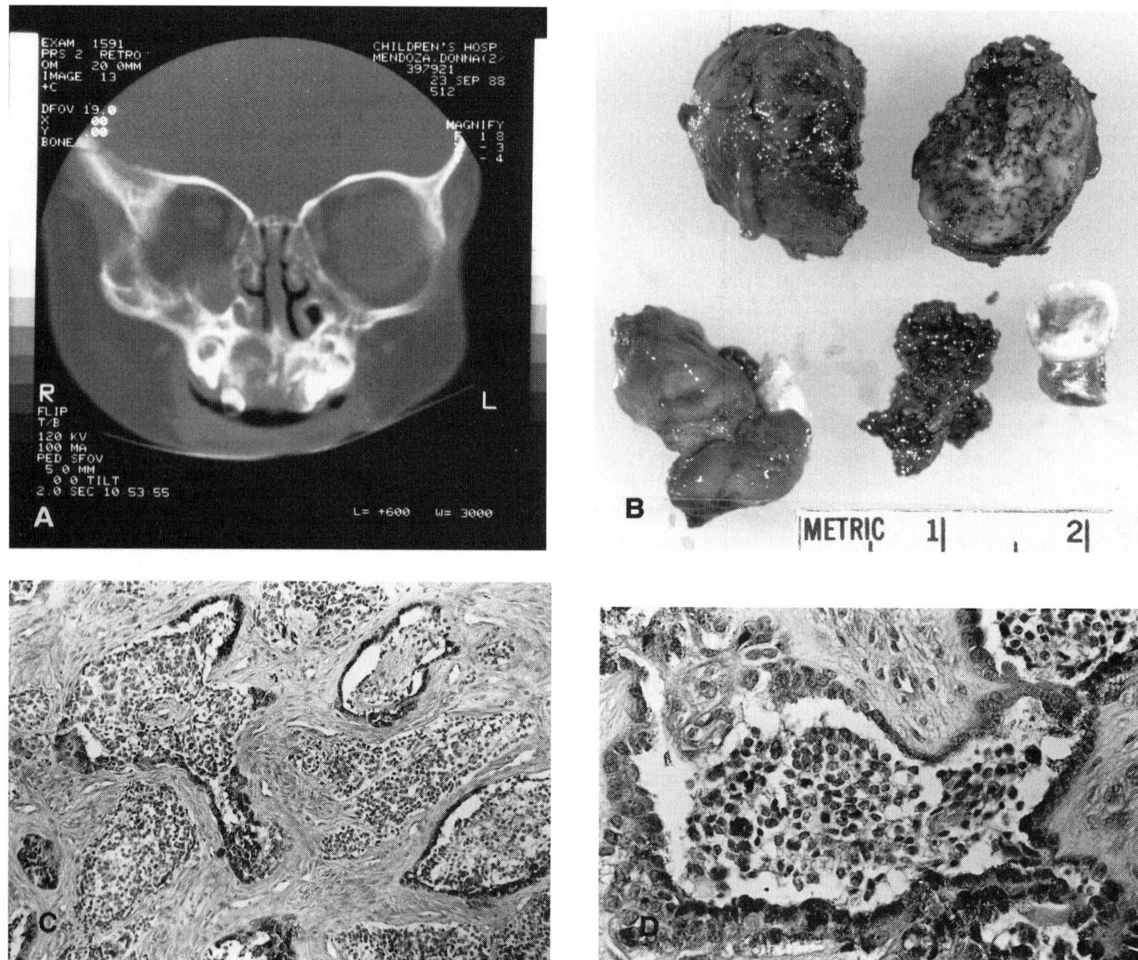

Figure 4–36. Pigmented (melanotic) primitive neuroectodermal tumor. *A,* Magnetic resonance imaging studies were done in a 6-month-old girl with a 2-month history of a mass in the hard palate. The imaging study shows a lytic lesion in the right maxilla and hard palate with erosion of the wall of the inferior orbit and displacement of teeth. *B,* The tumor, which is situated mostly in bone, is tan and firm, with irregular, black, pigmented areas. A tooth is part of the specimen. *C,* A low-power view shows irregular cystic structures containing nests of small, darkly staining cells (neuroblasts) and pigmented melanocytes lining the microcysts (hematoxylin-eosin, ×120). *D,* A view with higher magnification shows the neuroblasts and melanocytes in more detail (hematoxylin-eosin, ×480). (From Isaacs H Jr. Tumors of the Newborn and Infant. St. Louis: Mosby–Year Book, 1991.)

consistently elevated in patients with this tumor.[19,63,111,308]

Cutler and his colleagues collected and tabulated 138 examples of melanotic neuroectodermal tumor of infancy from the literature, including 2 cases of their own.[95] Of these, 54 patients were younger than 3 months of age. The distribution of lesions in this age group were as follows: maxilla (43 cases), mandible (4 cases), skull (3 cases), brain (2 cases), and one case each in the oropharynx and epididymis. Data derived from this study indicate that the tumor arises most often from the maxilla (80%) and seldom metastasizes in the perinatal period (2 of 53 cases, or 3.8%). One patient in the series, originally reported by Lindahl, was a stillborn infant with a maxillary tumor that had spread to the liver, adrenal, and lymph nodes.[237] Dehner et al. described a similar example of a 2-month-old male infant who had a maxillary melanotic neuroectodermal tumor that had not only extensively invaded the paranasal sinuses, orbit, cribriform plate, and floor of the anterior fossa, but also metastasized to the cervical, mediastinal, and periaortic lymph nodes, liver pleura, and peritoneum.[111] Urinary catecholamine levels were not elevated until the time of recurrence. At postmortem examination (and after irradiation and chemotherapy), the grayish-white tumor metastases were composed only of neuroblasts, without the larger melanocytic component.[111] In another report, Shira described a 2-month-old male infant with a maxillary primary tumor and regional lymph node metastases.[327] An additional maxillary melanotic neuroectodermal tumor that behaved in a malignant fashion in a 2-month-old male infant was reported by Shokry and colleagues.[329] The tumor recurred twice, destroying the floor of the right orbit and invading the nasopharynx and oropharynx. As with the case described by Dehner et al.[111] earlier, biopsy samples of the recurrent tumor showed only the neuroblastoma component. These two cases demonstrate the unpredictable nature of this neoplasm.

The Mayo Clinic reported seven patients with melanotic neuroectodermal tumor of infancy; three of these patients were younger than $3\frac{1}{2}$ months of age.[196] All three had maxillary lesions, were treated with surgery, and survived. Two had recurrences. Pettinato et al. reviewed 10 patients with this tumor, 6 of whom were age 3 months or younger at diagnosis.[288] Five of the six tumors arose from the maxilla, and one originated in the mandible. They were treated by local excision; three recurred within 3 months of the initial surgery, but eventually the patients were free of disease.[288] The AFIP reported 20 cases, 6 of which involved infants 3 months of age or younger; all had maxillary primaries treated by excision.[198] Although 5 of the 6 patients experienced recurrences as late as 10 years after the initial surgery, all survived.

The main clinical manifestation of the melanotic neuroectodermal tumor is a mass in the anterior maxilla (in 71% of patients) or in the mandible or anterior fontanelle.[111] Imaging studies reveal a cystic, radiolucent lesion with displacement or destruction of developing teeth (Fig. 4–36A). Occasionally, the tumor occurs outside the craniofacial bones (e.g., in the oropharynx or in the epididymis.[229,308,386] An oropharyngeal mass discovered in a 1-day-old, full-term female infant produced feeding problems and respiratory obstruction requiring a tracheostomy. The tumor involved the lateral pharyngeal wall, soft palate, and the tonsillar fossa. The specimen measured 3×2 cm and consisted mostly of brain tissue. On microscopic examination, astrocytes, oligodendroglia, and choroid plexus were present; in addition, the heterotropic brain tissue contained a nodule composed of neuroblasts and cuboidal epithelial cells with melanin pigment situated in alveolar spaces.[229] Lee et al. proposed that this lesion resulted from a pinching off of both the neural crest and medullary epithelium of the neural tube during the 25–30 somite stage.[229] Two examples of epididymal melanotic neuroectodermal tumor presenting as a scrotal mass have been described in newborns; neither recurrence nor metastases occurred after orchiectomy.[308,386]

Prior to 1985, there were seven known examples of epididymal melanotic neuroectodermal tumor reported in infants and children, all associated with a favorable outcome.[308] Two occurred in patients younger than 2 months of age and presented as asymptomatic scrotal masses.[308,386] Awareness of this infrequent anatomic site is important in the diagnosis of these neoplasms.[288]

On gross examination, the tumor varies in color from gray to black, depending upon the amount of melanin pigment present (Fig. 4–36B). One or more deciduous teeth may be included as part of the specimen when the tumor involves the alveolar process of either the maxilla or mandible.

Histologic examination reveals the melanotic neuroectodermal tumor to consist of two main types of cells situated in irregular, microcystic spaces: a small, dark, round cell resembling a neuroblast, and a slightly larger, paler cell containing melanin pigment (Fig. 4–36C and D). The tumor insidiously infiltrates bone and soft tissues and provokes an exuberant fibrotic and/or gliotic response, depending on its location.

Ultrastructural studies reveal that the small, dark, round cells have the morphologic features of neuroblasts containing neurosecretory granules and neurofilaments, whereas the larger, paler cells are related to melanocytes, as melanosomes are found in their cytoplasm.[63,111,288] Immunohistochemical studies show that the small neuroblastic cells and the larger melanocytic cells are reactive for NSE, synaptophysin, HMB45, and dopamine-β-hydroxylase, and are focally positive for vimentin and cytokeratin; the tumor is nonreactive for neurofilaments, S-100 protein, retinol binding protein, alpha-fetoprotein, and carcinoembryonic antigen (CEA).[198,288,344] Raju et al. examined four melanotic neuroectodermal tumors of infancy by immunohistochemical analysis and compared the results with those in 10 neuroblastomas, 5 retinoblastomas, and 5 retinas, thereby confirming the concept that the melanotic tumor belongs to the family of PNETs.[298] The authors demonstrated that melanotic neuroectodermal tumors display a polyphenotypic profile composed of epithelial antigens (epithelial membrane antigen [EMA], cytokeratin), melanoma-associated antigens (HMB45 and HMB50), and neural antigens (NSE, synaptophysin, neurofilament). In addition, myogenic markers (actin and desmin) are focally present in some of the tumors.[298]

The presence or absence of aneuploid DNA shows little or no correlation with recurrence.[288] Flow cytometric studies are inconclusive, and no definite conclusions can be drawn regarding the usefulness of this procedure in predicting recurrence or metastases.[198]

The clinical behavior of the melanotic PNET is not completely predictable, as was once thought, although previously it was regarded as an innocuous but troublesome lesion.[187] The prognosis of melanotic neuroectodermal tumor is relatively good, provided that it has been completely resected, preferably at the time of the initial surgical procedure.[102,128,288] According to Dehner, the recurrence rate is approximately 15%, and overt malignant behavior is noted in about 5% of cases.[102]

Ectomesenchymoma

Ectomesenchymoma is an unusual neoplasm of divergent differentiation thought to be derived from remnants of migratory pluripotential neural crest cells—the so-called ectomesenchyme—composed of both neuroectodermal and mesenchymal elements.[200,356] The former consists of ganglioneuroma and/or neuroblastoma and Schwann cells and the latter, embryonal rhabdomyosarcoma[207] (Fig. 4–37). Because of its biphasic pattern, it also has been termed gangliorhabdomyosarcoma.[212] Ectomesenchymomas occur predominantly in infants, in whom 77% of the cases are reported.[207]

The tumor is found in a variety of locations, but mainly involves the genitourinary system, perineum, retroperitoneum, and abdominal wall; less often, it is found in the head and neck region and brain (see Fig. 4–37).[186,200,207,212] Immunohistochemical studies reveal that the rhabdomyoblasts are positive for myoglobin, the Schwann cells for S-100 protein, and the ganglion cells and neuroblasts for NSE.[207,212] Ultrastructural studies confirm the presence of both neural and skeletal muscle elements.

Kawamoto et al. reviewed 13 examples of ectomesenchymoma, including 2 of their own cases.[207] Seven patients were younger than 1 year of age, and one was a newborn with a facial lesion who had fatal complications following chemotherapy. Five others survived, and one with a prostatic primary tumor who had been reported previously by Kodet et al. died with pulmonary metastases.[207,212] Patients whose localized tumors are resectable have the best prognosis, whereas those who have tumors that are unresectable or metastasize usually die of their disease.[207]

Polyphenotypic Small Cell Tumor

Even more exotic, complex phenotypic tumors with neural, rhabdoid, skeletal muscle, and epithelial components have been reported. These include the intra-abdominal small cell desmoplastic tumors found in older children[139,149,278] and the congenital temporofacial tumor with PNET, glial, and epithelial elements.[162] Dehner described a newborn with a massive malignant tumor involving the face, neck, and trachea that histologically was characterized by multiple components that he called "polyantigenic small cell tumor with PNET and rhabdoid-like features."[105] The small blue cell tumor was reactive to vimentin and cytokeratin antibodies, in addition to NSE and muscle-specific actin. Additional examples of congenital polyphenotypic small cell tumors include an orbitocranial primary tumor described by Lyon and associates[241] and a forearm tumor observed by this author (Fig. 4–38). The former patient died from extensive local invasion despite orbital exenteration and chemotherapy; the latter survived following disarticulation at the elbow and chemotherapy.

The congenital, 4.5 × 4.5 cm, temporofacial malignant tumor depicted by Hachitanda et al. was a densely cellular, small cell tumor containing both Homer-Wright and Flexner-Wintersteiner–type rosettes.[162] In addition, there were cytokeratin and EMA-positive atypical gland formations and epithelioid cells. Glial differentiation was demonstrated by the presence of cytoplasmic glial fibrillary acidic protein and S-100 protein–positive cells. Moreover, neurosecretory granules and intermediate filaments were found. The infant died of brain metastases 7 months after diagnosis.[162]

Triton Tumor

The triton tumor is yet another example of a neoplasm with divergent differentiation in

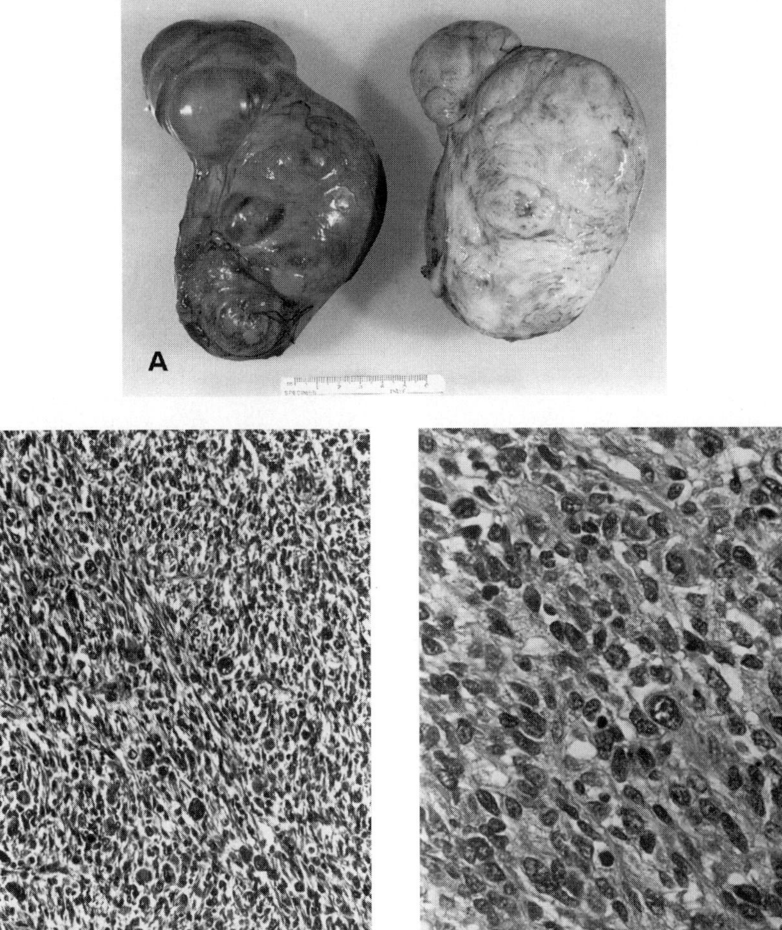

Figure 4–37. Ectomesenchymoma. The parents of a 6-month-old male infant noted an abdominal mass 2 months prior to the child's hospitalization. *A,* The mass, weighing 940 g and measuring 18 × 11 cm, is attached to the internal inguinal ring and has a white, bulging, whorled, lobular appearance. *B,* The tumor consists of spindle-shaped rhabdomyoblasts and larger, rounder ganglion cells (trichrome, ×150). *C,* A higher-power view of the rhabdomyoblasts and ganglion cells (hematoxylin-eosin, ×300). (From Isaacs H Jr. Tumors of the Newborn and Infant. St. Louis: Mosby–Year Book, 1991.)

which malignant nerve sheath tumor ("malignant schwannoma") and embryonal rhabdomyosarcoma components coexist.[50,51,128,379] The name triton, coined by Woodruff et al.,[379] is derived from the genus of salamander in which the growth of both neural and muscular elements were induced by nerve transplantation experiments. Neurofibromatosis type 1 is common in patients with this tumor.[96,128] Two examples of congenital triton tumor that involved the retroperitoneal area metastasized and proved fatal.[50,51]

The diagnosis of malignant triton tumor is established by identifying both malignant nerve sheath tumor and rhabdomyosarcoma components.[50,96,128,379] The former consists of spindle-

or comma-shaped cells with a scanty cytoplasm and elongated nuclei forming alternating bundles. In addition, Antoni type A and type B tissue growth patterns (positive for S-100 protein) are present. The latter component consists of rhabdomyoblasts demonstrated by the appropriate skeletal muscle markers (myoglobin, desmin, actin) and by electron microscopy, which reveals cells with basal lamina and filaments with Z-bands.[50,96] There are some histologic similarities between the triton tumor and ectomesenchymoma, but ganglion cells and neuroblasts are not observed in the triton tumor. Neither the site of origin nor the age of the patient apparently affect the outcome, for the prognosis of patients with malignant triton tu-

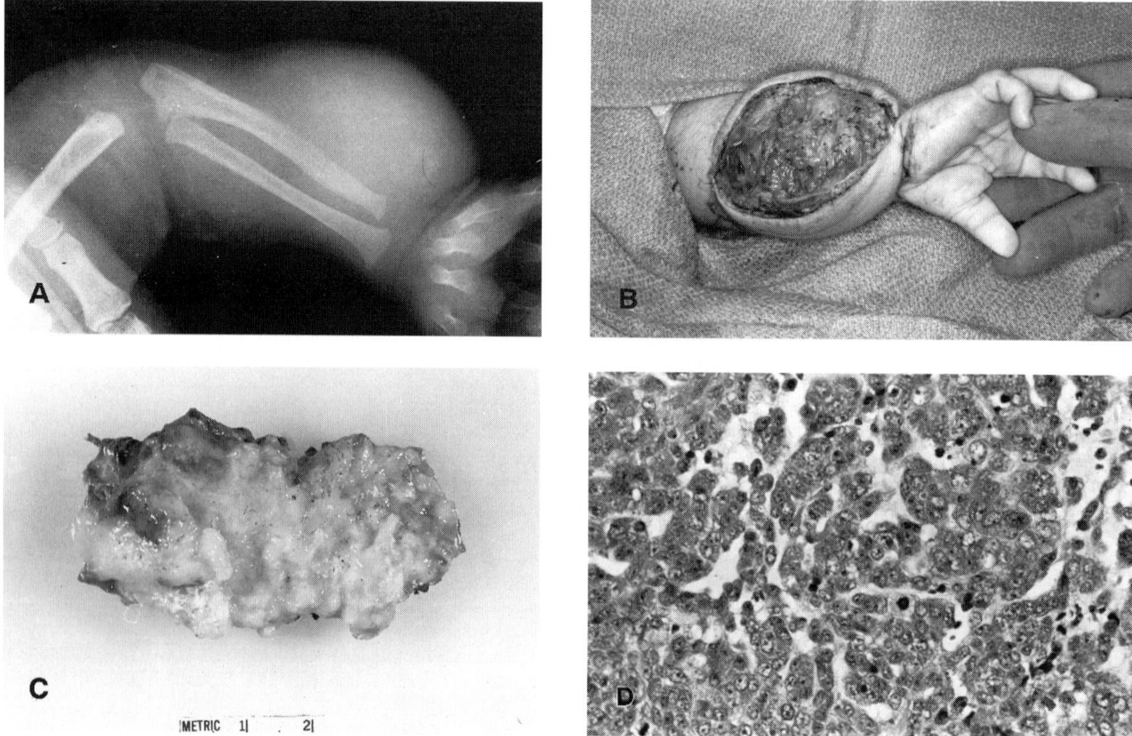

Figure 4–38. Polyphenotypic small cell tumor. A 2-month-old male infant presented with a rapidly growing neoplasm of the forearm that had been present since birth. *A,* An x-ray film reveals a large soft tissue mass. *B,* The tumor is exposed at surgery. *C,* The tumor exhibits a soft, gelatinous appearance. *D,* The tumor contains nests and cords of epithelial-like cells (hematoxylin-eosin, ×300). Immunoperoxidase staining was weakly positive for neuron-specific enolase, vimentin, cytokeratin, and actin.

mor is dismal.[50,96] Recurrence is common. The 5-year survival rate for one series of nine patients was only 12%.[50]

MESENCHYMOMA

Mesenchymoma, a controversial neoplasm of disputed histogenesis, is defined as a mixed tumor arising primarily in soft tissues composed of two or more mesenchymal components other than fibrous connective tissue.[128,272] Whether mesenchymomas are dysontogenetic growths (reflecting defective embryonic development), hamartomas, true neoplasms, or a variation of polyphenotypic tumors is open for debate. Benign and malignant forms have been described in patients of all ages.[53,128,177,187,203,228,272] The extremities are the most common primary site in the newborn, followed by the trunk and the head and neck.[53,203]

Bures and Barnes collected eight cases of benign mesenchymomas of the head and neck, four of which were present at birth.[53] Clinically, the lesions presented as enlarging, nontender, subcutaneous masses in the neck, cheek, or scalp. The major histologic component of the tumors, other than fibrous connective tissue, was smooth muscle, followed (in order) by adipose and vascular tissue. Minor components included skeletal muscle, cartilage, lymphoid tissue, and hemangiopericytoma. None of these tumors recurred after excision. LeBer and Stout described two congenital benign mesenchymomas arising from the tongue and the trapezius muscle, respectively.[228]

Over the years, the number of tumors diagnosed as benign mesenchymoma has declined considerably. On review, some of these lesions appear to be hemangiomas, hamartomas, or other vascular malformations situated in skeletal muscle and fat with lymphoid nodule formation. One notable exception is the chest wall mesenchymoma or hamartoma, which often appears at birth as an impressive chest wall mass.[184] The adjacent lung may be compressed,

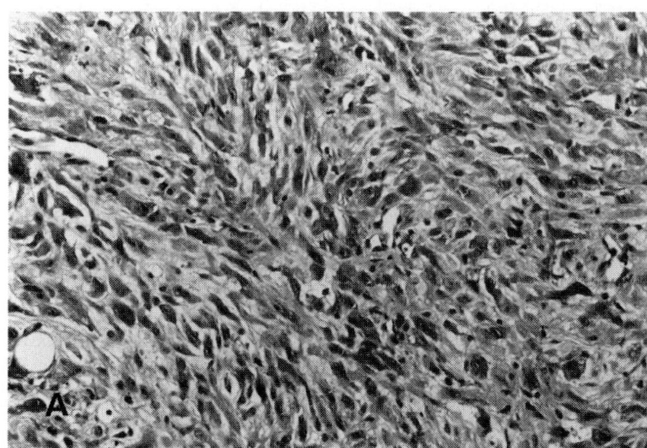
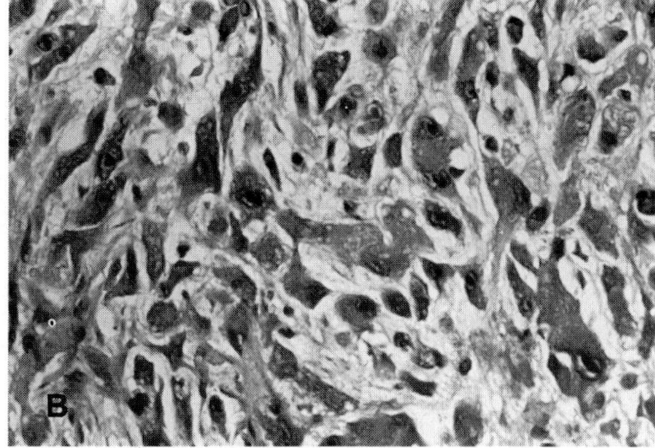

Figure 4–39. Proliferative fasciitis. *A,* Biopsy examination of a subcutaneous mass on the lower leg of a 3-month-old girl revealed fibroblasts and giant cells with vesicular nuclei, prominent nucleoli, and basophilic cytoplasms that resembled ganglion cells. In addition, there are a few scattered lymphocytes (hematoxylin-eosin, ×100). *B,* A higher-power view shows the ganglion-like cells in greater detail (hematoxylin-eosin, ×600). (The microscopic slides are courtesy of D. R. Dickson, MD, Santa Barbara Cottage Hospital, Santa Barbara, CA.) (From Isaacs H Jr. Tumors of the Newborn and Infant. St. Louis: Mosby–Year Book, 1991.)

producing respiratory symptoms. Two or more ribs and the adjacent intercostal muscles may be involved. Grossly and microscopically, the chest wall hamartoma has features of an aneurysmal bone cyst with a prominent cartilaginous component (see Figs. 18–1 and 18–2 in Chapter 18, "Bone Tumors").[29,86,116,184]

To qualify as a malignant mesenchymoma, two or more of the components must be malignant other than fibrosarcoma (e.g., rhabdomyosarcoma plus liposarcoma and/or chondrosarcoma).[203] Components found in childhood malignant mesenchymoma include smooth and skeletal muscle, adipose tissue, cartilage, and fibrous, vascular, and undifferentiated elements.[187,203] Tumors with rhabdomyosarcoma as one of the malignant components have the least favorable prognosis.[203] A malignant mesenchymoma of the axilla in a 1-year-old girl was found, on histologic examination, to consist of chondrosarcoma, liposarcoma, and rhabdomyosarcoma components, in addition to fibrosarcoma.[187] This child had an uneventful recovery following wide local excision.

PROLIFERATIVE MYOSITIS AND FASCIITIS

Proliferative myositis and fasciitis and cranial fasciitis are examples of non-neoplastic, reparative lesions that are infrequently encountered in the newborn but that should be considered in the differential diagnosis of a soft tissue mass.[187,226] They are more common in older children and adults, but their clinical behavior and histopathologic findings are similar.[36] The lesions appear suddenly and grow rapidly. They tend to be small (usually less than 5 cm in diameter), are well circumscribed, and are located in the subcutaneous tissue, most often in the extremities (Fig. 4–39).[347] Three neonates with proliferative ("nodular") fasciitis involving the neck, arm, and lower leg, respectively, have been described.[187,251,286,345]

Occasionally, these lesions have mistakenly been called sarcomas owing to their worrisome microscopic appearance.[72,79,104,128,251,347] On histologic examination, proliferative fasciitis is characterized by marked cellularity, a brisk mitotic rate, nuclear atypia, and a myxoid appearance.[104,128,251] Typically, it is composed of fibroblasts and giant cells with vesicular nuclei, prominent nucleoli, and basophilic cytoplasm resembling ganglion cells, which are pathognomonic (see Fig. 4–39).[187,251,264] The ganglion-like cells have myofibroblastic and histiocytic features, staining positively for vimentin and actin and focally positive with KP1 (CD68 antigen).[251,261] Keratin, desmin, and S-100 immunoperoxidase studies are negative. Electron microscopy shows cells with fibroblastic, myofibroblastic, and histiocytic differentiation. If biopsied early in the course of the disease, the lesion may recur at an alarming rate, recurring more rapidly than a sarcoma. The prognosis is excellent following local excision. Un-

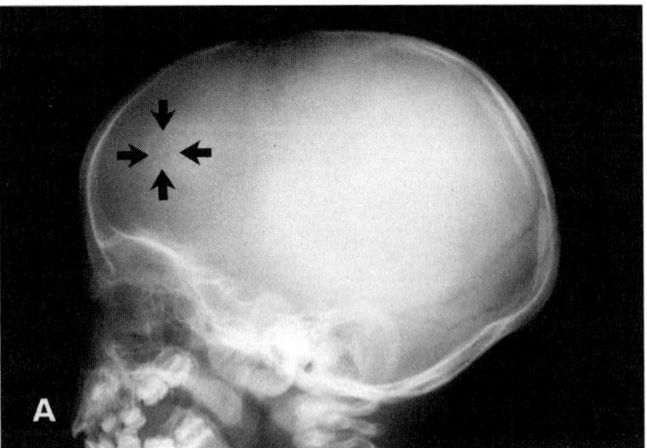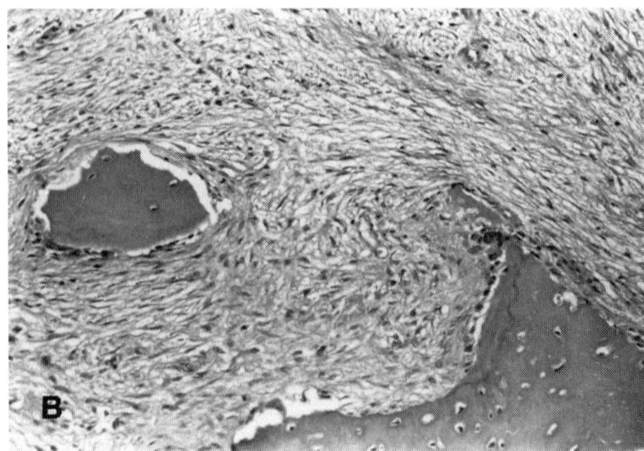

Figure 4–40. Cranial fasciitis. *A*, A skull x-ray film of a 1½-year-old boy with bilateral scalp masses reveals an irregular, punched-out lesion (*arrows*) in the left temporal bone. Langerhans cell histiocytosis has an identical roentgenographic appearance. *B*, Biopsy studies show fibroblastic reaction surrounding bone spicules (hematoxylin-eosin, ×300). (From Adler R, Wong CA. Cranial fasciitis simulating histiocytosis. J Pediatr 1986;109:85. Used by permission.)

necessarily aggressive therapy should not be considered.[128,187,251]

Cranial Fasciitis

Cranial fasciitis is another example of a reactive lesion that occasionally causes diagnostic problems in young children.[5,226] Typically, it occurs in infants ranging in age from birth to 2 years, but sometimes it affects older children. Two of nine children included in the AFIP study, both of whom were male patients, were younger than 2 months of age, and neither one experienced a recurrence after surgical excision.[226] The lesion usually begins as a rapidly growing, firm, soft tissue mass that may or may not be painful.[5,226] Imaging studies reveal an irregular, lytic lesion with a sclerotic rim, measuring 1.5 to 9 cm, situated in various locations in the cranium, and accompanied by an overlying soft tissue mass (Fig. 4–40).[5,187] Usually, the lesion only involves the outer table of the skull, with preservation of the inner table, and forms a saucer-like defect seen on tangential views.[5,226] Occasionally, the lesion extends through the inner table to the underlying dura.[226] Cranial fasciitis is seldom bilateral.[5] Clinically and on imaging studies, the lesion may be confused with Langerhans cell histiocytosis.[5]

On gross examination, the lesions are firm and grey-white and resemble dense fibrous connective tissue. If small spicules of bone are present, the lesion may have a gritty sensation on sectioning. Histologic findings include islands of cranial bone surrounded by spindle-shaped cells embedded in loose, myxoid-appearing connective tissue and alternating with dense fibrosis, not unlike that observed in proliferative fasciitis (Fig. 4–40*B*). Low mitotic activity and mild chronic inflammation are present. Sometimes, there is a storiform pattern.[226] Excisional biopsy and curettage are curative, but the lesion will recur if not adequately excised. The etiology is unknown. Birth trauma has been implicated, but this does not explain the occurrence of cranial fasciitis in older children.

Another variation of reactive, tumor-like processes is myositis ossificans. One of the youngest patients reported with myositis ossificans (heterotopic ossification in muscle and other soft tissues) occurred in a 5-month-old girl following minor trauma to the soft tissues of the posterior aspect of the right knee.[172]

MISCELLANEOUS SOFT TISSUE TUMORS AND TUMOR-LIKE CONDITIONS

For the sake of completeness, a few additional neoplasms that occur in the perinatal period should be mentioned. Malignant mesothelioma of the peritoneum was diagnosed in a 16-day-old male infant who died of disseminated metastases.[274] Congenital epithelioid sarcoma occurred in a 12-week-old female infant with a forehead lesion, stage I, who recovered after surgery and chemotherapy.[214] At Children's Hospital, Los Angeles, an umbilical myxoma was removed from a female infant with Beckwith-Wiedemann syndrome. This patient is described in Chapter 14 ("Pancreatic Tumors"). Nakamura et al. documented an example of a congenital peripheral medulloepithelioma originating in the sciatic nerve.[271] The tumor consisted of neuroepithelium composed of pseudostratified columnar cells forming tubular and papillary structures with prominent external and internal limiting membranes resembling the medullary plate and neural tube. In addition, the neoplasm displayed multiple divergent differentiation into astrocytoma, ependymoma, oligodendroglioma, and ganglioneuroma. The child was alive 7 years after amputation of the right leg and hemipelvis. This rare "embryoma" occurs more often in the cerebral hemispheres and eye (see Chapter 9, "Brain Tumors," and Chapter 10, "Tumors of the Eye").

REFERENCES

1. Abell MR, Hart WR, Olson JR. Tumors of the peripheral nervous system. Hum Pathol 1970;1:503.
2. Abramowicz JS, Warsof SL, Doyle DL, et al. Congenital cystic hygroma of the neck diagnosed prenatally: Outcome with normal and abnormal karyotype. Prenatal Diagn 1989;9:321.
3. Adam LR, Davison EV, Malcom AJ, et al. Cytogenetic analysis of a congenital fibrosarcoma. Cancer Genet Cytogenet 1991;52:37.
4. Adickes ED, Goodrich P, AuchMoedy J, et al. Central nervous system involvement in congenital visceral fibromatosis. Pediatr Pathol 1985;3:329.
5. Adler R, Wong CA. Cranial fasciitis simulating histiocytosis. J Pediatr 1986;109:85.
6. Allen MS Jr, Harrison W, Jahrsdoerfer RA. "Retinal anlage" tumors. Am J Clin Pathol 1969;51:309.
7. Allen PW. The fibromatoses: A clinicopathologic classification based on 140 cases, Part 1. Am J Surg Pathol 1977;1:255.
8. Allen PW. The fibromatoses: A clinicopathologic classification based on 140 cases, Part 2. Am J Surg Pathol 1977;1:305.
9. Alpers CE, Rosenau W, Finkbeiber WE, et al. Congenital (infantile) hemangiopericytoma of the tongue and sublingual region. Am J Clin Pathol 1984;81:377.
10. Altemani AM, Amstalden EI, Filho JM. Congenital generalized fibromatosis causing spinal cord compression. Hum Pathol 1985;16:1063.
11. Angel CA, Gant LL, Parham DM, et al. Leiomyosarcomas in children: Clinicopathologic characteristics. Pediatr Surg Int 1992;7:116.
12. Apter N, Chemke J, Hurwitz N, et al. Neonatal neurofibromatosis: Unusual manifestations with malignant clinical course. Clin Genet 1975;7:388.
13. Arceci RJ, Weinstein HJ. Neoplasia. *In* Avery GB, Fletcher MA, MacDonald MG (eds): Neonatology: Pathophysiology and Management in the Newborn, 4th ed, p 1211. Philadelphia: JB Lippincott, 1994.
14. Arean V, Marcial-Rojas RA. Rhabdomyosarcoma in children. Am J Surg 1957;93:143.
15. Argenyi ZB, Van Rybroek JJ, Kemp JD, et al. Congenital angiomatoid malignant fibrous histiocytoma: A light-microscopic, immunopathologic, and electron-microscopic study. Am J Dermatopathol 1988;10:59.
16. Argyle JC, Tomlinson GE, Stewart D, et al. Ultrastructural, immunocytochemical and cytogenetic characterization of a large congenital fibrosarcoma. Arch Pathol Lab Med 1992;116:972.
17. Arush MW, Arie YB, Bialik V, et al. Limb congenital fibrosarcoma: Report of two cases and review of the literature. Med Pediatr Oncol 1993;10:357.
18. Askin FB, Rosai J, Sibley RK, et al. Malignant small cell tumor of the thoracopulmonary region in childhood: A distinctive clinicopathologic entity of uncertain histogenesis. Cancer 1979;43:2438.
19. Atkinson GO Jr, Davis PC, Patrick LE, et al. Melanotic neuroectodermal tumor of infancy: MR findings and a review of the literature. Pediatr Radiol 1989;20:20.
20. Atkinson JB, Mahour GH, Isaacs H Jr, et al. Hemangiopericytoma in infants and children: A report of six patients. Am J Surg 1984;148:372.
21. Ayala AG, Ro JY, Goepfert H, et al. Desmoid fibromatosis: A clinicopathologic study of 25 children. Semin Diagn Pathol 1986;3:138.
22. Bader JL, Miller RW. Neurofibromatosis and childhood leukemia. J Pediatr 1978;92:925.
23. Bader JL, Miller RW. U.S. cancer incidence and mortality in the first year of life. Am J Dis Child 1979;133:157.
24. Bailey PV, Weber TR, Tracey TF Jr, et al. Congenital hemangiopericytoma: An unusual vascular neoplasm of infancy. Surgery 1993;114:936.
25. Baird PA, Worth AJ. Congenital generalized fibromatosis: An autosomal recessive condition? Clin Genet 1976;9:488.
26. Bale PM, Parsons RE, Stevens MM. Pathology and behavior of juvenile rhabdomyosarcoma. *In* Finegold M (ed): Pathology of Neoplasia in Children and Adolescents. Major Problems in Pathology, Vol 18, p 196. Philadelphia: WB Saunders, 1986.
27. Bale PM, Reye RDK. Rhabdomyosarcoma in childhood. Pathology 1975;7:101.
28. Balsalver AM, Butler JJ, Martin RG. Congenital fibrosarcoma. Cancer 1967;20:1607.
29. Baretton G, Stehr M, Nerlich A, et al. Chest wall hamartoma in infancy: A case report with immunohistochemical analysis of various interstitial collagen types. Pediatr Pathol 1994;14:3.
30. Batcup G: Cancer in the very young child—Pitfalls and problems for the pathologist. Br J Cancer 1992;66 (Suppl 18):S5.
31. Battifora H: Hemangiopericytoma: Ultrastructural study of five cases. Cancer 1973;31:1418.
32. Battifora H, Hines J. Recurring digital fibromas of childhood. Cancer 1971;27:1530.
33. Beckett JH, Jacobs AH. Recurring digital fibrous tumors of childhood: A review. Pediatrics 1977;59:401.
34. Bellman B, Wooming G, Landsman L, et al. Infantile myofibromatosis: A case report. Pediatr Dermatol 1991;8:306.
35. Benjamin SP, Mercer RD, Hawk WA. Myofibroblastic contraction in spontaneous regression of multiple, congenital mesenchymal hamartomas. Cancer 1977;40:2343.
36. Bernstein KE, Lattes R. Nodular (pseudosarcomatous) fasciitis, nonrecurrent lesion: Clinicopathologic study of 134 cases. Cancer 1982;49:1668.
37. Bernstein R, Zeltzer PM, Lin F, et al. Trisomy 11 and

other nonrandom trisomies in congenital fibrosarcoma. Cancer Genet Cytogenet 1994;78:82.

38. Bhawan J, Baccheta C, Joris I, et al. Infantile digital fibroma (recurrent digital fibrous tumor of childhood). A myofibroblastic tumor. Am J Pathol 1979; 94:19.

39. Blocker SH, Golladay ES, Baker GF. Congenital leiomyoma of the distal ileum associated with ileal atresia and malrotation. Pediatr Surg Int 1992;7:129.

40. Blocker S, Koenig J, Ternberg J. Congenital fibrosarcoma. J Pediatr Surg 1987;22:665.

41. Bolande RP, Towler WF. A possible relationship of neuroblastoma to von Recklinghausen's disease. Cancer 1970;26:162.

42. Bolen JW, Thorning D. Benign lipoblastoma and myxoid liposarcoma: A comparative light- and electron-microscopic study. Am J Surg Pathol 1980;4:163.

43. Bonneau R, Brochu P. Neuromuscular choristoma: A pathologic study of two cases. Am J Surg Pathol 1983; 7:521.

44. Borello ED, Gorlin RJ. Melanotic neuroectodermal tumor of infancy: A neoplasm of neural crest origin. Cancer 1966;19:196.

45. Botting AJ, Soule EH, Brown AL. Smooth muscle tumors in children. Cancer 1965;18:711.

46. Bozic C. Fetal rhabdomyoma of the parotid gland in an infant: Histological, immunohistochemical and ultrastructural features. Pediatr Pathol 1986;6:139.

47. Bracko M, Cindro L, Golou R. Familial occurrence of infantile myofibromatosis. Cancer 69:1294, 1992.

48. Brill PW, Yandow DR, Langer LO, et al. Congenital generalized fibromatosis. Case report and literature review. Pediatr Radiol 1982;12:771.

49. Briselli EH, Soule EH, Gilchrist GS. Congenital fibromatosis: Report of 18 cases of solitary and 4 cases of multiple tumors. Mayo Clin Proc 1980;55:554.

50. Brooks JSJ, Freeman M, Enterline HT. Malignant "triton" tumors. Natural history and immunochemistry of nine new cases with literature review. Cancer 1985; 55:2543.

51. Buck BE, Mahboubi S, Raney RB Jr. Congenital neurogenous sarcoma with rhabdomyosarcomatous differentiation. J Pediatr Surg 1977;12:581.

52. Bulas DI, Saal HM, Allen JF, et al. Cystic hygroma and congenital diaphragmatic hernia: Early prenatal sonographic evaluation of Fryns' syndrome. Prenatal Diagn 1992;12:867.

53. Bures C, Barnes L. Benign mesenchymomas of the head and neck. Arch Pathol Lab Med 1978;102:237.

54. Burgess LPA, Quilligan JJ, Moe RD, et al. Congenital multiple fibromatosis (infantile myofibromatosis). Arch Otolaryngol Head Neck Surg 1988;114:207.

55. Burke EC, Winklemann RK, Strickland MK. Disseminated hemangiomatosis: The newborn with central nervous system involvement. Am J Dis Child 1964;108: 418.

56. Burman D, Mansell PWA, Warin WP. Miliary haemangiomata in the newborn. Arch Dis Child 1967;42:193.

57. Burry AF, Kerr JFR, Pope JH. Recurring digital fibrous tumors of childhood: An electron microscopic and virological study. Pathology 1970;2:287.

58. Byard RW, Burrows PE, Izakawa T, et al. Diffuse infantile haemangiomatosis: Clinicopathologic features and management problems in five fatal cases. Eur J Pediatr 1991;150:224.

59. Byrne J, Blanc WA, Warburton D, et al. The significance of cystic hygroma in fetuses. Hum Pathol 1984; 15:61.

60. Campbell AN, Chan HSL, O'Brien A, et al. Malignant tumours in the neonate. Arch Dis Child 1987;62:19.

61. Canarelli JP, Pautard B, Ricard J, et al. Rhabdomyosarcome embryonaire de decouverte antenatale. Chir Pediatr 1988;29:349.

62. Cardia E, Molina D, Zaccone C, et al. Intracranial solitary-type infantile myofibromatosis. Childs Nerv System 1993;9:246.

63. Carpenter BF, Jimenez C, Robb IA. Melanotic neuroectodermal tumor of infancy. Pediatr Pathol 1985; 3:227.

64. Carson HJ, Taxy JB. Role of autopsy in congenital cystic hygroma. Pediatr Pathol 1994;14:183.

65. Cavazzana AO, Schmidt D, Ninfo V, et al. Spindle cell rhabdomyosarcoma: A prognostically favorable variant of rhabdomyosarcoma. Am J Surg Pathol 1992;16: 229.

66. Chami RG, Wang HS. Large congenital epulis of the newborn. J Pediatr Surg 1986;21:929.

67. Chan Y-F, Lau JHK, Tong CY. Congenital generalized fibromatosis with predominant osseous involvement in a Chinese newborn. J Pediatr Orthoped 1989;9:64.

68. Chang WWL, Griffith KM. Solitary intestinal fibromatosis: A rare cause of intestinal obstruction in the neonate and infant. J Pediatr Surg 1991;26:1406.

69. Chen KTK, Kassel SH, Medrano VA. Congenital hemangiopericytoma. J Surg Oncol 1986;31:127.

70. Chervenak FA, Isaacson G, Blakemore KJ, et al. Fetal cystic hygroma: Cause and natural history. N Engl J Med 1983;309:822.

71. Chervenak FA, Isaacson G, Tortora M. A sonographic study of fetal cystic hygromas. J Clin Ultrasound 1985; 13:317.

72. Chung EB. Pitfalls in diagnosing benign soft tissue tumors in infancy and childhood. Pathol Annu 1985;2: 323–386.

73. Chung EB, Enzinger FM. Benign lipoblastomatosis: An analysis of 35 cases. Cancer 1973;32:482.

74. Chung EB, Enzinger FM. Infantile fibrosarcoma. Cancer 1976;38:729.

75. Chung EB, Enzinger FM. Infantile myofibromatosis. Cancer 1981;48:1807.

76. Clarke BE, Parson H. An embryological tumor of retinal anlage involving the skull. Cancer 1951;4:78.

77. Coffin CM, Dehner LP. Congenital tumors. _In_ Stocker JT, Dehner LP (eds): Pediatric Pathology, Vol I, p 325. Philadelphia: JB Lippincott, 1992.

78. Coffin CM, Dehner LP: Fibroblastic-myofibroblastic tumors in children: A clinicopathologic study of 108 examples in 103 patients. Pediatr Pathol 1991;11:559.

79. Coffin CM, Dehner LP. Soft tissue neoplasms in childhood: A clinicopathologic overview in pathology of neoplasia in children and adolescents. _In_ Finegold M (ed): Major Problems in Pathology, Vol 18, p 397. Philadelphia: WB Saunders, 1986.

80. Coffin CM, Dehner LP. Soft tissue tumors in the first year of life. A report of 190 cases, Pediatr Pathol 10: 509, 1990.

81. Coffin CM, Dehner LP. Vascular tumors in children and adolescents: A clinicopathologic study of 228 tumors in 222 patients. Pathol Annu 1993;28(1):97.

82. Coffin CM, Jaszcz W, O'Shea PA, et al. So-called congenital-infantile fibrosarcoma: Does it exist and what is it? Pediatr Pathol 1994;14:133.

83. Coffin CM, Neilson KA, Ingels S, et al. Congenital generalized myofibromatosis (CGMF): A disseminated angiocentric myofibromatosis (abstract). Pediatr Pathol 1994;14:549.

84. Coffin CM, Neilson KA, Ingels S, et al. Congenital generalized myofibromatosis: A disseminated angiocentric myofibromatosis. Pediatr Pathol Lab Med 1995;15:571.

85. Coffin CM, Williams RA. Congenital lipoblastoma of the hand. Pediatr Pathol 12:857, 1992.

86. Cohen MC, Drut R, Garcia C, et al. Mesenchymal hamartoma of the chest wall: A cooperative study with review of the literature. Pediatr Pathol 1992;12:525.

87. Cohen MM, Schwartz S, Schwartz MF, et al. Antenatal detection of cystic hygroma. Obstet Gynecol Surv 1989;44:481.

88. Costa MJ, Weiss SW. Angiomatoid malignant fibrous histiocytoma: A follow-up study of 108 cases with evaluation of possible histologic predictors of outcome. Am J Surg Pathol 1990;14:1126.

89. Coventry MB, Harris LE, Bianco AJ Jr et al. Congenital muscular torticollis (wry neck). Postgrad Med 1960;28:383.

90. Craver RD, Heinrich S. Bone invasion by a recurrent digital fibroma of infancy in a child with Beckwith-Wiedemann syndrome. Pediatr Pathol Lab Med 1995;15:147.

91. Crawford AH. Neurofibromatosis in the pediatric patient. Orthoped Clin North Am 1978;9:11.

92. Crotty PL, Nakhleh RF, Dehner LP. Juvenile rhabdomyoma: An intermediate form of skeletal muscle tumor in children. Arch Pathol Lab Med 1993;117:43.

93. Crowe FW, Schull WJ, Neel JV. A Clinical, Pathological and Genetic Study of Multiple Neurofibromatosis. Springfield, IL: CC Thomas, 1956.

94. Currie BG, Schell D, Bowring AC. Giant hemangioma of the arm associated with cardiac failure and the Kasabach-Merritt syndrome in a neonate. J Pediatr Surg 1991;26:734.

95. Cutler LS, Chaudhry AP, Topazian R. Melanotic neuroectodermal tumor of infancy: An ultrastructural study, literature review and reevaluation. Cancer 1981;48:257.

96. Daimaru Y, Hashimoto H, Enjoji M. Malignant "triton" tumors. A clinicopathologic and immunohistochemical study of nine cases. Hum Pathol 1984;15:768.

97. Dardick I, Hammar S, Scheithauer BW. Ultrastructural spectrum of hemangiopericytoma: A comparative study of fetal, adult and neoplastic pericytes. Ultrastruct Pathol 1989;13:111.

98. Das L, Chang C, Cushing B, et al. Congenital primitive neuroectodermal tumor (neuroepithelioma) of the chest wall. Med Pediatr Oncol 1982;10:349.

99. Davies MRQ, Mogilner JG. Congenital malignant rhabdoid tumor of the skin: Case report. Pediatr Surg Int 1991;6:230.

100. Davis CF, Carachi R, Young DG. Neonatal tumors: Glasgow 1966–86. Arch Dis Child 1988;63:1075.

101. de Graaf JH, Timens W, Tamminga RYJ, et al. Deep juvenile xantogranuloma: A lesion related to dermal intermediate cells. Hum Pathol 1992;23:905.

102. Dehner LP. Neoplasms of the fetus and neonate. *In* Naeye RL, Kissane JM, Kaufman N (eds): Perinatal Diseases. International Academy of Pathology, Monograph number 22, p 286. Baltimore: Williams and Wilkins, 1981.

103. Dehner LP. Neuroepithelioma (primitive neuroectodermal tumor) and Ewing's sarcoma: At least a partial consensus. Arch Pathol Lab Med 1994;118:606.

104. Dehner LP. Pediatric Surgical Pathology, 2nd ed. Baltimore: Williams and Wilkins, 1987.

105. Dehner LP. Pediatric tumors. Lecture, Aspen Conference, 1993.

106. Dehner LP. Peripheral and central primitive neuroectodermal tumors: A nosologic concept seeking a consensus. Arch Pathol Lab Med 1986;110:997.

107. Dehner LP. Personal communication.

108. Dehner LP. Primitive neuroectodermal tumor and Ewing's sarcoma. Am J Surg Pathol 1993;17:1.

109. Dehner LP, Askin FB. Tumors of fibrous tissue origin in childhood. A clinicopathologic study of cutaneous and soft tissue neoplasms in 66 children. Cancer 1976;38:888.

110. Dehner LP, Enzinger FM, Font RL. Fetal rhabdomyoma: An analysis of nine cases. Cancer 1972;30:160.

111. Dehner LP, Sibley RK, Sauk JJ Jr, et al. Malignant melanotic neuroectodermal tumor of infancy: A clinical, pathologic, ultrastructural and tissue culture study. Cancer 1979;43:1389–1410.

112. Dimmick JE, Wood WS. Congenital multiple fibromatosis. Am J Dermatopathol 1983;5:289.

113. Dingman RP: Hemangiopericytoma. A report of 2 cases—One congenital in origin. Plast Reconstruc Surg 1958;21:393.

114. Di Sant'Agnese PA, Knowles DM. Extracardiac rhabdomyoma: A clinicopathologic study and review of the literature. Cancer 1980;46:780.

115. Doi O, Takada Y. Kasabach-Merritt syndrome in two neonates. J Pediatr Surg 1992;27:1507.

116. Dounies R, Chwals WJ, Lally KP, et al. Hamartomas of the chest wall in infants. Ann Thorac Surg 1994;57:868.

117. Drut R, Sapia S, Gril D, et al. Nonimmune hydrops fetalis, hydramnios, microcephaly, and intracranial meningeal hemangioendothelioma. Pediatr Pathol 1993;13:9, 1993.

118. Dymock RB, Allen PW, Stirling JW, et al. Giant cell fibroelastoma. A distinctive, recurrent tumor of childhood. Am J Surg Pathol 1987;11:263.

119. Ehrlich FE, Haas JE, Kieswetter WB. Rhabdomyosarcoma in infants and children: Factors affecting long term survival. J Pediat Surg 1971;6:571.

120. Eimoto T. Ultrastructure of an infantile hemangiopericytoma. Cancer 1977;40:2161.

121. Ellenbogen E, Lasky MA. Rhabdomyosarcoma of the orbit in the newborn. Am J Ophthalmol 1975;80:1024.

122. Enghardt MH, Warren RC. Congenital palpebral lipoblastoma: First report of a case. Am J Dermatopathol 1990;12:408.

123. Enterline HT. Histopathology of sarcomas. Semin Oncol 1981;8:133.

124. Enterline HT, Horn RC Jr. Alveolar rhabdomyosarcoma. A distinctive tumor type. Am J Clin Pathol 1958;29:356.

125. Enzinger FM. Angiomatoid malignant fibrous histiocytoma: A distinct fibrohistiocytic tumor of children and young adults simulating a vascular neoplasm. Cancer 1979;44:2147.

126. Enzinger FM. Fibrous hamartoma of infancy. Cancer 1965;18:241.

126a. Enzinger FM. Fibrous tumors of infancy. *In* Enzinger FM (ed): Tumors of Bone and Soft Tissue, p 375. Chicago: Year Book, 1965.

127. Enzinger FM, Smith MD. Hemangiopericytoma: An analysis of 106 cases. Hum Pathol 1976;7:61.

128. Enzinger FM, Weiss SW. Soft Tissue Tumors, 3rd ed. St Louis: CV Mosby, 1995.

129. Enzinger FM, Zhang R. Plexiform fibrohistiocytic tu-

mor presenting in children and young adults: An analysis of 65 cases. Am J Surg Pathol 1988;12:818.

130. Eppley BL, Sadove AM, Campbell A. Obstructive congenital epulis in a newborn. Ann Plastic Surg 1991; 27:152.

131. Erlandson RA, Woodruff JM. Peripheral nerve sheath tumors: An electron microscopic study of 43 cases. Cancer 1982;43:273.

132. Fletcher CDM, Achu P, Van Noorden S, et al. Infantile myofibromatosis: A light microscopic, histochemical and immunohistochemical study suggesting smooth muscle differentiation. Histopathology 1987;11:245.

132a. Fletcher CD, Powell G, Van Noorden S, McKee PH. Fibrous hamartoma of infancy: A histochemical and immunohistochemical study. Histopathology 1988; 12:65.

133. Fringes B, Thais H, Bohm N, et al. Identification of actin microfilaments in the intracytoplasmic inclusions present in recurring infantile digital fibromatosis (Reye tumor). Pediatr Pathol 1986;6:311.

134. Fromowitz FB, Hurst LC, Nathan J, et al. Infantile (desmoid type) fibromatosis with extensive ossification. Am J Surg Pathol 1987;11:66.

135. Fuzesi L, Heller R, Schreiber H, et al. Cytogenetics of Askin's tumour: Case report and review of the literature. Pathol Res Pract 189:235, 1993.

136. Gaffney EF, Vellios F, Hargreaves HK. Lipoblastomatosis: Ultrastructure of two cases and relationship to fetal white adipose tissue. Pediatr Pathol 1986;5: 207.

137. Galliani CA, Beatty JF, Grosfeld JL. Cavernous hemangioma of the lung in an infant. Pediatr Pathol 1992; 12:105.

138. Gehan EA, Glover FM, Mauer HM, et al. Prognostic factors in children with rhabdomyosarcoma. Natl Cancer Instit Monogr 1981;56:83.

139. Gerald WL, Rosai J. Case 2. Desmoplastic small cell tumor with divergent differentiation. Pediatr Pathol 1989;9:177.

140. Ghosh BC, Ghosh L, Huvos AG, et al. Malignant schwannoma: A clinicopathologic study. Cancer 1973; 31:184.

141. Gibos MK, Soule EH, Hayles AB, et al. Lipoblastomatosis: A tumor of children. Pediatrics 1977;60:235.

142. Goetsch E. Hygroma colli cysticum, and hygroma axillare. Arch Surg 1938;36:394.

143. Goh DW, Raafat F, Gornall P, et al. Intestinal leiomyoma in neonates. Pediatr Surg Int 1990;5:208.

144. Golden WL, Schneider BF, Gustashaw KM, et al. Prenatal diagnosis of Turner syndrome using cells cultured from cystic hygromas in two pregnancies with normal maternal serum alpha-fetoprotein. Prenatal Diagn 1989;9:683.

145. Golitz LE, Rudikoff J, O'Meara P. Diffuse neonatal hemangiomatosis. Pediatr Dermatol 1986;3:145.

146. Gonzalez-Crussi F. Ultrastructure of congenital fibrosarcoma. Cancer 1970;26:1289.

147. Gonzalez-Crussi F, Black-Schaffer S. Rhabdomyosarcoma of infancy and childhood. Problems of morphologic classification. Am J Surg Pathol 1979;3:157.

148. Gonzalez-Crussi F, Campbell RJ. Juvenile xanthogranuloma. Ultrastructural study. Arch Pathol 1970; 89:65.

149. Gonzalez-Crussi F, Crawford SE, Sun C-CJ. Intra-abdominal desmoplastic small-cell tumors with divergent differentiation: Observations on three cases of childhood. Am J Surg Pathol 1990;14:633.

150. Gonzalez-Crussi F, Goldschmidt RA, Hsueh W, et al. Infantile sarcoma with intracytoplasmic filamentous inclusions. Cancer 1982;49:2365.

151. Gonzalez-Crussi F, Noronha R. Solitary fibromatosis in the newborn. Rare cause of neonatal intestinal obstruction. Arch Pathol Lab Med 1985;109:97.

152. Gonzalez-Crussi F, Reyes-Mugica M. Cellular hemangiomas ("hemangioendotheliomas") in infants: Light microscopic, immunohistochemical and ultrastructural observations. Am J Surg Pathol 1991;15: 769.

153. Gonzalez-Crussi F, Wiederhold MD, Sotelo-Avila C. Congenital fibrosarcoma: Presence of a histiocytic component. Cancer 1980;46:77.

154. Good TA, Carnazzo SF, Good RA. Thrombocytopenia and giant hemangioma in infants. Am J Dis Child 1955;90:260.

155. Gorenstein A, Katz S, Rein A, et al. Giant cystic hygroma associated with venous aneurysm. J Pediatr Surg 1992;27:1504.

156. Gormley PD, Thompson J, Aylward GW, et al. Congenital undifferentiated sarcoma of the orbit. J Pediatr Ophthalmol Strabismus 1994;31:59.

157. Greco MA, Garcia RL, Vuletin JC. Benign lipoblastomatosis. Ultrastructure and histogenesis. Cancer 1980;45:511.

158. Greco MA, Schinella RA, Vuletin JC. Fibrous hamartoma of infancy: An ultrastructural study. Hum Pathol 1984;15:717.

159. Grier HE, Perez-Atayde AR, Weinstein HJ. Chemotherapy for inoperable infantile fibrosarcoma. Cancer 1985;56:1507.

160. Grosfeld JL, Clatworthy HW, Newton WA. Combined therapy in childhood rhabdomyosarcomas: An analysis of 42 cases. J Pediatr Surg 1969;4:637.

161. Gutierrez-Ortega P, Hierro-Orozco S, Sanchez-Cisneros R, et al. Kaposi's sarcoma in a 6-day-old infant with human immunodeficiency virus. Arch Dermatol 1989;125:432.

162. Hachitanda Y, Tsuneyoshi M, Enjoji M, et al. Congenital primitive neuroectodermal tumor with epithelial and glial differentiation: An ultrastructural and immunohistochemical study. Arch Pathol Lab Med 1990;114:101.

163. Hagerman LJ, Czapek EE, Donnellan WL, et al. Giant hemangioma with consumption coagulopathy. J Pediatr 1975;87:766.

163a. Hart PS, Bodurtha J, Redwine FO, et al. Prenatal detection of non-cardiac rhabdomyosarcoma. Prenatal Diagn 10:169, 1990.

164. Hashimoto H, Enjoji M, Nakajima T, et al. Malignant neuroepithelioma (peripheral neuroblastoma): A clinicopathologic study of 15 cases. Am J Surg Pathol 1983;7:309.

165. Hawkins DB, Luxford WM. Schwannomas of the head and neck in children. Laryngoscope 1980;90:1921.

166. Hawkins HK, Camacho-Velasquez JV. Rhabdomyosarcoma in children: Correlation of form and prognosis in one institution's experience. Am J Surg Pathol 1987;11(7):531.

167. Hayashi K, Ohtsuki Y, Takahashi K, et al. Congenital alveolar rhabdomyosarcoma with multiple skin metastases. Acta Pathol Jpn 1988;38:241.

168. Hayashi Y, Inaba T, Hanada R, et al. Translocation 2; 8 in a congenital rhabdomyosarcoma. Cancer Genet Cytogenet 1988;30:343.

169. Hayashi Y, Spitz L, Kiely E, et al. Fibrous tissue tumors. Prog Pediatr Surg 1989;22:121.

170. Hays DM, Mirabal VQ, Karlan MS, et al. Fibrosarcomas in infants and children. J Pediatr Surg 1970;5:176.

171. Hayward PG, Orgill DP, Mulliken JB, et al. Congenital fibrosarcoma masquerading as lymphatic malformation: Report of two cases. J Pediatr Surg 1995;30:84.

172. Heifetz SA, Galliani CA, DeRosa GP. Myositis (fasciitis) ossificans in an infant. Pediatr Pathol 1992;12:223.

173. Hendrickson MR, Ross JC. Neoplasms arising in congenital giant nevi. Morphologic study of seven cases and review of the literature. Am J Surg Pathol 1981;5:109.

174. Hijazi YM, Axiotis CA, Navarro S, et al. Immunohistochemical detection of P-glycoprotein in Ewing's sarcoma and primitive neuroectodermal tumors before and after chemotherapy. Am J Clin Pathol 1994;102:61.

175. Himmel S, Siegel H. Congenital embryonal orbital rhabdomyosarcoma in a newborn. Arch Ophthalmol 1967;77:662.

176. Holden KR, Alexander F. Diffuse neonatal hemangiomatosis. Pediatrics 1970;46:411.

177. Holdsworth Mayer CM, Favara BE, Holton CP, et al. Malignant mesenchymoma in infants. Am J Dis Child 1974;128:847.

178. Horn RC, Enterline HT. Rhabdomyosarcoma: A clinicopathologic study of 39 cases. Cancer 1958;11:181.

179. Horowitz ME, DeLaney TF, Malawer MM, et al. Ewing's sarcoma family of tumors: Ewing's sarcoma of bone and soft tissue and the peripheral primitive neuroectodermal tumors. *In* Pizzo PA, Poplack DG (eds): Principles and Practice of Pediatric Oncology, 2nd ed, p 795. Philadelphia: JB Lippincott, 1993.

180. Humar S, Chou S, Carpenter B. Fibromatosis in infancy and childhood: The spectrum. J Pediatr Surg 1993;28:1446.

181. Inwards CV, Unni KK, Beabout JW, et al. Solitary congenital fibromatosis (infantile myofibromatosis) of bone. Am J Surg Pathol 1991;15:935.

182. Isaacs H Jr. Congenital malignant tumors. *In* Reed GB, Claireaux AE, Bain AD (eds): Diseases of the Fetus and Newborn: Pathology, Radiology and Genetics, p 131. London: Chapman Hall, 1989.

183. Isaacs, H Jr. Congenital and neonatal malignant tumors: A 28-year experience at Children's Hospital of Los Angeles. Am J Pediatr Hematol/Oncol 1987;9:121.

184. Isaacs H Jr. Neoplasms in infants: A report of 265 cases. *In* Sommers SC, Rosen PP (eds): Pathol Annu 1983;18(2):165.

185. Isaacs H Jr. Perinatal (congenital and neonatal) neoplasms: A report of 110 cases. Pediatr Pathol 1985;3:165.

186. Isaacs H Jr. Tumors. *In* Gilbert-Barness E (ed): Potter's Pathology of the Fetus and Infant, Vol 2, p 1242. St. Louis: Mosby–Year Book, 1996.

187. Isaacs H Jr. Tumors of the Newborn and Infant. St. Louis: Mosby–Year Book, 1991.

188. Iwasaki H, Kikuchi M, Ohtsuki I, et al. Infantile digital fibromatosis: Identification of actin filaments in cytoplasmic inclusions by heavy meromyosin binding. Cancer 1983;52:1653.

189. Jacobs AH, Walton RG. The incidence of birthmarks in the neonate. Pediatrics 58:218, 1976.

190. James CL, Bramwell NH, Davey RB, et al. Two unusual congenital tumors with long-term follow-up after local surgical resection. Pediatr Surg Int 1993;8:270.

191. Janney CG, Hurt MA, Santa Cruz DJ. Deep juvenile xanthogranuloma: Subcutaneous and intramuscular forms. Am J Surg Pathol 1991;15:150.

192. Jenkins HR, Hill CM. Spontaneous regression of congenital epulis of the newborn. Arch Dis Child 1989;64:145.

193. Jenkins JJ. Congenital malignant hemangiopericytoma. Pediatr Pathol 1987;7:119.

194. Jennings TA, Duray PH, Collins FS, et al. Infantile myofibromatosis. Evidence for an autosomal dominant disorder. Am J Surg Pathol 1984;8:259.

195. Jimenez JF, Seibert RW, Char F, et al. Melanotic neuroectodermal tumor of infancy and fetal hydantoin syndrome. Am J Pediatr Hematol Oncol 1981;3:9.

196. Johnson RE, Scheithauer BW, Dahlin DC. Melanotic neuroectodermal tumor of infancy. A review of seven cases. Cancer 1983;52:661.

197. Jones CJ. Unusual hamartoma of the lung in a newborn infant. Arch Pathol 1949;48:150.

198. Kapadia SB, Frisman DM, Hitchcock CL, et al. Melanotic neuroectodermal tumor of infancy: Clinicopathological, immunohistochemical and flow cytometric study. Am J Surg Pathol 1993;17:566.

199. Kapadia SB, Meis JM, Frisman DM, et al. Fetal rhabdomyoma of the head and neck: A clinicopathologic and immunophenotypic study of 24 cases. Hum Pathol 1993;24:754.

200. Karcioglu Z, Somerin A, Mathes SJ. Ectomesenchymoma. A malignant tumor of migratory neural crest (ectomesenchyme) remnants showing ganglionic, schwannian, melanocytic and rhabdomyoblastic differentiation. Cancer 1977;39:2486.

201. Kasabach HH, Merritt KK. Capillary hemangioma with extensive purpura: Report of a case. Am J Dis Child 1940;59:1063.

202. Katz VL, Watson WJ, Thorp JM Jr, et al. Prenatal sonographic findings of massive lower extremity lymphangioma. Am J Perinatol 1992;9:127.

203. Kauffman SL, Stout AP. Congenital mesenchymal tumors. Cancer 1965;18:460.

204. Kauffman SL, Stout AP. Hemangiopericytoma in children. Cancer 1960;13:695.

205. Kauffman SL, Stout AP. Histiocytic tumors in children. Cancer 1961;14:469.

206. Kauffman SL, Stout AP. Lipoblastic tumors of children. Cancer 1959;59:512.

207. Kawamoto EH, Weidner N, Agostini RM, et al. Malignant ectomesenchymoma of soft tissue. Report of two cases and review of the literature. Cancer 1987;59:1791.

208. Keeling JW. Fetal hydrops. *In* Keeling JW (ed): Fetal and Neonatal Pathology, 2nd ed, p 253. Berlin: Springer-Verlag, 1993.

209. Khoury EN, Speer FD. Rhabdomyosarcoma of the urinary bladder: A clinicopathological case report with a review of the literature, including a tabulation of rhabdomyosarcoma of the prostate. J Urol 1944;51:505.

210. Kingston JE, McElwain TJ, Malpas JS. Childhood rhabdomyosarcoma: Experience of the Children's Solid Tumor Group. Br J Cancer 1983;48:195.

211. Kodet R, Fajstavr J, Kabelka, et al. Is fetal cellular rhabdomyoma an entity or a differentiated rhabdomyosarcoma?: A study of patients with rhabdomyoma of the tongue and sarcoma of the tongue enrolled in the Intergroup Rhabdomyosarcoma Studies I, II, and III. Cancer 1991;67:2907.

212. Kodet R, Kasthuri N, Marsden HB, et al. Ganglio-rhabdomyosarcoma: A histopathological and immunohistochemical study of three cases. Histopathology 1986;10:181.

213. Kodet R, Newton WA Jr, Sachs N, et al. Rhabdoid tumors of soft tissues: A clinicopathologic study of 26 cases enrolled in the Intergroup Rhabdomyosarcoma Study. Hum Pathol 22:674, 1991.

214. Kodet R, Smelhaus V, Newton WA Jr, et al. Epithelioid sarcoma in childhood: An immunohistochemical, electron microscopic and clinicopathologic study of 11 cases under 15 years of age and review of the literature. Pediatr Pathol 1994;14:433.

215. Konrad EA, Meister P, Hubner G. Extracardiac rhabdomyoma: Report of different types with light microscopic and ultrastructural studies. Cancer 1982;49:898.

216. Koscieiniak H, Harms D, Schmidt, et al. Soft tissue sarcomas in infants younger than 1 year of age: A report of the German Soft Tissue Sarcoma Study Group (CSW-81). Med Pediatr Oncol 1989;17:105.

217. Krugly M, Emanuel B, Smallberg W, et al. Retroperitoneal xanthogranuloma. Pediatr 1962;30:608.

218. Krumerman MS, Stingle W. Synchronous malignant glandular schwannomas in congenital neurofibromatosis. Cancer 1978;41:2444.

219. Kurjak A, Zalud I, Jurkovic Z, et al. Ultrasound diagnosis and evaluation of fetal tumors. J Perinat Med 1989;17:173.

220. Kynaston JA, Malcolm AJ, Craft AW, et al. Chemotherapy in the management of infantile fibrosarcoma. Med Pediatr Oncol 1993;21:488.

221. Lack EE. Leiomyosarcomas in childhood: A clinical and pathologic study of 10 cases. Pediatr Pathol 1986;6:181.

222. Lack EE, Perez-Atayde AR, McGill TJ. Gingival granular cell tumor of the newborn (congenital "epulis"): Ultrastructural observations relating to histiogenesis. Hum Pathol 1982;13:686.

223. Lack EE, Worsham GF, Callihan MD, et al. Gingival granular cell tumors of the newborn (congenital "epulis"): A clinical and pathologic study of 21 patients. Am J Surg Pathol 1981;5:37.

224. Landing BH, Farber S. Tumors of the Cardiovascular System. *In* Atlas of Tumor Pathology. Washington, DC: Armed Forces Institute of Pathology, 1956.

225. Larsen EC, Zinkham WH, Eggleston JC, et al. Kasabach-Merritt syndrome: Therapeutic considerations. Pediatrics 1987;79:971.

226. Lauer D, Enzinger FM. Cranial fasciitis of childhood. Cancer 1980;45:401.

227. Lawrence W Jr, Gehan EA, Hays DM, et al. Prognostic significance of staging factors of the UICC staging system in childhood rhabdomyosarcoma: A report of the Intergroup Rhabdomyosarcoma Study (IRS-II). J Clin Oncol 1987;5:46.

228. LeBer MS, Stout AP. Benign mesenchymomas in children. Cancer 1962;15:598.

229. Lee SC, Henry MM, Gonzalez-Crussi F. Simultaneous occurrence of melanotic neuroectodermal tumor and brain heterotopia in the oropharynx. Cancer 1976;38:249.

230. Lemos LB, Hamoudi AB. Malignant thymic tumor in an infant (malignant histiocytoma). Arch Pathol Lab Med 1978;102:84.

231. Leuschner I, Newton WA Jr, Schmidt D, et al. Spindle cell variants of embryonal rhabdomyosarcoma in the paratesticular region: A report of the Intergroup Rhabdomyosarcoma Study. Am J Surg Pathol 1993;17:221.

232. Lever WF, Schaumburg-Lever G. Histopathology of the Skin, 7th ed. Philadelphia: JB Lippincott, 1990.

233. Li FP, Fraumeni JF Jr. Rhabdomyosarcoma in children: Epidemiologic study and identification of a familial cancer syndrome. J Natl Cancer Inst 1969;43:1365.

234. Liew S, Haynes M. Localized form of congenital generalized fibromatosis. A report of three cases with myofibroblasts. Pathology 1981;13:257.

235. Lifshitz MS, Flotte TJ, Greco MA. Congenital granular cell epulis. Immunohistochemical and ultrastructural observations. Cancer 1984;53;1845.

236. Lin JJ, Svoboda DJ. Multiple congenital mesenchymal tumors—Multiple vascular leiomyomas in several organs of a newborn. Cancer 1971;28:1046.

237. Lindahl F. Malignant melanotic progonoma: One case. Acta Pathol Microbiol Scand 1970;78A:532.

238. Lobe TE, Wiener ES, Hays DM, et al. Neonatal rhabdomyosarcoma: The IRS experience. J Pediatr Surg 1994;29:1167.

239. Lundgren L, Angervall L, Stenman G, et al. Infantile rhabdomyofibrosarcoma: A high grade sarcoma distinguishable. Hum Pathol 1993;24:785.

240. Lynch HT, Shurin SB, Dahms BB, et al. Paravertebral malignant rhabdoid tumor in infancy: In vitro studies of a familial tumor. Cancer 1983;52:290.

241. Lyon DB, Dortzbach RK, Gilbert-Barness E. Polyphenotypic small-cell orbitocranial tumor. Arch Ophthalmol 1993;111:1402.

242. MacDonald D. Sternomastoid tumor and muscular torticollis. J Bone Joint Surg 1969;51B:432.

243. Madarikan BA, Thompson EN, Lari J. Neonatal colorectal spindle cell sarcoma. J Pediatr Surg 26:1416, 1991.

244. Madden NP, Spicer RD, Allibone EB, et al. Spontaneous regression of neonatal fibrosarcoma. Br J Cancer 66 (Suppl 18):S72, 1992.

245. Mahour GH, Bryan BJ, Isaacs H Jr. Lipoblastoma and lipoblastomatosis—A report of six cases. Surgery 1988;104:577.

246. Mahour GH, Soule EH, Mills SD, et al. Rhabdomyosarcoma in infants and children: A clinicopathologic study of 75 cases. J Pediatr Surg 1967;2:402.

247. Martell JR Jr, Busnardo MS, Barja RH, et al. Congenital fibrosarcoma of the forearm: A case report. J Bone Joint Surg 1986;68A:620.

248. Matsui I, Tanimura M, Kobayashi N, et al. Neurofibromatosis type 1 and childhood cancer. Cancer 1993;72:2746, 1993.

249. Maurer HM, Ragab AH. Rhabdomyosarcoma. *In* Fernbach DJ, Vietti TJ (eds): Clinical Pediatric Oncology, 4th ed, p 491. St. Louis: Mosby–Year Book, 1991.

250. McKeen EA, Bodurtha J, Meadows AT, et al. Rhabdomyosarcoma complicating multiple neurofibromatosis. J Pediatr 1978;93:992.

251. Meis JM, Enzinger FM. Proliferative fasciitis and myositis of childhood. Am J Surg Pathol 1992;16:364.

252. Meis JM, Enzinger FM, Martz KL, et al. Malignant peripheral nerve sheath tumors (malignant schwannomas) in children. Am J Surg Pathol 1992;16:694.

253. Meis-Kindblom JM, Enzinger FM. Plexiform malignant peripheral nerve sheath tumor of infancy and childhood. Am J Surg Pathol 1994;18:479.

254. Mentzel T, Calonje E, Fletcher CDM. Lipoblastoma and lipoblastomatosis: A clinicopathologic study of 14 cases. Histopathology 1993;23:527.

255. Mentzel T, Calonje E, Nascimento AG, et al. Infantile hemangiopericytoma versus infantile myofibromatosis: Study of a series suggesting a continuous spectrum of infantile myofibroblastic lesions. Am J Surg Pathol 1994;18:922.

256. Michel M, Ninane J, Claus D, et al. Major malformations in a case of infantile myofibromatosis. Eur J Pediatr 1990;149:251.

257. Mitchell ML, Di Sant'Agnese PA, Gerber JE. Fibrous hamartoma of infancy. Hum Pathol 1982;13:586.

258. Modi N: Congenital generalized fibromatosis. Arch Dis Child 1982;57:881.

259. Moerman P, Goddeeris P, Fryns J, et al. Primitive neuroectodermal tumor: A newly recognized cause of early fetal death. Pediatr Pathol 1985;4:137.

260. Mohan KK, Lal A. Congenital embryonal rhabdomyosarcoma of the tongue (letter). Anesth Analg 1992;74:930.

261. Montgomery EA, Meis JM. Nodular fasciitis: Its morphologic spectrum and immunohistochemical profile. Am J Surg Pathol 1991;15:942.

262. Moore JB, Waldenmaier N, Potchen EJ. Congenital generalized fibromatosis. A new management strategy provided by magnetic resonance imaging. Am J Dis Child 1987;141:714.

263. Moore KL. The Developing Human: Clinically Oriented Embryology, 5th ed. Philadelphia: WB Saunders, 1993.

264. Morgan K, Batcup G, Aparicio S, et al. Proliferative fasciitis in childhood: A case report. Pediatr Pathol 1990;10:431.

265. Morgan R, Evboumwan I. Congenital haemangiopericytoma of the face with early distant metastases. JR Coll Surg Edinb 1983;28:123.

266. Morison JE. Foetal and Neonatal Pathology, 3rd ed, p 119. New York: Appleton-Century-Crofts, 1970.

267. Mukai M, Torikata C, Hisami I, et al. Immunohistochemical identification of aggregated actin filaments in formalin-fixed, paraffin embedded sections. I. A study of infantile digital fibromatosis by a new pretreatment. Am J Surg Pathol 1992;16:110.

268. Muraskas JK, Gianopoulos JG, Husain A, et al. Mediastinal cystic hygroma: Prenatal decompression with neonatal resection and recurrence at 19 months of age. J Perinatol 1983;13:381.

269. Nagase H, Yamaguchi Y, Morinaga H, et al. Multicentric infantile myofibromatosis with spontaneous regression. Pediatr Surg Int 1993;8:84.

270. Nagaya M, Tsuda M, Ishiguro Y. Leiomyosarcoma of the transverse colon in a neonate: A rare cause of meconium peritonitis. J Pediatr Surg 1989;24:1177.

271. Nakamura Y, Becker LE, Mancer K, et al. Peripheral medulloepithelioma. Acta Neuropathol 1982;57:137.

272. Nash A, Stout AP. Malignant mesenchymomas in children. Cancer 1961;14:524.

273. Ninane J, Gosseye S, Panteon E, et al. Congenital fibrosarcoma: Preoperative chemotherapy and conservative surgery. Cancer 1986;58:1400.

274. Nishioka H, Furusho K, Yasunaga T, et al. Congenital malignant mesothelioma: A case report and electron-microscopic study. Eur J Pediatr 1988;147:428.

275. Nixon HH, Scobie WG. Congenital lipomatosis: A report of four cases. J Pediatr Surg 1971;6:742.

276. Nunnery EW, Kahn LB, Reddick RL, et al. Hemangiopericytoma: A light microscopic and ultrastructural study. Cancer 1981;47:906.

277. Ober WB, Smith JA, Rouillard FC. Congenital sarcoma botryoides of the vagina—Report of two cases. Cancer 1958;11:620.

278. Ordonez NG, El-Naggar AK, Ro JY, et al. Intra-abdominal desmoplastic small cell tumor: A light microscopic, immunocytochemical, and flow cytometric study. Hum Pathol 1993;24:850.

279. Ordonez NG, Mackay B, El-Naggar AK, et al. Congenital hemangiopericytoma: An ultrastructural, immunocytochemical and flow cytometric study. Arch Pathol Lab Med 1993;117:934.

280. Pappo AS, Douglass EC, Meyer WH, et al. Use of HBA 71 and anti-β2-microglobulin to distinguish peripheral neuroepithelioma from neuroblastoma. Hum Pathol 1993;24:880.

281. Parham DM. The molecular biology of childhood rhabdomyosarcoma. Semin Diagn Pathol 11:39, 1994.

281a. Parham DM, Shapiro DN, Downing JR, et al. Solid alveolar rhabdomyosarcomas with the t(2;13): Report of two cases with diagnostic implications. Am J Surg Pathol 1994;18:474.

282. Parham DM, Weeks DA, Beckwith JB. The clinicopathologic spectrum of putative extrarenal rhabdoid tumors: An analysis of 42 cases studied with immunohistochemistry or electron microscopy. Am J Surg Pathol 1994;18:1010.

283. Park SH, Kim TJ, Je GC. Congenital granular cell tumor with systemic involvement: Immunohistochemical and ultrastructural study. Arch Pathol Lab Med 1991;115:934.

284. Parkes SE, Muir KR, Southern L, et al. Neonatal tumours: A thirty-year population based study. Med Pediatr Oncol 1994;22:309.

285. Parry DM, Mulvihill JJ, Miller RW, et al. Sarcomas in a child and her father. Am J Dis Childh 1979;133:130.

286. Pasquel P, Salazar M, Marvan E. Proliferative myositis in an infant: Report of a case with electron microscopic observations. Pediatr Pathol 1988;8:545.

287. Peace RJ. A congenital neoplasm of the brain of a newborn infant. Report of a case with necropsy. Am J Clin Pathol 1954;24:1272.

288. Pettinato G, Manivel C, d'Amore SG, et al. Melanotic neuroectodermal tumor of infancy: A reexamination of a histogenetic problem based on immunohistochemical, flow cytometric and ultrastructural study. Am J Surg Pathol 1991;15:233.

289. Pierce RN, Dunn L, Knisely AS. Consumptive coagulopathy in utero associated with multiple vascular malformations. Pediatr Pathol 1992;12:67.

290. Pijpers L, Renss A, Stuart PA, et al. Fetal cystic hygroma: Prenatal diagnosis and management. Obstet Gynecol 1988;72:233.

291. Pleasure J, Geller SA. Neurofibromatosis in infancy presenting with congenital stridor. Am J Dis Child 1967;113:390.

292. Potter EL, Craig JM. Pathology of the Fetus and Infant, 3rd ed, p 177. Chicago: Year Book Medical Publishers, 1975.

293. Potter EL, Parrish JM. Neuroblastoma, ganglioneuroma and fibroneuroma in a stillborn fetus. Am J Pathol 1942;18:141.

294. Qualman SJ, Green WR, Brovall C, et al. Neurofibromatosis and associated neuroectodermal tumors: A congenital neurocristopathy. Pediatr Pathol 1986;5:65.

295. Quinn FMJ, Brown S, O'Hara D. Hemangiopericytoma of the stomach in a neonate. J Pediatr Surg 1991;26:101.

296. Ragab AH, Heyn R, Tefft M, et al. Infants younger than 1 year of age with rhabdomyosarcoma. Cancer 1986;58:2606–2610.

297. Rainey JB, Smith IJ. Congenital epulis of the newborn. J Pediatr Surg 1985;19:305.

298. Raju U, Zarbo RJ, Regezi JA, et al. Melanotic neuroectodermal tumors of infancy: Intermediate filament-, neuroendocrine- and melanoma-associated antigen profiles. Applied Immunohistochem 1993;1:69.

299. Raney RB, Allen A, O'Neil J, et al. Malignant fibrous histiocytoma of soft tissue in childhood. Cancer 1986; 57:2198.

300. Raney RB Jr, Hays DM, Tefft M, et al. Rhabdomyosarcoma and the undifferentiated sarcomas. *In* Pizzo PA, Poplack DG (eds): Principles and Practice of Pediatric Oncology, 2nd ed, p 769. Philadelphia: JB Lippincott, 1993.

301. Reddick RL, Michelitch H, Triche TJ. Malignant soft tissue tumors (malignant fibrous histiocytoma, pleomorphic liposarcoma, and pleomorphic rhabdomyosarcoma): An electron microscopic study. Hum Pathol 1979;10:327.

302. Reece EA: Fetal neoplasm. *In* Reece EA, Hobbins JC, Mahoney MJ, Petrie RH (eds): Medicine of the Fetus and Mother, p 617. Philadelphia: JB Lippincott, 1992.

303. Reese V, Frieden IJ, Paller AS, et al. Association of facial hemangiomas with Dandy-Walker and other posterior fossa malformations. J Pediatr 1993;122:379.

304. Resnick SD, Lacey S, Jones G. Hemorrhagic complications in a rapidly growing, congenital hemangiopericytoma. Pediatr Dermatol 1993;10:267.

305. Reye RDK. Considerations of certain subdermal "fibromatous tumors" of infancy. J Pathol Bact 1956;72:149.

305a. Reye RDK. Recurring digital fibrous tumors of childhood. Arch Pathol 1965;80:228.

306. Rhodin JAG. Histology: A Text and Atlas, p 354. New York: Oxford University Press, 1974.

307. Riccardi VM, Eichner JE. Neurofibromatosis: Phenotype, natural history, and pathogenesis. Baltimore: Johns Hopkins University Press, 1986.

308. Ricketts RR, Majmudarr B. Epididymal melanotic neuroectodermal tumor of infancy. Hum Pathol 1985;16:416.

309. Robinson W, Crawford AH. Infantile fibrosarcoma: Report of a case with long-term follow-up. J Bone Joint Surg 1990;72-A:291.

310. Roggli VL, Kim HS, Hawkins E. Congenital generalized fibromatosis with visceral involvement. A case report. Cancer 1980;45:954.

311. Romero R, Oilu G, Jeanty P, Ghidini A, Hobbins JC: Prenatal Diagnosis of Congenital Anomalies. Norwalk, CT: Appleton & Lange, 1988.

312. Rootman J, Carvounis EE, Dolman CL, et al. Congenital fibrosarcoma metastatic to the choroid. Am J Ophthalmol 1979;87:632.

313. Rosenberg HS, Stenback WA, Spjut HJ. The fibromatoses of infancy and childhood. *In* Rosenberg HS, Bolande RP (eds): Perspectives in Pediatric Pathology, Vol 4, p 269. Chicago: Year Book Medical Publishers, 1978.

314. Rothe MJ, Rowse D, Grant-Kels JM. Benign neonatal hemangiomatosis with aggressive growth of cutaneous lesions. Pediatr Dermatol 1991;8:140.

315. Ruymann FB, Newton W, Ragab A, et al. Congenital anomalies in rhabdomyosarcoma. Proceedings of the Conference on Congenital Birth Defects. Memphis, TN, June 9–11, 1977.

316. Salamah MM, Hammoudi SM, Sadi ARM. Infantile myofibromatosis. J Pediatr Surg 1988;23:975.

317. Salloum E, Flamant F, Caillaud JM, et al. Diagnostic and therapeutic problems of soft tissue tumors other than rhabdomyosarcoma in infants under 1 year of age: A clinicopathological study of 34 cases treated at the Institut Gustave-Roussy. Med Pediatr Oncol 1990: 18:37, 1990.

318. Schechheimer K, Kuhl G. Arteriovenous angioma of the vein of Galen causing cardiac failure in the neonate. Report on clinical and pathological findings in two cases. Neuropediatrics 1983;14:184.

319. Schmidt D, Harms D. Fibromatosis of infancy and childhood—Histology and ultrastructure and clinicopathologic correlation. Z Kinderchir 1985;40:40.

320. Schmidt D, Harms D, Burdach S. Malignant peripheral neuroectodermal tumours of childhood and adolescence. Virch Arch [Pathol Anat] 1985;406:351.

321. Schmookler BM, Enzinger FM. Liposarcoma occurring in children: An analysis of 17 cases and review of the literature. Cancer 1983;52:567.

322. Schofield DE, Fletcher JA, Grier HE, et al. Fibrosarcoma of infants and children: Application of new techniques. Am J Surg Pathol 1994;18:14.

323. Seemayer TA, Thelmo WL, Bolande RP, et al. Peripheral neuroectodermal tumors. *In* Rosenberg HS, Bolande RP (eds): Perspectives in Pediatric Pathology, Vol 2, p 151. Chicago: Year Book Medical Publishers, 1975.

324. Seibert JJ, Seibert RW, Weisenburger DS, et al. Multiple congenital hemangiopericytomas of the head and neck. Laryngoscope 1978;88:1006.

325. Shamberger RC, Grier HE, et al. Chest wall tumors in infancy and childhood. Cancer 63:774, 1989.

326. Shearer WT, Schreiner RL, Ward SP, et al. Benign nasal tumor appearing as neonatal respiratory distress: First reported case of nasopharyngeal fibrous histiocytoma. Am J Dis Child 1973;126:238.

327. Shira RA: Pigmented neuroectodermal tumor of infancy: An example of rarely expressed malignant behavior. Oral Surg 1980;49:279.

328. Shnitka TK, Asp DM, Horner RH. Congenital generalized fibromatosis. Cancer 1958;11:627.

329. Shokry A, Briner J, Makek M. Malignant melanotic neuroectodermal tumor of infancy: A case report. Pediatr Pathol 1986;5:217.

330. Small EJ, Gordon GJ, Dahms BB. Malignant rhabdoid tumor of the heart in an infant. Cancer 55:2850, 1985.

331. Sonoda T, Hashimoto H, Enjoji M: Juvenile xanthogranuloma: Clinicopathologic analysis and immunohistochemical study of 57 patients. Cancer 1985;56: 2280.

332. Sonoda T, Itami S, Seguchi S, et al. Infantile myofibromatosis: Report of two cases. J Dermatol 1994;21: 508.

333. Soper JR, De Silva M. Infantile myofibromatosis: A radiological review. Pediatr Radiol 1993;23:189.

334. Sotelo-Avila C, Bale PM. Subepidermal fibrous hamartoma of infancy: Pathology of 40 cases and differential diagnosis. Pediatr Pathol 1994;14:39.

335. Sotelo-Avila C, Gonzalez-Crussi F, deMello D, et al. Renal and extrarenal rhabdoid tumors in children: A clinicopathologic study of 14 patients. Semin Diagn Pathol 1986;3:151.

336. Soule EH, Pritchard DJ. Fibrosarcoma in infants and children. A review of 110 cases. Cancer 1977;40: 1711.

337. Spaeth EB, Cleveland AF. Rhabdomyosarcoma in infancy and childhood. Am J Ophthalmol 1962;53:463.

338. Speleman F, Dal Cin P, De Potter K, et al. Cytogenetic investigation of a case of congenital fibrosarcoma. Cancer Genet Cytogenet 1989;39:21.

339. Spraker MK, Stack C, Esterly NB. Congenital generalized fibromatosis: A review of the literature and report of a case associated with porencephaly, hemiatrophy, and cutis marmorata telangiectatica congenita. J Am Acad Dermatol 1984;10:365.

340. Srigley JR, Mancer K. Solitary intestinal fibromatosis with perinatal bowel obstruction. Pediatr Pathol 1984; 2:249.

341. Stay EJ, Vawter G. The relationship between nephroblastoma and neurofibromatosis (von Recklinghausen's disease). Cancer 1977;39:2550.

342. Stenninger E, Schollin J. Diffuse neonatal haemangiomatosis in a newborn child. Acta Paediatr 1993;82: 102.

343. Stillman AE, Hansen RC, Hallinan V, et al. Diffuse neonatal hemangiomatosis with severe gastrointestinal involvement: Favorable response to steroid therapy. Clin Pediatr 1983;22:589.

344. Stirling RW, Powell G, Fletcher CDM. Pigmented neuroectodermal tumor of infancy: An immunohistochemical study. Histopathology 1988;12:425.

345. Stout AP. Fibrosarcoma in infants and children. Cancer 1962;15:1028.

346. Stout AP. Juvenile fibromatoses. Cancer 1954;7:953.

347. Stout AP. Pseudosarcomatous fasciitis in children. Cancer 1961;14:1216.

348. Stout AP, Murray MR. Hemangiopericytoma. A vascular tumor featuring Zimmermann's pericytes. Ann Surg 1942;116:26.

349. Stowens D, Lin T-H. Melanotic progonoma of the brain. Hum Pathol 1974;5:105.

350. Swanson PE, Wick MR, Dehner LP. Leiomyosarcoma of somatic soft tissues in childhood: An immunohistochemical analysis of six cases with ultrastructural correlation. Hum Pathol 1991;22:569.

351. Teng P, Warden MJ, Cohn WL. Congenital generalized fibromatosis (renal and skeletal) with complete spontaneous regression. J Pediatr 1963;62:748.

352. Thomas RL. Prenatal diagnosis of giant cystic hygroma: Prognosis, counselling, and management: Case presentation and review of the recent literature. Prenatal Diagn 1992;12:919.

353. Tracy TJR, Neifield JP, DeMay RM, et al. Malignant fibrous histiocytoma in children. J Pediatr Surg 1984; 19:81.

354. Ts'o TOT, Teoh TB. Fibromatosis in an infant. J Pathol Bacteriol 1963;85:521.

355. Tsokos M. The diagnosis and classification of childhood rhabdomyosarcoma. Semin Diagn Pathol 1994; 11:26.

356. Tsokos M. Peripheral primitive neuroectodermal tumors: Diagnosis, classification and prognosis. Perspect Pediatr Pathol 16:27, 1992.

357. Tsokos M, Kouraklis G, Chandra RS, et al. Malignant rhabdoid tumor of the kidney and soft tissues: Evidence for a diverse morphological and immunocytochemical phenotype. Arch Pathol Lab Med 1989;113: 115.

358. Tsokos M, Webber BL, Parham DM, et al. Rhabdomyosarcoma: A new classification scheme related to prognosis. Arch Pathol Lab Med 1992;116:847.

359. Tsui HN, Lore JM. Congenital subglottic fibroma in the newborn. Laryngoscope 1976;86:571.

360. Tsuneyoshi M, Daimaru Y, Hashimoto H, et al. Malignant soft tissue neoplasms with the histologic features of renal rhabdoid tumors: An ultrastructural and immunohistochemical study. Hum Pathol 1985;16:1235.

361. Tucker MC, Rusnock EJ, Azumi N, et al. Gingival granular cell tumors of the newborn: An ultrastructural and immunohistochemical study. Arch Pathol Lab Med 1990;114:895.

362. Tulenko JF. Congenital hemangiopericytoma: Case report. Plastic Reconstruct Surg 1968;41:276.

363. van Baarlen J, Bax NMA. Congenital hemangiopericytoma: Report of a case. Pediatr Pathol 1988;8:109.

364. Variend S, Bax NMA, Van Gorp J. Are infantile myofibromatosis, congenital fibrosarcoma and congenital haemangiopericytoma histogenetically related? Histopathology 1995;26:57.

365. Virden CP, Lynch FP. Infantile hemangiopericytoma: A rare cause of a soft tissue mass. J Pediatr Surg 1993; 28:741.

366. Voss BL, Pysher TJ, Humphrey GB. Peripheral neuroepithelioma in childhood. Cancer 1984;54:3059.

367. Walts AE, Asch M, Raj C. Solitary lesion of congenital fibromatosis. Am J Surg Pathol 1982;6:255.

368. Wee A, Pho RWH, Ong LB. Infantile fibrosarcoma: Report of cases. Arch Pathol Lab Med 1979; 103:236.

369. Weeks DA, Beckwith JB, Mierau GW, et al. Rhabdoid tumor of the kidney: A report of 11 cases from the National Wilms' Tumor Study Pathology Center. Am J Surg Pathol 1989;13:439.

370. Weiss SW, Enzinger FM. Malignant fibrous histiocytoma: An analysis of 200 cases. Cancer 1978;41: 2250.

371. Welborn JL, Timm NS. Trisomy 21 and cystic hygromas in early gestational age fetuses. Am J Perinatol 1994;11:19.

372. Wharan M, Beltangady M, Hays DM, et al. Localized orbital rhabdomyosarcoma: An interim report of the Intergroup Rhabdomyosarcoma Study Committee. Ophthalmology 1987;94:251.

373. White W, Garen P. Juvenile xanthogranuloma of the paravertebral soft tissue in infancy: A report of two cases. Pediatr Pathol 1991;11:105.

374. Whitten RO, Benjamin DR. Rhabdomyoma of the retroperitoneum: A report of a tumor with both adult and fetal characteristics. A study by light and electron microscopy, histochemistry and immunochemistry. Cancer 1987;59:818.

375. Wigger JH, Mitsudo SM. Fibrous histiocytoma simulating congenital fibromatosis: A light-, electron microscopic and tissue culture study. Virchow Arch [A] 1976;370;255.

376. Willis RA. The Borderland of Embryology and Pathology, 2nd ed, p 422. London: Butterworths, 1962.

377. Wiswell TE, Davis J, Cunningham BE, et al. Infantile myofibromatosis: The most common fibrous tumor of infancy. J Pediatr Surg 1988;23:314.

378. Wood GS, Beckstead JH, Turner RR, et al. Malignant fibrous histiocytoma tumor cells resemble fibroblasts. Am J Surg Pathol 1986;10:323.

379. Woodruff JM, Chernik NL, Smith MC, et al. Peripheral nerve tumors with rhabdomyosarcomatous differentiation (malignant "triton" tumors). Cancer 1973; 32:426.

380. Yannopoulos K, Stout AP. Smooth muscle tumors in children. Cancer 1962;15:958.

381. Young JL, Miller RW. Incidence of malignant tumors in U.S. children. J Pediatr 1975;86:254.

382. Young S, Crocker D. Congenital midline bilateral ganglioneuromas associated with hydrops fetalis and neurofibromatosis. Pediatr Pathol 1993;13:115.

383. Yun K. Infantile digital fibromatosis: Immunohistochemical and ultrastructural observations of cytoplasmic inclusions. Cancer 1988;61:500.

384. Zalel Y, Shalev E, Ben-Ami M, et al. Ultrasonic diagnosis of mediastinal cystic hygroma. Prenat Diagn 1992;12:541.

385. Zelger B, Cerio R, Orchard G, et al. Juvenile and adult xanthogranuloma: A histological and immunohistochemical comparison. Am J Surg Pathol 1994;18:126.

386. Zone RM. Retinal anlage tumor of the epididymis. A case report. J Urol 1970;103:106.

387. Zuniga S, Las Heras J, Benveniste S. Rhabdomyosarcoma arising in a congenital giant nevus associated with neurocutaneous melanosis in a neonate. J Pediatr Surg 1987;22:1036.

388. Zuppan CW, Mierau GW, Wilson HL. Malignant fibrous histiocytoma in childhood: A report of two cases and review of the literature. Pediatr Pathol 1987;7:303.

5

TUMORS AND TUMOR-LIKE CONDITIONS OF THE SKIN

Tumors and tumor-like conditions of the skin occur frequently in the fetus and newborn and include a wide variety of entities (Table 5–1). The vascular lesions hemangioma and lymphangioma are the most prevalent of such tumors, but other conditions, such as congenital melanocytic nevi, cutaneous hamartomas, and neoplastic-like infiltrations occur as well (see Table 5–1).[2,21,53,62,74] In the differential diagnosis of a cutaneous nodular infiltrate, leukemia cutis, neuroblastoma, and other neoplasms that are metastatic to the skin (as listed in Table 5–1) should be considered.

The term nevus is a common but rather nebulous term applied to many different kinds of cutaneous nodules and birthmarks. Generally, it refers to a localized malformation of the skin, consisting of mature or nearly mature elements, which may or may not be present at birth.[62] The term is frequently used in two ways: (1) as a name for a lesion composed of nevus cells (e.g., a congenital melanocytic nevus) and (2) as a name for a non-nevus cell condition, such as one consisting of vascular, epidermal, adnexal, connective tissue, or neural elements. Whether nevi actually represent true tumors, hamartomas, or hyperplasias is open for debate, but most appear to be hamartomas, which are classically defined as proliferations of cellular elements normally found in the location of origin. The term birthmark is defined as a skin lesion existing at birth or appearing within the first week of life.[56]

EMBRYOLOGY

At the end of the first month of development, the embryo is covered by a single layer of cells—the periderm—which is derived from the ectoderm.[70,76] These cells gradually proliferate and, by the fourth month, a superficial keratinized layer, an intermediate transitional zone, and a basal germinal layer can be recognized. The dermis arises from the mesoderm situated beneath the periderm. In the early months, the junction between the epidermis and underlying dermal connective tissue is a smooth plane. As the epidermis thickens, the junction becomes irregular, and the mesenchyme of the dermis projects into the epidermis, forming the vascular connective tissue of the dermal papillae.[70,76]

The primordia of hair follicles and sebaceous glands appear during the third and fourth months of gestation. Hairs are not visible above the body surface until late in the sixth or early part of the seventh month. The first hairs are fine, are set close together, and form a downy coat called lanugo. Most of these hairs are shed before or soon after birth and are replaced by coarser hairs that arise from new follicles.[76]

Sebaceous glands form concomitantly with hair follicles. They are actively secreting by the seventh month, and at the normal time of birth, the fetus is usually irregularly coated with a thin layer of white, cheesy material known as vernix caseosa. It is a mixture of sebum,

Table 5–1. Tumors and Tumor-like Conditions of the Skin in the Fetus and Newborn

Hemangioma
Pyogenic granuloma
Lymphangioma
Neurofibroma
Digital fibromatosis
Myofibromatosis
Fibrous hamartoma of infancy
Smooth muscle hamartoma
Nevus lipomatosis
Granular cell tumor
Melanocytic nevus
Malignant melanoma
Epidermal nevus
Sebaceous nevus
Papilloma
Langerhans cell histiocytosis (Letterer-Siwe disease)
Urticaria pigmentosa (mast cell disease)
Juvenile xanthogranuloma
Dermal extramedullary erythropoiesis
Tumors metastatic to the skin
   Neuroblastoma
   Leukemia
   Rhabdomyosarcoma
   Rhabdoid tumor
   Adrenocortical carcinoma

desquamated squamous epithelium, and lanugo.[76]

Sweat glands begin to develop slightly later than the sebaceous glands. They appear first as solid cords of cells extending from the epidermis into the underlying connective tissue. They begin to develop lumina during the seventh month, but there is no proof of secretion before birth.[76]

Early in the second month of gestation, melanoblasts derived from neural crest cells migrate into the dermis around vessels and nerves; slightly later, they migrate into the epidermis. The differentiation of melanoblasts into mature melanocytes involves the development of pigment granules, termed melanosomes, from premelanosomes. Melanosomes are evident in epidermal melanocytes at about 8 weeks.[66]

In the first trimester, at approximately 12 weeks, Langerhans cells, derived from the monocyte-macrophage system, migrate into the epidermis.[66] They are involved in the presentation of antigens and cooperate with T lymphocytes in the skin to initiate cell-mediated responses against foreign antigens. Although Langerhans cells are not observed on sections of the skin stained with hematoxylin-eosin, they are readily identified by their reactivity with S-100 protein and T6 thymocyte antigen and by the presence of cytoplasmic, tennis racket–shaped Birbeck granules on electron microscopic studies (see Figs. 5–11 and 8–1).[50] Langerhans cells constitute 2% to 8% of the total number of epidermal cells and are found in relatively smaller numbers in the dermis.[66]

Dermal myelopoiesis and erythropoiesis are normally present from the first to fifth month of gestation.

VASCULAR CONDITIONS

Hemangioma and lymphangioma are the main vascular lesions involving the skin of newborns and infants. Hemangiomas are noted much more frequently than lymphangiomas and are operated upon less often than the latter, presumably because most of them regress or disappear spontaneously by adolescence.[50,76]

Hemangioma

Hemangioma is the most common tumor-like condition and birthmark of the newborn and infant, and it may be found on any part of the skin, most often on the neck and face, as one or, sometimes, as multiple lesions.[2,12,27,51,52,56,76] These lesions are observed in 10% of infants, compared to only 2% to 4% of newborns, as many of them are not apparent at birth.[2,52,56] Of the various vascular lesions, the capillary hemangioma and the port wine nevus are the ones that are seen most often during the first year of life.[76]

Hemangiomas are classified into two main histologic types—capillary and cavernous—on the basis of the caliber of the blood vessels involved[27,76] (see Chapter 4, "Soft Tissue Tumors"). Clinically, the capillary hemangioma may produce a pink to purple, noncompressible area on the skin surface; it forms no tumor mass. An example is the nevus flammeus, or port wine stain (nevus venosus). Other findings may include bluish, elevated nodules of various sizes within the skin and subcutaneous tissue. The term strawberry nevus or hemangioma is applied to raised, verrucous, cutaneous, vascular lesions that are reddish-purple. They are composed of both a cavernous component at the surface and a capillary component in the deeper underlying soft tissues (Fig. 5–1). At least 70% of strawberry hemangiomas regress or disappear completely by the age of 7 years.[66]

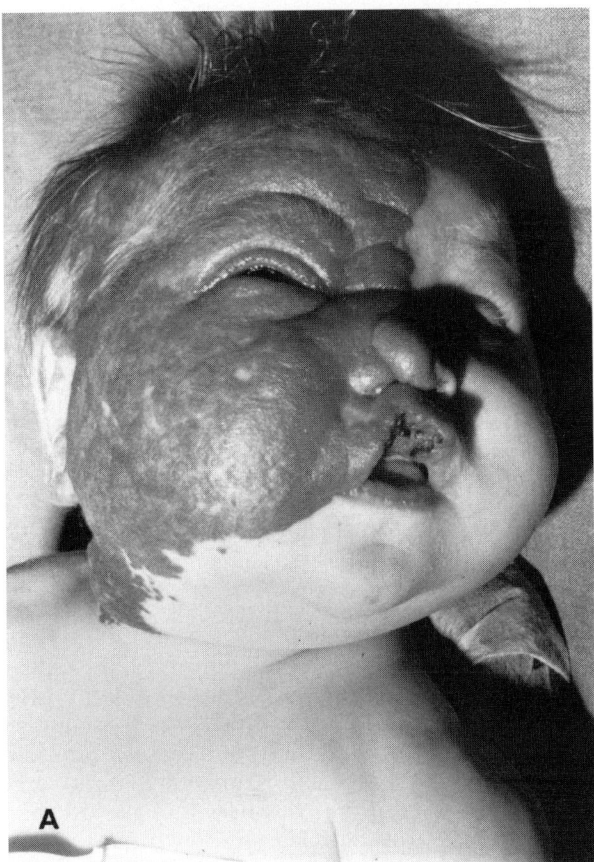
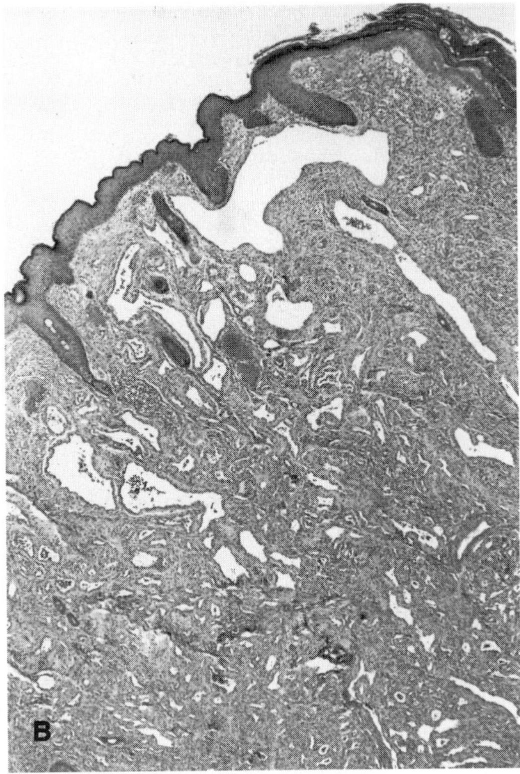

Figure 5–1. Strawberry hemangioma. *A,* A newborn with an extensive capillary and cavernous ("strawberry") hemangioma distributed over the scalp, face, and neck. In addition, the baby had a hemangioma of the larynx that was causing respiratory distress. *B,* A low-power view of a strawberry hemangioma shows the cavernous component within the dermis and the capillary component in the subcutaneous tissue (hematoxylin-eosin, ×30). (From Isaacs H Jr. Tumors of the Newborn and Infant. St. Louis, Mosby–Year Book, 1991.)

However, the cavernous hemangioma component of the blue rubber bleb nevus does not regress.[71] Conservative management of the hemangiomas is recommended.

Macular Stains

Both port wine stain and nevus flammeus are usually present at birth and are situated most often on the face and neck.[12,62,76] They have an incidence of approximately 3 births per 1000.[56] Initially, they have a pink appearance, but with age, the port wine stain develops a bluish-red to purple tone, becoming darker, irregular, thickened, and nodular. In contrast to the port wine stain, the nevus flammeus generally resolves with time; some, however, may persist, becoming lighter. Microscopic findings reveal dilated capillaries in the dermis or no recognizable abnormality at all.[62,76]

Syndromes Associated with Vascular Conditions

Occasionally, cutaneous vascular lesions—particularly, hemangioma, vascular malformations, and macular stains—indicate a more serious underlying dysmorphic condition. This depends on the location of the birthmark and whether or not the structures beneath it are affected.[12,52,62,76] In Sturge-Weber syndrome, there is involvement of the forehead and upper eyelid (the distribution of the first branch of the trigeminal nerve) and the underlying meninges and brain (see Fig. 9–13).

In at least 50% of the patients with this syn-

Table 5–2. Differential Diagnosis of the "Blueberry Muffin Baby" (Cutaneous Blue Nodules)

Dermal extramedullary erythropoiesis
  Congenital infection
    Rubella
    Cytomegalovirus
    Toxoplasmosis
  Hemolytic disease of the newborn
  Twin transfusion syndrome
  Hereditary spherocytosis
Blue rubber bleb nevus syndrome
Neoplastic infiltrations of the skin
  Neuroblastoma
  Leukemia
  Rhabdomyosarcoma

Modified from Gottesfeld E, Silverman RA, Coccia PF, et al. Transient blueberry muffin appearance of a newborn with congenital monoblastic leukemia. J Am Acad Dermatol 1989;21:347. Used by permission.

drome, the associated leptomeningeal hemangiomatosis is manifested clinically by a constellation of findings, including mental retardation, seizures, and hemiplegia with or without cerebral calcification.[52,62] Glaucoma is a serious complication of the disease. When an individual has a hemangioma and/or a port wine stain on an extremity, and when that lesion is accompanied by focal gigantism of the affected part and, often, a bone deformity, the diagnosis of Klippel-Trenaunay-Weber syndrome should be considered.[27]

Diffuse neonatal hemangiomatosis is an uncommon condition characterized by multiple hemangiomas in the skin, liver, gastrointestinal tract, lungs, and central nervous system.[10,11,13,37,45,97,98] Multiple cutaneous hemangiomas, in the absence of visceral or brain lesions, are associated with a more favorable outcome, as compared with those with visceral and central nervous system involvement (see Chapter 4, "Soft Tissue Tumors"). Another variation is the blue rubber bleb nevus syndrome, an unusual disorder characterized by multiple cavernous hemangiomas of the skin, stomach, and intestines.[62,71] Numerous cutaneous lesions may be present at birth and may resemble the "blueberry muffin" lesions seen in other disorders (Table 5–2). These hemangiomas do not resolve spontaneously. Severe anemia occurs as the result of multiple bleeds into the gastrointestinal tract.

Pyogenic Granuloma

Pyogenic granuloma occurs during the first year of life and in the older individual, typically as a single polypoid cutaneous nodule that bleeds easily on palpation (Fig. 5–2). The face, lip, and umbilicus are common sites in the infant. Although this lesion appears in areas of trauma or infection, some believe that this tumor-like condition should be considered to be a form of capillary hemangioma, as it is practically indistinguishable from this entity on microscopic examination.[27,62] Histologically, the lesion consists of lobules of proliferating capillaries and fibroblasts that often resemble granulation tissue. There is a characteristic epithelial collarette at the base of the nodule, a diagnostic feature that is helpful in distinguishing this lesion from some of the other vascular conditions described earlier (see Fig. 5–2).

Lymphangioma

Lymphangiomas occur as superficial cutaneous and deep-seated soft tissue lesions that histologically consist of dilated lymphatic channels lined by a single layer of regular endothelial cells.[27,49,76] The superficial ones—namely, lymphangioma circumscriptum—are composed of one or more small skin vesicles and are seen infrequently in the neonatal period, being more prevalent later on in infancy. The deeply situated cavernous lymphangiomas present as rubbery, skin-colored nodules that may enlarge rapidly, producing a palpable mass in an extremity. Alternatively, they may form a large sac filled with lymph fluid (e.g., in the neck, axilla, or mesentery), in which case they are called a cystic hygroma (see Chapter 4, "Soft Tissue Tumors") (Figs. 4–20, 4–21, and 4–23).

Miscellaneous Vascular Conditions

Congenital glomus tumors are very rare but have been described in the literature.[59,76] According to Landthaler et al., a few cases have been reported in newborns.[59] Multiple glomus tumors are less common in the neonate than are solitary ones, and they present as cutaneous nodules. These authors also describe a variant consisting of plaque-like lesions measuring up to 13 cm in diameter.[59] On histologic examination, the findings are those of a glomus tumor—namely, the presence of numerous, dilated vascular channels lined by a single layer of endothelial cells that is adjacent to collections of glomus cells embedded in a fibrous stroma. Immunohistochemical testing reveals

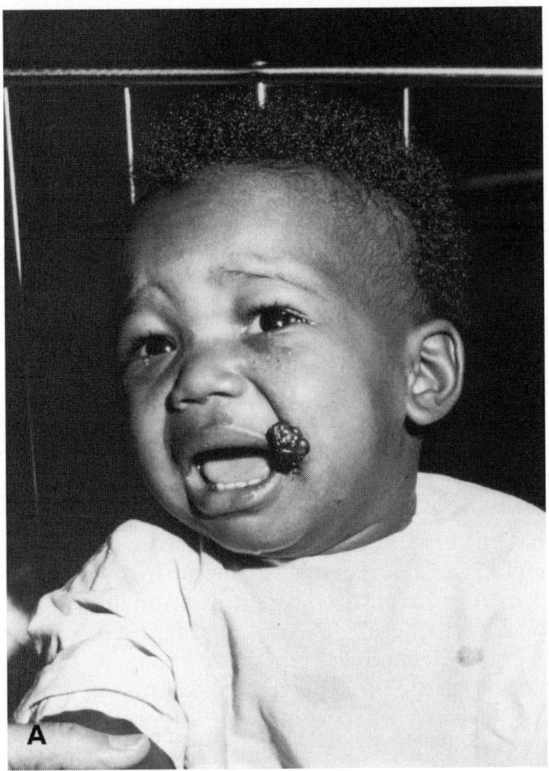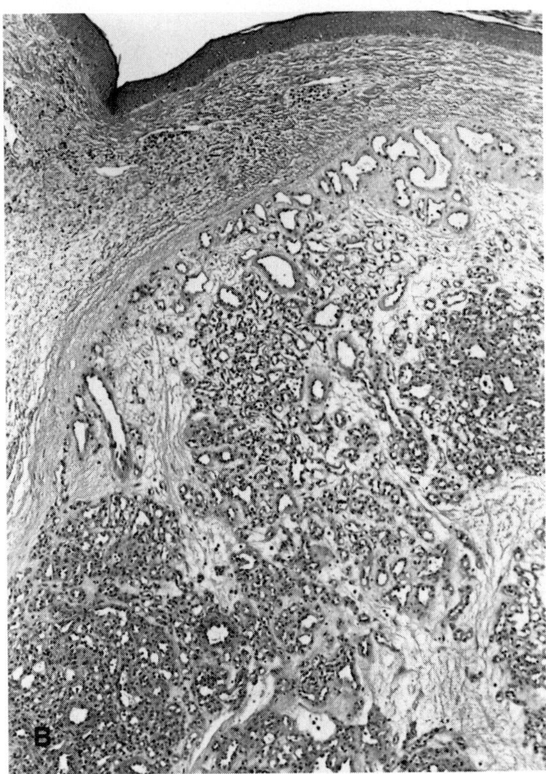

Figure 5–2. Pyogenic granuloma. *A,* A 1-year-old boy with a rapidly growing, polypoid mass on the left side of the cheek. The excised specimen measures 1.5 × 1.5 cm and has a red, fleshy-appearing cut surface. *B,* Lobules of capillaries are separated by fibrous connective tissue. There is a notch in the skin, suggestive of an epithelial collarette, which is situated in the upper left corner of the photograph (hematoxylin-eosin, ×120). Notice the similarity between the histologic features of the pyogenic granuloma and those of the capillary hemangioma depicted in Figure 4–17. (From Isaacs H Jr. Tumors of the Newborn and Infant. St. Louis: Mosby–Year Book, 1991.)

that the tumor glomus cells are characterized by reactivity with vimentin and α-smooth muscle actin. Ultrastructural examination reveals a thick basal lamina, dense bodies, and attachment plaques.[59]

EPIDERMAL BIRTHMARKS

The two principal epidermal birthmarks are the epidermal nevus (linear or verrucous epidermal nevus) and the sebaceous nevus, each of which has an indicence of about 0.2%.[53] The Becker nevus is a more uncommon member of this group.

Epidermal Nevus

Epidermal nevi occur as local or systematized lesions that may be noted at birth or that may develop later in childhood. They present as flesh-colored to yellow-brown, verrucous, oval,

or linear plaques that continue to enlarge and spread until puberty. On microscopic examination, they have the appearance of a papilloma with papillomatosis, hyperkeratosis, and acanthosis (Fig. 5–3).[62] The epidermal nevus is associated not only with benign and malignant tumors that arise from within the nevus, but also with an increased frequency of noncutaneous malformations within the central nervous system, eye, and skeleton. Moreover, the epidermal nevus syndrome, as the name implies, is characterized by large epidermal nevi, skeletal anomalies, vascular malformations, and mental retardation.[52,85,94]

Sebaceous Nevus

Sebaceous nevi present in the neonate as flat or slightly raised, yellow-brown to pink, hairless plaques distributed over the scalp or forehead. The nevi tend to regress after birth, only to enlarge again at puberty. A biopsy study of the

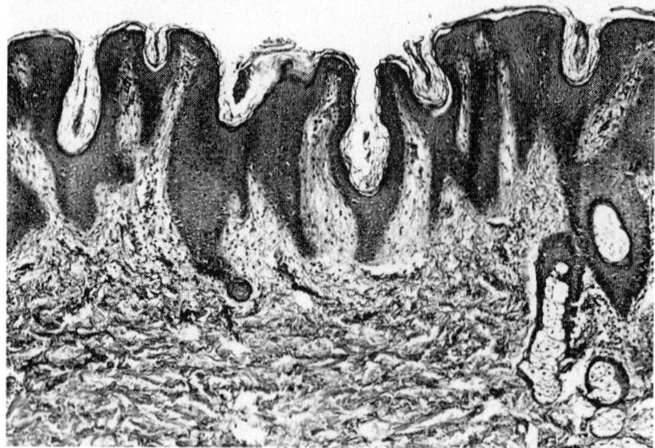

Figure 5–3. Giant linear epidermal nevus. The epidermal nevus has a verrucous appearance and appears darker than the surrounding skin. There is papillomatosis, hyperkeratosis, and acanthosis, which are features of a papillomatous process (hematoxylin-eosin, ×100). (From Isaacs H Jr. Tumors of the Newborn and Infant. St. Louis: Mosby–Year Book, 1991.)

lesion during the first year of life may show no diagnostic abnormality, but later on, the skin appendages will appear to be malformed and irregular, and the sebaceous glands are increased in size and number (Fig. 5–4).[62] Papillomatosis, acanthosis, sebaceous gland hypertrophy, and hair follicle hyperplasia may be evident at birth.[75] Older individuals with sebaceous nevi are susceptible to basal cell carcinoma and adnexal tumors arising from the lesion, thus warranting surgical removal. Moreover, some patients with nevus sebaceus have central nervous system or other anomalies in common with both the epidermal nevus syndrome and tuberous sclerosis.[61–63]

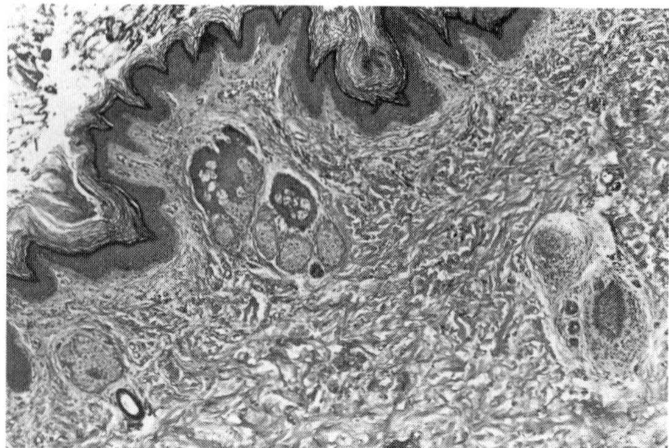

Figure 5–4. Nevus sebaceus. This lesion usually presents at birth as a flat, yellowish, hairless plaque on the scalp, forehead, or neck. Hyperkeratosis, irregular papillomatosis, and acanthosis are evident. Skin appendages are malformed, consisting of sebaceous glands without hair follicles (hematoxylin-eosin, ×48).

Becker Nevus

The pigmented variant of epidermal nevus, called the Becker nevus, usually appears in childhood or adolescence, but it may be found at birth.[16] Clinically, the lesion presents as a pigmented macule containing many hairs. On microscopic examination, it shows acanthosis and diffuse, heavy pigmentation of epidermal cells. Moreover, Becker's nevus has been described in association with smooth muscle hamartoma and neurofibroma.[16]

MELANOCYTIC NEVI

Pigmented Nevi

The term nevus is used in a broad sense to include all abnormal growths involving the skin. A more restricted definition includes only lesions containing nevus cells. Pigmented nevi are also called melanocytic or nevocellular nevi. Because most nevus cells contain melanin, the majority of true nevi are pigmented, with the color varying from light brown to black. It has been estimated that they are present in the skin of at least 90% of the adult population.[62]

Although melanocytic nevi are common among adults, they are not often visible at birth. Roughly 1% of melanocytic nevi are congenital.[62,66] Nevi that measure less than 2 cm at their greatest dimension are far more common than the giant pigmented nevi, which are noted in less than 1 in 20,000 newborns.[66] In a Finnish study of newborn infants, the incidence of congenital melanocytic nevi was 1.5%, which is in agreement with the figure just cited; however, only 1 in 4346 newborns (0.023%) had a giant melanocytic nevus.[56]

Giant pigmented nevi are regarded as cutaneous developmental abnormalities of the neural crest because they contain both melanocytic (nevus cells) and neural elements similar to those observed in association with neurofibromatosis.[19,42,78] Most occur sporadically, although familial occurrence has occasionally been observed.[106] The presence of an extra chromosome 7 (trisomy 7) is one of the chromosomal defects found in both individuals with giant pigmented nevi and those with melanoma.[3]

The nevi may be located on the face, trunk, or extremities and may involve extensive areas of the skin, sometimes affecting an entire segment of the body (Fig. 5–5). Giant pigmented nevi have a variable gross appearance that

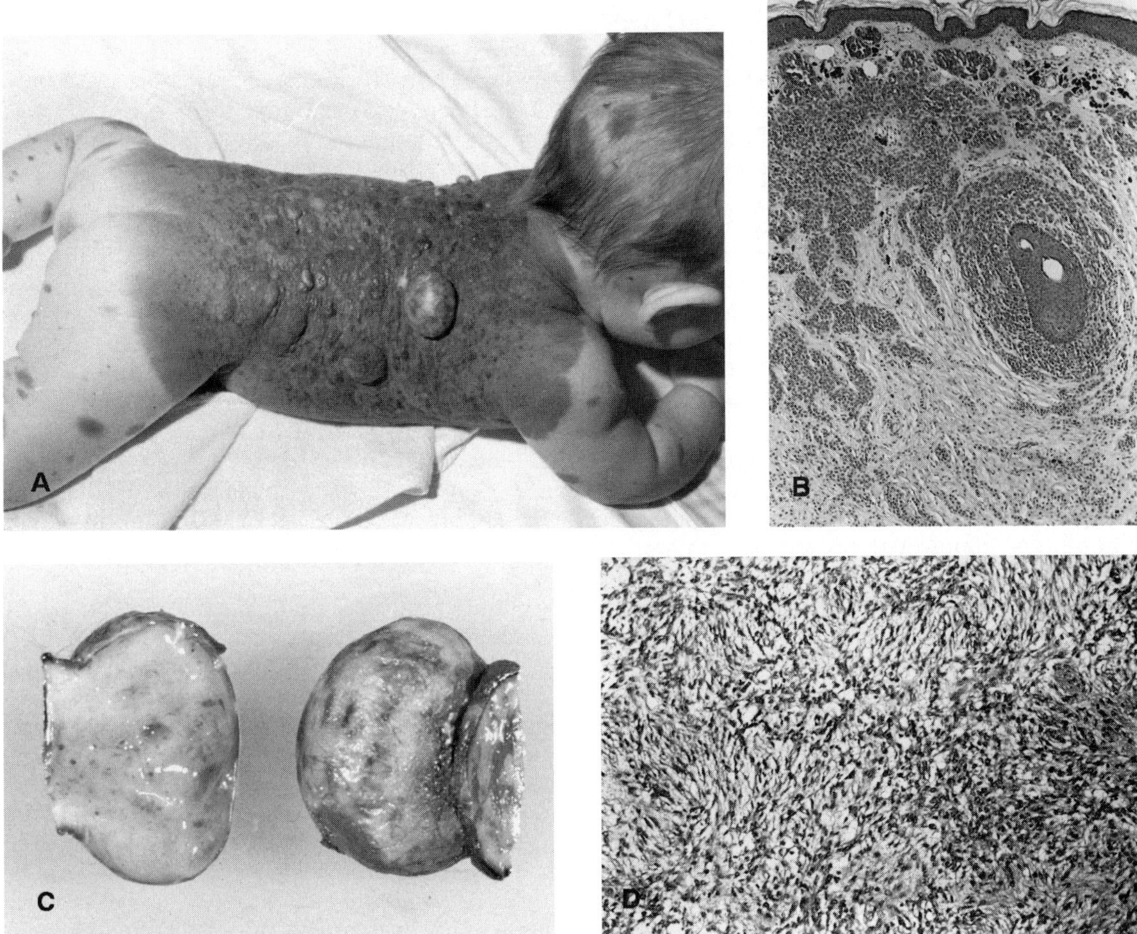

Figure 5–5. Giant congenital melanocytic nevus. *A,* A 3-month-old boy with a giant pigmented nevus involving most of the back, thorax, and abdomen. In addition, there are multiple other pigmented nevi located on the extremities and scalp. *B,* A biopsy reveals nests of pigmented and nonpigmented nevus cells situated in the dermis and deep in the subcutaneous tissue surrounding skin appendages, which is a characteristic feature of congenital melanocytic nevi (hematoxylin-eosin, ×100). *C,* The cut surface of a large nodule, taken from the right side of the back and measuring 3 cm in diameter, has a pale white gelatinous cystic appearance. *D,* In addition to nevus cells, sections of the nodule show pallisades of spindle-shaped cells suggestive of a neuroid component (hematoxylin-eosin, ×240). (From Isaacs H Jr. Tumors of the Newborn and Infant. St. Louis: Mosby–Year Book, 1991.)

ranges from flat to nodular to rough and verrucous. The amount of pigmentation and hair that are present differs with each lesion and with the age of the patient. Generally, the color is dark brown or black. When present on the trunk, countless other small, nonelevated nevi are usually scattered over the surrounding skin. Lesions on the extremities are more apt to occur singly. The hair in these nevi is always black, even in blond patients.[76]

Reyes-Mugica et al. have described a form of giant pigmented nevus that presents as a large, tumor-like mass in the perineum.[81] Clinically, the tumor resembles a sacrococcygeal teratoma, being covered by darkly pigmented skin

and measuring 10 cm or more in diameter. In addition to the prominent nevocytic and neural components, numerous pseudofollicular structures lined by nevus cells are noted; a malignant melanoma component has not been reported. Angelucci et al. have described a similar example.[4]

The histologic features of congenital melanocytic nevi, giant or not, differ in some respects from those of acquired nevi.[21,22] In the neonate, most congenital nevi are classified histologically as compound; that is, nevus cells are situated in the epidermis, epidermal-dermal junction, and dermis. Later in childhood, the nevus cells tend to be more intradermal in location, at least in the author's experience. The main finding observed in the congenital melanocytic nevus that distinguishes it from the acquired nevus is the extension of the nevus cells deep into the dermis, subcutaneous fat, and connective tissue, where they surround skin appendages, blood, and lymphatic vessels in an infiltrative fashion (Fig. 5–5*B*). The cells, which are triangular or polyhedral, are arranged in small groups that are isolated by narrow connective tissue fasciculi. Some contain melanin. The amount of melanin, both in normal skin and in nevi, increases after birth, causing deepening of the color of the nevi or making them visible for the first time. Maturation of nevus cells (i.e., when they become smaller and rounder as they migrate deeper into the dermis) is an important histologic feature of benign nevi. In addition to the melanocytic component mentioned earlier, the congenital nevus may contain blue nevus and neural elements, such as Schwann cells, Meissner's corpuscles, Verocay bodies, and neurofibroma[78] (Figs. 5–5*C* and *D*, and 5–6).

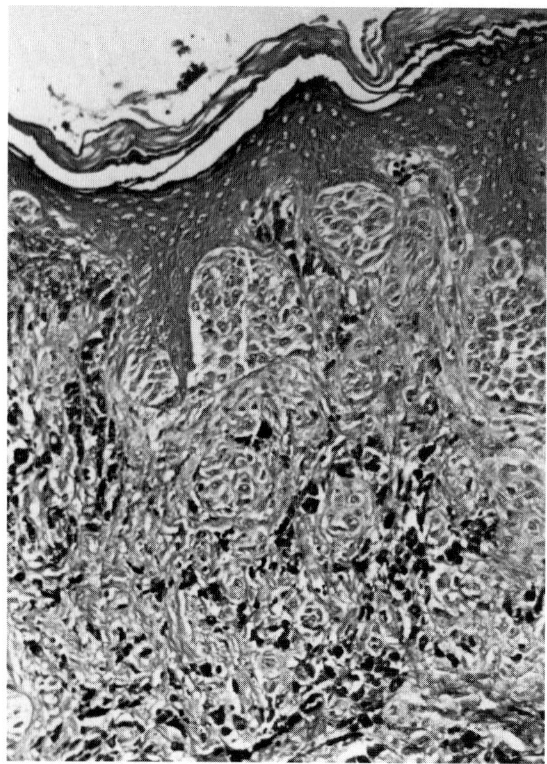

Figure 5–6. Congenital melanocytic nevus with a blue nevus component. In addition to clusters of round to oval nevus cells within the epidermal-dermal junction, dermis, and subcutis, collections of darkly staining spindle cells are present (hematoxylin-eosin, ×120).

Malignant Melanoma

Nearly all nevi seen at birth are benign and grow only as the body grows; however, a few have been reported that were considered to have been malignant even before birth.[14,31,49,100] The exact incidence of malignant melanoma arising from a giant pigmented nevus is difficult to ascertain from the literature, but according to the studies of Rhodes and Melski[82] and Lanier and colleagues,[60] it appears to be approximately 6%. Gari and co-workers reviewed 460 patients with giant congenital nevocytic nevi who had been culled from eight different series.[35] Of these, 36 (7.8%) developed melanoma and 18 died of malignant disease (50% survival). A much lower figure—13 of 451 (3%)—was cited by Williams and Pennella, based on a review of 13 childhood cases; the overall mortality rate was reported to be 40%.[106]

Congenital malignant melanoma can be divided into three main categories: (1) that which is transplacentally acquired from the mother; (2) primary malignant melanoma that develops antenatally; and (3) melanoma originating from giant melanocytic nevi[8,14] (Tables 5–3 through 5–5). In the first category, the fetus develops malignant melanoma as a result of advanced maternal disease and transplacental metastases. The affected mothers are usually primiparous, conceive within 4 years of their diagnosis and treatment, and have a high rate of recurrence and a 100% mortality[14] (see Table 5–3). The involved placentas have a mottled, brownish-black appearance and vary in size from normal to enlarged.[14] Tumor cells are present within the intervillous space and, rarely, in the chorionic villi per se. Fetal melanoma is not usually apparent at birth, but becomes manifest several months post partum. One exception noted by Brodsky et al. was a newborn in whom tumor cells were found in the cord blood and cutaneous lesions appeared in the neonatal period.[9] Table 5–3, which lists six cases of transplacentally acquired melanoma, shows only 1 infant survivor (reported by Cavell).[15] The other five patients died by 11 months of age.

The malignant melanoma may arise from giant or smaller pigmented nevi in the fetus during gestation, and it may metastasize (see Tables 5–4 and 5–5).[8,14,89,100] Cutaneous malignant melanoma associated with a giant nevus has been detected by antenatal sonography.[14,89] Placental, but not maternal, metastases were reported in this case by Campbell et al.[14] Placental

Table 5–3. Six Examples of Congenital Transplacental Malignant Melanoma

Case No.	Age at Diagnosis	Infant Findings	Maternal Findings	Placenta Involved	Age of Child at Death	Reference
1	8 mo	Hepatosplenomegaly; disseminated metastatic melanoma at necropsy	Died of metastatic melanoma 3 months after delivery	+	10 mo	Weber et al.[105]
2	5 mo	Hepatosplenomegaly; mass in left upper quadrant	Died of metastatic melanoma of the neck 5 weeks after delivery	?	5 mo	Gottron & Gertler[39]
3	8 mo	Hepatosplenomegaly; subcutaneous nodules; disseminated visceral metastases	Died with metastatic malignant melanoma 3 months after delivery	+	10 mo	Holland[46]
4	7.5 mo	Mass in ear canal; preauricular swelling; facial palsy; disseminated metastases at necropsy	Died of malignant melanoma of the leg, with metastases, 4 days after delivery	?	11 mo	Dargeon et al.[20]
5	2 mo	Tumors in thigh, legs, buttocks, & lungs	Died 4 days after delivery with metastatic malignant melanoma	?	Alive	Cavell[15]
6	11 d	Hepatomegaly; skin nodules; disseminated metastases	Died with disseminated malignant melanoma 17 days after delivery	+	48 d	Brodsky et al.[9]

transmission of melanoma to the mother from an affected fetus has not been documented.

Table 5–4 lists nine newborns with primary cutaneous malignant melanoma. The sites of involvement are as follows: head, 4; extremities, 4; and abdomen, 1. Metastases occurred in 7 patients; 6 of 9 survived, including 4 who had metastases to regional nodes and distant sites. All patients were treated by surgery and, in addition, three received chemotherapy. Two of the three patients who received both surgery and chemotherapy survived. The mortality rate in this small series was 3 of 9 (33%), which is comparable to the overall mortality rate of 40% reported by Williams and Pennella in their analysis of 13 pediatric surveys.[106]

Patients with melanomas arising from giant pigmented nevi have an intermediately poor outcome compared to those with transplacental metastatic disease and those with primary melanomas. Table 5–5 lists six patients, two of whom survived. The two survivors were the only

Table 5–4. Nine Examples of Cutaneous Primary Malignant Melanomas of the Fetus and Infant

Case No.	Age at Diagnosis	Primary Site	Metastases	Therapy	Age at Death	Reference
1	8 wk*	Forehead	Cervical lymph nodes	S	4 months	Coe[17]
2	12 mo*	Finger	Axillary lymph nodes	S, CT	Alive	Lyall[64]
3	Birth	Thigh	—	S	Alive	Oldhoff & Koudstall[72]
4	4 mo	Cheek	Cervical lymph nodes	S	Alive	Trozak et al.[101]
5	4 mo*	Mastoid process	Retroauricular lymph nodes	S	Alive	Stromberg[99]
6	2 mo	Scalp	Skull, scalp, abdomen, lymph nodes	S	2 years	Pratt et al.[76a]
7	Birth	Leg	Skin, inguinal lymph nodes, liver	S, CT	Alive	Hayes & Green[40a]
8	6 wk	Abdomen	—	S	Alive	Prose et al.[77]
9	Birth	Thigh	Skin, lung, bone, liver	S, CT	18 months	Ishii et al.[51]

*Present at birth
S = surgery; CT = chemotherapy.

Table 5–5. Six Examples of Congenital Malignant Melanomas Arising from Giant Melanocytic Nevi

Case No.	Age at Diagnosis	Cutaneous Primary Site	Metastases	Therapy	Age at Death	Reference
1	Birth	Genital area	Disseminated (including liver & brain)	—	17 d	Sweet & Connerty[100]
2	Birth	Buttocks, back	? (no necropsy)	—	2 yr	Hendrix[43]
3	Birth	Back, buttocks, thighs	—	S	Alive	Mompoint & Blumberg[69]
4	Birth	Back, buttocks, thighs, lower abdomen	Skin (disseminated), inguinal lymph nodes	—	5 wk	Ahmed[1]
5	Birth	Temporal area with invasion of skull & dura	—	S	Alive	Stromberg[99]
6	Birth	Back*	Lungs, liver, spinal cord, meninges, placenta	—	17 min	Campbell et al.[14] and Schneiderman et al.[89]

*Detected by antenatal sonography at 30 weeks' gestation; hydrocephalus present.
S = surgery.

ones treated (i.e., by surgery). Metastases were documented in three patients, all of whom died in the neonatal period. In comparing the results of this study with those of Williams and Pennella, the mortality rate was 67%, much higher than the latter's figure of 44%.[106]

Neurocutaneous Melanosis

Neurocutaneous melanosis (melanocytosis) is a rare congenital disorder in which giant or multiple congenital melanocytic nevi occur in conjunction with benign or malignant melanocytic tumors of the leptomeninges.[35,55,76,78,80] Touraine's syndrome is another term for this usually fatal condition. Normally, melanin-containing cells are present in the leptomeninges of individuals, particularly over the brain stem.[78] Dandy-Walker malformation and Sturge-Weber syndrome have also been reported in patients with this disorder.[55,80] Cytologic examination of the cerebrospinal fluid of patients with neurocutaneous melanosis is an important diagnostic procedure, revealing pigmented nevus cells with hyperchromatic nuclei and cytoplasmic projections.[80]

Of 55 patients with giant hairy nevi who were investigated by Reed et al., 20 had leptomeningeal involvement.[78] The nevus cells in the leptomeninges were histologically similar to those found in the overlying skin. All 20 patients had scalp or posterior midline involvement, yet only 13% were considered to have truly metastatic melanoma. Twelve of 20 patients had so-called bathing trunk nevi; 10 died in infancy. Ten had hydrocephalus, and almost all had epilepsy.

Patients with cutaneous melanosis become symptomatic before 2 years of age. Touraine's syndrome is characterized by increased intracranial pressure, seizures, developmental delay, and a generally poor prognosis.[106] Eventually, 50% of affected children develop leptomeningeal melanoma.

In one striking case reported by Sweet and Connerty and quoted by Potter and Craig, a patient had widespread, darkly pigmented, moderately indurated, elevated cutaneous lesions on the head, trunk, and all extremities; the largest of the lesions were covered by hair.[76,100] A diffuse, gray-brown lesion covered the diaper region and extended down the right leg to below the knee. The external genitalia were replaced by large, fungating growths, and similar masses arose from the perineal and perianal regions. During the infant's 17 days of life, the color of the lesion deepened visibly. Necropsy revealed numerous, nonpigmented nodules of tumor tissue in the liver, as well as masses of tumor cells containing pigment in the pons and cerebral cortex, in the subcutaneous tissue, and in the tumor masses arising from the perineal region.

Nevus cell aggregates have been described in the placentas of newborns with giant pigmented nevi.[21,24,96] The interstitium of placental villi is infiltrated by numerous nevus cells. Melanin pigment is present within both the nevus cells and the interstitium. Neither the umbilical cord nor the fetal membranes are usually affected. An aberrant migration of neural crest elements is suggested as an explanation for this unusual placental finding.[24,96] Nevus cell aggregates resulting from lymphatic spread have been noted in the lymph nodes of patients with giant congenital nevi.[40] During resection of an abdominal giant nevus in a 2-year-old boy, three enlarged, black, inguinal lymph nodes were removed. Neurocutaneous melanosis was also suspected in this child. Histologic examination of the lymph nodes revealed collections of pigmented nevus within the extranodal lymphatic vessels and marginal sinuses. Both ordinary and atypical nevus cells were found in the lymph nodes, which were positive for S-100 protein and variably positive for HMB-45, and which had melanosomes and other ultrastructural features of melanocytes.[40]

Hendrickson and Ross documented several different types of malignant neoplasms arising from giant melanocytic nevi other than melanoma.[42] Liposarcoma, rhabdomyosarcoma, malignant blue nevus, and spindle cell tumors, presumably of neural origin, were some of the ones mentioned. It is significant that three of the seven patients with congenital giant cell nevi included in the study developed one or more of the malignant tumors just mentioned by the age of 7 months.[42] An additional example of rhabdomyosarcoma arising from a giant melanocytic nevus was reported by Schmitt and co-workers.[87] These studies confirm the widely held view that, because of the definite risk of developing malignant disease, congenital melanocytic nevi should be excised by staged plastic surgical procedures if those are what are required to remove the lesion. The management of this complex problem is discussed by Williams and Pennella.[106]

INFANTILE DIGITAL FIBROMATOSIS

Digital fibromatosis manifests clinically as one or more nodular swellings on the sides or dorsal surfaces of the distal or middle aspects of the fingers or toes.[47,48] The tumor occurs almost exclusively in neonates and infants. Most of these tumors eventually resolve at puberty, although there is a high incidence of recurrence after excision (see Fig. 4–4).[47,48]

A Children's Hospital, Los Angeles study conducted over a 25-year period revealed three patients with congenital digital fibromatosis.[50] One was born with symmetric lesions on the lateral aspect of the fourth finger of both hands, another had a lesion on the thumb, and a third had a single nodule on the toe. The patients with the single tumors did not have recurrences after resection. However, the infant with the

bilateral nodules experienced several recurrences despite attempts at conservative surgery (i.e., simply "whittling away" at them when they recurred). All the lesions eventually resolved at puberty (see Fig. 4–4). Histologically, the digital fibromatoses are characterized by a proliferation of uniform, spindle-shaped cells within the dermis and subcutaneous tissue (see Fig. 4–4). Nuclear atypia and increased mitotic activity are not observed. Not all tumors contain the eosinophilic, cytoplasmic, filamentous inclusions demonstrated by trichrome staining and electron microscopy. Based on ultrastructural studies, the tumor cells are considered to be of myofibroblastic origin.[27] The reader is referred to Chapter 4, "Soft Tissue Tumors," for further discussion.

FIBROUS HAMARTOMA OF INFANCY

Under the term fibrous hamartoma of infancy, Enzinger included poorly circumscribed, rapidly infiltrating tumors of the dermis and subcutaneous tissue that were present at birth or that appeared in the first year of life (average age of 5½ months), occurring almost exclusively in male patients.[26] Most frequently involving the region of the shoulder, axilla, and upper arm, these tumors consist of loosely arranged, myxoid-appearing, cellular connective tissue; tendon-like bands of fibrous connective tissue; and fat (see Figs. 4–7 through 4–9). Some lesions spread or recur locally following removal, but distant metastases do not occur.[26,68]

Two male neonates with fibrous hamartomas of the scalp that mimicked encephaloceles have been described by Madden and Cudmore.[65] One tumor measured 6 cm in diameter and was situated over the left side of the lambdoid suture; the other, a lesion measuring 5 cm in diameter, was located in the parietal region. Both tumors were easily excised without recurrence. This subject is covered in more detail in Chapter 4, "Soft Tissue Tumors."

NEUROFIBROMATOSIS

Neurofibromatosis includes several entities that are usually transmitted as an autosomal dominant trait.[83,93] The main forms of neurofibromatosis recognized at birth are NF-1, also called the classic form or von Recklinghausen's disease, which is responsible for most cases; NF-2, which is associated with bilateral acoustic neurofibromas; NF-5, which is the localized or segmental form; and NF-6, which is associated only with café au lait spots.

The gene locus for NF-1 has been localized to chromosome 17, whereas the locus for NF-2 is chromosome 22. The frequency of neurofibromatosis is about 1 in 3000 live births.[83,93]

The cutaneous manifestations in newborns with neurofibromatosis types 1, 2, and 6 usually consist of a few café au lait spots that increase in number as the child grows older.[83] However, one or more cutaneous neurofibromas may be present at birth. Multiple cutaneous lesions were present in a 1650-g premature female infant reported by Tveten; the infant died 28 hours after delivery as a result of respiratory distress.[102] The baby had a large, ulcerated, subcutaneous neurofibroma in the supraclavicular area and multiple smaller ones in the subcutis of the trunk and limbs, which were situated in groups along the course of peripheral nerves. The cut surfaces of the tumors were depicted as greyish-white or pink with central yellow patches. Similar tumors were found in the pancreas and within the wall of the stomach. Moreover, fusiform enlargement of the spinal nerve roots and multiple tumors were found along the lumbar and sacral nerve trunks, which, on microscopic examination, showed proliferation of spindle-shaped neurites and Schwann cells. Although focal necrosis and increased mitotic activity were noted, there was no evidence of malignant disease.[102] The subject of neurofibromas is discussed in greater detail in Chapter 4, "Soft Tissue Tumors."

TUBEROUS SCLEROSIS

Four main cutaneous lesions are associated with tuberous sclerosis: facial angiofibroma, fibroma, and flat white shagreen patch and leaf-shaped areas of hypopigmentation.[62,92] The earliest cutaneous manifestation of the disease is a maple leaf–shaped area of white hypopigmentation, which may be present at birth.[62] Later in childhood, when mental deficiency and seizures become apparent, the characteristic facial angiofibromas and other hamartomatous lesions begin to appear. Adenoma sebaceum, the former term used for facial angiofibroma, is a misnomer because the lesion does not arise from sebaceous glands but instead consists of concentric layers of dense fi-

brous connective tissue surrounding pilosebaceous structures.[62] Central nervous system and cardiac lesions associated with tuberous sclerosis are discussed in Chapters 9 and 16, respectively.

CUTANEOUS HAMARTOMAS

Smooth Muscle Hamartoma

Smooth muscle hamartoma is often noted at birth, presenting as an irregular, elevated patch with hypertrichosis and mild hyperpigmentation.[54,62,107] The incidence of this lesion is about 1:2600. It is located primarily over the lumbar area. On microscopic examination, the main feature is a haphazard proliferation of smooth muscle bundles within the lower dermis. When hypertrichosis is present, prominent hair follicles are attached to well-defined bundles of smooth muscle fibers (Fig. 5–7). An association with Becker's melanosis has been suggested.[54,62]

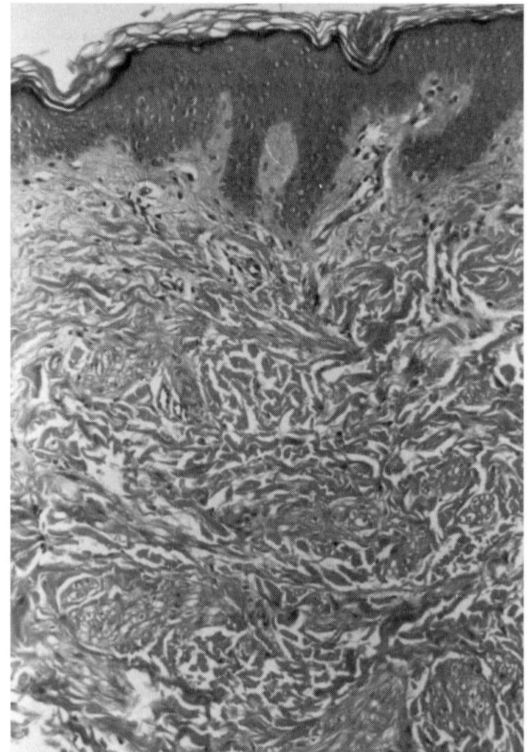

Figure 5–7. Smooth muscle hamartoma. Probably representing overgrowths of arrector pili smooth muscle, hamartomas typically occur in the lumbosacral region. Bundles of smooth muscle are noted within the dermis (hematoxylin-eosin, ×120).

Glover and colleagues describe a newborn with the "Michelin-tire baby syndrome," which is characterized by dermatomegaly (excessive folding of the skin) and hypertrichosis.[36] The histologic findings revealed diffuse smooth muscle hamartomas.

Nevus Lipomatosus

Nevus lipomatosus is a rare, often congenital, hamartoma of adipose tissue characterized by ectopic adipose tissue in the dermis.[41a] The clinical features include large, irregular papules and nodules that are situated most often in the skin of the hip and gluteal region. The Michelin-tire–like appearance may also result from an underlying lipomatous nevus.[36]

Other kinds of so-called mesenchymal hamartomas have also been described in the newborn. Connective tissue hamartomas, neural hamartomas composed of Schwann cells, and facial rhabdomyomatous mesenchymal hamartomas consisting of mature skeletal muscle and fat are a few examples.[5,62,67,103]

TUMORS AND TUMOR-LIKE INFILTRATIONS OF THE SKIN

Malignant neoplasms may appear in the fetus and newborn as cutaneous metastases, which may be the initial manifestation of a tumor.[49] Neuroblastoma and leukemia are prime examples (see Tables 5–1 and 5–2).

Congenital Leukemia

Leukemia cutis occurs in about one third of infants with leukemia[79] (see Chapter 7, "Leukemia"). Resnik and Brod documented 41 examples of leukemia cutis collected from 175 reported cases of congenital leukemia.[79] When extensively involved, the skin has a nodular, indurated appearance. About 1% of infants with congenital leukemia have mouth lesions. The natural course of congenital leukemia is not changed by the presence of leukemia cutis.[79] Skin biopsy studies reveal infiltrates of immature lymphoid, monocytic, or myeloid cells (depending on the type of leukemia) within the

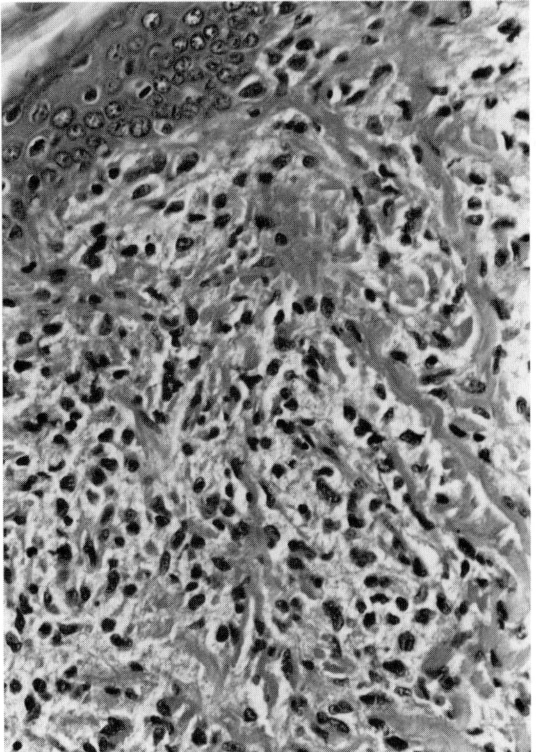

Figure 5–8. Leukemia cutis. A 1-month-old girl with acute myeloid leukemia had a peripheral leukocyte count of 118,000 and several raised, purplish nodules on the scalp. Biopsy of a scalp nodule revealed a dense cellular infiltrate composed of small, round tumor cells in the dermis and subcutaneous tissue. The cells consist of round, oval, or indented nuclei, some with prominent nucleoli (hematoxylin-eosin, ×250). (From Isaacs H Jr. Tumors of the Newborn and Infant. St. Louis: Mosby–Year Book, 1991.)

dermis and subcutaneous tissues (Fig. 5–8). Occasionally, ultrastructural and immunocytochemical studies are required to rule out other conditions that have a similar presentation, such as Langerhans histiocytosis, mastocytosis, or metastatic neuroblastoma. Bone marrow examination is not a helpful diagnostic tool in all instances. The newborn's leukemia and leukemia cutis may spontaneously resolve[49] (see Fig. 7–2).

Neuroblastoma

Multiple, bluish, cutaneous nodules, producing the so-called "blueberry muffin" baby, may be the initial manifestation of metastatic neuroblastoma in the neonate; like leukemia, this disease is seen in about one third of

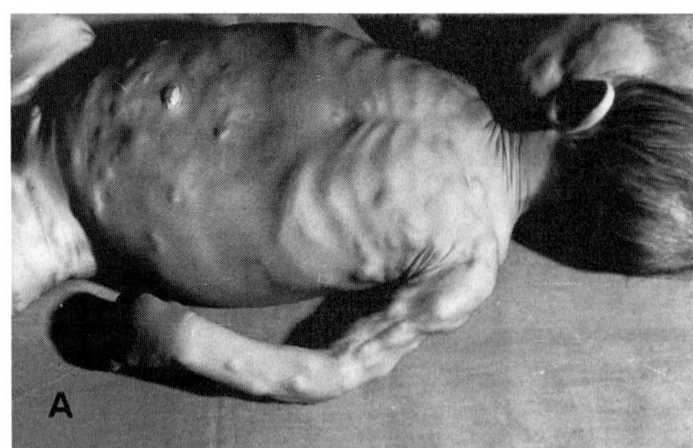
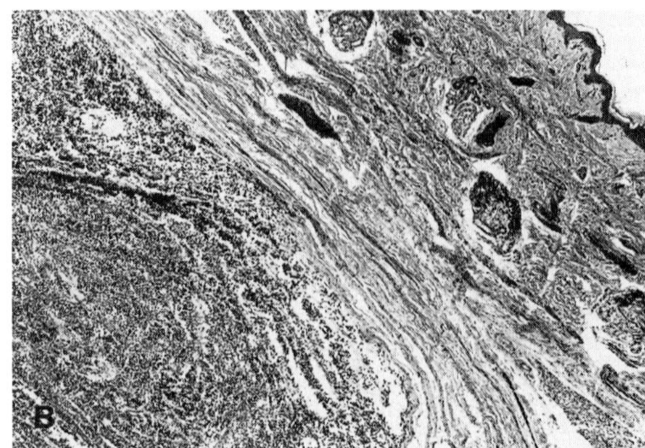

Figure 5–9. Skin nodules are the initial manifestation in patients affected by congenital neuroblastoma ("blueberry muffin babies"). *A,* A 3-month-old boy with stage IV-S neuroblastoma and multiple cutaneous nodules distributed over the body. *B,* A subcutaneous nodule reveals a partially autolyzed, small cell malignant tumor (hematoxylin-eosin, ×100). (Figure 5–9*B* from Isaacs H Jr. Tumors of the Newborn and Infant. St. Louis: Mosby–Year Book, 1991.)

cases (Fig. 5–9).[7,88] Strangely enough, most of these babies have stage IV-S neuroblastoma, which is frequently associated with a favorable clinical outcome (see Chapter 6, "Neuroblastoma").[29,30] In addition to the skin lesions, affected patients typically have a small primary tumor, which is usually situated in the adrenal, along with multiple metastases to the liver and bone marrow, which tend to resolve spontaneously.[29,30] Histologic examination of the cutaneous nodule reveals a uniform, small cell, malignant tumor, with or without Homer-Wright pseudorosettes (see Fig. 5–9). The tumor cells show nonspecific enolase (NSE) reactivity by immunoperoxidase staining and neurosecretory (dense core) granules by electron microscopy (see Chapter 6, "Neuroblastoma," and Table 4–5).

Rhabdomyosarcoma

Both primary and metastatic rhabdomyosarcoma of the skin are unusual. In a study of 682 cases of rhabdomyosarcoma collected from two institutions, Schmidt and co-workers found 5 primary and 2 metastatic alveolar rhabdomyosarcomas of the skin.[86] Two patients with primary neoplasms (of the nose) were younger than 3 months of age, and one of two with metastatic disease was a neonate with a retroperitoneal primary tumor. The three alveolar rhabdomyosarcomas were composed of medium-sized cells with rounded nuclei and scant cytoplasm arranged in an alveolar pattern. All tumors were immunoreactive with vimentin, desmin,

and muscle actin. Two infants who were treated with chemotherapy died of their disease. One newborn with a cutaneous primary was lost to follow-up. Rhabdomyosarcoma metastasizes to the skin, forming bluish cutaneous nodules that resemble those found in "blueberry muffin babies" with neuroblastoma[86] (Fig. 5–10), in dermal erythropoiesis associated with Rh hemolytic disease of the newborn,[41] or in congenital monocytic leukemia (Table 5–2).[38]

Rhabdoid Tumor

An example of primary subcutaneous rhabdoid tumor of the face and scalp in a newborn was described by Dominey and colleagues.[25] A firm, 13 × 7 cm, subcutaneous tumor involved the right maxillary and right temporal areas, producing marked proptosis of the right eye. Computed tomography (CT) scans revealed invasion of the base and right side of the skull. Metastases to the skin were found in other sites.[25] In addition to rhabdomyosarcoma and rhabdoid tumor, Dominey and co-workers noted that fibrosarcoma and leiomyosarcoma can occur also in the skin and subcutaneous tissue of the newborn.[25]

Perez-Atayde et al. have described a congenital "neurovascular hamartoma" of the skin associated with rhabdoid tumor; the authors consider it to be a cutaneous marker for this malignant disease.[74] The skin lesions present as focally raised and papillomatous erythematous plaques distributed over the back, scapula, and buttock. One patient, a 4-month-old boy, had

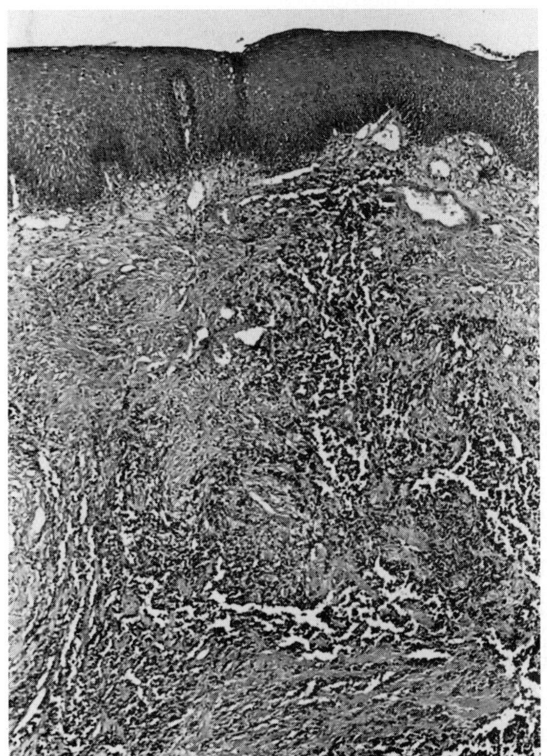

Figure 5–10. Rhabdomyosarcoma presenting as skin metastasis. A 7-month-old boy underwent a biopsy examination for what was thought to be a pyogenic granuloma of the lip. The excised specimen measured 2.5 cm in diameter and had a pale, tan-gray cut surface. The biopsy results show a dense infiltrate of small, darkly staining, neoplastic cells in the submucosa and underlying soft tissue. The tumor has a suggestive alveolar pattern (hematoxylin-eosin, ×100). (See Figure 4–31 for other findings.) (From Isaacs H Jr. Tumors of the Newborn and Infant. St. Louis: Mosby–Year Book, 1991.)

a rhabdoid tumor of the kidney and a synchronous primitive neuroectodermal tumor of the brain. Another patient, a 1-month-old boy, had a scapular hamartoma with a contiguous rhabdoid tumor beneath, which had metastasized widely. Histologically, the neurovascular hamartomas consist of papillary formations covered by epidermis with vascular and spindle-cell components, the latter of which stain positively with the neural markers NSE and S-100 protein. Parham and colleagues reviewed 42 patients with putative extrarenal rhabdoid tumor who were referred to them for consultation.[73] Four were infants, 3 months of age or younger, with cutaneous primary tumors. Case number 40 appears to be identical to the second one depicted earlier by Perez-Atayde et al.[74]

Langerhans Cell Histiocytosis

Skin lesions are important manifestations of disseminated Langerhans cell histiocytosis (histiocytosis X) in the newborn and infant.[47,48,58] Typically, these patients present with a salmon-colored, maculopapular rash that is refractory to therapy, accompanied by anemia, thrombocytopenia, hepatosplenomegaly, lymphadenopathy, and, generally, failure to thrive[48,58] (Fig. 5–11) (see Chapter 8, "Histiocytoses"). Although the disease is considered to be a non-neoplastic proliferation of Langerhans cells, which normally are present in small numbers in the skin, infants with disseminated Langerhans histiocytosis (Letterer-Siwe) disease generally die within 1 year of diagnosis, often with extensive lung involvement.[47,48] On the other hand, sporadic cases have been reported of spontaneous regression of pure congenital cutaneous Langerhans cell histiocytosis.[21]

The diagnosis is established following a skin biopsy of a representative lesion, which on microscopic examination, shows variable numbers of Langerhans histiocytes infiltrating the subcutaneous tissue and dermis, and extending through the epidermis into the stratum corneum, a helpful diagnostic feature (see Fig. 5–11). Ultrastructural studies reveal the presence of diagnostic tennis racket–shaped Birbeck granules in the cytoplasm of the Langerhans cells, which react to S-100 protein and T6 (CD1) thymocyte antigen on immunocytochemical staining[6,33] (Fig. 8–1).

Juvenile Xanthogranuloma

Juvenile xanthogranuloma is a self-limited, benign disorder of histiocytes that is found more often in newborns and infants than in older children and adolescents.[18,27,62,95] One fifth of infants with juvenile xanthogranuloma are affected at birth, and two thirds have onset of lesions prior to the age of 3 months.[18] Whether the lesion represents a neoplasm or a peculiar reactive process has not been resolved completely; however, because of its tendency to regress spontaneously, as well as the findings of several recent studies, it probably represents the latter.[62,90]

Clinically, xanthogranuloma presents as one or more yellow to reddish-brown cutaneous nodules that usually are less than 1 cm in diameter. However, some nodules arising from the skin of an extremity measure larger than 3 cm

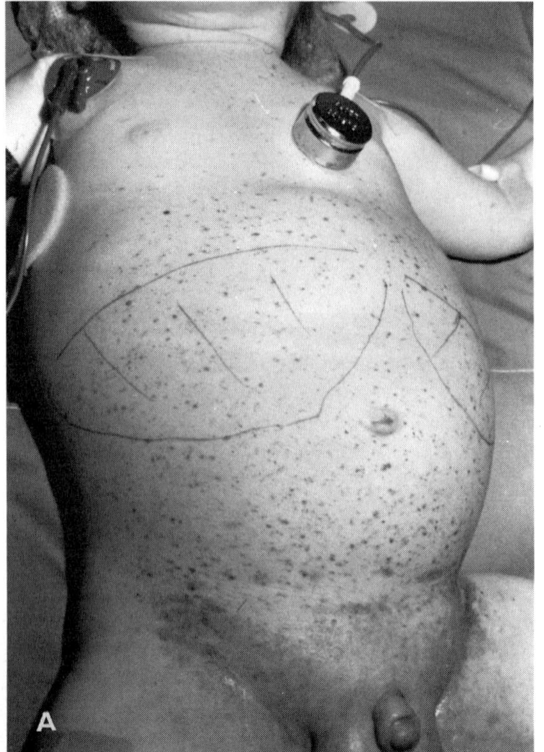
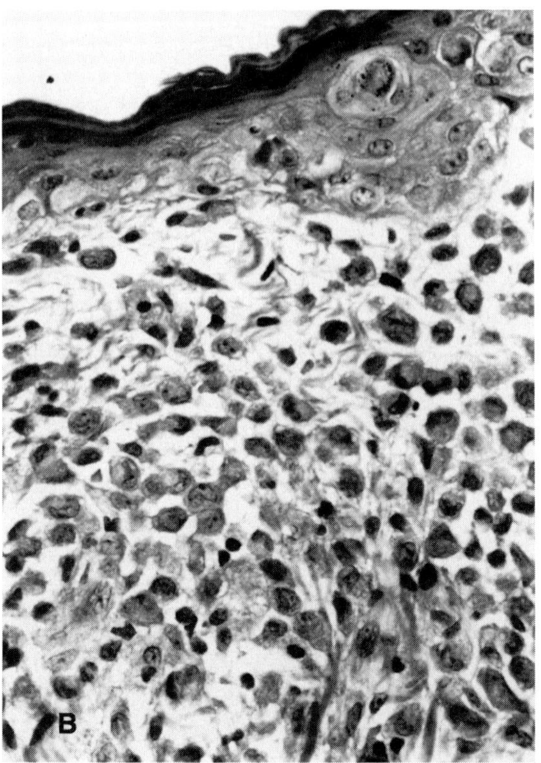

Figure 5–11. Disseminated Langerhans histiocytosis (Letterer-Siwe disease). An 11-month-old boy with a salmon-colored, maculopapular rash; anemia; thrombocytopenia; and hepatosplenomegaly. *A,* The maculopapular rash is particularly heavy over the diaper area. The enlarged liver and spleen are outlined on the abdomen. *B,* Biopsy examination of one of the skin lesions shows a dense cellular infiltrate composed of Langerhans histiocytes with characteristic folded nuclei and prominent eosinophilic cytoplasms. The histiocytes typically extend into the epidermis, which is in contrast to urticaria pigmentosa and xanthogranuloma, in which the infiltrates stop abruptly at the epidermal junction (hematoxylin-eosin, ×250). Langerhans histiocytes demonstrate positive reactivity to S-100 protein and T6 thymocyte antigen and contain Birbeck granules, as shown by electron microscopy; these characteristics contrast with those of the entities just mentioned (hematoxylin-eosin, ×250). (From Isaacs H Jr. Tumors of the Newborn and Infant. St. Louis: Mosby–Year Book, 1991.)

(Fig. 5–12). Most occur on the head and neck and extremities, spontaneously regressing within 2 years or less after diagnosis.[18,22,27,62] Cutaneous xanthogranulomas may be associated with similar lesions in other sites, such as the eye or, less frequently, the lung and deep soft tissues.[22,27,62] Ocular involvement is the most serious complication. The histiocytic infiltrates may invade the iris, ciliary body, sclera, or entire orbit.[44] Glaucoma, hyphema, uveitis, heterochromia iridis, or proptosis are the usual clinical manifestations.

Typically, microscopic examination reveals a subcutaneous nodule composed chiefly of proliferating histiocytes, which are often vacuolated, and fibroblasts (Fig. 5–12*B*). The presence of multinucleated Touton giant cells on hematoxylin-eosin staining is helpful diagnostically as these cells distinguish the lesion from Langerhans histiocytosis. Ultrastructural and immunocytochemical studies reveal that the cells are histiocytic in origin and that they lack the characteristic diagnostic features of the Langerhans cell—namely, reactivity with S-100 protein and thymocyte antigen, as well as the presence of Birbeck granules.[90,95] Favara and coworkers have described an invasive, atypical xanthogranuloma of the scalp in a 7-week-old boy that involved the underlying fascia and skeletal muscle and that displayed a high mitotic rate and an aneuploid DNA pattern.[32] Although the lesion recurred, it was cured by wide re-excision.

Urticaria Pigmentosa (Mast Cell Disease)

In urticaria pigmentosa, bullous or nodular lesions, associated with focal nodular or diffuse

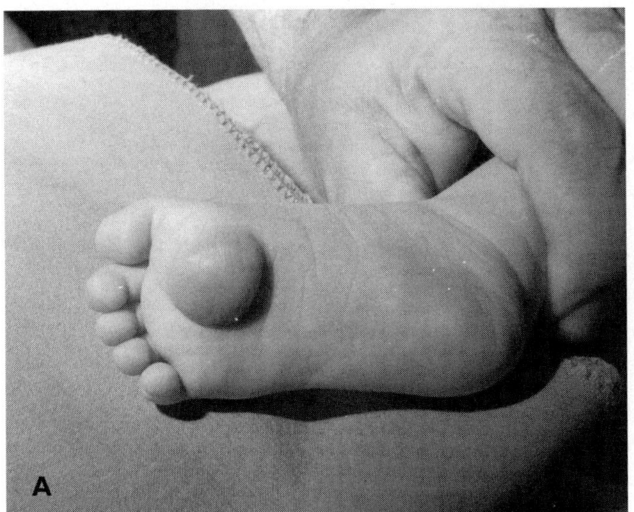
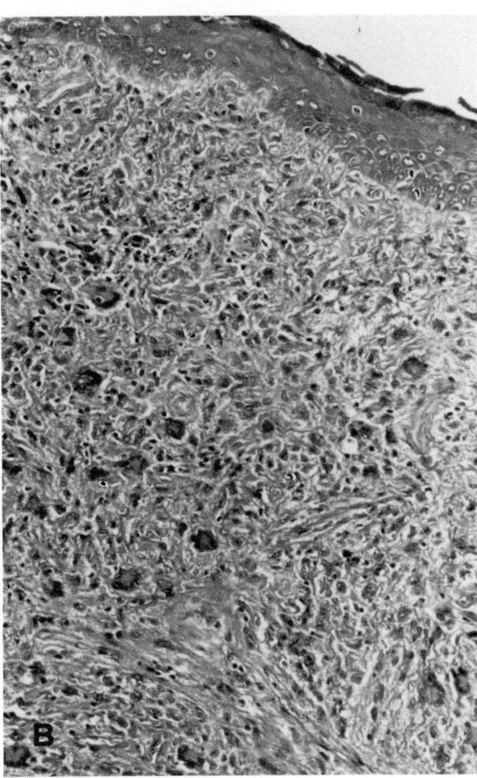

Figure 5–12. Juvenile xanthogranuloma. *A,* A 5-month-old boy with a mass on the plantar aspect of the right foot since birth. The specimen measures 3 cm in diameter and has a uniform, smooth, tan-yellow cut surface. *B,* A photomicrograph displays a mixed cellular infiltrate, involving the dermis and subcutaneous tissue, that is composed of round to oval histiocytes, spindle-shaped fibroblasts, and scattered Touton multinucleated giant cells. Some histiocytes appear to be vacuolated. Fibrosis is present (hematoxylin-eosin ×300). (From Isaacs H Jr. Tumors of the Newborn and Infant. St. Louis: Mosby–Year Book, 1991.)

infiltration of mast cells in the skin, appear in infants, usually before 6 months of age and sometimes at birth (Fig. 5–13). Mast cell proliferations may be preceded by a pink macular rash and fever; later, plaques may develop in the dermis. The solitary mast cell tumor is the most common form present at birth, and the maculopapular and nodular eruptions appear later in infancy.[28]

The lesions consist of infiltrates of mast cells within the upper dermis. The overlying epidermis is essentially normal except for increased melanin in the basal layers. Mast cells are round to spindle-shaped, with round, regular nuclei demonstrated on hematoxylin-eosin staining. They cannot be identified definitively without a Giemsa or toluidine blue stain, which are required to demonstrate the purple metachromatic granules (see Fig. 5–13).[50,62] When focally nodular, the lesions tend to disappear in childhood. When diffuse, they may persist throughout life, the disease may be generalized, and the

liver, spleen, and bone marrow may become involved. In rare instances, leukemia may eventually develop.[22,57,84,104] Mastocytoma arising as a separate nodule from within a congenital melanocytic nevus has been described.[91]

MISCELLANEOUS TUMORS

Ferreiro and Carney reported 22 examples of external ear myxomas, two of which were noted at birth, in patients with a familial (autosomal dominant) syndrome consisting of myxomas, spotty pigmentation, endocrine tumors, and schwannomas.[34] Detection of this rare tumor is important in that it should initiate investigation for other components of the syndrome, particularly cardiac myxoma. Myxomas of the external ear present as lobulated, polypoid masses protruding from the ear canal. Microscopically, they consist of scattered spindle cells with fusiform, plump, and elongated nu-

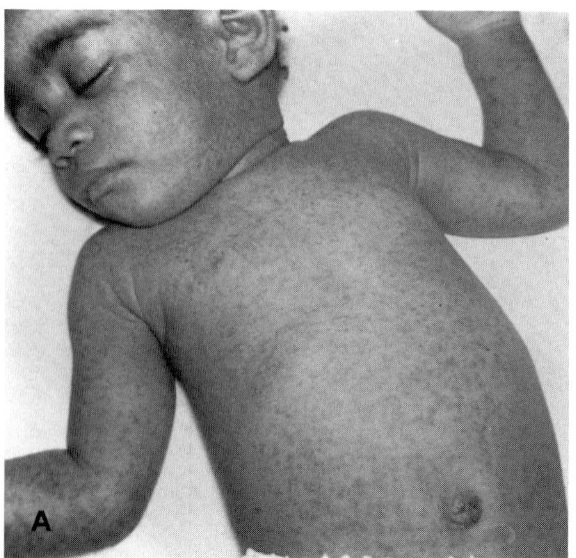

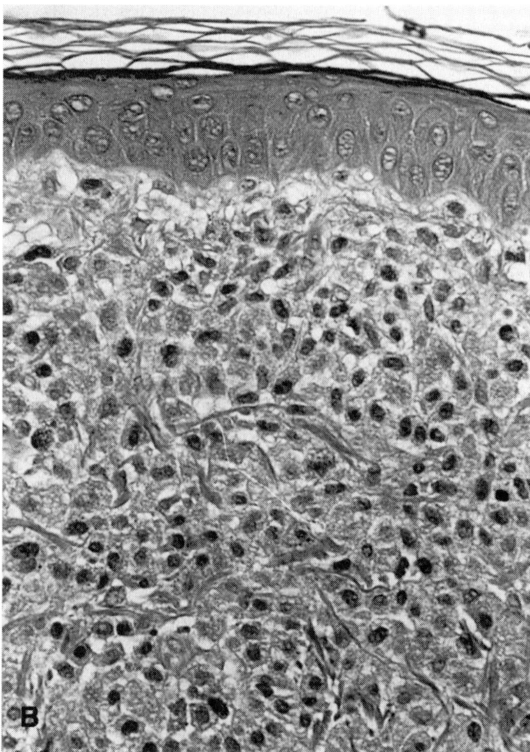

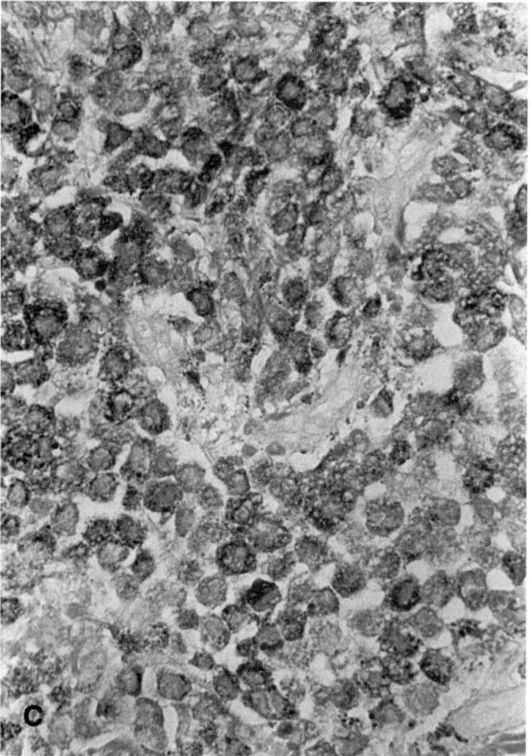

Figure 5–13. Urticaria pigmentosa. *A,* A 1-year-old male infant with a generalized brown, maculopapular rash that urticated (formed wheals) upon stroking. *B,* A skin biopsy reveals a dermal infiltrate composed of rather uniform, cuboidal mast cells (hematoxylin-eosin, ×600). *C,* A Giemsa-stained section demonstrates the mast cell granules that cannot be seen with ordinary hematoxylin-eosin staining (Giemsa, ×600). (From Isaacs H Jr. Tumors of the Newborn and Infant. St. Louis: Mosby–Year Book, 1991.)

clei and intranuclear vacuoles. Abundant collagen fibers surround the cells in a myxoid stroma. The tumor is cured by surgical resection, but in one study, 6 of 42 patients had recurrences following simple excision.[34]

Papillomas may be found at birth as localized outgrowths of skin and connective tissue. They are present on any part of the body, but are most common on the side of the face in front of the ear, where they arise by anomalous growth of tissue surrounding the first branchial cleft. The ear is also abnormal in shape. In one infant, multiple papillomas resulted from adhesions attaching the skin to the amnion. The amnion enclosed only the upper half of the fetus and, where it encircled the waist, it had caused papillomatous elevations of several areas.[76]

REFERENCES

1. Ahmed R. Congenital malignant melanoma in a newborn. Indian Pediatr 1979;16:723.
2. Alper JC, Holmes LB. The incidence and significance of birthmarks in a cohort of 4,641 newborns. Pediatr Dermatol 1983;1:58.
3. Alvarez-Franco M, Vicari FA, Reyes-Mugica M, et al. Extra chromosome 7 is present in congenital pigmented nevi (Abstract). Pediatr Pathol 1994;14:539.
4. Angelucci D, Natali PG, Amerio PL, et al. Rapid perinatal growth mimicking malignant transformation in a giant congenital melanocytic nevus. Hum Pathol 1991;22:297.
5. Argenyi ZB, Goodenberger ME, Strauss JS. Congenital neural hamartoma (''fascicular Schwannoma''): A light microscopic, immunohistochemical and ultrastructural study. Am J Dermatol 1990;12:283.
6. Beckstead JH, Wood GS, Turner RR. Histiocytosis X cells and Langerhans cells: Enzyme histochemical and immunologic similarities. Hum Pathol 1984;15:826.
7. Broadbent VA: Malignant disease in the neonate. *In* Roberton NRC (ed): Textbook of Neonatology, 2nd ed, p 879. Edinburgh: Churchill Livingstone, 1992.
8. Broadway D, Lang S, Harper J, et al. Congenital malignant melanoma of the eye. Cancer 1991;67:2642.
9. Brodsky I, Baren M, Kahn SB, et al. Metastatic malignant melanoma from mother to fetus. Cancer 1965;18:1048.
10. Burke EC, Winklemann RK, Strickland MK. Disseminated hemangiomatosis: The newborn with central nervous system involvement. Am J Dis Child 1964;108:418.
11. Burman D, Mansell PWA, Warin WP. Miliary haemangiomata in the newborn. Arch Dis Child 1967;42:193.
12. Burns AJ, Kaplan LC, Mulliken JB. Is there an association between hemangioma and syndromes with dysmorphic features? Pediatrics 1991;88:1257.
13. Byard RW, Burrows PE, Izakawa T, et al. Diffuse infantile haemangiomatosis: Clinicopathologic features and management problems in five fatal cases. Eur J Pediatr 1991;150:224.
14. Campbell WA, Storlazzi E, Vintzileos AM, et al. Fetal malignant melanoma: Ultrasound presentation and review of the literature. Obstet Gynecol 1987;70:434.
15. Cavell B. Transplacental metastasis of malignant melanoma. Acta Paediatr Suppl 1963;146:37.
16. Chapel TA, Tavafoghi V, Mehregan AH, et al. Becker's melanosis: An organoid hamartoma. Cutis 1981;27:405.
17. Coe HE. Malignant pigmented mole in an infant. Northwest Med 1925;24:181.
18. Cohen BA, Hood A. Xanthogranuloma: Report on clinical and histologic findings in 64 patients. Pediatr Dermatol 1989;6:262.
19. Cramer SF. The origin of epidermal melanocytes: Implications for the histogenesis of nevi and melanomas. Arch Pathol Lab Med 1991;115:115.
20. Dargeon HW, Eversole JW, Del Duca V. Malignant melanoma in an infant. Cancer 1950;3:299.
21. Dehner LP. Neoplasms of the fetus and neonate. *In* Naeye RL, Kissane JM, Kaufman N (eds): Perinatal Disease, International Academy of Pathology Monograph No. 22, p 286. Baltimore: Williams and Wilkins, 1981.
22. Dehner LP. Pediatric Surgical Pathology, 2nd ed. Baltimore: Williams and Wilkins, 1987.
23. Dehner LP, Bamford JT, McDonald EC. Spontaneous regression of congenital cutaneous histiocytosis X: Report of a case with discussion of nosology and pathogenesis. Pediatr Pathol 1983;1:99.
24. Demian SDE, Donnell WH, Frias JL, et al. Placental lesions in congenital giant pigmented nevi. Am J Clin Pathol 1974;61:438.
25. Dominey A, Paller AS, Gonzalez-Crussi. Congenital rhabdoid sarcoma with cutaneous metastases. J Am Acad Dermatol 1990;22:969.
26. Enzinger FM. Fibrous hamartoma of infancy. Cancer 1965;18:241.
27. Enzinger FM, Weiss SW: Soft Tissue Tumors, 3rd ed. St Louis: CV Mosby, 1995.
28. Esterly NB, Solomon LM. The skin. *In* Fanaroff AA, Martin RJ (ed): Neonatal-Perinatal Medicine: Diseases of the Fetus and Infant, 5th ed, p 1328. St. Louis: Mosby–Year Book, 1992.
29. Evans AE, Baum E, Chard R. Do infants with stage IV-S neuroblastoma need treatment? Arch Dis Child 1981;56:271.
30. Evans AE, Chatten J, D'Angio JG, et al. A review of 17 IV-S neuroblastoma patients at the Children's Hospital of Philadelphia. Cancer 1980;45:833.
31. Everet MA. Histopathology of congenital pigmented nevi. Am J Dermatopathol 1989;11:11.
32. Favara BE, Caldwell S, Steele A, et al. Case 3. Atypical juvenile xanthogranuloma. Pediatr Pathol 1995;15:169.
33. Favara BE, McCarthy RC, Mierau GW. Histiocytosis X. Hum Pathol 1983;14:663.
34. Ferreiro JA, Carney JA. Myxomas of the external ear and their significance. Am J Surg Pathol 1994;18:274.
35. Gari LM, Rivers JK, Kopf AW. Melanomas arising in large congenital nevocytic nevi: A prospective study. Pediatr Dermatol 1988;5:151.
36. Glover MT, Malone M, Atherton DJ. Michelin-tire baby syndrome resulting from diffuse smooth muscle hamartoma. Pediatr Dermatol 6:329, 1989.
37. Golitz LE, Rudikoff J, O'Meara P. Diffuse neonatal hemangiomatosis. Pediatr Dermatol 1986;3:145.
38. Gottesfeld E, Silverman RA, Coccia PF, et al. Transient blueberry muffin appearance of a newborn with

congenital monoblastic leukemia. J Am Acad Dermatol 1989;21:347.

39. Gottron H, Gertler W. Zur frage des ubertritts von melanogen von der mutter auf den saugling uber der muttermilch. Arch Dermatol Syph 1941;181:91.

40. Hara K. Melanocytic lesions in lymph nodes associated with congenital naevus. Histopathology 1993;23:445.

40a. Hayes FA, Green AA. Malignant melanoma in childhood: Clinical course and response to therapy. J Clin Oncol 1984;2:1229.

41. Hebert AA, Esterly NB, Gardner TH. Dermal erythropoiesis in Rh hemolytic disease of the newborn. J Pediatr 1985;107:799.

41a. Hendricks WM, Limber GK. Nevus lipomatosus cutaneous superficialis. Cutis 1982;29:183.

42. Hendrickson MR, Ross JC. Neoplasms arising in congenital giant nevi. Morphologic study of seven cases and review of the literature. Am J Surg Pathol 1981;5:109.

43. Hendrix RC. Juvenile melanomas benign and malignant: Fatal melanoblastoma in a 2-year-old boy. Arch Pathol 1954;58:636.

44. Hogan MJ, Zimmerman LE: Ophthalmic Pathology: An Atlas and Textbook, 2nd ed. Philadelphia: WB Saunders, 1962.

45. Holden KR, Alexander F. Diffuse neonatal hemangiomatosis. Pediatrics 1970;46:411.

46. Holland E. A case of transplacental metastasis of malignant melanoma from mother to fetus. J Obstet Gynecol Br Emp 1949;56:529.

47. Isaacs H Jr. Neoplasms in infants: A report of 265 cases. In Sommers SC, Rosen PP (eds): Pathol Annu 1983;18(2):165.

48. Isaacs H Jr. Perinatal (congenital and neonatal) neoplasms: A report of 110 cases. Pediatr Pathol 1985;3:165.

49. Isaacs H Jr. Tumors. In Gilbert-Barness E (ed): Potter's Pathology of the Fetus and Infant, Vol 2, p 1242. St. Louis: Mosby–Year Book, 1996.

50. Isaacs H Jr. Tumors of the Newborn and Infant. St. Louis: Mosby–Year Book, 1991.

51. Ishii N, Ichiyama S, Saito S, et al. Congenital malignant melanoma. Br J Dermatol 1991;124:492.

52. Jacobs AH. Vascular nevi. Pediatr Clin North Am 1983;30:465.

53. Jacobs AH, Walton RG. The incidence of birthmarks in the neonate. Pediatrics 1976;58:218.

54. Johnson MD, Jacobs AH. Congenital smooth muscle hamartoma. A report of six cases and review of the literature. Arch Dermatol 1989;125:820.

55. Kadonaga JN, Barkovich AJ, Edwards MSB, et al. Neurocutaneous melanosis in association with the Dandy-Walker complex. Pediatr Dermatol 1992;9:37.

56. Karvonen S-L, Vaajalahti P, Marenk M, et al. Birthmarks in 4346 Finnish newborns. Acta Derm Venereol (Stockh) 1992;72:55.

57. Klaus SN, Winkelmann RK. Course of urticaria pigmentosa in children. Arch Dermatol 1962;86:68.

58. Ladisch S, Jaffe ES. The histiocytoses. In Pizzo PA, Poplack DG (eds): Principles and Practice of Pediatric Oncology, 2nd ed, p 617. Philadelphia: JB Lippincott, 1993.

59. Landthaler M, Braun-Falco O, Eckert F, et al. Congenital multiple plaque-like glomus tumors. Arch Dermatol 1990;126:1203.

60. Lanier VC, Pickrell KL, Georgiade NG. Congenital giant nevi: Clinical and pathologic considerations. Plast Reconstruct Surg 1976;58:48.

61. Lansky LL, Funderburk S, Cuppage FE, et al. Linear sebaceous nevus syndrome: A hamartoma variant. Am J Dis Child 1972;123:587.

62. Lever WF, Schaumburg-Lever G. Histopathology of the Skin, 7th ed. Philadelphia: JB Lippincott, 1990.

63. Lovejoy FH Jr, Boyle WE Jr. Linear nevus sebaceous syndrome: Report of two cases and review of the literature. Pediatrics 1973;52:382.

64. Lyall D. Malignant melanoma in infancy. JAMA 1967;202:93.

65. Madden NP, Cudmore RE. Scalp tumours mimicking encephaloceles. Arch Dis Child 1991;66:884.

66. Millard PR. The skin. In Keeling JW (ed): Fetal and Neonatal Pathology, 2nd ed, p 641. Berlin: Springer-Verlag, 1993.

67. Mills AE. Rhabdomyomatous mesenchymal hamartoma of skin. Am J Dermatopathol 1989;11:58.

68. Mitchell ML, di Sant' Agnese PA, Gerber JE. Fibrous hamartoma of infancy. Hum Pathol 1982;13:536.

69. Mompoint O, Blumberg ML. Congenital malignant melanoma. NY State J Med 1972;72:1629.

70. Moore, KL. The Developing Human: Clinically Oriented Embryology, 5th ed. Philadelphia: WB Saunders, 1993.

71. Munkvad M. Blue rubber nevus syndrome. Dermatologica 1983;167:307.

72. Oldhoff J, Koudstall J. Congenital papillomatous malignant melanoma of the skin. Cancer 1968;21:1193.

73. Parham DM, Weeks DA, Beckwith JB. The clinicopathologic spectrum of putative extrarenal rhabdoid tumors. An analysis of 42 cases studied with immunohistochemistry or electron microscopy. Am J Surg Pathol 1994;18:1010.

74. Perez-Atayde AR, Newbury R, Fletcher JA, et al. Congenital "neurovascular hamartoma" of the skin. A possible marker of malignant rhabdoid tumor. Am J Surg Pathol 1994;18:1030.

75. Pierini A-M, Lopez-Ramos N, Siminovich M, et al. Exophytic scalp tumor in a newborn. Pediatr Dermatol 1991;8:84.

76. Potter EL, Craig JM. Pathology of the Fetus and Infant, 3rd ed. Chicago: Year Book Medical Publishers, 1975.

76a. Pratt CB, Palmer MK, Thatcher N, et al. Malignant melanoma in children and adolescents. Cancer 1981;47:392.

77. Prose NS, Laude TA, Heilman ER, et al. Congenital malignant melanoma. Pediatrics 1987;79:967.

78. Reed WB, Becker SW Sr, Becker SW Jr, et al. Giant pigmented nevi, melanoma, and leptomeningeal melanocytosis. A clinical and histopathological study. Arch Dermatol 1965;91:100.

79. Resnik KS, Brod BB. Leukemia cutis in congenital leukemia. Arch Dermatol 1993;129:1301.

80. Reyes-Mugica M, Chou P, Byrd S, et al. Nevomelanocytic proliferations in the central nervous system of children. Cancer 1993;72:2277.

81. Reyes-Mugica M, Gonzalez-Crussi F, Bauer BS, et al. Bulky naevocytoma of the perineum: A singular variant of congenital giant pigmented naevus. Virchows Arch [A] 1992;420:87.

82. Rhodes AR, Melski J. Small congenital nevocellular nevi and the risk of cutaneous melanoma. J Pediatr 1982;100:219.

83. Riccardi VM, Eichner JE. Neurofibromatosis: Phenotype, Natural History and Pathogenesis. Baltimore: Johns Hopkins University Press, 1986.

84. Rider TL, Stern AA, Abbuhl JW. Generalized mast cell disease and urticaria pigmentosa. Pediatrics 1957;19:1203.
85. Rogers M, McCrossin I, Commens C. Epidermal nevi and the epidermal nevus syndrome. J Am Acad Dermatol 1989;20:476.
86. Schmidt D, Fletcher CDM, Harms D. Rhabdomyosarcomas with primary presentation in the skin. Pathol Res Pract 1993;189:422.
87. Schmitt FC, Bittencourt A, Mendonca N. Rhabdomyosarcoma in a congenital pigmented nevus. Pediatr Pathol 1992;12:93.
88. Schneider KM, Becker JM, Krasna IH. Neonatal neuroblastoma. Pediatrics 1965;36:359.
89. Schneiderman H, Wu AY-Y, Campbell WA, et al. Congenital melanoma with multiple prenatal metastases. Cancer 1987;60:1371.
90. Seo S, Min KW, Mirkin LD. Juvenile xanthogranuloma: Ultrastructural and immunocytochemical studies. Arch Pathol Lab Med 1986;110:911.
91. Silverman RA, Zaim MT. Mastocytoma arising from within a congenital nevocellular nevus. Arch Dermatol 1988;124:1016.
92. Simopoulos AP, Breslow A. Tuberous sclerosis in the newborn. Am J Dis Child 1966;111:313.
93. Solomon LM, Esterly NB. Nevi and cutaneous tumors. *In* Taeusch HW, Ballard RA, Avery ME (eds): Schaffer and Avery's Diseases of the Newborn, 6th ed. Philadelphia: WB Saunders, 1991.
94. Solomon LM, Fretzin DF, Dewald RI. The epidermal nevus syndrome. Arch Dermatol 1968;97:273.
95. Sonoda T, Hashimoto H, Enjoji M. Juvenile xanthogranuloma: Clinicopathologic analysis and immunohistochemical study of 57 patients. Cancer 1985;56:2280.
96. Sotelo-Avila C, Graham M, Hanby DE, et al. Nevus cell aggregates in the placenta: A histochemical and electron microscopic study. Am J Clin Pathol 1988;89:395.
97. Stenninger E, Schollin J. Diffuse neonatal haemangiomatosis in a newborn child. Acta Paediatr 1993;82:102.
98. Stillman AE, Hansen RC, Hallinan V, et al. Diffuse neonatal hemangiomatosis with severe gastrointestinal involvement: Favorable response to steroid therapy. Clin Pediatr 1983;22:589.
99. Stromberg BV. Malignant melanoma in children. J Pediatr Surg 1979;14:465.
100. Sweet LK, Connerty HV. Congenital melanoma: Report of cases in which antenatal metastases occurred. Am J Dis Child 1941;62:1029.
101. Trozak DJ, Rowland WD, Hu F. Metastatic malignant melanoma in prepubertal children. Pediatrics 1975;55:191.
102. Tveten L. Congenital neurocutaneous syndromes. A clinico-pathological report of neurofibromatosis in a newborn and a fully developed tuberous sclerosis in a 20-month-old girl. Acta Pathol Microbiol Immunol Scand 1965;63:11.
103. Uitto J, Santa Cruz DJ, Eisen AZ. Connective tissue nevi of the skin. J Am Acad Dermatol 1980;3:441.
104. Waters WJ, Lacson PS. Mast cell leukemia presenting as urticaria pigmentosa. Pediatrics 1957;19:1033.
105. Weber FP, Schwarz E, Hellenschmied R. Spontaneous inoculation of melanotic sarcoma from mother to fetus. Br Med J 1930;1:537.
106. Williams ML, Pennella R. Melanoma, melanocytic nevi, and other risk factors in children. J Pediatr 1994;124:833.
107. Zvulunov A, Rotem A, Merlob P, et al. Congenital smooth muscle hamartoma: Prevalence, clinical findings and follow-up in 15 patients. Am J Dis Child 1990;144:782.

NEUROBLASTOMA

Neuroblastoma is the most common malignant neoplasm of the fetus and newborn (see Table 1–1).[6,7,17,18,28,34,36–38,77,81,89,97,107,145,146] The tumor arises from neural crest cells, which migrate to form the adrenal medulla and sympathetic ganglia; therefore, the tumor can originate anywhere along the sympathetic chain from the pelvis to the cranium.[14]

EMBRYOLOGY

During the fifth week of gestation, neural crest cells migrate along each side of the spinal cord, forming nodular longitudinal cell columns situated dorsolateral to the aorta.[99] The columns are the anlage of the ganglion cells of the sympathetic nervous system. The sympathetic ganglia are connected by longitudinal nerve fibers that form chains extending cephalad to the cervical area and caudad to the lumbosacral region.

The cortex and medulla of the adrenal gland are derived embryologically from two different sources. The cortex is mesodermal in origin and is first noted at 6 weeks' gestation as a condensation of coelomic mesothelium situated between the root of the mesentery and the developing gonad.[99] At approximately the same time, cells originating from the adjacent sympathetic chain congregate at the medial aspect of the adrenal gland and then become surrounded by cells of the fetal cortex. Subsequently, these neural crest–derived cells develop into the chromaffin cells of the adrenal medulla (Fig. 6–1).[99] Neuroblastoma is considered to be a tumor consisting of primitive nerve cells or neuroblasts derived from migratory neural crest cells.[14]

INCIDENCE

Neuroblastoma is the leading congenital malignant tumor (see Table 1–1).[6,7,17,18,28,34,38,79,107] Indeed, the Third United States National Cancer Survey (1969–1971) recorded a frequency rate of 19.7 neuroblastoma cases per million live births per year in the neonate as compared to a rate of 4.7 for both leukemia and renal tumors.[6] Neuroblastoma constituted 21 (54%) of the 39 malignant tumors recorded in the Survey for the neonatal period and 67 (34%) of the 196 malignant tumors for infants.[6] Table 1–1 is a compilation of 11 surveys consisting of 795 fetal and newborn tumors. It shows that neuroblastoma (219 [27.5%]) is the most common tumor, followed by teratoma (195 [24.7%]).

The Childhood Cancer Research Group, Oxford survey, 1978–84, as quoted by Broadbent, revealed that neuroblastoma constituted 30 (39%) of the total 77 neonatal malignant tumors, occurring at a rate of 0.61 per 100,000 live births.[22] Parkes et al. published another study, which included 170 cases of benign and malignant neonatal tumors culled from the files of the Midlands Regional Children's Tumour Research Group from 1957.[107] Following teratoma, neuroblastoma was second in frequency with cases numbering 49 (18%); moreover, it was the most common malignant tumor. According to the Evans classification, 10 patients had stage 1 or 2 disease, 12 had stage 3 or 4, and 9 were classified as having stage IV-S disease. Half were diagnosed within the first month of life, and the survival rate was 35%.[107]

The neonatal tumor study from the Institute Gustave-Roussy in France again showed that neuroblastoma was the leading cancer, com-

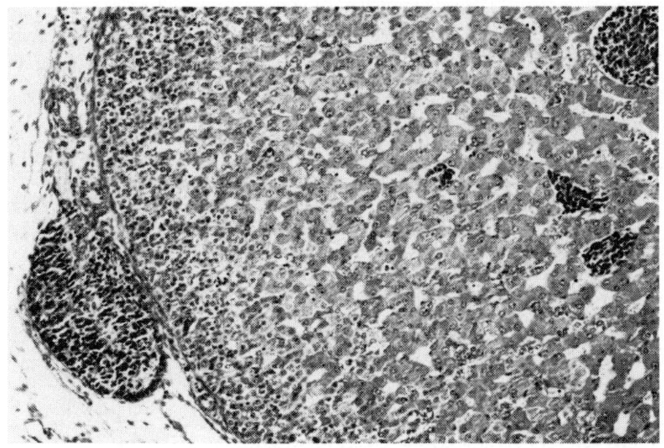

Figure 6–1. Developing adrenal gland. The developing adrenal gland and sympathetic ganglia of an aborted fetus of unknown gestation. Nests of small cells with darkly staining nuclei and scant cytoplasms are situated within and adjacent to the adrenal and in the region of the sympathetic ganglia. Compare the morphology of the developing neuroblasts in this photomicrograph to the ones in Figure 6–13 (neuroblastoma in situ) and in Figure 6–3 (congenital neuroblastomatosis) (hematoxylin-eosin, ×240). (From Isaacs H Jr. Tumors of the Newborn and Infant. St. Louis: Mosby–Year Book, 1991.)

prising 47 (62%) of 75 neoplasms; 42 of the 47 patients (89%) survived.[121] Neuroblastoma also constituted the majority of the cancers affecting newborns (i.e., 19 of 34, or 56%) in the St. Jude Children's Research Hospital review; it was followed in frequency by leukemia (6 cases), retinoblastomas (3 cases) and Wilms' tumor (2 cases).[34] Most patients with neuroblastoma were classified as having clinical stage III disease (11 patients), 7 were diagnosed with stage II disease, and 1 had stage IV disease; the overall survival was 74%.

Neuroblastoma was also the leading malignant tumor in the Hospital for Sick Children, Toronto study, as it accounted for almost 50% of the neonatal malignant tumors in this series.[28] The Children's Hospital, Los Angeles review of 110 perinatal neoplasms showed that neuroblastoma followed teratoma and soft tissue tumors in order of frequency, constituting one third of the total of 44 neonatal malignant tumors and comprising 8% of the neuroblastomas occurring at all ages, as compared to 12% for the Toronto study.[79]

The Melbourne, Australia survey of 17,417 perinatal necropsies revealed 46 tumors, yielding an incidence of 1 in 379.[146] Again, neuroblastoma was the predominant malignant tumor (6 cases) and was third in order of frequency following teratoma and vascular tumors. Four of these six neuroblastomas were confined to the adrenal, a fifth was a 70-g adrenal primary with metastases to the liver, and the last one was an extra-adrenal (paravertebral) neuroblastoma.

CLINICAL FINDINGS

Familial neuroblastoma occurs among siblings and identical twins and is associated with multiple primary tumors.[21,25,29,65,90,93,109,143] Most familial cases occur in the first 18 months of life at ages that fall within 1 year of the age at diagnosis of the affected sibling. Boyd and Schofield described a set of monozygotic twins concordant for neuroblastoma.[21] One twin who had an abdominal mass and hydronephrosis detected on antenatal sonography died 1 week post partum. Stage IV neuroblastoma and placental metastases were found at necropsy. The cotwin subsequently developed stage IV-S disease, which proved to be rapidly fatal despite irradiation and chemotherapy. Bilateral adrenal tumors and massive neoplastic hepatomegaly were noted at necropsy at 1 month of age. Further studies showed two unfavorable characteristics as far as prognosis is concerned: diploidy and N-myc amplification. The authors propose that one of the twins developed neuroblastoma in utero, which then metastasized to the cotwin through placental anastomoses. In their study, the authors reviewed the findings of six sets of monozygotic twins that were discordant and six sets of monozygotic twins, including this case, that were concordant for neuroblastoma.[21]

The occurrence of neuroblastoma with neurofibromatosis;[16] severe hypoglycemia in the neonate secondary to nesidioblastosis;[59] central hypoventilation (Ondine's curse);[19] Hirschsprung's disease, including total aganglionosis;[29,96] and ganglioneuroblastoma of the myenteric plexus of the large intestine[88] suggests that the tumor is part of a complex neurocristopathy, or a maldevelopment of neural crest tissues.[14] Severe eye defects—namely, bilateral microphthalmia, cataract, coloboma of the optic disc, and retinal dystrophy—have been reported in a newborn with stage IV-S neuroblastoma.[66]

Occasionally, neuroblastoma is described in association with other apparently non-neural crest–related syndromes, such as the Beckwith-Wiedemann syndrome,[30,43] the CHARGE association (choanal atresia, heart defects, growth retardation, mental deficiency, hypogonadism, ear anomalies),[70] DiGeorge anomaly,[108] and the fetal hydantoin and fetal alcohol syndromes.[110,126,128] A wide variety of developmental defects without a specific pattern occur in association with neuroblastoma.[4,104]

Antenatal sonography has allowed the detection of tumors before birth.[120] The primary sonographic findings of a fetal adrenal neuroblastoma are a cystic and/or solid mass located at the upper pole of the kidney; hydrops and hydramnios also may be present, particularly in association with extensive hepatic metastases.[48,54,56,71,82,86,120] Metastatic disease in the fetus without an identifiable primary tumor has also been revealed by prenatal imaging studies.[82]

Neuroblastoma has been discovered on prenatal sonography as an unsuspected finding.[35,49,51,54,57,73,84,107] For example, Janetschek et al. detected a neuroblastoma of the right adrenal in a fetus of 34 weeks' gestation, and Fowlie et al. reported a left adrenal lesion in a fetus of 28 weeks' gestation.[49,84] Moreover, Gadwood and Reynes detected a solid cervical neuroblastoma at 32 weeks' gestation by sonography; ultimately the pregnancy terminated in stillbirth.[51] At necropsy, the diagnosis was confirmed and, in addition, multiple metastases were found. Three cases of antenatally diagnosed neuroblastomas have been described by Forman et al.[48] Only the adrenal gland was involved in two patients who were diagnosed with stage I and II disease (see Table 6–3) and who underwent successful postnatal surgical excision. They were asymptomatic at birth and no masses were palpable. The third patient, who had bilateral adrenal primary tumors with extension into the paravertebral area (stage III),

hydrops, and congestive heart failure, was treated only with chemotherapy. All three patients survived.[48] Jaffa et al. reported a large, partially calcified, solid liver metastasis as the initial sonographic finding in a fetus of 32 weeks' gestatation; at the time, there was no discernible primary tumor.[82] The newborn survived for 36 hours; a retroperitoneal neuroblastoma, which was presumed to be the primary tumor, was discovered at necropsy.

Jennings et al. described five fetuses with adrenal neuroblastoma detected by prenatal sonography at 26 to 39 weeks' gestation.[86] The tumors were successfully resected following delivery, and the patients, all of whom had had stage I disease, remained free of disease. One mother in the study had obstetrical complications (i.e., preeclampsia) at 36 weeks. In addition, Jennings et al. reviewed 16 other published cases of fetal neuroblastomas detected by sonography between 29 and 38 weeks' gestation. The adrenal was the most common primary site in this series, as well; the two extra-adrenal tumors involved the neck and thorax, respectively.[86] Most were diagnosed with stage I disease, although not all were staged. One was classified as having stage II disease, and three were diagnosed with stage IV or IV-S disease, including a stillborn reported by Gadwood et al.[51] It is significant that four mothers, three of whose newborns had liver metastases and hydrops, had hypertension or preeclampsia.

An adrenal cyst detected by antenatal or postnatal sonography may be the initial finding (Figs. 6–2 and 13–7). Atkinson and colleagues described three examples of cystic neuro-

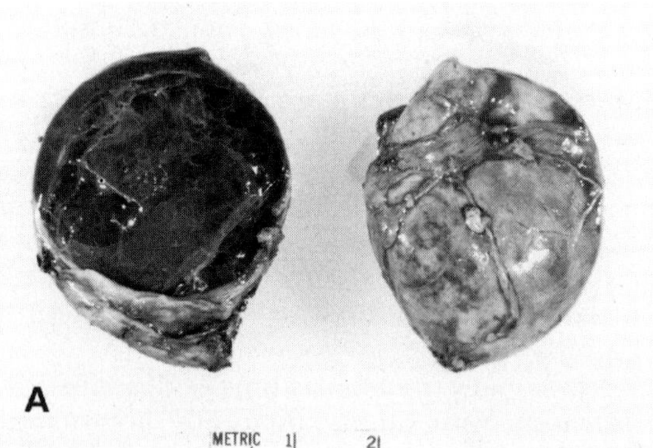
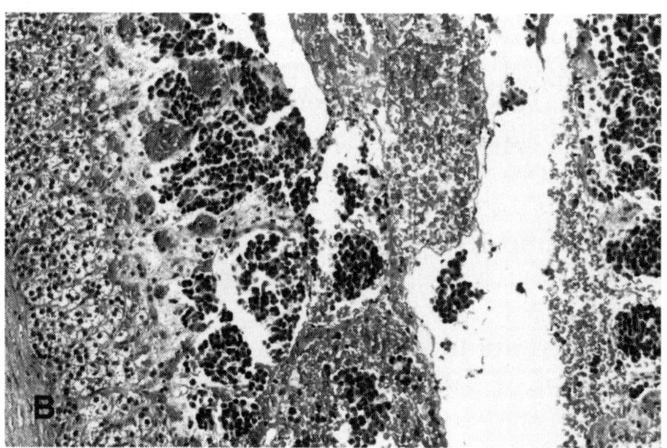

Figure 6–2. Cystic adrenal hemorrhage with neuroblastoma. An adrenal cystic lesion thought to be the result of hemorrhage was detected by antenatal sonography. *A,* The gross specimen, which was excised when the patient was 1 month of age, reveals the hemorrhagic cut surface (on left). *B,* The adrenal capsule and cortex are on the left, adjacent to nests of neuroblasts surrounded by hemorrhage (hematoxylin-eosin, ×150).

Table 6–1. Neuroblastoma Catecholamine Metabolism

Phenylalanine
↓
Tyrosine
↓
Dihydroxyphenylalanine (DOPA) ⟶ Dihydroxyphenylethylamine (DOPAMINE) ⟶ Norepinephrine
↓   ↓   ↓
3-Methoxytyrosine   3-Methoxytyramine   Normetanephrine
↓   ↓   ↓
Vanillylpyruvic acid ⟶ |
↓   ↓   ↓
Vanillylacetic acid (VLA)*   Homovanillic acid (HVA)*   Vanillylmandelic acid (VMA)*

*Metabolites measured in the urine of patients with neuroblastoma.
From Isaacs H Jr: Tumors of the Newborn and Infant. St. Louis: Mosby–Year Book, 1991.

blastoma in infants younger than 3 months of age.[5] In two of the infants, the cystic masses were demonstrated by antenatal sonography. The differential diagnosis of adrenal cysts in the newborn includes hemorrhage (by far the most common), abscess, and neuroblastoma (see Chapter 13, "Adrenocortical Tumors"). The sonographic findings of neuroblastoma and adrenal hemorrhage are similar, and differentiating between the two by imaging studies alone may be difficult.[33] Croitoru and co-workers described a premature female who had respiratory distress syndrome and a left upper quadrant mass at birth. Sonography revealed a thick-walled, cystic adrenal mass that was initially regarded as an adrenal hemorrhage. However, during the patient's evaluation, elevated urinary catecholamine levels were noted, and the diagnosis of stage I neuroblastoma was established following exploratory laparotomy and histologic examination.[33] The child survived. The authors recommend serial sonographic examinations and urinary catecholamine analysis in all neonates with adrenal masses as part of the clinical evaluation (Table 6–1).[33]

Weber and associates reported an example of a newborn with a right-sided abdominal mass.[144] A computed tomography (CT) scan revealed a cystic lesion in the right adrenal which, upon removal, proved to be a neuroblastoma. The child showed no evidence of tumor after a 3-year follow-up period. A hemorrhagic adrenal cyst rimmed by neuroblastoma was an incidental postmortem finding in a newborn with meconium aspiration syndrome who died following a massive intracerebral hemorrhage.[81] In addition, the baby had liver metastases.

The Children's Hospital, Boston group re-viewed 11 patients with neuroblastoma that was initially detected prenatally by sonography during the years 1982 to 1992.[71] The earliest diagnosis was established at 30 weeks' gestation. Nine patients had adrenal primaries and two had thoracic paraspinal tumors. Nine were classified as having stage I disease, two had stage IV-S disease, and one had stage IV disease; all survived following postnatal surgical resection. Only one received multiagent chemotherapy. Interestingly enough, Ho et al. found that 7 of these 11 patients had a cystic neuroblastoma with small collections of neuroblasts in the wall of the cyst, similar to those found in neuroblastoma in situ. Moreover, they considered the cystic tumor to be a form of neuroblastoma associated with a favorable outcome. The authors pointed out that the natural history of fetal neuroblastoma in situ is characterized by spontaneous regression, which probably would explain the favorable outcome in these patients.[71] In addition, many of the neonates in this study had other favorable prognostic indicators, namely, a low stage of disease (stage I) and tumor cells with aneuploid DNA and absence of N-myc amplification (Table 6–2; see also Fig. 6–6).[33]

One of the fascinating aspects of the biology of neuroblastoma is the tumor's diverse clinical manifestations in the perinatal period.[10,22,28,37,81,112] Nonimmune fetal hydrops with or without hydramnios, accompanying extensive placental metastases, may be evident at birth (Fig. 6–3).[15,81,100,105,141,146] Neonates with neuroblastoma may have clinical findings similar to those of hemolytic disease of the newborn—namely, hydrops, anemia, hepatosplenomegaly, jaundice, and increased numbers of nucleated erythrocytes on the peripheral blood smear.[3] Disseminated neuro-

Table 6–2. Laboratory Findings Associated with an Unfavorable Prognosis in Neuroblastoma

---

N-myc oncogene amplification
Diploid DNA
Serum ferritin increased
Neuron-specific enolase (NSE) increased
E rosette inhibition increased
Nerve growth factor receptor decreased
Lactic dehydrogenase (LDH) increased
Urinary VMA/HVA < 1.5
Urinary cystathionine increased

---

blastoma is responsible for intrauterine death and stillbirth in some cases.[3,4,9,12,54,93,113,135,141] Strauss and Driscoll, as well as Smith et al., described neuroblastomas in four neonates with simultaneous involvement of the placentas.[132,135] Neuroblasts in the placentas are situated almost entirely within blood vessels, particularly in the villous capillaries (Fig. 6–3C). The placentas are histologically immature, and their gross appearances suggest erythroblastosis secondary to Rh incompatibility, for they weigh more than 1000 g and have a bulky, edematous appearance. van der Slikke and Balk reported a similar example of a primigravida with hydramnios and acute toxemia who delivered a hydropic stillborn male infant with an adrenal neuroblastoma that metastasized to the liver, placenta, and other organs.[141] Anders et al. described two newborns, one of whom was stillborn, with metastases to the liver and placenta who were thought to have erythroblastosis fetalis. The diagnosis of neuroblastoma was first established in the stillborn after histologic examination of the placenta.[3] In most reported cases of neuroblastoma metastatic to the placenta, the tumor cells are confined to the chorionic villous vessels; however, Garth et al. have also reported infiltration of the villous stroma.[55] Placental involvement by congenital malignant tumors may be more common than actually realized because placentas in cases of stillbirth and hydrops fetalis are frequently discarded without first being examined.[132]

In the differential diagnosis of an abnormally large placenta, a congenital malignant tumor should be considered in addition to infection, maternal diabetes, and erythroblastosis fetalis, which are seen more often.[132] Involvement of the placenta by fetal tumors other than neuroblastoma is very unusual. Assuming the non-neoplastic conditions just described have been ruled out, congenital leukemia and hepato-

blastoma are the other diagnostic considerations.[81,117]

Neuroblastoma is the malignant tumor most often found in the fetus and newborn, presenting as an abdominal mass owing to either an adrenal-retroperitoneal primary or to hepatomegaly secondary to extensive metastases (Fig. 6–4; see also Figs. 6–7 and 6–8).[13,37,79,112,124,144] More than 50% of neuroblastomas are noted in the abdominal cavity.[22,25,28,35,58,124,148] Less frequently, the neoplasm occurs as a mass lesion in the mediastinum or neck, with the former being more prevalent than the latter (see also Fig. 6–9).[79]

Multifocal primary neuroblastoma, either synchronous or metachronous, has been described.[32,79] The tumors may arise from both adrenals or from other locations in which neuroblastomas usually are found. Generally, there are two primary sites, but more than two can occur. Multifocal tumors are associated with an increased familial incidence.[21,29,79,93,143]

Progressive respiratory distress and pneumonia are presenting signs, with bronchial obstruction secondary to mediastinal neuroblastoma and paralysis or weakness occurring in those patients with spinal cord compression.[1,72,74,101,114] Airway problems, which occasionally are incorrectable and fatal, can occur with large primary tumors in the neck.[79] Other clinical manifestations in the perinatal period include metastasis to the umbilical cord leading to intrauterine death,[4] hemoperitoneum from spontaneous rupture of tumor,[23,102] neurogenic bladder,[101] congenital chylothorax with a mediastinal neuroblastoma involving the thoracic duct,[42,72] cervical sympathetic ganglia involvement with Horner syndrome with or without heterochromia (difference in color between the two irides),[28,83,106] myoclonic encephalopathy,[40] leukoerythroblastic anemia secondary to replacement of the bone marrow by tumor,[17] a visible dorsal paravertebral mass secondary to a retroperitoneal abdominal neuroblastoma invading the dorsal musculature,[50,133] intestinal tumor associated with omphalocele and ileal atresia,[88] metastases to the eye (bilateral involvement of the iris or bilateral choroidal metastases followed by spontaneous regression),[20,31] or a metastatic scrotal mass (as the initial clinical manifestation).[150] Hrabovsky and Jones described 12 cases of intraspinal "dumbbell" neuroblastoma in newborns in whom partial or complete paralysis of both lower extremities was present at birth.[74] Most had urinary incontinence or retention. Although 11 of 12

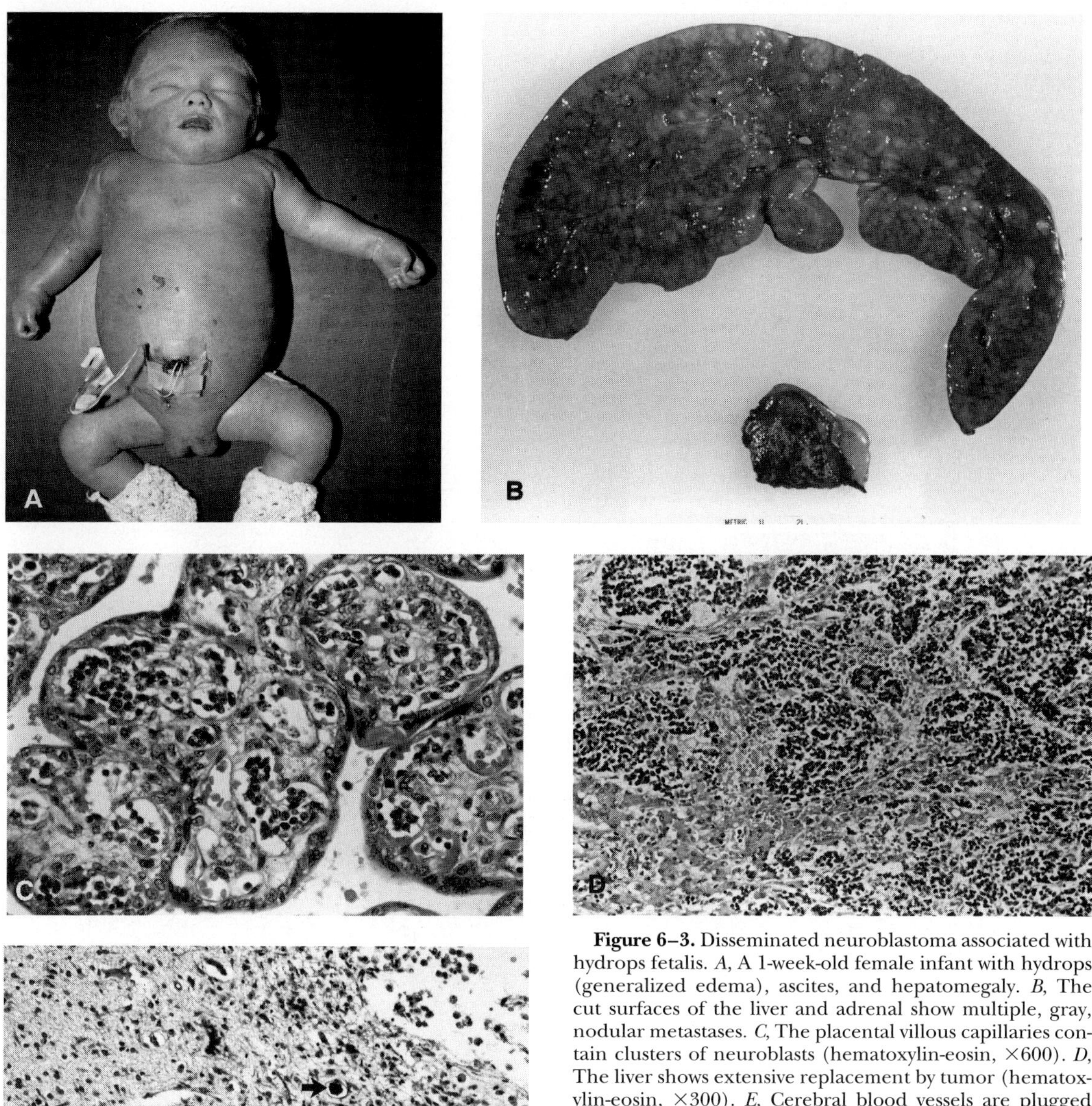

Figure 6–3. Disseminated neuroblastoma associated with hydrops fetalis. *A,* A 1-week-old female infant with hydrops (generalized edema), ascites, and hepatomegaly. *B,* The cut surfaces of the liver and adrenal show multiple, gray, nodular metastases. *C,* The placental villous capillaries contain clusters of neuroblasts (hematoxylin-eosin, ×600). *D,* The liver shows extensive replacement by tumor (hematoxylin-eosin, ×300). *E,* Cerebral blood vessels are plugged with tumor emboli (*arrows*), and there is infarction of the adjacent cortical white matter. A cystic infarct is noted in the upper right hand corner (hematoxylin-eosin, ×300). (*A–C:* From Isaacs H Jr. Congenital malignant tumors. *In* Reed GB, Claireaux AE, Bain AD (eds): Diseases of the Fetus and Newborn: Pathology, Radiology and Genetics, p 131. London: Chapman Hall, 1989. Used by permission. *D* and *E:* From Isaacs H Jr. Tumors of the Newborn and Infant. St. Louis: Mosby–Year Book, 1991.)

survived, their neurologic deficit showed slight or no improvement, regardless of the form of therapy.

In addition to the three patients with antenatally diagnosed neuroblastoma who were just mentioned, Forman et al. described the clinical features of 9 neonates with this tumor.[48] These infants had clinical signs at birth, usually hepatomegaly or a palpable abdominal mass, which appeared on sonography as solid, echogenic, adrenal masses. Six of these neonates had stage IV-S disease arising from the adrenal; there was

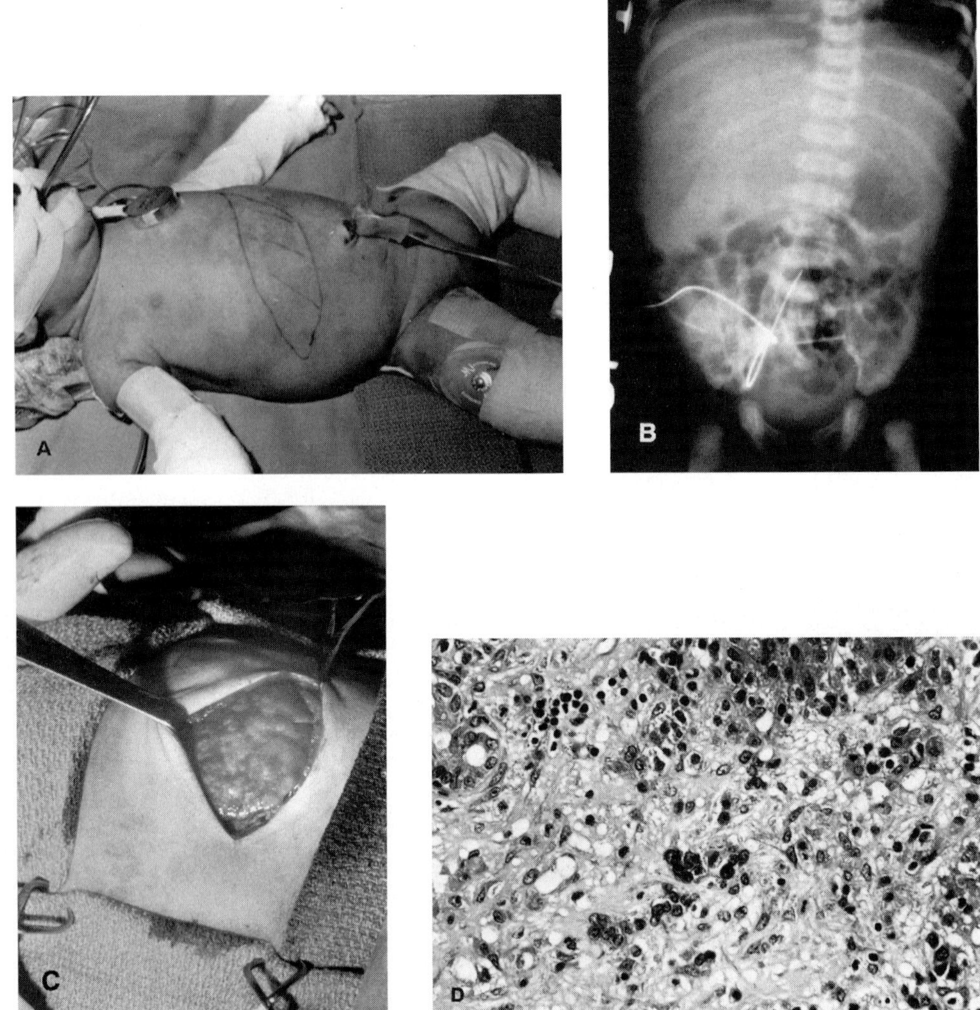

Figure 6–4. Congenital neuroblastoma, stage IV-S, presenting as an abdominal mass due to neoplastic hepatomegaly. *A*, A 6-day-old female infant with an enlarged liver (outlined). *B*, Massive hepatomegaly was noted on an abdominal x-ray film. *C*, Exploratory laparotomy revealed multiple tumor nodules replacing most of the liver. *D*, Liver biopsy revealed extensive fibrosis, parenchymal loss, and tiny nests of neuroblasts, many of which are necrotic (hematoxylin-eosin, ×600). (From Isaacs H Jr. Tumors of the Newborn and Infant. St. Louis: Mosby–Year Book, 1991.)

one death secondary to neoplastic hepatomegaly and liver failure. Two neonates with adrenal and retroperitoneal tumors, stages II and III, respectively, were treated with surgery and chemotherapy and survived. One with stage IV disease and an adrenal primary died at the age of 5 days following chemotherapy. The overall survival, including the prenatally diagnosed cases, was 10 of 12, or 83%.[48]

Stage IV-S disease is a special pattern of metastatic neuroblastoma unique to the first year of life; in many instances, it is associated with a favorable outcome (Table 6–3).[44–46,61,134] Patients diagnosed with stage IV-S disease have a small or undetectable primary neuroblastoma with metastases in one or more of the following sites: liver, skin, or bone marrow (not bone). The adrenal is the most common primary site, but other locations that may be affected include the retroperitoneal area, mediastinum, and pelvis; there may also be multiple primary tumors or no discernible primary site (see Figs. 6–4 and 6–7).[44,58,94] Multiple bluish cutaneous nodules producing "blueberry muffin" babies are noted in about one third of patients with stage IV-S neuroblastomatosis metastatic to the skin (see Table 5–2 and Fig. 5–9).[22,41,58,67,130] When present, these nodules almost always are

Table 6–3. International Staging System for Neuroblastoma

Stage	Description
I	Localized tumor confined to the area of origin; complete gross excision with or without microscopic residual disease; identifiable ipsilateral and contralateral lymph nodes negative microscopically
IIA	Unilateral tumor with incomplete gross excision; identifiable ipsilateral and contralateral lymph nodes negative microscopically
IIB	Unilateral tumor with complete or incomplete gross removal, with positive ipsilateral regional lymph nodes; identifiable contralateral lymph nodes negative microscopically
III	Tumor infiltrating across the midline with or without regional lymph node involvement; or, midline tumor with bilateral regional lymph node involvement
IV	Dissemination of tumor to distant lymph nodes, bone, bone marrow, liver, and/or other organs (except as defined in stage IV-S)
IV-S	Localized primary tumor as defined for stage I or II with dissemination limited to liver, skin, and/or bone marrow

From Brodeur GM, Seeger RC, Barrett A, et al. International criteria for diagnosis, staging and response to treatment in patients with neuroblastoma. J Clin Oncol 1988;6:1874. Used by permission.

associated with liver metastases and usually, but not always, herald a favorable prognosis.[149] The nodules blanch on palpation or rubbing. This color change is thought to be attributable to the release of catecholamines from the tumor.[41] Spontaneous regression and histologic maturation have been documented in patients with stage IV-S neuroblastoma (see Fig. 6–12).[61,81,131]

It should be mentioned that there are some conflicting reports regarding the optimistic prognosis for the newborn with stage IV-S neuroblastoma. The study from the Hospital for Sick Children, Toronto, which consisted of 18 infants younger than 6 months of age with IV-S neuroblastoma, suggests that stage IV-S disease represents a biologically heterogeneous group of patients without a uniformly favorable prognosis.[149] Ten of these infants were younger than 3 months of age, and only 50% survived. The babies who died probably had extensive metastatic organ involvement. Three died from respiratory failure secondary to neoplastic hepatomegaly, and one with tumor N-myc amplification succumbed to progressive disease. The two neonates with cutaneous metastases survived.

Some newborns with neuroblastoma do not die from the spread of the tumor per se, but from complications arising directly from either the treatment or from the effects of neoplastic hepatomegaly or liver failure. One explanation as to why the liver is so extensively involved with metastases in some fetuses and newborns is that the organ may be massively reseeded from the placenta by way of the umbilical vein.[147] The neonate with extensive liver metastases is susceptible to mechanical problems produced by a massively enlarged liver.[27,44,45,134] The problems described by Evans and colleagues[44] include pulmonary compromise as the result of an elevated diaphragm; compression of the vena cava and renal vessels, producing renal failure; gastric compression that contributes to feeding problems; and bleeding diatheses secondary to liver failure resulting from replacement of the parenchyma by extensive tumor deposits. Infants with massive metastatic hepatomegaly have died from this complication; in one series, four of five infants with stage IV-S disease died because of this problem.[184] Maternal dystocia caused by gigantic neoplastic hepatomegaly with fetal hydrops has also been reported.[63,91,135]

DIAGNOSTIC TESTS

Most neuroblastomas are biochemically active, secreting varying quantities of catecholamines, such as vanillylmandelic acid (VMA) and homovanillic acid (HVA), which can be analyzed by blood and urine studies (see Table 6–1).[92] Apparently, it is not the levels, per se, but the ratios of these two metabolites that are important for estimating prognosis. According to the studies of Laug and colleagues, infants and children with a low VMA:HVA ratio and increased vanillylacetic acid and cystathionine excretion generally have an unfavorable prognosis.[92,119] Urinary catecholamine analysis is important, not only for establishing the diagnosis and perhaps for predicting prognosis, but also for follow-up evaluation to detect recurrence or metastatic disease. Furthermore, the diagnosis of neuroblastoma can be confirmed in a neonate, without resorting to an exploratory operation, by the findings of elevated urinary catecholamine levels and the typical, small, round tumor cell syncytia in a bone marrow aspirate (Fig. 6–5).[78] If the syncytia exhibit catecholamine fluorescence, then the diagnosis is confirmed with certainty.[116] Biopsy examination of the primary tumor is indicated if the urinary catecholamine determination and the bone marrow aspirate yield negative or equivocal results.[22]

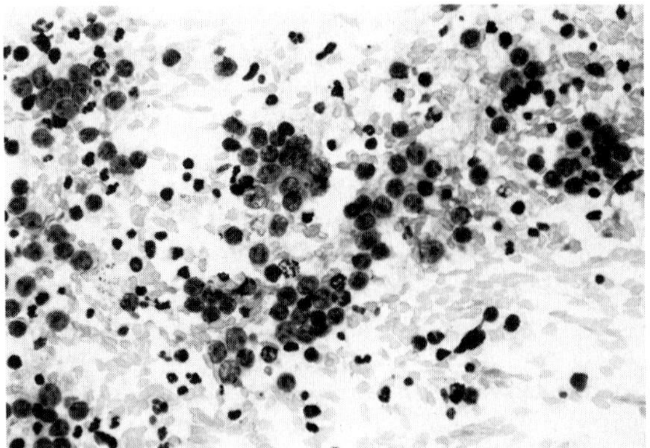

Figure 6–5. Bone marrow smear with neuroblastoma metastases. A Giemsa-stained smear reveals small, round, darkly staining tumor cells forming syncytia (Giemsa, ×600). The bone marrow aspirate was from a neonate with stage IV-S neuroblastoma who had significantly elevated urinary VMA and HVA levels (see Table 6–1). The bone marrow cytologic and urinary catecholamine findings were sufficient to establish the diagnosis of neuroblastoma without resorting to a biopsy. Catecholamine fluorescence, performed directly on tumor cells in bone marrow smears, is a rapid method for establishing the diagnosis.[116] (From Isaacs H Jr. Tumors of the Newborn and Infant. St. Louis: Mosby–Year Book, 1991.)

Mass screening programs introduced in Japan measuring the urinary levels of VMA and HVA in 6-month-old infants revealed numerous cases of neuroblastoma, but despite this, the number of cases in older children has not decreased.[11,68,122,123] Sawada uncovered 170 cases by the urinary catecholamine screening program, and 165 (96%) of these patients survived.[123] The findings resulting from these studies suggest that the cases found by early catecholamine screening represent neuroblastomas that undergo spontaneous regression and do not appear clinically; because of this phenomenon, patients identified by catecholamine screening generally have a good prognosis.

Additional tests are available that are of prognostic significance (see Table 6–2).[46] Elevated levels of serum ferritin and inhibition of E rosette formation by the patient's T lymphocytes are unfavorable prognostic indicators that often correlate with advanced disease (stages III and IV) (see Table 6–3).[46,64] It is proposed that neuroblastoma cells produce ferritin, which interferes with lymphocyte immune function. Ferritin-labeled immunoperoxidase testing yields positive results in neuroblastoma cells showing a high mitotic karyorrhexis index (MKI) and N-myc amplification. Normal serum

levels of neuron-specific enolase (NSE) are associated with a more favorable outcome than when these levels are elevated.[46] Serial serum lactic dehydrogenase (LDH) measurements are helpful for monitoring tumor activity.[115] Patients whose LDH levels return to normal generally have a favorable prognosis, whereas those whose levels begin to rise have recurrences and, often, a fatal outcome. Nerve growth factor receptor, which is expressed by the TRK proto-oncogene, is a transmembrane glycoprotein (a tyrosine kinase) that is produced in the developing nervous system and is believed to be responsible for neuronal differentiation. High levels of expression of the nerve growth factor receptor are associated with a good prognosis in patients with neuroblastoma.[3]

Clinical manifestations of circulating vasoactive compounds in the fetus, infant, or mother may be the first sign of a neuroblastoma.[105,112,142] Newton et al. reported a case of a 28-year-old gravida 2, para 1 who presented at 33 weeks' gestation with severe preeclampsia and symptoms of catecholamine excess.[105] An ultrasonogram revealed a cystic right adrenal mass. Following cesarean section, a hydropic infant and placenta were delivered, and the baby expired at 4 hours of age. Necropsy revealed bilateral adrenal neuroblastomas with extensive metastases to the liver, lungs, brain, placenta, and other organs. Voute and colleagues described pheochromocytoma-like symptoms consisting of headaches, paroxysmal hypertension, pallor, sweating, and tingling sensations in the hands and feet of six mothers during the last 2 months of pregnancy who gave birth to infants with disseminated neuroblastoma.[142] The authors thus recommend that babies born to mothers having these symptoms in the last trimester should be investigated for a congenital neuroblastoma. Moreover, maternal urine should be examined for elevated VMA and HVA levels. An extra-adrenal neuroblastoma in a newborn was associated with clinical and pathologic evidence of norepinephrine release, including flushing, extreme tachycardia, and pulmonary edema. Histologically, there was massive hemorrhagic necrosis and complete necrosis of the fetal fat owing to lipolytic activity of the secretion. No metastases were present.[112] Instances of neuroblastoma presenting as chronic, watery diarrhea are attributed to vasoactive intestinal peptides produced by the tumor in the first year of life.[75] Of the 31 cases of diarrhea associated with sympathetic nervous system tumors reviewed by Iida and colleagues, only 4 were younger than 1 year of age; the youngest in the study was 7 months of age.[75]

DNA cytometric analysis performed on neuroblastoma specimens show that a favorable outcome is associated with aneuploidy and a low percentage of tumor cells in the S, G2, and M phases of the cell cycle.[53] Aneuploidy in neuroblastoma cells correlates with a better prognosis than diploidy, which is surprisingly different from what is observed with most other malignant tumors.

CYTOGENETICS

Specific chromosomal defects are found in neuroblastomas. The tumor cells show deletions of the short arm of chromosome 1 (band 1p36), extrachromosomal double minute chromatin bodies, and homogeneously staining regions.[24,25,47] The 1p deletion represents a loss of a suppressor gene involved in neuroblastoma, and the double minutes and homogeneously staining regions are a manifestation of gene amplification. Both the N-myc and ras oncogenes are found in neuroblastomas, and both are highly amplified in some tumor specimens.[24,25,47] A definite relationship exists between N-myc amplification and loss of heterozygosity for chromosome 1p.[47] N-myc genomic amplification correlates with prognosis, the extent of disease at the time of diagnosis, and histologic findings.[25] Tumors from patients with stage I and stage IV-S disease show single copies of N-myc gene, whereas stages III and IV neuroblastomas have multiple copies of the gene (genomic amplification) (Fig. 6–6).[47,69,125] N-myc amplification is associated with an unfavorable histologic pattern, namely, high mitotic activity. N-myc amplification has been analyzed in a few neonatal neuroblastoma specimens.[54,71,73,86] Most of the tumors studied showed no N-myc amplification, which perhaps would explain the generally favorable prognosis in this age group.

Neuroblastoma cell lines show defects in the nerve growth factor receptor pathway, which may play a role in the initiation or maintenance of the undifferentiated state of the tumor.[24,103] The nerve growth factor is the product of the proto-oncogene TRK, a transmembrane protein tyrosine kinase that is expressed in the developing nervous system.[103] TRK is expressed in many neuroblastomas and correlates inversely with N-myc amplification. In other words, a

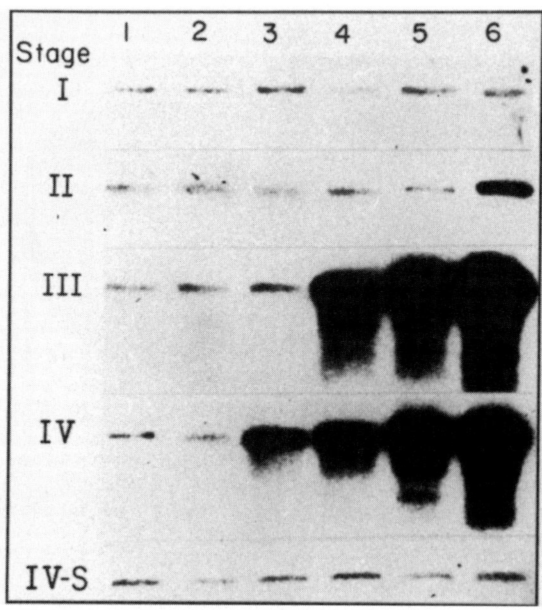

Figure 6–6. Relationship between N-myc amplification and clinical stage. Autoradiograms of DNA from untreated primary neuroblastoma specimens show the high levels of N-myc in tumors from patients with advanced disease (stages III and IV). Note the absence of amplification in the stage IV-S tumors. (From Seeger RC, Brodeur GM, Sather H, et al. Association of multiple copies of the N-myc oncogene with rapid progression of neuroblastomas. N Engl J Med 1985;313:1111. Used by permission of the Massachusetts Medical Society.)

high level of TRK expression correlates with a low clinical stage and a favorable outcome.

PATHOLOGY

Gross and microscopic findings of neuroblastoma in the fetus and newborn are similar to those seen in the older child.[13,37–39,78,79,112] The size of neonatal primary neuroblastomas varies considerably, with the adrenal masses ranging from 1 cm to 15 cm or more in greatest dimension and from 4 g to 750 g in weight.[79] The cervical and mediastinal tumors average 5 cm in greatest dimension. Neuroblastomas have a tan-gray, bosselated, capsular surface and a light gray or red-brown to dark red cut surface, depending upon the amount of hemorrhage, which is often considerable. They may be solid or cystic (Figs. 6–7A, 6–8C, and 6–9B). The cortical tissue of the adrenal gland usually persists and may surround the tumor or be visible only on one surface; the remainder is so attenuated that it cannot be distinguished on gross examination. The solid portions of the tumor are

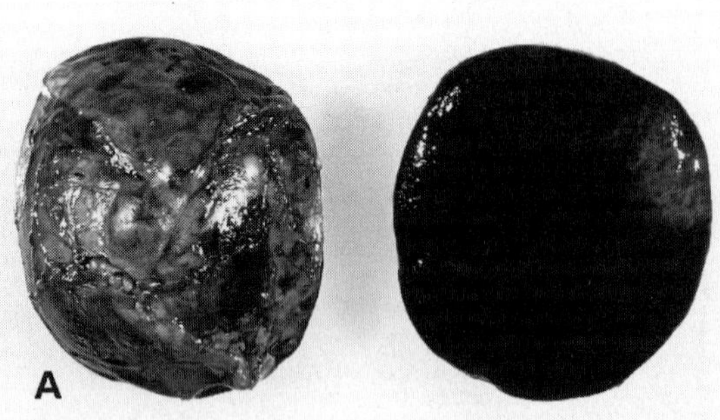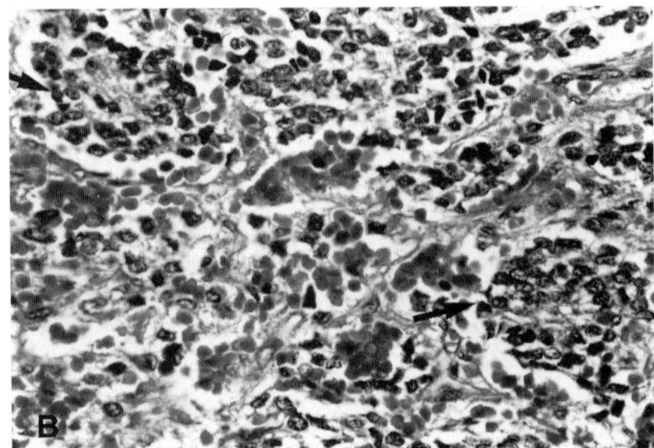

Figure 6–7. Differentiated neuroblastoma. *A,* A tumor measuring 8 × 6 cm and weighing 143 g was found to have replaced the left adrenal, which was removed from a 3-day-old male infant with stage IV-S disease. The specimen has a hemorrhagic cut surface, which is on the right. *B,* The tumor consists of small, round, darkly staining cells forming Homer-Wright rosettes (*arrows*) with fibrillary material (neuropil), in addition to extensive hemorrhage (hematoxylin-eosin, ×750). (From Isaacs H Jr. Tumors of the Newborn and Infant. St. Louis: Mosby–Year Book, 1991.)

light gray to red-brown, depending on the amount of hemorrhage, and soft and somewhat granular in appearance. Some lesions from other sites are tan-gray and lighter in color, firmer, and with much less hemorrhage than the adrenal primaries; this appearance may be related to the degree of tumor maturation.[79] Nevertheless, tiny white to yellow foci of calcification are noted, especially in specimens removed at follow-up or "second look" operations performed after a course of therapy during which maturation and/or regression has occurred (see Fig. 6–12).

Microscopically, the tumor consists of small cells with poorly demarcated boundaries whose round or oval hyperchromatic nuclei are proportionately large in relation to total cell volume (Figs. 6–3, 6–5, and 6–7 through 6–11). Fine fibrils either form a delicate interlacing network between the cells or are found in areas almost devoid of cells. Rosettes, consisting of a small, pale, finely granular central area surrounded by a petal-like arrangement of cells (Homer-Wright rosettes), are common (see Figs. 6–7 through 6–9). Hemorrhagic necrosis and calcification are often present in larger tumors.[38,79]

Neuroblastomas displaying an organoid histologic pattern, which consists of individual small tumor cell nests regularly surrounded by a meshwork of thin fibrovascular septae, are associated with a good prognosis in the newborn.[62] Three patients in Hachitanda and Tsuneyoshi's study who were 4 months of age or younger had adrenal primaries; two were staged as IV-S and one as stage III, and all survived. The tumors had low MKI values and S-100 protein reactivity, the latter of which suggested Schwann cell differentiation, which was confirmed by ultrastructural studies. Parenthetically, according to the authors, this unique pattern was observed in 86% of patients found by mass screening in Japan.[62]

Neuroblastoma is a classic example of one of the small blue cell tumors of infancy and childhood (see Fig. 6–10). The pathologic features and differential diagnoses of neuroblastoma and the small blue cell tumors have been discussed thoroughly by Dehner and by Tsokos (see Table 4–5).[38,139]

Shimada et al.[129] proposed a histopathologic classification for neuroblastoma that correlates certain histologic patterns and prognosis. The histologic criteria are based primarily on the evaluation of maturation of both neuroblastic and stromal elements and of nuclear morphology. Neuroblastomas are divided into two main categories: stroma-rich and stroma-poor categories. The MKI of the neuroblasts is evaluated, and this index appears to be the most important factor for prognosis, particularly in children younger than 1½ years of age.[129] These authors' data suggest that a low MKI is more significant in this age group for survival than maturation. Infants with stage I and IV-S disease, the most favorable prognostic groups, usually have, in addition to a stroma-poor pattern, a low MKI and usually, no N-myc amplification. The stroma-rich pattern is usually not observed in neuroblastomas removed from newborns.[81,129]

Joshi et al. proposed a more simplified histo-

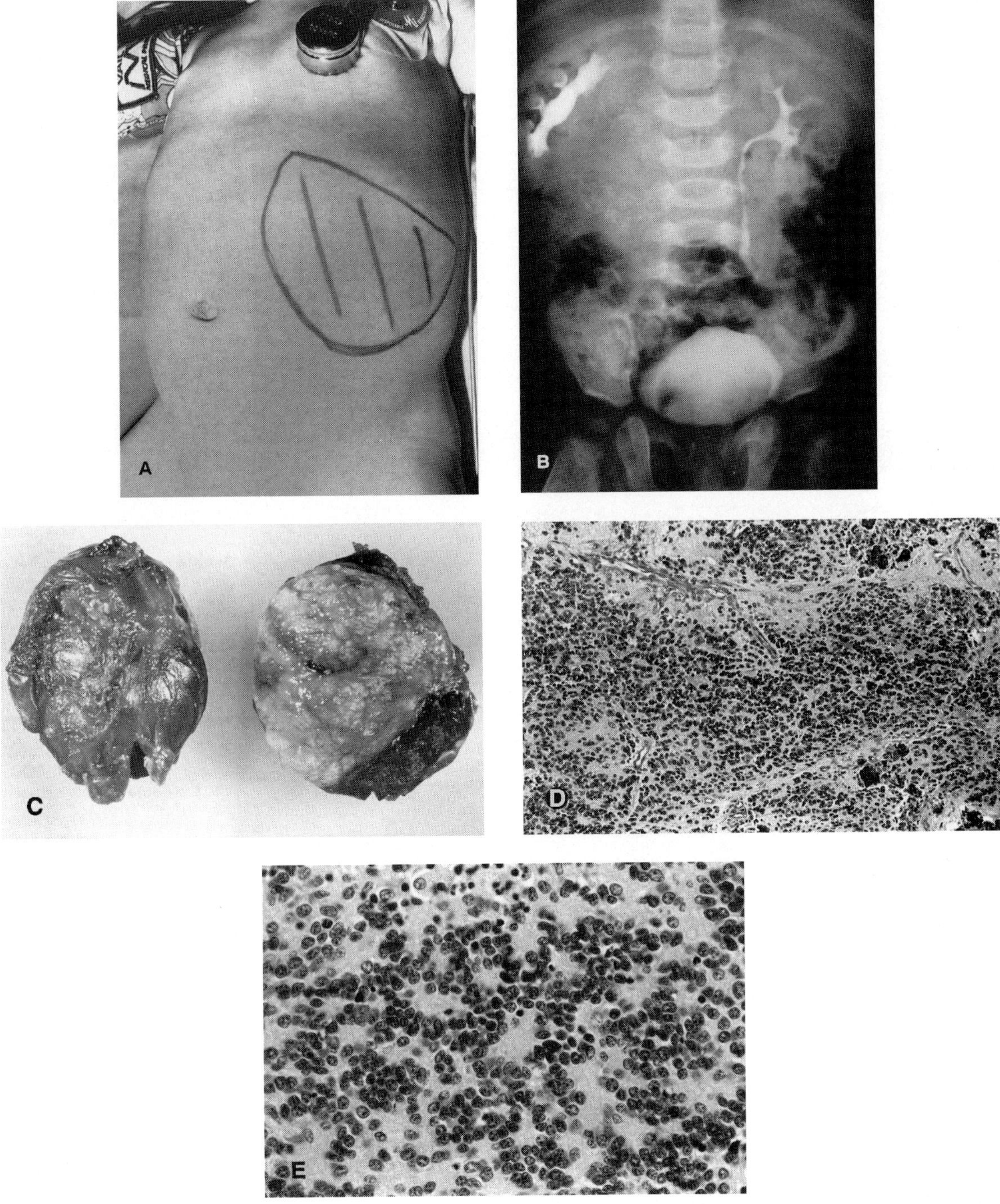

Figure 6–8. Retroperitoneal neuroblastoma, stage III, manifesting as an abdominal mass. *A*, A 5-month-old boy with a left abdominal mass (outlined). *B*, Intravenous pyelography showed a left retroperitoneal tumor with tiny foci of calcification displacing the adjacent kidney upward. *C*, A retroperitoneal tumor measuring 8 × 7 cm and weighing 118 g was removed, along with several paraaortic lymph nodes. A cross section of the adrenal shows a tan, soft tumor with multiple foci of yellow calcification. *D*, A moderately well-differentiated neuroblastoma is composed of small, dark, round cells separated by pink fibrillar material and scattered, irregular, black-staining areas of calcification, which can be seen on the right side of the photomicrograph (hematoxylin-eosin, ×120). *E*, A higher-power view reveals several Homer-Wright pseudorosettes with central fibrillar material (hematoxylin-eosin, ×600). (From Isaacs H Jr. Tumors of the Newborn and Infant. St. Louis: Mosby–Year Book, 1991.)

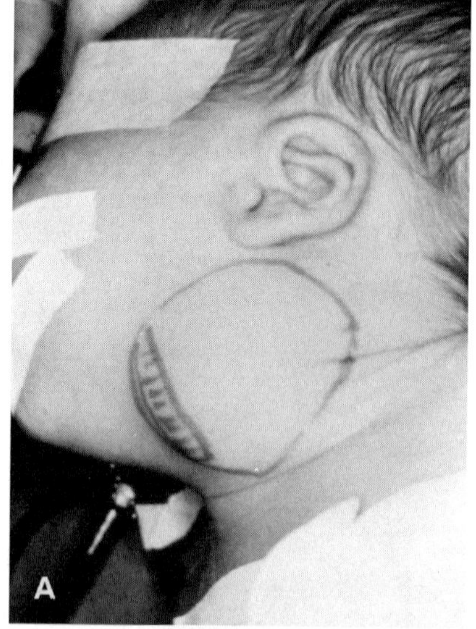
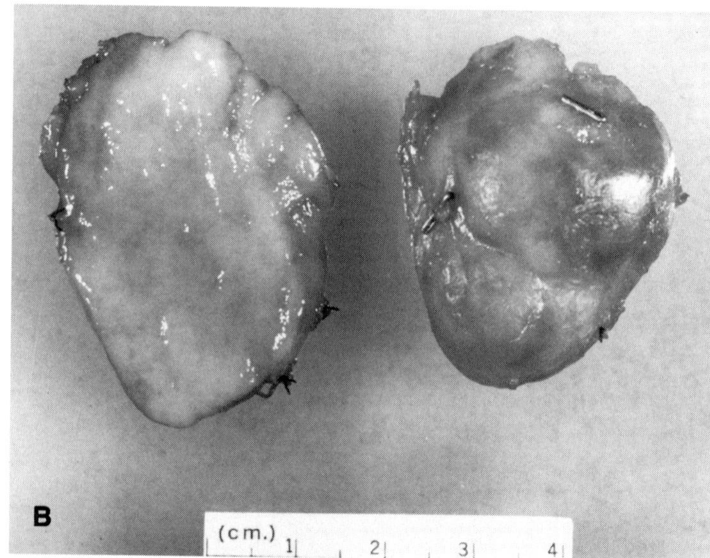

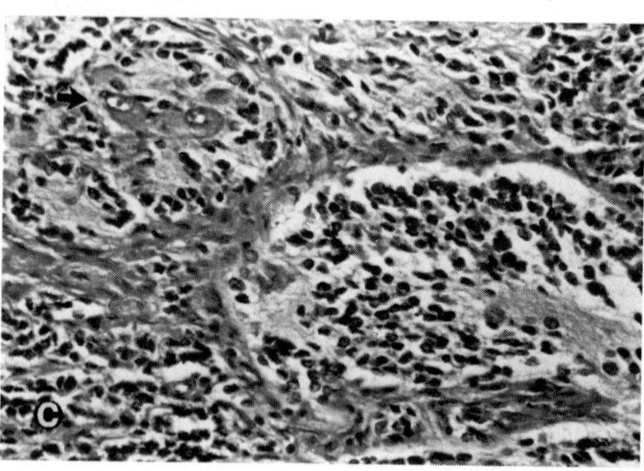

Figure 6–9. Differentiating cervical neuroblastoma, stage I. *A,* A 2-month-old boy with a cervical mass and noisy respirations noted 1 month prior to hospitalization. The tumor, presumably arising from the cervical sympathetic ganglia, is outlined. *B,* The specimen, measuring 4.5 × 3.5 cm and weighing 20 g, has a rather uniform, light tan cut surface, which is on the left. *C,* The tumor displays the histologic features of a typical neuroblastoma. In addition, focal differentiation is demonstrated by the presence of ganglioneuroblasts having a large vesicular nucleus, prominent nucleolus, and abundant cytoplasm (*arrow*) (hematoxylin-eosin, ×600). (From Isaacs H Jr. Tumors of the Newborn and Infant. St. Louis: Mosby–Year Book, 1991.)

logic grading system.[87] In their grading system, the more familiar terms neuroblastoma and ganglioneuroblastoma are retained and used instead of stroma-poor neuroblastoma and stroma-rich neuroblastoma.[129] Undifferentiated neuroblastoma is regarded as a subtype separate from poorly differentiated neuroblastoma, and the term ganglioneuroblastoma is reserved for a predominant ganglioneuroma component in addition to the minor neuroblastoma component.[87] Calcification and a low mitotic rate of less than 10 mitoses per high-power field are the two most important prognostic histologic indicators.[87] Histologic grades 1, 2, and 3 are determined on the basis of the presence of both, any one, or none of these two histologic indicators, respectively. Similar to the Shimada classification, age (older or younger than 1 year of age) is a separate significant prognostic factor that is combined with the histologic grade to yield a final interpretation of high- and low-

risk categories. Infants with low-grade tumors (grades 1 and 2) are categorized as a low-risk group and have the best prognosis.[87] Joshi et al. further recommend that, in the histologic grading of neuroblastomas, the karyorrhectic index can be used instead of the mitotic rate because it can be determined more readily and it is more reproducible.[87a]

Practically all the initial biopsy specimens taken from 17 neonates with neuroblastoma in the Children's Hospital, Los Angeles study[81] showed a stroma-poor histologic pattern according to the criteria of Shimada and colleagues;[129] these tumors were judged to be grade 1 or 2 by Joshi et al.'s classification system.[87] Low MKI values were noted in specimens obtained from the one patient with stage I and the 10 patients with stage IV-S disease. Focal cytodifferentiation—that is, the presence of tumor cells with more abundant eosinophilic cytoplasms and larger and more numerous

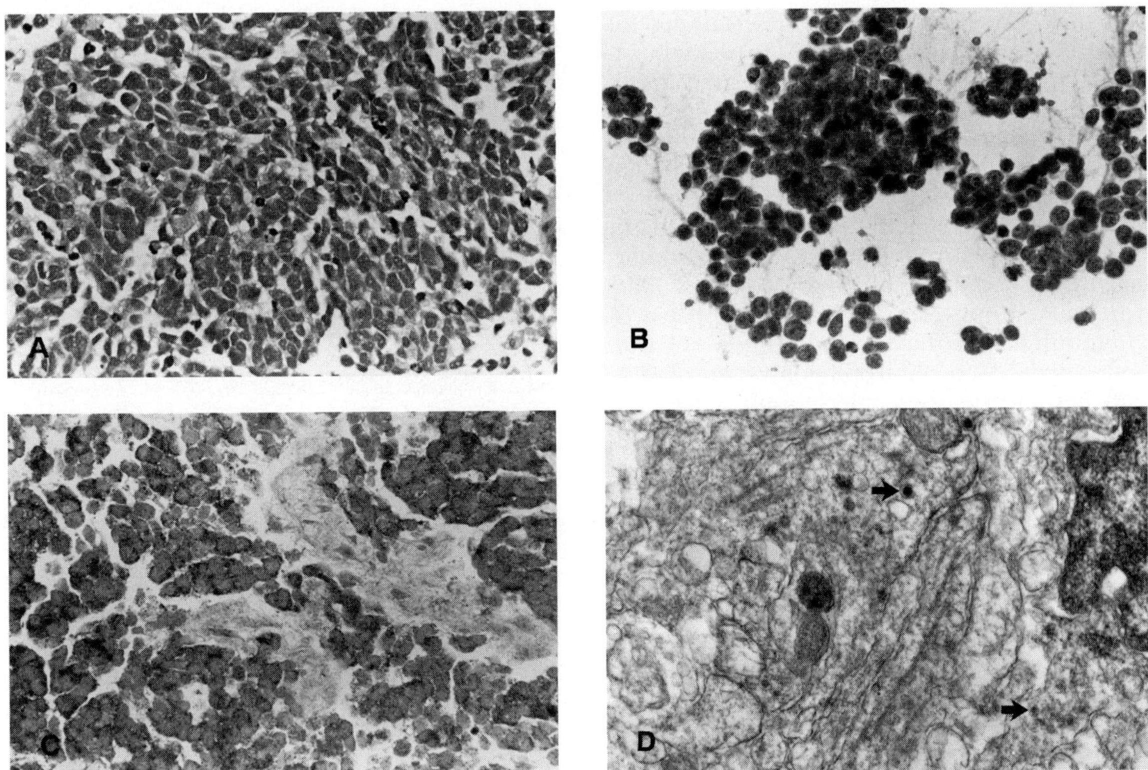

Figure 6–10. Poorly differentiated neuroblastoma. *A*, Microscopic examination reveals a small cell malignant tumor without rosettes or neuropil (hematoxylin-eosin, ×150). *B*, An imprint ("touch preparation") of the tumor. The cells are round to oval with a high nuclear:cytoplasmic ratio. A fine "peppery" chromatin pattern and one or more tiny nucleoli are noted (hematoxylin-eosin, ×300). *C*, The cells stain positively with neuron-specific enolase (NSE) immunoperoxidase, are reactive with synaptophysin, are focally reactive with S-100 protein, but stain negatively with desmin, actin, leukocyte common antigen, anti-β_2-microglobulin, and HBA71 antibodies. The tumor exhibited N-myc amplification (NSE, ×300). *D*, An electron photomicrograph reveals microtubules and dense core (neurosecretory) granules (*arrows*) (×42,000). (Electron microscopy courtesy of Ann Peters, Children's Hospital, San Diego, CA.)

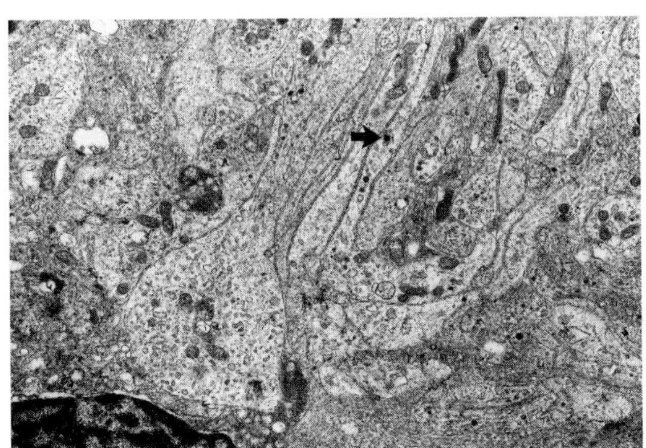

Figure 6–11. Ultrastructural analysis of a more differentiated neuroblastoma. Neuropil, composed of a network of neurites containing neurotubules and neurosecretory granules (*arrow*), are present. One neurite directly adjacent to the nucleus has a bulbous swelling suggestive of synaptic bouton ×20,000 (Courtesy of Darkin Chan, Children's Hospital, Los Angeles, CA). (From Isaacs H Jr. Tumors of the Newborn and Infant. St. Louis: Mosby–Year Book, 1991.)

vesicular nuclei—were observed in 2 of the 17 tumors (see Fig. 6–9*C*). Furthermore, serial biopsy studies were performed on two infants diagnosed as having stage IV-S disease. Both of the initial biopsies showed neuroblastoma; the second biopsy revealed ganglioneuroblastoma, and the third biopsy study also showed small foci of ganglioneuroma or no identifiable tumor, or areas of fibrosis with or without calcification. Haas and colleagues reported similar microscopic findings in serial biopsies performed on untreated patients with stage IV-S disease.[61] Although several other examples of maturation of neuroblastoma to ganglioneuroma have been cited,[2,131] the frequency of this event is unknown.

The ultrastructural features of neuroblastoma have been reported by several investigators.[39,81,98,118,119,136,138,139] Most agree that the findings depend upon the degree of cytologic differentiation. Neuroblastomas with a densely cellular, primitive, "small blue cell tumor" appearance on hematoxylin-eosin staining of thick sections may be difficult to distinguish by electron microscopy from other small cell malignant tumors, such as the primitive neuroectodermal tumor (PNET), undifferentiated sarcomas, rhabdomyosarcoma, and leukemia. The presence of dense core or neurosecretory granules, which incidentally are found in small numbers in the primitive neuroectodermal tumor, establishes the diagnosis by electron microscopy (see Fig. 6–10*D*).[38,119,136,138,139] The more differentiated tumors show, in addition, a network or neuropil composed of cells with neural processes, microtubules, neurofilaments, and cell attachments, with some resembling synapses (see Fig. 6–11).[119,136]

Immunoperoxidase techniques are requisite for establishing the diagnosis. The tumor cells test positive for NSE, synaptophysin, and neurofilament, and are focally positive for S-100 protein but stain negatively for desmin, actin, leukocyte common antigen, and cytokeratin (see Fig. 6–10*C*) (Table 4–5).[38,81,138,139] In contrast to the primitive neuroectodermal tumor, the anti-β_2-microglobulin and HBA71 antigens are nonreactive, which also are helpful distinguishing features (see Table 4–5).

METASTASIS

In more than half the cases of neuroblastoma in newborns, the first clinical manifestations are usually the result of metastatic disease.[95] Regardless of the extent of disseminated disease in stage IV-S disease, the prognosis is surprisingly favorable. Both the Children's Hospital of Philadelphia and the Children's Hospital, Los Angeles neonatal studies revealed that neuroblastoma metastasizes most often to the liver, bone marrow, skin, and regional lymph nodes, in that order.[45,79] In a review of 60 patients with congenital neuroblastoma by Schneider and co-workers, the adrenal was the leading primary site; 31 patients (51.7%) had metastases at the time of diagnosis, and the sites of metastases were similar to those just described except that the skin was involved more often than the bone marrow.[124] In one 3925-g stillborn fetus examined by Potter and Craig,[112] the liver was enormously enlarged, weighing 390 g. The liver parenchyma was almost entirely replaced by islands of neuroblasts separated by sinusoidal endothelium. The adrenal glands, although not appreciably enlarged, showed replacement of the fetal zone by cells similar to those in the

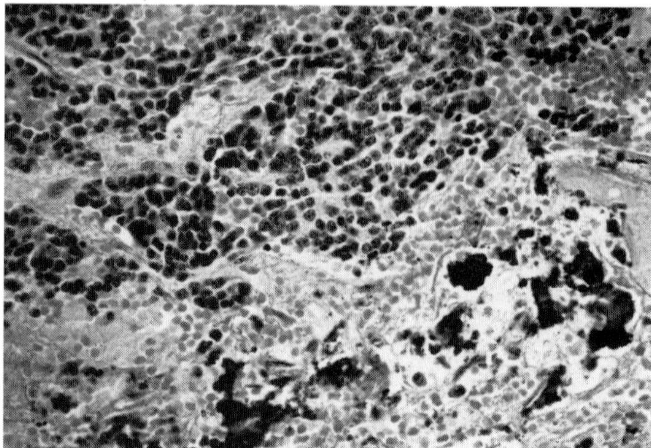

Figure 6–12. Spontaneous regression of congenital neuroblastoma, stage IV-S. Extensive necrosis, hemorrhage, and calcification provide evidence of tumor regression (hematoxylin-eosin, ×600). (From Isaacs H Jr. Tumors of the Newborn and Infant. St. Louis: Mosby–Year Book, 1991.)

liver, but the definitive cortex was uninvolved. Small islands of tumor cells were also present in the lungs and kidneys.[112]

SPONTANEOUS REGRESSION

Apparently spontaneous regression of neuroblastomas is not uncommon.[13,37,61,81,131] Neonatal neuroblastoma is characterized by an exceptional natural inclination to regress spontaneously or disappear, which is noted usually within 2 to 6 months after the initial diagnosis and is heralded clinically by a decrease in liver size.[13,37] Spontaneous regression of this tumor occurs more often than for any other malignant neoplasm, but the exact frequency of this event is unknown.[13,61] As would be anticipated, spontaneous regression is related to an increased survival rate, which is reported to be as high as 85% in the newborn as compared to only 19% in the second year of life and 5% after the age of 2 years, by which time this phenomenon is rarely seen.[13,71] According to Bolande, spontaneous regression is characterized histologically by three main events: (1) necrosis followed by fibrosis and calcification (Fig. 6–12); (2) disappearance of tumor by cytolysis; and (3) cytodifferentiation (maturation) to ganglioneuroma.[13] These findings are observed particularly in serial biopsies performed in patients with stage IV-S neuroblastoma. Similar trends are observed among patients with congenital retinoblastomas.

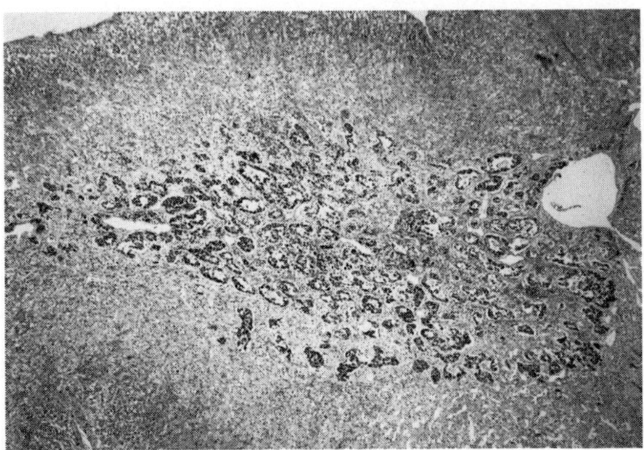

Figure 6–13. Neuroblastoma in situ. The adrenal contains a central area of neuroblasts not invading the capsule. This was an incidental postmortem microscopic finding in a 2-day-old, 3-kg male neonate who died from hypoplastic left heart syndrome (hematoxylin-eosin, ×60). (From Isaacs H Jr. Tumors of the Newborn and Infant. St. Louis: Mosby–Year Book, 1991.)

NEUROBLASTOMA IN SITU

Neuroblastoma in situ occurs exclusively in the fetus and young infant and is defined as microscopic, incidentally found nests of neuroblastic cells situated in the adrenal medulla and not associated with either grossly visible tumor or metastases (Fig. 6–13).[8] The frequency with which small collections of neuroblasts are found in newborns suggests that maturation and cessation of growth of potentially lethal tumors are relatively common occurrences.[8,15,60,79,127] The reported frequency of neuroblastoma in situ differs considerably, varying from 1 in 10 to 1 in 500 necropsies.[8,15,60,79] Most agree that the lesion is a precursor of neuroblastoma,[37,118,124] whereas others suggest that the cell clusters represent a phase in the natural embryologic development of neuroblastoma cells.[140] Nevertheless, it should be pointed out that congenital malformations, such as congenital heart disease, tracheoesophageal fistula, and genitourinary tract anomalies, are found in fetuses and newborns at postmortem examination in as many as 73% of patients with neuroblastoma in situ.[8,37,60,79] Such collections of cells have been observed frequently in infants with trisomy 18 and those with cystic adrenal neuroblastomas.[5,71,81,112]

According to Romansky and associates, normal neural crest aggregates in the developing fetal adrenal can be distinguished from in situ neuroblastoma cells. The former, on ultrastructural examination, are composed of two cell types, neuroblasts and pheochromoblasts (chromaffin cells), whereas the latter is composed of only one cell type (i.e., neuroblasts).[118]

PROGNOSIS

The age of the patient and the stage of the disease are the two most important factors in determining the outcome of infants and children with neuroblastoma. The prognosis for infants and newborns is far better than that for older children, mainly because they present more often with a treatable localized lesion (lower stage disease) as compared to the older child (see Table 6–3).

In addition, more infants and newborns have stage IV-S disease, which exhibits a tendency to regress spontaneously with little or no therapy.[17,44–46,61,71] Survival in several series was 100% for those with stages I, II, and III disease; approximately 80% for patients with stage IV-S disease; and 50% for those with stage IV disease.[58] Other than the age of the patient and the stage at the time of diagnosis, improved survival is attributed to one or more of the following: spontaneous regression, favorable histologic findings, normal chromosome 1, aneuploidy, low N-myc oncogene expression, and normal serum ferritin values (see Table 6–2).[58]

An awareness that multifocal primary neuroblastoma can occur may prevent errors in diagnosis and staging.[32] Familial screening for this tumor should be performed if multifocal tumors are found, and investigation for a second primary tumor should be performed in the child with a diagnosis and family history of neuroblastoma. Oddly enough, newborns and infants with multifocal tumors seem to have a similar outcome as those with stage IV-S disease.[32]

Garmel et al. recommend the use of serial ultrasonography to assess tumor size, amniotic fluid volume, and fetal well-being as part of pregnancy management.[54] In addition, the presence of metastases and clinical staging should be determined by this procedure if possible. Extensive liver metastases are correlated with the development of hydrops and placentomegaly, which usually ends in fetal or neonatal death.[12,54,82] Delivery is recommended if hydrops occurs because of the poor prognosis.[54] Moreover, sonography should be performed toward the end of the third trimester to evaluate the possibility of dystocia and the necessity for cesarean section.

The studies of Ho et al. show that patients

with neuroblastoma that is detected by antenatal sonography usually (but not always) survive when surgical resection is curative.[71] They recommend not using chemotherapy unless significant progression of disease occurs.

REFERENCES

1. Adams GA, Shochat SJ, Smith EI, et al. Thoracic neuroblastoma: A Pediatric Oncology Group study. J Pediatr Surg 1993;28:372.
2. Alterman K, Schuller EF. Maturation of neuroblastoma to ganglioneuroma. Am J Dis Child 1970;120:217.
3. Anders D, Kindermann G, Pfeifer U. Metastasizing fetal neuroblastoma with involvement of the placenta simulating fetal erythroblastosis. Report of two cases. J Pediatr 1973;82:50.
4. Andersen HJ, Hariri J. Congenital neuroblastoma in a fetus with multiple malformations: Metastasis in the umbilical cord as a cause of intrauterine death. Virch Archiv [A] 1983;400:219.
5. Atkinson GO, Zaatari GS, Gay BB, et al. Cystic neuroblastoma in infants: Radiographic and pathologic features. Am J Radiol 1986;146:113.
6. Bader JL, Miller RW. U.S. cancer incidence and mortality in the first year of life. Am J Dis Child 1979;133:157.
7. Barson AJ. Congenital neoplasia. The Society's experience, abstracted. Arch Dis Child 1978;53:436.
8. Beckwith JB, Perrin EV. In situ neuroblastomas: A contribution to the natural history of neural crest tumors. Am J Pathol 1963;43:1089.
9. Benirschke K, Kaufmann P. The Pathology of the Human Placenta, 2nd ed. New York: Springer-Verlag, 1990.
10. Berry PJ. Congenital tumours. In Keeling JW (ed): Fetal and Neonatal Pathology, 2nd ed, p 273. Berlin: Springer-Verlag, 1993.
11. Bessho F, Hashizume K, Nakajo T, et al. Mass screening in Japan increased the detection of infants with neuroblastoma without a decrease in cases in older children. J Pediatr 1991;119:237.
12. Birner WF. Neuroblastoma as a cause of antenatal death. Am J Obstet Gynecol 1961;81:1388.
13. Bolande RP. Developmental pathology. Am J Pathol 1979;94:627.
14. Bolande RP. The neurocristopathies. A unifying concept of diseases arising in neural crest maldevelopment. Hum Pathol 1974;5:409.
15. Bolande RP. Neoplasia of early life and its relationships to teratogenesis. In Rosenberg HS, Bolande RP (eds): Perspectives in Pediatric Pathology, Vol 3, p 145. Chicago: Year Book–Medical Publishers, 1976.
16. Bolande RP, Towler WF. A possible relationship of neuroblastoma to von Recklinghausen's disease. Cancer 1970;26:162.
17. Bond JV. Neuroblastoma in infants. In Pochedly C (ed): Neuroblastoma: Clinical and Biological Manifestations, p 1. New York: Elsevier Biomedical, 1982.
18. Borch K, Jacobsen T, Olsen JH, et al. Neonatal cancer in Denmark 1943–1985. Pediatr Hematol Oncol 1992;9:209.
19. Bower JR, Adkins JC. Ondine's curse and neurocristopathy. Clin Pediatr 1980;19:665.
20. Bowns GT, Walls RP, Murphree AL, et al. Neonatal neuroblastoma metastatic to the iris. Cancer 1983;52:929.
21. Boyd TK, Schofield DE. Monozygotic twins concordant for congenital neuroblastoma: Case report and review of the literature. Pediatr Pathol 1995;15:931.
22. Broadbent VA. Malignant disease in the neonate. In Roberton NRC (ed): Textbook of Neonatology, 2nd ed, p 879. Edinburgh: Churchill Livingstone, 1992.
23. Brock CE, Ricketts RR. Hemoperitoneum from spontaneous rupture of neonatal neuroblastoma. Am J Dis Child 1982;136:370.
24. Brodeur GM, Azar C, Brother M, et al. Neuroblastoma: Effect of genetic factors on prognosis and treatment. Cancer 1992;70:1685.
25. Brodeur GM, Castleberry RP. Neuroblastoma. In Pizzo PA, Poplack DG (eds): Principles and Practice of Pediatric Oncology, 2nd ed, p 739. Philadelphia: JB Lippincott, 1993.
26. Brodeur GM, Seeger RC, Barrett A, et al. International criteria for diagnosis, staging and response to treatment in patients with neuroblastoma. J Clin Oncol 1988;6:1874.
27. Butler H, Bick R, Morrison S. Unsuspected adrenal masses in the neonate: Adrenal cortical carcinoma and neuroblastoma: Report of two cases. Pediatr Radiol 1988;18:237.
28. Campbell AN, Chan HSL, O'Brien A, et al. Malignant tumours in the neonate. Arch Dis Child 1987;62:19.
29. Chatten J, Voorhess M. Familial neuroblastoma. N Engl J Med 1967;277:1230.
30. Chitayat D, Friedman JM, Dimmick JE. Neuroblastoma in a child with Wiedemann-Beckwith syndrome. Am J Med Genet 1990;35:433.
31. Cibis GW, Freeman AI, Pang V, et al. Bilateral choroidal neonatal neuroblastoma. Am J Ophthalmol 1990;109:445.
32. Cohen MD, Auringer ST, Grosfeld JL, et al. Multifocal primary neuroblastoma. Pediatr Radiol 1993;23:463.
33. Croituru DP, Sinsky AB, Laberge J-M. Cystic neuroblastoma. J Pediatr Surg 1992;27:1320.
34. Crom DB, Wilimas JA, Green AA, et al. Malignancy in the neonate. Med Pediatr Oncol 1989;17:101.
35. Crombleholme TM, Murray TA, Harris BH. Diagnosis and management of fetal neuroblastoma. Curr Opin Obstet Gynecol 1994;6:199.
36. Davis CF, Carachi R, Young DG. Neonatal tumors: Glasgow 1966–86. Arch Dis Child 63:1075,1988.
37. Dehner LP. Neoplasms of the fetus and neonate. In Naeye RL, Kissane JM, Kaufman N (eds): Perinatal Diseases, International Academy of Pathology, Monograph No. 22, p 286. Baltimore: Williams and Wilkins, 1981.
38. Dehner LP. Pathologic anatomy of classic neuroblastoma: Including prognostic features and differential diagnosis. In Pochedly C (ed): Neuroblastoma: Tumor Biology and Therapy, p 112. Boca Raton, FL: CRC Press, 1990.
39. Dehner LP: Pediatric Surgical Pathology, 2nd ed. Baltimore: Williams and Wilkins, 1987.
40. Delalieux C, Ebinger G, Maurus R, et al. Myoclonic encephalopathy and neuroblastoma. N Engl J Med 1975;292:46.
41. Dominey AM, Hawkins H, Levy ML. Congenital cutaneous and subcutaneous nodules. Pediatr Dermatol 9:301;1992.
42. Easa D, Balaraman V, Ash K, et al. Congenital chylo-

thorax and mediastinal neuroblastoma. J Pediatr Surg 1991;26:96.

43. Emery LG, Shields N, Narayan R, et al. Neuroblastoma associated with Beckwith-Wiedemann syndrome. Cancer 1983;52:176.

44. Evans AE, Baum E, Chard R. Do infants with Stage IV-S neuroblastoma need treatment? Arch Dis Child 1981;56:271.

45. Evans AE, Chatten J, D'Angio JG, et al. A review of 17 IV-S neuroblastoma patients at the Children's Hospital of Philadelphia. Cancer 1980;45:833.

46. Evans AE, D'Angio GJ, Propert K, et al. Prognostic factors in neuroblastoma. Cancer 1987;59:1853.

47. Fong C, Dracopoli NC, White PS, et al. Loss of heterozygosity for the short arm of chromosome 1 in human neuroblastomas: Correlation with N-myc amplification. Proc Natl Acad Sci USA 1989;86:3753.

48. Forman HP, Leonidas JC, Berdon WE, et al. Congenital neuroblastoma: Evaluation with multimodality imaging. Radiology 1990;175:365.

49. Fowlie F, Giacomantonio M, McKenzie E, et al. Antenatal sonographic diagnosis of adrenal neuroblastoma. J Can Assoc Radiol 1986;37:50.

50. Freud E, Mares AJ, Finaly R, et al. Visible dorsal paravertebral mass: An unusual presentation of neuroblastoma in infancy. Pediatr Surg Int 1988;3:193.

51. Gadwood KA, Reynes CJ. Prenatal sonography of metastatic neuroblastoma. J Clin Ultrasound 1983;11:512.

52. Gale GB, D'Angio GJ, Uri A, et al. Cancer in neonates: The experience at the Children's Hospital of Philadelphia. Pediatrics 1982;70:409.

53. Gansler T, Chatten J, Varello M, et al. Flow cytometric DNA analysis of neuroblastoma: Correlation with histology and clinical outcome. Cancer 1986;58:2453.

54. Garmel SH, Crombleholme TM, Semple JP, et al. Prenatal diagnosis and management of fetal tumors. Semin Perinatol 1994;18:350.

55. Garth D, Perkins DG, Kopp CM, et al. Placental infiltration in congenital neuroblastoma: A case study with ultrastructure. Histopathology 1980;4:383.

56. Giulian BB, Chang CNC, Yoss BS. Prenatal ultrasonographic diagnosis of fetal adrenal neuroblastoma. J Clin Ultrasound 1986;14:225.

57. Goldstein I, Gomez K, Copel JA. The real-time and color Doppler appearance of adrenal neuroblastoma in a third-trimester fetus. Obstet Gynecol 1994;83:584.

58. Grosfeld JL, Rescoria FJ, West KW, et al. Neuroblastoma in the first year of life: Clinical and biologic factors influencing outcome. Semin Pediatr Surg 1993;2:37.

59. Grotting JC, Kassel S, Dehner LP. Nesidioblastosis and congenital neuroblastoma. Arch Pathol Lab Med 1979;103:642.

60. Guin HG, Gilbert FE, Jones B. Incidental neuroblastoma in infants. Am J Clin Pathol 1969;51:126.

61. Haas D, Ablin AR, Miller C, et al. Complete pathologic maturation and regression of stage IVS neuroblastoma without treatment. Cancer 1988;62:818.

62. Hachitanda Y, Tsuneyoshi M. Neuroblastoma with a distinct organoid pattern: A clinicopathologic, immunohistochemical and ultrastructural study. Hum Pathol 1994;25:67.

63. Hagstrom HT. Fetal dystocia due to metastatic neuroblastoma of the liver. Am J Obstet Gynecol 1930;19:673.

64. Hann H-WL, Evans AE, Cohen IJ, et al. Biologic differences between neuroblastoma Stage IVS and Stage IV, measurement of serum ferritin and E-rosette inhibition in 30 children. N Engl J Med 1981;305:425.

65. Hardy PC, Nesbit ME. Familial neuroblastoma: Report of a kindred with a high incidence of infantile tumors. J Pediatr 1972;80:74.

66. Haupt R, Dolci A, Nantron M, et al. Neuroblastoma IV-S in a patient with bilateral microphthalmia. Acta Paediatr 1993;82:1085.

67. Hawthorne HC, Nelson JS, Witzleben CL, et al. Blanching subcutaneous nodules in neonatal neuroblastoma. J Pediatr 1970;77:297.

68. Hayashi Y, Hanada R, Yamamoto K. Biology of neuroblastomas in Japan found by screening. Am J Pediatr Hematol Oncol 1992;14:342.

69. Hiyama E, Hiyama K, Yokoyama T, et al. Immunohistochemical analysis of N-myc protein expression in neuroblastoma: Correlation with prognosis of patients. J Pediatr Surg 1991;26:838.

70. Hiyama E, Yokoyama T, Ichikawa T, et al. CHARGE association with neuroblastoma. Pediatr Surg Int 1990;5:463.

71. Ho PTC, Estroff JA, Kozakewich H, et al. Prenatal detection of neuroblastoma: A ten year experience from the Dana-Farber Cancer Institute and Children's Hospital. Pediatrics 1993;92:358.

72. Holgerson LO, Santulli TV, Schullinger JN, et al. Neuroblastoma with intraspinal (dumbbell) extension. J Pediatr Surg 1983;18:406.

73. Hosoda Y, Miyano T, Kimura K, et al. Characteristics and management of patients with fetal neuroblastoma. J Pediatr Surg 1992;27:623.

74. Hrabovsky E, Jones B. Congenital intraspinal neuroblastoma. Am J Dis Child 1979;133:73.

75. Iida Y, Nose O, Okada A, et al. Watery diarrhoea with a vasoactive intestinal peptide producing ganglioneuroblastoma. Arch Dis Child 1980;55:929.

76. Isaacs H Jr. Congenital malignant tumors. *In* Reed GB, Claireaux AE, Bain AD (eds): Diseases of the Fetus and Newborn: Pathology, Radiology and Genetics, p 131. London: Chapman Hall, 1989.

77. Isaacs H Jr. Congenital and neonatal malignant tumors: A 28-year experience at Children's Hospital of Los Angeles. Am J Pediatr Hematol/Oncol 1987;9:121.

78. Isaacs H Jr. Neoplasms in infants: A report of 265 cases. Pathol Annu 1983;18(2):165.

79. Isaacs H Jr. Perinatal (congenital and neonatal) neoplasms: A report of 110 cases. Pediatr Pathol 1985;3:165.

80. Isaacs H Jr. Tumors. *In* Gilbert-Barness E (ed): Potter's Pathology of the Fetus and Infant, Vol 2, p 1242. St. Louis: Mosby–Year Book, 1996.

81. Isaacs H Jr. Tumors of the Newborn and Infant: St. Louis: Mosby–Year Book, 1991.

82. Jaffa AJ, Many A, Hartoov J, et al. Prenatal sonographic diagnosis of metastatic neuroblastoma: Report of a case and review of the literature. Prenatal Diagn 1993;13:73.

83. Jaffe N, Cassady JR, Filler RM, et al. Heterochromia and Horner syndrome associated with cervical and mediastinal neuroblastoma. J Pediatr 1975;87:75.

84. Janetschek G, Weitzel D, Stein W, et al. Prenatal diagnosis of neuroblastoma by sonography. Urology 1984;24:397.

85. Jansen-Goemans A, Engelhardt J. Intractable diarrhea in a boy with vasoactive intestinal peptise-producing ganglioneuroblastoma. Pediatrics 1977;59:710.

86. Jennings RW, LaQuaglia MP, Leong K, et al. Fetal

neuroblastoma: Prenatal diagnosis and natural history, J Pediatr Surg 28:1168,1993.

87. Joshi VV, Cantor AB, Altshuler G, et al. Age-linked prognostic categorization based on a new histologic grading system of neuroblastomas. Cancer 1992;69:2197.

87a. Joshi VV, Rao PV, Cantor AB, et al. Modified histologic grading of neuroblastomas by replacement of mitotic rate with mitosis karyorrhexis index: A clinicopathologic study of 223 cases from the Pediatric Oncology Group. Cancer 1996;77:1582.

88. Kapur RJ, Shepard TH. Intestinal ganglioneuroblastoma in a 22-week fetus. Pediatr Pathol 1992;12:583.

89. Koop CE. Abdominal mass in the newborn infant. N Engl J Med 1973;289:569.

90. Kushner BH, Gilbert F, Helson L. Familial neuroblastoma. Cancer 1986;57:1887.

91. Larimer RC. Neuroblastoma (sympathicogonioma) of the adrenal in a newborn infant. J Pediatr 1949;34:365.

92. Laug WE, Siegel SE, Shaw KNF, et al. Initial urinary catecholamine concentrations and prognosis in neuroblastoma. Pediatrics 1978;62:77.

93. Mancini AF, Rosito P, Faldella G, et al. Neuroblastoma in a pair of identical twins. Med Pediatr Oncol 1982;10:45.

94. Mancini AF, Rosito P, Vitelli A, et al. IV-S neuroblastoma: A cooperative study of 30 children. Med Pediatr Oncol 1984;12:155.

95. Matthay KK. Congenital malignant disorders. *In* Taeusch HW, Ballard RA, Avery ME (eds): Schaffer and Avery's Diseases of the Newborn, 6th ed, p 1025. Philadelphia: WB Saunders, 1991.

96. Michna BA, McWilliams NB, Krummel TM, et al. Multifocal ganglioneuroblastoma coexistent with total colonic aganglionosis. J Pediatr Surg 1988;23:57.

97. Miller RW, Dalager NA. U.S. childhood cancer deaths by cell type, 1960–1968. J Pediatr 1974;85:664.

98. Misugi K, Misugi N, Newton WAS. Fine structural study of neuroblastoma, ganglioneuroblastoma, and pheochromocytoma. Arch Pathol 1968;86:160.

99. Moore KL: The Developing Human—Clinically Oriented Embryology, 5th ed. Philadelphia: WB Saunders, 1993.

100. Moss TJ, Kaplan L. Association of hydrops fetalis with congenital neuroblastoma. Am J Obstet Gynecol 1987;132:905.

101. Munro FD, Carachi R, Fyfe AHB. Congenital neuroblastoma presenting with paraplegia. Arch Dis Child 1991;66:1246.

102. Murthy TVM, Irving IM, Lister J. Massive adrenal hemorrhage in neonatal neuroblastoma. J Pediatr Surg 13:31, 1978.

103. Nakagawara A, Arima-Nakagawara M, Scavarda NJ, et al. Association between high levels of expression of the TRK gene and favorable outcome in human neuroblastoma. N Engl J Med 1993;328:847.

104. Nakissa N, Constine LS, Rubin P, et al. Birth defects in three common pediatric malignancies: Wilms' tumor, neuroblastoma and Ewing's sarcoma. Oncology 1985;42:358.

105. Newton ER, Lewis F, Dalton ME, et al. Fetal neuroblastoma and catecholamine induced maternal hypertension. Obstet Gynecol 1985;65(Suppl): 49S.

106. Ogita S, Tokiwa K, Takahashi T, et al. Congenital cervical neuroblastoma associated with Horner syndrome. J Pediatr Surg 1988;23:991.

107. Parkes SE, Muir KR, Southern L, et al. Neonatal tumours: A thirty-year population based study. Med Pediatr Oncol 1994;22:309.

108. Patrone PM, Chatten J, Weinberg P. Neuroblastoma and DiGeorge anomaly. Pediatr Pathol 1990;10:425.

109. Pegelow C, Ebbin AJ, Powars D, et al. Familial neuroblastoma. J Pediatr 1975;87:763.

110. Pendergrass TW, Hanson JW. Fetal hydantoin syndrome and neuroblastoma. Lancet 1976;2:150.

111. Perkins DG, Kopp CM, Haust MD. Placental infiltration in congenital neuroblastoma: A case study with ultrastructure. Histopathology 1980;4:383.

112. Potter EL, Craig JM: Pathology of the Fetus and Infant, 3rd ed, p 177. Chicago: Year Book Medical Publishers, 1975.

113. Potter EL, Parish JM. Neuroblastoma, ganglioneuroma and fibroneuroma in a stillborn fetus. Am J Pathol 1942;18:181.

114. Punt J, Pritchard J, Pincott JR, Till K. Neuroblastoma: A review of 21 cases presenting with spinal cord compression. Cancer 1980;45:3095.

115. Quinn JJ, Altman AJ, Frantz CN. Serum lactic dehydrogenase, an indicator of tumor activity in neuroblastoma. J Pediatr 1980;97:89.

116. Reynolds CP, German DC, Weinberg AG, et al. Catecholamine fluorescence and tissue culture morphology. Techniques in the diagnosis of neuroblastoma. Am J Clin Pathol 1981;75:275.

117. Robinson HB, Bolande RP. Fetal hepatoblastoma with placental metastases. Pediatr Pathol 1985;4:163.

118. Romansky SG. Neural crest aggregates in the human fetal adrenal gland (Abstract). Lab Invest 1979;40:309.

119. Romansky SG, Crocker DW, Shaw KNF. Ultrastructural studies on neuroblastoma: Evaluation of cytodifferentiation and correlation of biochemical survival data. Cancer 1978;42:2392.

120. Romero R, Oilu G, Jeanty P, Ghidini A, Hobbins JC. Prenatal Diagnosis of Congenital Anomalies. Norwalk, CT: Appleton & Lange, 1988.

121. Rubie H, Baunin C, Guitard J, et al. Tumeurs neonatales malignes. Rev Prat (Paris) 1993;43(17):2208.

122. Sawada T. Outcome of 25 neuroblastomas revealed by screening in Japan. Lancet 1986;1:377.

123. Sawada T. Present status of mass screening for neuroblastoma. Pediatr Rev 1989;22:336.

124. Schneider KM, Becker JM, Krasna IH. Neonatal neuroblastoma. Pediatrics 1965;36:359.

125. Seeger RC, Brodeur GM, Sather H, et al. Association of multiple copies of the N-myc oncogene with rapid progression of neuroblastomas. N Engl J Med 1985;313:1111.

126. Seeler RA, Israel JN, Royal JE, et al. Ganglioneuroblastoma and fetal hydantoin-alcohol syndromes. Pediatrics 1979;63:524.

127. Shanklin DR, Sotelo-Avila C. In situ tumors in fetuses, newborns and young infants. Biol Neonatol 1969;14:286.

128. Sherman S, Roizen N. Fetal hydantoin syndrome and neuroblastoma. Lancet 1976;2:517.

129. Shimada H, Chatten J, Newton WA Jr, et al. Histopathologic prognostic factors in neuroblastic tumors: Definition of subtypes of ganglioneuroblastoma and an age-linked classification of neuroblastomas. J Natl Cancer Inst 1984;73:405.

130. Shown TE, Durfee, MF. Blueberry muffin baby: Neonatal neuroblastoma with subcutaneous metastases. J Urol 1970;104:193.

131. Sitarz AL, Santulli TV, Wigger HJ, et al. Complete

maturation of neuroblastoma with bone metastases in documented stages. J Pediatr Surg 1975;10:533.

132. Smith CR, Chan HSL, DeSa DJ. Placental involvement in congenital neuroblastoma. J Clin Pathol 1981;34: 785.

133. Souid A, Seidberg N, Sadowitz PD, et al. Congenital neuroblastoma (Radiological Cases of the Month). Arch Pediatr Adolesc Med 1994;148:525.

134. Stephenson SR, Cook BA, Mease AD, Ruymann FB. The prognostic significance of age and pattern of metastases in stage IV-S neuroblastoma. Cancer 1986;58: 372.

135. Strauss L, Driscoll SG. Congenital neuroblastoma involving the placenta: Reports of two cases. Pediatrics 1964;34:23.

136. Taxy JB. Electron microscopy in the diagnosis of neuroblastoma. Arch Pathol Lab Med 1980;104:355.

137. Tovar JA, Arena J, Trecet J, et al. Prenatal diagnosis of adrenal neuroblastoma. Pediatr Surg Int 1988;3:195.

138. Triche TJ. Pathology of pediatric malignancies. *In* Pizzo PA, Poplack DG (eds): Principles and Practice of Pediatric Oncology, 2nd ed, p 115. Philadelphia: JB Lippincott, 1993.

139. Tsokos M. Peripheral primitive neuroectodermal tumors: Diagnosis, classification and prognosis. Perspect Pediatr Pathol 1992;16:27.

140. Turkel SB, Itabashi HH. The natural history of neuroblastic cells in the fetal adrenal gland. Am J Pathol 1974;76:225.

141. van der Slikke, Balk AG. Hydramnios with hydrops fetalis and disseminated fetal neuroblastoma. Obstet Gynecol 1980;55:250.

142. Voute PA, Wadman SK, Van Putten WJ. Congenital neuroblastoma: Symptoms in the mother during pregnancy. Clin Pediatr 1970;9:206.

143. Wagget J, Aherne G, Aherne W. Familial neuroblastoma: Report of two sib pairs. Arch Dis Child 1973;48:63.

144. Weber T, Sotelo-Avila C, Gale G. Cystic neuroblastoma in a newborn. J Pediatr Surg 1993;28:1603.

145. Wells HG. Occurrence and significance of congenital malignant neoplasms. Arch Pathol 1940;30:535.

146. Werb P, Scurry J, Ostor A, et al. Survey of congenital tumors in perinatal necropsies. Pathology 1992;24: 247.

147. Wieberdink J. Metastases in neonatal neuroblastoma. *In* Pochedly C (ed): Neuroblastoma: Clinical and Biological Manifestations, p 13. New York: Elsevier Biomedical, 1982.

148. Willis RA. The Borderland of Embryology and Pathology, 2nd ed. London: Butterworths, 1962.

149. Wilson PCG, Coppes MJ, Solh H, et al. Neuroblastoma stage IV-S: A heterogeneous disease. Med Pediatr Oncol 1991;19:467.

150. Yamashina M, Kayan H, Katayama I, et al. Congenital neuroblastoma presenting as a paratesticular tumor. J Urol 1988;139:796.

LEUKEMIA

7

The leukemias are a heterogeneous group of hematologic neoplasms characterized by the infiltration of abnormal hematopoietic cells in the bone marrow, peripheral blood, and various organs and tissues. Following this clonal overgrowth of leukemic cells, the patient eventually develops the hematologic sequelae of bone marrow failure manifested by anemia, neutropenia, and thrombocytopenia.

Leukemia occurs infrequently in the perinatal period as compared to later in childhood.* Although it is not as common as neuroblastoma, leukemia is the malignant disease responsible for the greatest mortality secondary to neoplastic disease in the newborn.[9,45,60] The clinical findings and biological features of congenital leukemia are distinctively different from those of older children and adults. The disease in the newborn has an unexplained natural tendency to undergo spontaneous remissions lasting months or sometimes years.[29,72,96,101,121] The prognosis for newborns with either acute nonlymphoblastic or lymphoblastic leukemia, regardless of the course of therapy, is generally poor.[19,24,26,28,31,32,60,65,66,94,97,101,103]

With few exceptions, congenital leukemias are classified as acute because they have a predominance of immature myeloid, monocytic, or lymphoid precursors. Most are classified as acute nonlymphoblastic leukemia (ANLL), accounting for as many as 90% of the cases in some series as compared to acute lymphoblastic leukemia (ALL).[21,54,69,91,101,111,129] Congenital chronic myelogenous leukemia is reported infrequently.[30,57,86]

INCIDENCE

Data from the Third National Cancer Survey reveal that the incidence of malignant tumors in newborns is 36.5 per million live births per year, and that neuroblastoma ranks first, with an incidence of 19.7 per million live births (54% of cases), and leukemia ranks second, with an incidence of 4.7 per million live births (13%).[9] However, the mortality from leukemia (2.6 per million live births) exceeds that of neuroblastoma by 1.5 times (1.8 per million).

The frequency of leukemia in fetuses and newborns is much less than in older children. During the years 1983 through 1987, there were 224 children recorded in the Children's Hospital of Los Angeles Surgical Pathology files as having the diagnosis of leukemia, only three of whom (1.3%) were newborns.[63] The frequency of leukemia was much lower in the St. Jude Children's Hospital, Memphis neonatal cancer study, in which only 6 of 2569 (0.2%) children affected were neonates.[32] In this study, leukemia ranked second in frequency (6 of 34 [18%]) following neuroblastoma, which accounted for 56% of the cases of cancer. Of the six patients with leukemia, four were diagnosed as having ALL and two as having ANLL. Skin nodules were the initial manifestation in four, all had petechiae, and two had central nervous system involvement; only one patient survived.[32] The Hospital for Sick Children, Toronto group reported a higher incidence figure for leuke-

The author wishes to express his appreciation and gratitude to Dr. William Roberts, Hematology Oncology Division, Children's Hospital, San Diego, for kindly reviewing this chapter and for his helpful suggestions.

*References: 1, 2, 16, 20–22, 24, 26, 28, 31, 34, 37, 41, 45, 46, 48, 55, 58, 61, 63, 69, 72, 73, 75, 78, 81, 85, 91, 97–99, 104–106, 109, 112, 115, 118, 120, 125, 126, 129.

mia: 8 of 1609 or 0.5%.[22] Leukemia ranked fifth following neuroblastoma, retinoblastoma, and renal and liver tumors, in that order.

Pierce reviewed 45 cases of congenital leukemia, including one of her own reported prior to 1959, of which 37 were myelocytic, 5 were lymphocytic, and 3 were unclassified as to type.[97] The Children's Hospital, Los Angeles study of 224 infants and children with leukemia mentioned earlier revealed an ANLL:ALL ratio, for both infants and neonates, of 2:1 and a reciprocal ratio for the older child and adolescent whereby ALL accounted for more than 75% of the leukemias.[63] A St. Jude Children's Hospital study later than the one previously described consisted of 27 infants with acute leukemia; it, too, showed a ratio of 2:1 for both the infants and the nine patients younger than 3 months of age.[101] The six ANLL cases were subclassified as follows: two myeloblastic, two myelomonocytic, and two monocytic. The three ALL cases lacked the common ALL antigen (CALLA) and B and T cell markers and, therefore, were assigned to the category of "null" ALL. The Children's Hospital of Michigan reported an incidence of congenital leukemia of 4 in 500 (0.8%).[123] Patients with the transient leukemia of Down syndrome were excluded from the review. The ANLL:ALL ratio in this study was 1:1, and one of four neonates experienced spontaneous remission without treatment. Allan et al. analyzed 12 cases of erythroleukemia in infants, including one of their own.[2] Six patients were younger than 3.5 months of age at diagnosis. Liver disease was a prominent feature in all but one.

In the Children's Hospital, Birmingham, U.K. study, which consisted of 170 neonatal tumors, leukemia was ranked third in frequency (21 cases [12%]) following teratoma (29%) and neuroblastoma (18%).[94] Of the 21 leukemias, 3 were classified as ALL, 8 as acute myeloid leukemia (AML), 2 as megakaryoblastic, and 8 as unspecified as to type. The only survivor was a child with Down syndrome who had acute megakaryoblastic leukemia (AMKL) and a spontaneous remission. The Danish study reported similar findings as those just described. Again, neuroblastoma was the leading neonatal cancer, accounting for 20 of 76 cases (26%), followed by leukemia (12 of 76 [16%]) and soft tissue sarcomas (11 of 76 [14%]).[19] No patient with leukemia survived. Three of 22 (14%) neonatal malignant tumors diagnosed as ALL, AML, and acute monocytic leukemia, respectively, in the Children's Hospital of Philadel-

phia study were leukemias; all were fatal.[46] The Hospital for Sick Children, Toronto series consisted of eight neonates with leukemia (7.8% of the total number malignant cases); four were classified as undifferentiated leukemia, three as ANLL, and one as ALL; none survived.[24]

EMBRYOLOGY

Development of blood and blood vessels begins within the blood islands of the yolk sac and, to a lesser extent, in the chorion, body stalk, and allantois, at approximately 19 days.[99,117a] Cells within the center of the blood islands become the blood-forming cells, or the hematopoietic stem cells (hemocytoblasts), whereas those at the periphery form the endothelial cells, which line vessels. Hematopoietic stem cells are carried in the blood from the yolk sac to populate the liver, bone marrow, spleen, lymph nodes, and other sites (e.g., thymus and kidney). Blood formation begins in the liver during the fifth week, and this organ becomes the main source of erythrocytes until near the end of fetal life (see Fig. 12–1). By the end of the third month, hematopoiesis is noted in the bone marrow, which becomes the major site of erythropoiesis during the latter part of the third trimester.[99,117a]

Blood cells formed within the yolk sac and in the liver during the second trimester are predominantly erythropoietic elements, and many are large and nucleated, having a megaloblastic appearance. Leukocytes (granulocytes, histiocytes, lymphocytes, and megakaryocytes) appear in the liver and yolk sac at about 5 weeks' gestation and a few weeks later in the spleen, lymph nodes, and bone marrow.[117a]

CYTOGENETICS

Chromosomal abnormalities, syndromes, and malformations are often found in association with congenital leukemia.[5,6,26,47,81,89,116,119,126,131] The most common chromosomal anomaly occurs in patients with Down syndrome. Occasionally, other chromosomal defects are described, such as trisomy 8, 19, and 13; Turner's syndrome; Klinefelter syndrome (47 XXY); X; 1;6, 9;11, 8;16 translocations, monosomy 7, mosaic trisomy 9, and chromosome 11 anomalies.[25,26,28,47,89,103,126] Examples of presumably nonchromosomally derived congenital anomalies or syndromes associated with leukemia are

Bloom's syndrome, Diamond-Blackfan anemia, Klippel-Feil syndrome, Fanconi's anemia, Ellis-van Creveld syndrome, neurofibromatosis I, Schwachman syndrome, TAR syndrome (thrombocytopenia and absent radii), Marfan's syndrome, and certain cardiac malformations.[8,9,16,35,54,116,125] The interesting association of neurofibromatosis type I, monosomy 7, and juvenile chronic myelomonocytic leukemia has been noted in a 9-month-old boy.[67]

The St. Jude Children's Hospital group analyzed 27 infants with acute leukemia for chromosomal defects.[101] Twenty-five had an abnormal karyotype, and chromosomal translocations were found in 67% of those with ANLL and 78% of those with ALL. These authors found that leukemic cell abnormalities involving 11q23 were present in most patients, and that t(9;11)(p21;q23) translocations were detected in both ANLL and ALL. Pui et al. concluded from their study that the large leukemic cell burden, the unfavorable immunophenotype, and chromosomal translocations are factors responsible for the poor outcome for infants with leukemia.[101] Their results were in accord with an earlier study by Abe et al., in which 10 of 13 (77%) leukemic patients younger than 4 months of age were found to have chromosomal anomalies involving 11q22-23.[1]

Other studies implicating chromosome 11 include the one conducted by Kaneko et al., who reviewed the clinical, cytogenetic, and immunophenotypic findings in 34 infants with leukemia, demonstrating that most had an 11q23 translocation (65). Moreover, four of five infants 3 months of age or less had this chromosomal anomaly. Most of the infants with the 11q23 translocation had a high leukocyte count at the time of diagnosis. Four were diagnosed as having ALL and one was diagnosed as having monocytic leukemia; all had an HLA/DR (Ia)-positive and CALLA-negative phenotype. Coexpression of myeloid and lymphoid antigens was noted in one of the five patients in the newborn-to-3-months-of-age group, and according to the authors, this finding is characteristic of the 11q23 translocation. The frequency of the 11q23 translocation in Japanese infants with leukemia is comparable to that reported in the American St. Jude Children's Hospital study.[65,101] An additional example of coexpression of myeloid and pre-B antigens in the cells of a 16-day-old male neonate with undifferentiated leukemia and a t(11;17) anomaly was reported by Umiel et al.[120]

Ludwig et al. analyzed the immunophenotypic and genotypic findings in 35 German infants with ALL, 12 of whom were younger than 3 months of age.[79] Their findings were similar to those of previous studies mentioned earlier[65,101] in that they found a high frequency of coexpression of lymphoid and myeloid associated antigens in their patient's leukemic cells. More than 50% (21 of 35) of the patients in whom the karyotypes were determined had an 11q23 translocation, and five had a mixed pre-B/myeloid phenotype. On the basis of their findings, these authors proposed that, because of the mixed myeloid/pre-B lineage and the 11q23 translocation, the leukemic cell of congenital ALL may represent a multipotential progenitor cell.[79] Concurrently, the Hospital for Sick Children, London group published their data on infant "null" ALL and arrived at similar conclusions.[66] They defined the null ALL phenotype as blast cells unreactive for T, B, and CALLA antigens and reactive for HLA/DR and terminal deoxynucleotidyl transferase (TdT).[31] Eight infants comprised the study, three of whom were 2 months of age or less; none survived. The leukemic cells of all infants displayed a chromosomal rearrangement of band 11q23. Hyperleukocytosis, organomegaly, and central nervous system involvement were the initial clinical findings. Immunophenotyping showed early B-cell markers, negative results for CALLA, positive results for HLA/DR and CD19 (B4), and rearrangement of the immunoglobulin heavy chain genes without evidence of κ light chain rearrangement. Two of the three newborns coexpressed myeloid markers CD33 (MY9) and CD15(TG1). Ultrastructural studies revealed a mixed population of leukemic cells consisting of lymphoblasts and monoblasts. Katz et al. concluded from their data that infant leukemias with the 11q23 translocation are heterogeneous with respect to the major cell type involved—that is, lymphoid, myeloid, or monocytic—suggesting a derivation from a common precursor "stem" cell having characteristics of both B lymphoid and myeloid progenitor cells.[66]

Although AMKL is considered to be one of the main forms of leukemia in newborns with Down syndrome, another important chromosomal anomaly has recently been detected in infants with AMKL. A Pediatric Oncology Group Study (1991) reported by Carroll et al. analyzed 252 cases of acute myeloid leukemia in children without Down syndrome and demonstrated a specific chromosomal translocation t(1;22) (p13;q13), which was found only in infants with AMKL.[26] Of the 252 patients in the study, 6 (2.4%) were younger than 10 months of age, including 3 neonates with AMKL and t(1;22). This translocation was not found in any other morphologic subtype of AML or ALL. The authors suggested that t(1;22) translocation is useful as a marker for AMKL.[26] Three of six newborns had hepatosplenomegaly and one had ascites. Lymphadenopathy, central nervous system or testicular involvement were not observed. Laboratory studies in these three neonates revealed leukocyte counts ranging from 21 to 52×10^9/L, hemoglobin levels ranging from 7 to 16 g/dL, and platelet counts ranging from 41 to 140×10^9/L. The bone marrow showed 7% to 30% blasts accompanied by myelofibrosis. All three newborns died.

Subsequently, Chan et al. reported the t(1;22) abnormality in six additional infants with AMKL.[28] Four of these infants were younger than 3 months of age, and two were in remission at the time of writing. Hepatosplenomegaly, anemia, and thrombocytopenia were the initial findings. Visceral fibrosis was a prominent feature, but in contrast to neonates with both Down syndrome and AMKL, extensive bone marrow fibrosis was present. The unusual histopathologic features in the patients with this t(1;22) chromosomal anomaly were emphasized. It was pointed out that the striking hepatosplenomegaly and tumor infiltrates with cohesive cells situated in the lymph node sinuses and liver sinusoids can easily be mistaken for other small cell malignant neoplasms, particularly metastatic neuroblastoma.[28]

Frequently, trisomy 21 is associated with erythroleukemia during the first year of life.[2] Trisomies 8 and 19 are also noted by cytogenetic analysis in this form of leukemia. Translocations t(9;11) (p21;q23) and t(8;16) (p11;p13) occur with acute monocytic leukemia.[14,17,56,87] Diffuse leukemic cell infiltration of the skin and central nervous system are characteristic of acute monocytic leukemia in newborns.[17]

CLINICAL FEATURES

There are rare case reports of congenital leukemia occurring in a newborn of a mother who had leukemia during pregnancy. The mother, described by Bernard et al.,[15] had leukemia at the time of birth, and the baby developed leukemia at 5 months of age. However, no specific fetal or maternal risk factor has been impli-

cated in this disease.[33,51,81,97] Campbell and Macafee described a family with congenital leukemia in siblings, which suggests that heredity may play a role in this malignant disease.[23] The male and female siblings died at 10 and 8 weeks of age, respectively, of acute myeloid leukemia (probably the myelomonocytic type according to the author's description) and a third male sibling died at 4 weeks of age after a similar clinical course. No chromosomal anomaly was identified in the siblings. Occurrence of leukemia in identical twins suggests also a genetic predisposition to the disease.[80] Data from a Children's Cancer Group study suggest that a maternal reproductive history of previous fetal loss is associated with an increased risk of leukemia in subsequent offspring at a young age.[132]

The prenatal diagnosis of leukemia is established by fetoscopy and fetal blood sampling.[38,42,92,133] The diagnosis should come to mind when hepatosplenomegaly, hydrops, and hydramnios are detected by ultrasonography.[92] Zerres et al. described two hydropic fetuses with ANLL and Down syndrome diagnosed by umbilical blood sampling at 33 and 36 weeks of gestation, respectively.[133] In both fetuses, umbilical blood smears showed numerous blasts with enlarged nuclei and prominent nucleoli and a thin rim of basophilic cytoplasm; the diagnosis of leukemia was confirmed after birth following examination of the bone marrow and peripheral blood smears. During the same period, 25 cases of Down syndrome, including the two depicted earlier, were diagnosed following sonography and chromosomal analysis. In other words, 8% of the fetuses in the series with Down syndrome developed leukemia or leukemic-like manifestations in the perinatal period. Other cases of Down syndrome with leukemia diagnosed in utero have been reported. Fourcar et al. documented the occurrence of transient AMKL in two fetuses with Down syndrome following sonography and percutaneous umbilical blood sampling.[42] Nicolaides et al. reported another example of antenatal leukemia detected by this method in a fetus with unexplained hydrops and a normal karyotype.[92] The fetal blood smear showed a high proportion of erythroid precursors and a dyserythropoietic process in the bone marrow that was consistent with the diagnosis of erythroleukemia.

Several examples of congenital leukemia as a cause of stillbirth have been described.[12,51,59,63,73,97] The affected stillborn infants are hydropic and are often macerated, and their placentas are significantly enlarged and edematous, not unlike the placentas of erythroblastosis fetalis. Gray et al. suggest that the general lack of recognition of congenital leukemia is the result of inadequate microscopic examination (or no examination at all) of the stillborn infant and placenta.[51]

The clinical signs and symptoms of neonatal leukemia are variable. Generally, the disease is characterized by a rapid downhill course, but it may be unpredictable. Some neonates show signs of leukemia at birth and die shortly thereafter, whereas others appear normal following delivery but develop clinical and hematologic problems later. In another group, leukemia is not discovered until the third to sixth week of life, despite a history suggestive of hematologic abnormalities dating back a few weeks earlier.[20,60]

Multiple petechiae and ecchymoses, hepatosplenomegaly, and leukemic cutaneous infiltrates (leukemia cutis) are characteristic clinical manifestations of perinatal leukemia.[24,97] Cutaneous involvement is observed in stillborns with the disease and is the initial presenting sign in less than 50% of newborns, particularly those with acute monocytic leukemia. Leukemia cutis may precede other signs of leukemia by as much as 4 months.[106] However, lymphadenopathy is seldom noted. When respiratory distress is present at birth, it is attributable to either pulmonary hemorrhage secondary to thrombocytopenia and/or extensive leukemic infiltration complicated by atelectasis.[60,81] A bulging fontanelle may be a sign of meningeal involvement or an intracranial bleed secondary to thrombocytopenia.[21] In patients whose leukemia is discovered toward the end of the neonatal period or later in infancy, the signs and symptoms tend to be more vague; for example, the infant may have a low-grade fever, pallor, lethargy, hepatosplenomegaly, a bleeding tendency, diarrhea, or generally "failure to thrive."[81,91] As in older children, sepsis and hemorrhage are the most common causes of death in the perinatal period.[41,53,58,60]

Newborns with either ANLL or ALL have a constellation of clinical findings usually associated with an unfavorable outcome. Hyperleukocytosis, hepatosplenomegaly, central nervous system involvement, hypogammaglobulinemia, and thrombocytopenia are seen more often in this age group than in older children with ALL.[103,104] As compared to the rest of the pediatric age group, the young child with ALL has a very high bone marrow and central nervous system relapse rate (see Fig. 7–4).[54] Moreover,

neonates with ANLL also have, at the time of diagnosis, higher leukocyte counts and an increased incidence of central nervous system leukemia and skin infiltration compared to older children.[71]

DIFFERENTIAL DIAGNOSIS

The predominance of ANLL during the perinatal period contributes to the difficulty in distinguishing the disease from the more common conditions causing leukemoid reactions.[5] Infections and hemolytic disease of the newborn stimulate both erythroid and myeloid hematopoiesis in the sites where they normally occur in fetal life; therefore, exclusion of leukemoid (leukoerythroblastic) reactions and blood group incompatibility is important, but sometimes difficult.[88]

Leukocytosis, thrombocytopenia, and hepatosplenomegaly often accompany congenital infections, such as rubella, cytomegalovirus, toxoplasmosis, syphilis, and bacterial sepsis. Severe hemolytic disease of the newborn (immune erythroblastosis fetalis) may masquerade as leukemia. If this disorder is severe enough, affected neonates will have hepatosplenomegaly, skin nodules, numerous erythroblasts in the peripheral blood smear, and, sometimes, thrombocytopenia (Fig. 7–1).[5] Hepatosplenomegaly and cutaneous nodules are seen in newborns with disseminated neuroblastoma, stage IV-S. Peripheral blood counts are usually normal, but if the bone marrow is involved, bone marrow aspirates will reveal characteristic, small syncytia of neuroblastoma cells, which are distinguishable from the bone marrow replaced by leukemic cells (Fig. 7–2).[5] Moreover, urinary catecholamine levels are usually elevated. Dermal erythropoiesis with a "blueberry muffin" appearance is found more often with congenital infections (i.e., rubella and cytomegalovirus) and hemolytic disease of the newborn than with either leukemia or neuroblastoma (see Table 5–2).[50]

Congenital human immunodeficiency virus (HIV) infection may be mistaken for leukemia.[81] Clonal B-cell proliferations in these patients may be responsible for lymphadenopathy and worrisome marrow findings. Voelkerding et al. described a newborn with HIV infection who presented with petechiae and thrombocytopenia.[122] The bone marrow contained collections of large lymphocytes with scant cytoplasms and dense, homogeneously staining

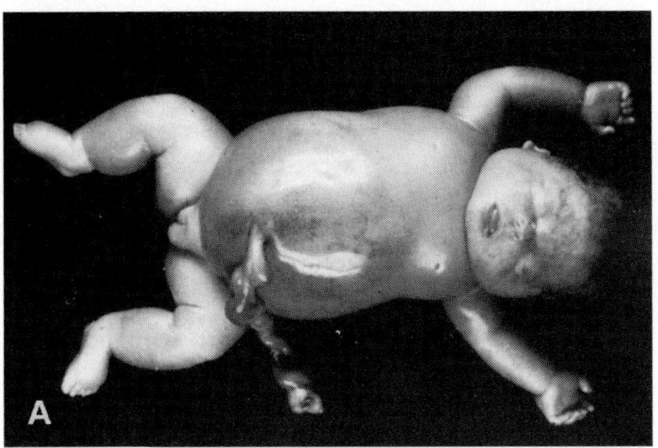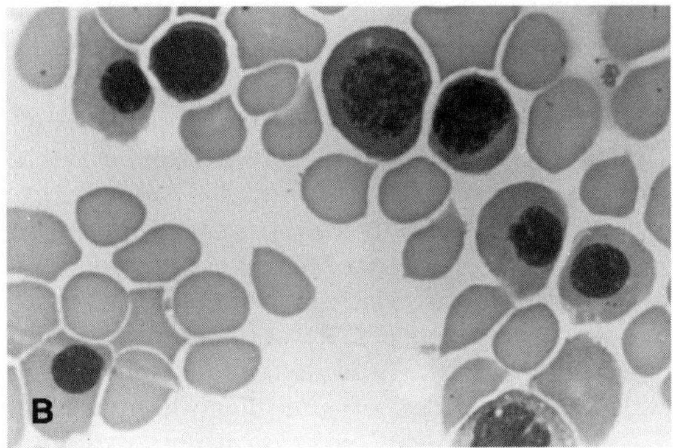

Figure 7–1. Erythroblastosis due to Rh incompatibility. *A,* A stillborn with hydrops fetalis. *B,* A peripheral smear from a newborn with erythroblastosis fetalis shows immature erythrocytes consisting of erythroblasts and normoblasts. Anisocytosis, poikilocytosis, and polychromasia are evident. (Wright-Giemsa, ×1200). Hematologic values were as follows: hemoglobin, 10 g/dL; leukocyte count, 39,000/mm³; platelet count, 158,000. (Peripheral smear courtesy of Glenn Billman, MD.)

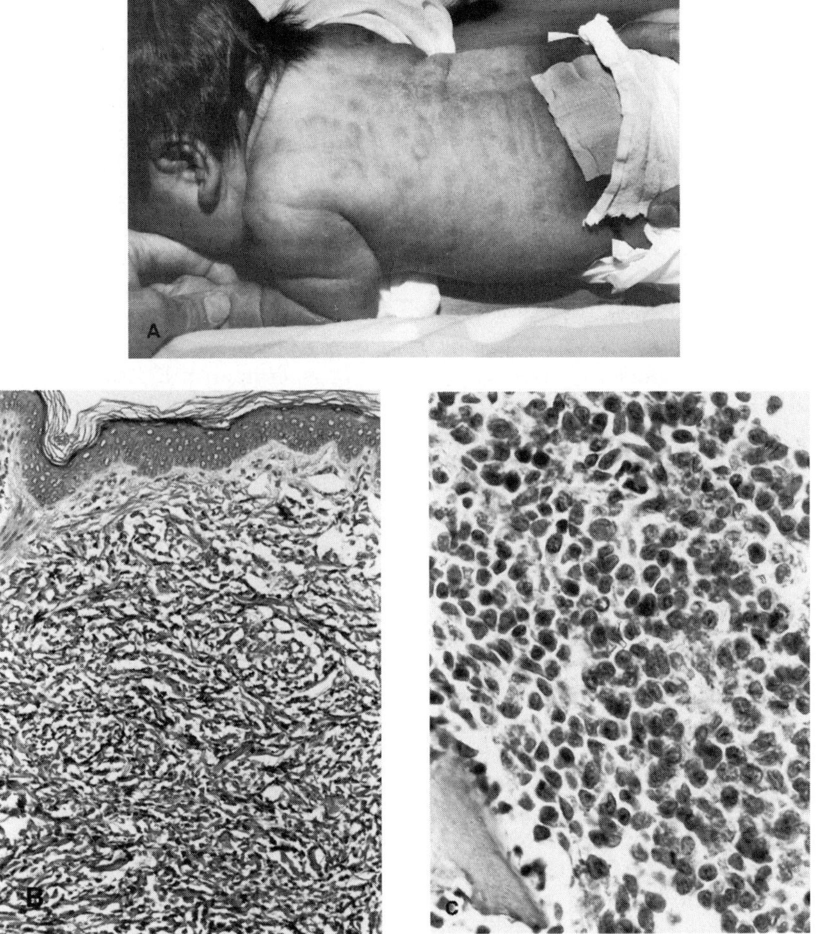

Figure 7–2. Transient congenital leukemia. *A,* A newborn male infant with multiple, raised, cutaneous nodules distributed over most of his body. The initial leukocyte count was 117,000, the hemoglobin value was 12.7 g/dL, and the karyotype was normal. *B,* A skin biopsy study of one of the nodules reveals diffuse dermal and subcutaneous leukemic cell infiltration (hematoxylin-eosin, ×300). *C,* The bone marrow has been replaced by myeloblasts (hematoxylin-eosin, ×970). (*A:* From Pediatr Pathol 1985;3:165, Isaacs H Jr, Taylor & Francis, Inc., Washington, DC. Reproduced with permission. All rights reserved. *B* and *C:* From Isaacs H Jr. Tumors of the Newborn and Infant. St. Louis: Mosby–Year Book, 1991.)

nuclei with clefts that were of B-cell lineage and CALLA-positive. Southern blot analysis of bone marrow DNA showed gene rearrangements in both the immunoglobulin light and heavy chain loci, establishing the presence of a clonal B-cell lymphoid proliferation. At 1 year of age, the child was clinically well without evidence of a malignant lymphoproliferative disorder.

Three main criteria must be met before the diagnosis of congenital leukemia can be definitively established: (1) immature hematopoietic cells present in the peripheral blood and bone marrow; (2) infiltration of nonhematopoietic tissues by these cells; and (3) the exclusion of conditions that should be considered in the differential diagnosis in this age group, namely, hemolytic disease of the newborn, congenital infections, and neuroblastoma.[93,97]

CONGENITAL LEUKEMIA AND DOWN SYNDROME

Down syndrome is associated with an increased frequency of leukemia in infants and in children. The Childhood Cancer Research Group, Oxford study (1990) showed that the frequency of leukemia is 14 times greater among individuals with Down syndrome than among the general population, and it is even greater in newborns.[76] This association has been noted in 25% of neonates with ANLL and Down syndrome.[21]

Newborns with Down syndrome may develop an enigmatic myeloproliferative disorder clinically which is morphologically indistinguishable from true leukemia. This disorder has been called by a variety of terms, including transient leukemia, transient myeloproliferative disorder, transient congenital leukemia, and ineffective regulation of myelopoiesis.[10,39,110,111,130] The peripheral leukocyte counts in these patients range from 25,000 to several hundred thousand, and bone marrow examination reveals 30% to 70% blasts. Hepatosplenomegaly and thrombocytopenia are present also. The hematologic picture usually returns to normal after 1 to 4 months with only supportive care. Some patients with this so-called "transient leukemia," who die of other conditions related to the Down syndrome (e.g., cardiac or pulmonary disease), lack microscopic evidence of leukemia at necropsy, whereas others may relapse and die months or years later.

Ross and colleagues[112] have proposed that this transient disorder represents a defect in the regulation of granulocyte multiplication

and maturation. By contrast, Lazarus and associates,[74] on the basis of marker chromosome studies, believe that this transient leukocytosis actually represents leukemia that spontaneously regresses. The question as to whether this disorder represents leukemia or a disorder in the regulation of myelopoiesis still has not been resolved.[11]

Zipursky and colleagues have suggested that practically all cases of ANLL in the newborn with Down syndrome can be classified as an unusual form of leukemia, AMKL.[134] None of 19 newborns and infants in the Oxford Registry carried the diagnosis of ALL, which occurs only in older children with Down syndrome. The leukemic cells in most neonates with Down syndrome are characterized as megakaryoblasts on the basis of their morphologic characteristics on light and electron microscopy and by immunohistochemical markers.[18,68,134] Moreover, Zipursky et al. propose that the AMKL cell is a hematopoietic progenitor cell capable of differentiating into three cell lines: megakaryocytic, erythrocytic, and basophilic.[134] In fact, some neonates with Down syndrome develop erythroid abnormalities, such as dyserythropoiesis and erythroleukemia, and one patient in Zipursky et al.'s series had basophilia while recovering from transient leukemia at 3 weeks of age.[134] Moreover, there is an increased frequency of neonatal polycythemia in Down syndrome.[124]

It is conceivable that the biological properties of the AMKL megakaryoblast—that is, its ability to differentiate into other hematopoietic cell lines—are analogous to the pre-B lymphoblast, in which both myeloid and lymphoid differentiation can occur. If this analogy is valid, then the early blast cells of some forms of perinatal leukemia could be regarded loosely as "embryonic hematopoietic tumors" or "embryomas," as described initially by Willis.[127]

A great deal of controversy persists over the natural history and treatment of transient leukemia in the newborn with Down syndrome. In most instances, the megakaryoblasts disappear from the blood within the first 2 months of life and the blood picture returns to normal.[134] However, about 25% of these infants develop AMKL 5 to 30 months later.[78,134] Therefore, one could conclude that the proliferation of megakaryoblasts in transient leukemia also represents a preleukemic process. The main problems for the clinician are predicting the outcome in such cases of transient leukemia and determining the best course of treatment for these patients. In other words, the clinician must try to determine whether or not the leukemia is transient. From what has been said earlier, it is practically impossible to determine with any accuracy what the outcome will be in a newborn with Down syndrome (or even the outcome in those newborns without Down syndrome and normal chromosomes) and leukemia. Therefore, conservative, watchful management is definitely indicated.[82]

Spontaneous remissions are uncommon in neonates who have leukemia and normal karyotypes, but this unusual event has been described.[24,50,64,70,72,77,96,113,121] One newborn in the Children's Hospital, Los Angeles series (see Fig. 7–2), had multiple, firm skin nodules which, on biopsy, showed myeloblasts and myeloid cells in various stages of maturation. The child's initial leukocyte count was 117,000 cells/mm^3, and his bone marrow had been replaced by leukemic cells that were morphologically similar to those in the skin. Chromosomal studies revealed a normal karyotype in both the leukemic cells and in the patient. The infant recovered uneventfully from transient leukemia a few months later (without chemotherapy) and has been in remission for more than 5 years.

Some cases of phenotypically normal infants with mosaic trisomy 21 karyotypes associated with transient leukemia in the neonate have been documented.[107,114] Seibel and co-workers described two neonates with ANLL and trisomy 21 mosaicism detected in the leukemic cells, but not in the cells of the patient who achieved a spontaneous remission, and Ridgway et al. have described two similar cases.[107,114] Penchansky et al. reported another child with a normal karyotype and a remission lasting 11 years.[96] Apparently, the traditional criteria used for the diagnosis of leukemia in the older child—namely, the presence of large numbers of leukemic blasts in the peripheral blood and bone marrow—are not always valid for the young infant.[96] Because of the uncertainty of the outcome of the neonate with leukemia, chemotherapy should be withheld until the disease becomes manifest.[72]

HEMATOLOGIC FINDINGS

Initially, hemoglobin values in the neonate with leukemia are normal or slightly decreased, but subsequently, they drop to very low levels. Thrombocytopenia, anemia, and leukocytosis are typical findings, with some leukocyte counts approaching 1 million/mm^3. Before death, the leukocyte counts progressively rise. The peripheral smear and bone marrow aspirates show a predominance of blast cells, including erythroblasts, and, depending on the type of leukemia, increased numbers of immature cells of the myeloid, monocytic, megakaryocytic, or lymphoid series may be noted (Figs. 7–3 through 7–5).[63,93]

ANLL is much more prevalent in the neonate than ALL. Acute myelomonocytic leukemia, particularly monocytic leukemia, is the form of ANLL that is most commonly found in this age group (see Figs. 7–3 and 7–5). In addition to AML, erythroleukemia and basophilic leukemia sometimes are described.[2,51,54,70,72,77,115,119] AMKL is the form of ANLL that typically occurs in newborns with Down syndrome and transient leukemia.[134]

Most acute lymphoblastic leukemias of childhood are characterized by leukemic cells having either T-cell–associated antigens or B-cell surface immunoglobulins, and older children with either T- or B-cell leukemia usually experience long-term disease-free survivals.[36,118] By contrast, monoclonal antibody studies performed on leukemic cells from infants with ALL often show a lack of expression of T-cell antigens, B-cell antigens, or CALLA, and may express only HLA/DR (see Fig. 7–4).[31,36,48,118] The Pediatric Oncology Group study reported by Pullen et al. revealed that infants with ALL generally have unfavorable lymphoblast immunophenotypes.[102] Moreover, specific lymphoid markers were found in only 38% of the patients, and 76% had CALLA-negative blasts. The investigations by Dinndorf and Reaman, Spier et al., Felix et al., and Garewal et al. suggest that infant ALL arises from cells at the earliest stage of B-cell differentiation.[36,40,48,118] As was mentioned earlier, the most common chromosomal defect in leukemic cells found in more than 30% of infants with ALL involves chromosome 11 (11q23), taking the form of a translocation, t(4;11), which is associated also with an unfavorable prognosis.[103] Moreover, most infants with ALL have clinical findings associated with a poor prognosis—namely, high leukocyte counts, hepatosplenomegaly, and central nervous system leukemia at presentation.[31,36,104]

PATHOLOGY

Leukemic involvement of placentas from fetuses with this disease has been described.[2,12,43,51,73] The placenta is usually enlarged, weigh-

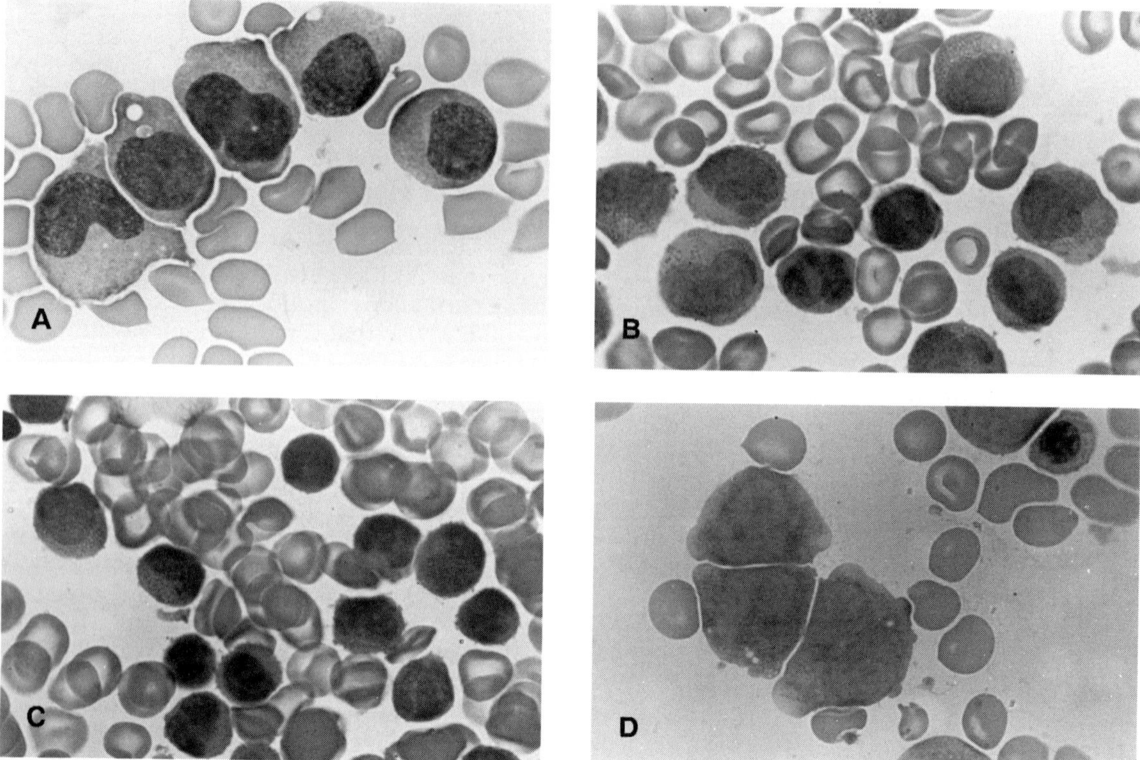

Figure 7–3. Acute myelomonocytic leukemia. A 1-month-old female infant had leukocytosis (50,400 cells/mm³) with 84% blasts and a hemoglobin value of 10.6 g/dL. *A,* A bone marrow smear reveals myeloid and large monocytoid forms, the latter having abundant (pale gray-blue) cytoplasm, nuclear lobulations and folds, chromatin varying from delicate to coarse, occasional nucleoli, and cytoplasmic vacuoles and pseudopodia (FAB, M4–M5) (Wright-Giemsa, ×1200). *B,* Non-specific esterase testing yields positive results (×1500). *C,* Chloroacetate esterase testing yields positive results (×1200). *D,* Acid phosphatase testing yields positive results (×1500). Negative results were obtained with histochemical testing with peroxidase and Sudan black. Positive myeloid markers included CD14, CD15, and CD33. CD4, an antigen found on monocytes and T-helper lymphocytes, was also reactive. The B-cell marker CD19 was positive (93% of blasts), whereas other B-cell markers and TdT were unreactive. Chromosome analysis revealed a t(11;9) balanced translocation. The data suggest an acute myelomonocytic leukemia with B-cell coexpression.

ing more than 700 g, pale, and edematous, and has a gross and microscopic appearance similar to erythroblastosis fetalis. Microscopically, the uniformly enlarged villi are composed of fetal blood vessels and villous stroma filled with leukemic blast cells, which usually do not invade the intervillous space of the maternal circulation. Because leukemia, neuroblastoma, and hepatoblastoma—the fetal tumors known to involve the placenta—are small cell malignant tumors, it may be difficult to distinguish between the various entities in this group based on hematoxylin-eosin staining alone, particularly if the affected fetus is hydropic, macerated, or stillborn. If the tissue is well preserved, the problem can usually be resolved by ultrastructural and immunohistochemical studies, such as leukocyte common antigen (leukemias in general), platelet peroxidase and platelet glyco-

protein GPIIIa (AMKL), epithelial membrane antigen (hepatoblastoma), and neuron-specific enolase (NSE) (neuroblastoma) (see Table 4–5). Wright-Giemsa–stained touch preparations are examined for cellular morphology; surface markers and chromosomal analysis are definitely indicated if the material is fresh.

At necropsy, the external examination of a newborn with leukemia reveals signs of anemia, namely, pallor and manifestations of bleeding, such as petechiae and ecchymoses and oozing from needle puncture sites, various orifices, and the umbilicus. The stigmata of Down syndrome—epicanthal folds, transverse palmar creases, and clinodactyly of the fifth finger—are observed in those patients with this chromosomal abnormality.[49] Significant organomegaly is present; indeed, the liver may weigh more than double its normal expected weight and

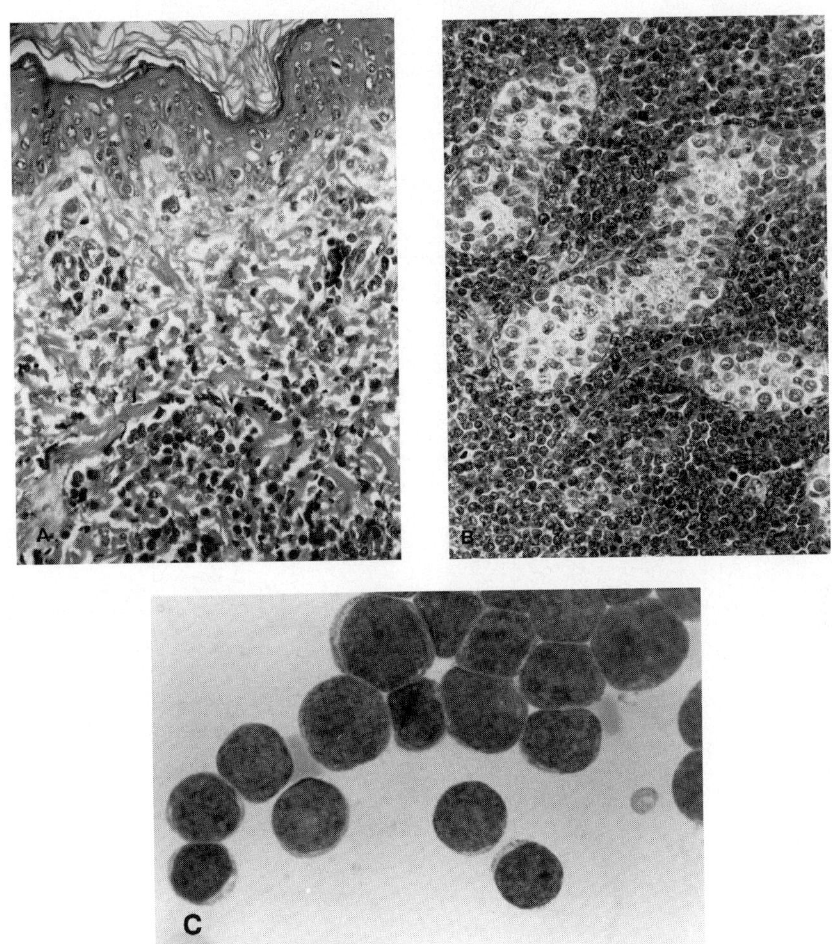

Figure 7–4. Acute lymphoid leukemia (ALL). A 3-month-old boy had anemia (hemoglobin of 5.8 g/dL) and a leukocytosis of 25,700 mm³ with a differential of 96% lymphoblasts and 4% neutrophils. The platelet count was 104,000. Scattered, bluish-purple nodules measuring less than 1 cm in diameter were distributed over the chest, back, groin, and scalp, and bilateral testicular enlargement was noted on physical examination. His karyotype was normal. *A,* A skin biopsy revealed leukemic cells in the dermis and subcutaneous tissue (hematoxylin-eosin, ×600). *B,* A testicular biopsy demonstrated extensive interstitial leukemic cell infiltrates (hematoxylin-eosin, ×600). *C,* An imprint ("touch preparation") of the testicular biopsy specimen revealed small lymphoblasts with a high nuclear:cytoplasmic ratio, a clumped chromatin pattern, and 1 or 2 small nucleoli, a pattern consistent with FAB L1 morphology (Giemsa, ×800). Similar cells found in the bone marrow contained PAS-positive granules, but were negative for CALLA, peroxidase, Sudan black, and α-naphthyl esterase. The anti-DR antibody test was positive, but no T-cell antibodies were detected. The findings were interpreted as indicating that the lymphoblasts were of early pre-B cell lineage, thereby belonging to the so-called pre-B cell ALL category. (From Isaacs H Jr. Tumors of the Newborn and Infant. St. Louis: Mosby–Year Book, 1991.)

the spleen may be larger than four times its normal size, with these organs appearing to occupy much of the abdominal cavity (see Fig. 7–5).[62] Renomegaly secondary to leukemic infiltration is a common feature of the disease. The kidneys weigh as much as twice their normal expected weight and have tense, tan-gray, smooth capsules, characteristic peripelvic hemorrhage, and bulging cut surfaces with partial or total obliteration of the normal corticomedullary architecture by gray to tan infiltrates (see Fig. 7–

5E). Grossly, the enlarged spleen shows a swollen, purple-gray smooth capsule and tan to redbrown bulging cut surfaces without either welldefined trabecular markings or white pulp lymphoid nodules, which are absent in the newborn (see Fig. 7–5D). Irregular, dark red, splenic infarcts may be present. Typically, the liver has a pale, tan, smooth capsule and a similar cut surface, with gray to red markings representing leukemic infiltrates and hemorrhage, respectively (see Fig. 7–5C). Rarely, lymphad-

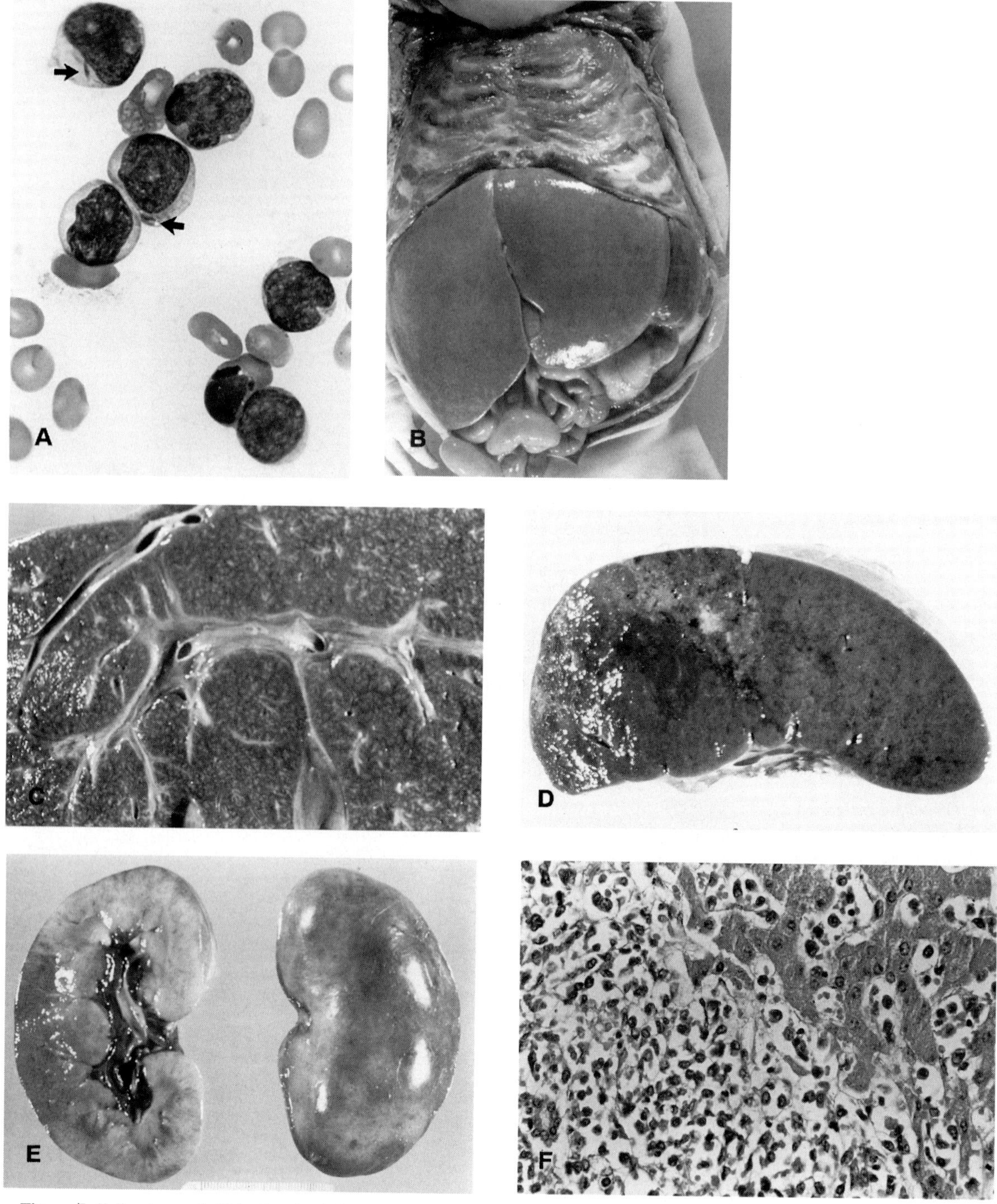

Figure 7–5. Acute myeloid leukemia. A 6-month-old boy presented with a 1-week history of fever and lethargy. Laboratory findings revealed anemia (hemoglobin value of 5.6 g/dL), leukopenia (white blood cell count of 2800 mm³; 94% blasts and 6% neutrophils), and thrombocytopenia (platelet count of 32,000). *A,* A bone marrow aspirate with myeloblasts is seen to have features consistent with an M-2 FAB morphology; the leukemic cells have a relatively low nuclear:cytoplasmic ratio, nuclei with a fine chromatin pattern, and two to three prominent nucleoli. Auer rods are present in two cells (*arrows*) (Giemsa, ×800). Cytochemical findings revealed positivity for Sudan black, myeloperoxidase, and nonspecific esterase and negativity for PAS. *B,* Postmortem examination revealed multiple petechiae and ecchymoses over the skin and viscera, hepatosplenomegaly, renomegaly, and lymphadenomegaly. This photograph displays the hepatosplenomegaly. *C,* A cross section of the liver shows extensive, whitish, leukemic infiltrates. *D,* The cut surface of the spleen shows diffuse leukemic infiltration and an infarct on the left (*dark area*). *E,* The capsular and cut surfaces of the kidney demonstrate central peripelvic hemorrhage and blurring of the corticomedullary architecture by leukemic infiltrates. *F,* A microscopic section of the liver reveals expansion of the portal tract by leukemic cells (on the right); these cells are also noted within the adjacent sinusoids (hematoxylin-eosin, ×600). (From Isaacs H Jr. Tumors of the Newborn and Infant. St. Louis: Mosby–Year Book, 1991.)

enomegaly is present in the untreated or partially treated infant. When involved, the lymph nodes are light tan to gray and swollen, with small foci of hemorrhage.

Grossly, the brain displays varying degrees of meningeal involvement (sometimes minimal), which is manifested by a white, milky appearance of the leptomeninges. Perivascular hemorrhage and gross evidence of leukemic infiltration involving Virchow-Robin spaces and the adjacent parenchyma are occasionally noted. One of 13 neonates with leukemia in the Children's Hospital, Los Angeles study died following a massive parietal-occipital lobe bleed.[60]

Histologic findings reveal varying degrees of infiltration of the involved organs and tissues by immature lymphoid or myeloid elements, depending on the type of leukemia and whether treatment was given. The lymph nodes, spleen, and bone marrow show mild to extensive diffuse infiltration by immature lymphoid or myeloid cells with variable numbers of young erythroid elements, namely, normoblasts and erythroblasts. Extramedullary organs, such as the lungs, kidneys, skin, and gastrointestinal tract, are similarly involved. Varying degrees of atrophy are noted in normal lymphoid tissue.

The infiltrates of lymphoid leukemia tend to be heavier in the hepatic periportal zones than in the sinusoids, but in myeloid and monocytic leukemia, the situation is reversed, with tumor cells tending to involve the hepatic sinusoids more extensively than the portal areas. However, in instances in which there is massive leukocytosis, as well as diffuse organ infiltration by blasts, this distinction clearly cannot be made; therefore, the pattern of infiltration is not a reliable criterion in establishing whether the leukemia is ALL or ANLL (see Fig. 7–5*F*).

One must be cautious in making the histologic diagnosis of perinatal leukemia based solely on the finding of hematopoietic infiltrates in the liver, spleen, and lymph nodes, as these organs are normally the sites of extramedullary hematopoiesis in the fetus and newborn.[88] Moreover, infiltrates of immature hematopoietic cells occur also in leukemoid reactions and in hemolytic disease of the newborn. Demonstration of blast cells in tissues that are not usually the sites of fetal extramedullary hematopoiesis is requisite for the diagnosis.[88]

Stillborns and neonates with Down syndrome and leukemia have variable degrees of visceral fibrosis, which can be extensive, and which particularly involves the liver and pancreas.[11,49,84,90,134] The finding occurs also in congenital syphilis, which should be considered in the differential diagnosis. Moreover, hepatic fibrosis occurs in neonates with erythroleukemia.[2,49,134] The fibrosis may be responsible for liver failure in infants with AMKL and erythroleukemia.[2,20] Myelofibrosis is found in older children and adults, but not in the newborn with Down syndrome; however, bone marrow fibrosis is seen in infants with the t(1;22) translocation and AMKL.[11,28] The lymph nodes in infants with AMKL and t(1;22) translocation show tumor cell clusters in sinusoids, accompanied by fibrosis and effacement of the nodal architecture, which mimics a metastatic small cell malignant tumor, such as neuroblastoma.[28] The explanation given for the fibrosis found in various sites in patients with AMKL and megakaryocytosis is that megakaryoblasts stimulate fibroblastic proliferation and fibrosis.[11,49]

Multiple petechiae and ecchymoses and nodular leukemic infiltrates are the cutaneous manifestations of congenital leukemia (see Fig. 7–2).[44,97] Leukemia cutis is noted in about 50% of newborns, and may be the first sign of the disease.[44,55,105] Skin involvement is particularly common with acute monocytic leukemia, which is the most frequent form of ANLL in the newborn.[34] The firm, red-brown to gray-blue, nodular infiltrates may involve more than 50% of the body and may range in size from a few millimeters to several centimeters in diameter, giving the baby a "blueberry muffin" appearance (see Table 5–2). The histologic findings consist of infiltrates of myeloid, lymphoid, or monocytic cells (depending on the type of leukemia) within the middle and deep dermis. In contrast to Langerhans cell histiocytosis, the epidermis usually is not invaded by leukemic cells.[63]

Neuropathologic findings include collections of leukemic cells in the leptomeninges and, depending on the amount of leukocytosis, distention of meningeal gray and white matter capillaries by blast cells; however, perivascular parenchymal involvement per se is seen infrequently. The histopathologic findings of central nervous system leukemia and complications of therapy have been discussed by Price.[100] Leukoencephalopathy and mineralizing microangiopathy, the sequelae of radiation therapy, are specifically mentioned.

Ocular involvement is described occasionally in congenital leukemia.[24,109] Rodgers et al. reviewed the ocular findings in a 5-week-old female infant with acute myeloid leukemia who presented with tachypnea, tachycardia, multiple hematomas, and a distended abdomen secondary to hepatosplenomegaly.[109] At necropsy, there was extensive organ infiltration by leukemic cells and significant atelectasis. Except for focal, fluffy, white retinal deposits, the eyes were grossly normal. Histologic examination, however, revealed leukemic infiltration of the ocular muscles, conjunctiva, uveal tract (iris, ciliary body, and choroid), and optic nerve. Retinal hemorrhage was present also. According to Rodgers et al., leukemia can involve almost any ocular structure by direct infiltration, hemorrhage, or infarction.[109] The choroid is the most common site of leukemic infiltration. Usually, the leukemic cells tend to be more numerous in well-vascularized locations within the eye.

The Children's Hospital, Los Angeles perinatal tumor study spanned a 28-year period (1958–1985) and included 13 cases of leukemia consisting of one stillborn case, three diagnosed at birth, and nine diagnosed later on in the neonatal period.[60] Two newborns had Down syndrome; one required immediate surgical correction of duodenal atresia and died 1 month later with sepsis, and the other presented with multiple petechiae and pneumonia and died 3 weeks following diagnosis. The third neonate had transient congenital leukemia cutis at birth, bone marrow that had been replaced by myeloblasts, and a normal karyotype. This patient experienced spontaneous remission without chemotherapy and was free of disease at 6 years of age (see Fig. 7–2).

Hemorrhagic manifestations—namely, petechiae, bleeding from needle puncture sites, and internal hemorrhage—were the most frequent clinical findings in the nine patients whose leukemia was diagnosed later. Congenital leukemia cutis was noted in three, and hepatomegaly was specifically mentioned in three. Lymphadenomegaly was not one of the physical findings. Some initial leukocyte counts were very high, with the entire group averaging 160,000 mm^3 (range of 9800 to 530,000 mm^3), and the presenting hemoglobin values were low, averaging 8.9 g/dL (range of 3.3 to 12.7 g/dL). There were twice as many infants with the diagnosis of acute myeloid leukemia as compared to ALL (8 and 4 cases, respectively; 1 unclassified).

Neither the leukocyte count nor the hemoglobin values had any prognostic significance. One newborn with an initial leukocyte count of 117,000 cm^3 and a hemoglobin of 12.7 g/dL had a spontaneous remission. Another infant with an initial count of 530,000 mm^3 and a hemoglobin of 3.3 g/dL lived for 7 months. Four patients experienced a fulminating downhill clinical course and expired within 4 days of diagnosis. Sepsis was considered to be the immediate cause of death in four, extensive hemorrhage or bleeding diathesis in three, and *Pneumocystis carinii* pneumonia in two.

CYTOLOGIC DIAGNOSIS

The hematologic evaluation of a patient with leukemia begins with performing a complete blood count (CBC) and examination of the peripheral smear.[3,4] Although these tests can be performed on umbilical cord blood, they alone are often insufficient for either diagnosis or classification. Moreover, the presence of leukocytosis and blasts in the peripheral smear does not necessarily establish the diagnosis of leukemia, as erythroblastosis fetalis, infections, and certain metastatic malignant diseases can cause an increased leukocyte count and release immature hematopoietic elements (see Fig. 7–1). In addition to the CBC and peripheral smear, bone marrow aspiration and biopsy are required to study cellular morphology and to rule out infections and the other entities mentioned earlier. Normally, there are less than 5% blasts in the bone marrow; greater than 25% blasts is required to establish the diagnosis.[3,98] Blood and bone marrow cultures are an important part of the work-up.

When the diagnosis of acute leukemia is established, it is important, particularly for therapeutic and prognostic reasons, to determine whether the leukemia is lymphocytic or non-lymphocytic.[3,4] Following this, the next step is to decide the subclassification—ALL or ANLL—to which the leukemia belongs. ALL and ANLL are diagnosed and classified on the basis of morphologic findings, according to the presence of granules or Auer rods, the nuclear, nucleolar, and cytoplasmic appearance, and by cytochemical stains. Traditionally, the international French-American-British (FAB) classification, which is based on these findings, is used to classify the leukemias (Table 7–1).[13] The FAB classification subdivides ALL into three groups: L1, L2, and L3; it categorizes ANLL into 7 groups designated as M1 to M7 (see Table 7–1).[13,54,98] Most infant cases of ALL fall into the L1 or L2 FAB morphologic classification.

Table 7–1. Morphologic and Cytochemical Features of ALL and ANLL

Type of Leukemia	FAB	Wright-Giemsa Stain Morphology	Cytochemistry							
			PAS	Sudan	MP	NSE	Glyc	VIII	PPO	IIb
Acute lymphoid	L1	Predominantly small cells; high N:C ratio; 1 to 2 nucleoli, which are indistinct; coarse nuclear chromatin; blue cytoplasm	+	−	−	−	−	−	−	−
	L2	Large cells, which vary in size; lower N:C ratio than L1; prominent nucleoli; stippled chromatin; blue cytoplasm	+	−	−	−	−	−	−	−
Acute myeloid	M1–M3	Low N:C ratio; Auer rods ±; 2 to 5 nucleoli; granules present; fine nuclear chromatin; blue-gray cytoplasm	−	+	+	+	−	−	−	−
Acute myelomonocytic	M4	Myeloblasts and monoblasts*	−	+	+	+	−	−	−	−
Acute monocytic	M5	Low N:C ratio; lobular or reniform nuclei; cells resembling monocytes; fine nuclear chromatin	−	±	±	+	−	−	−	−
Acute erythroleukemia	M6	Bizarre erythroblasts; multiple lobation of nucleus; multiple nuclei; blast cells with ragged cytoplasmic borders; vacuolated blue cytoplasms	±	±	−	−	+	−	−	−
Acute megakaryoblastic leukemia	M7	Blasts with high N:C ratio; cytoplasmic blebs	+	−	−	−	−	+	+	+

*See the description for both acute myeloid and acute monocytic leukemias.

FAB = French-American-British morphologic classification; N:C = nuclear to cytoplasmic; PAS = periodic acid-Schiff; Sudan = Sudan black B fat stain; MP = myeloperoxidase; NSE = nonspecific esterase; Glyc = glycophorin A; VIII = factor VIII; PPO = platelet peroxidase (by electron microscopy); IIb = glycoprotein IIb/IIIa.

From Allan,[2] Altman,[3] Bennett et al.,[13] Chan et al.,[28] Greaves et al.,[52] Grier and Weinstein,[54] Penchansky et al.,[95] Poplack,[98] and Windebank et al.[128]

Occasionally, leukemic blast cells are so poorly differentiated that it is impossible to determine whether the leukemia belongs to the ALL or ANLL category based only on morphologic and cytochemical findings. Therefore, the final interpretation of the type of leukemia depends on the use of a combination of supplemental methods, such as cytogenetic studies, surface marker analysis, or flow cytometric studies, which may assist in identifying the cellular lineage.[4]

Surface marker analysis accurately characterizes the cell types in leukemias.[54,98] Monoclonal antibodies for myeloid and lymphoid surface antigens are used to distinguish ANLL from ALL and to further subtype the leukemic cells. For example, the My, Mo, glycophorin A, and glycoprotein IIb/IIIa antibodies differentiate leukemic cells with granulocytic differentiation from those with monocytic, erythrocytic, or megakaryocytic differentiation, respectively (see Table 7–1).[54]

Most newborn and infant ALL cells have an early pre–B-cell phenotype manifested by HLA/DR (Ia) positivity and negativity for CALLA and T-cell and B-cell antigens.[31,36,40,79,81,118] L1 and/or L2 FAB morphology is noted most often in this age group (see Fig. 7–4). According to Grier and Weinstein, acute monocytic leukemia (M5) (52%) is the most common form of ANLL in infants, followed by acute myelomonocytic leukemia (M4) (30%) and acute myeloblastic leukemia (M1) (17%).[54]

Darbyshire and colleagues found that differentiating monocytic leukemia from malignant histiocytosis and Langerhans cell histiocytosis in extramedullary sites, such as the skin, can be difficult.[34] Malignant histiocytosis is characterized by polymorphous infiltrates, marked nuclear atypia, erythrophagocytosis, positive lysozyme (though variable), and extension of the infiltrates into the epidermis. Langerhans cell histiocytosis cells react with S-100 protein and contain Birbeck granules. Monocytic leukemic cells show neither one of these findings. The presence of glycophorin A in leukemic cells is considered to be pathognomonic for erythroleukemia.[2,52]

Because immature cells of the megakaryocytic series in smears and in tissues frequently lack distinctive morphologic features that aid in their recognition, some cases of AMKL have been classified as acute undifferentiated leukemia.[128] The diagnosis of AMKL is established on the basis of the appearance of the blasts on Wright-Giemsa–stained smears, the platelet peroxidase reaction by electron microscopy (which is also positive in erythroleukemic blasts), and reactivity with monoclonal platelet-specific antibodies.[28,69,95,128] Megakaryoblasts in Wright-Giemsa–stained smears display a variable morphology conforming to the M7 category according to the FAB classification.[28,95] Small and large cell blasts with cytoplasmic projections or blebs are considered to be diagnostic. The former have round nuclei, prominent nucleoli, stippled chromatin, and a moderate basophilic cytoplasm without granules, whereas the latter have a scant cytoplasm, a round nucleus with stippled chromatin, and an inconspicuous nucleolus.

Megakaryoblasts in blood and marrow smears react with platelet glycoprotein GPIIb/IIIa antibody.[28] Moreover, factor VIII (von Willebrand factor), CD43, and lectin Ulex europaeus I are expressed even in paraffin section material.[28] However, the blasts are nonreactive for CALLA (CD10), TdT, OKM1, myeloperoxidase, and α-naphthyl butyrate esterase.[128] The syncytial appearance of AMKL cells in the marrow and the infiltrative nature in other organs, accompanied by fibrosis, suggest a nonhematopoietic metastatic malignant disease. Markers, such as neuron-specific enolase (NSE), synaptophysin, desmin, and cytokeratin, may be required in some instances to exclude neuroblastoma, rhabdomyosarcoma, primitive neuroectodermal tumor (PNET), and other small cell malignant tumors.[28,95,128]

Cytogenetic analysis for chromosomal anomalies in leukemic cells plays an important role in subclassification and prognosis for both patients with ALL and ANLL.[81,98] Specific structural chromosomal defects have been described in newborn leukemias.[26,31,65,66,79,101,118] Translocations and rearrangements are associated, in some instances, with specific immunophenotypes. For example, 11q23 translocation occurs in more than 50% of neonatal leukemias (both ALL and ANLL) and is observed in ALL with phenotypic positivity to Ia and negativity to CALLA, T-cell, and B-cell antigens.[65,101] Moreover, the 11q23 anomaly is observed in null cell leukemias with mixed pre–B-cell and myeloid markers.[66,79] Neonates with AMKL who do not have Down syndrome have a specific chromosomal anomaly, t(1;22)(p13;q13), which is considered to be diagnostic.[261] Both the 11q23 and t(1;22) translocations are associated with a poor prognosis (see the previous Cytogenetics section).

PROGNOSIS

Historically, the natural history of congenital leukemia is characterized by an inexorably fatal, progressively downhill clinical course.[97] The life expectancy of the newborn and infant without treatment is brief, and few long-term survivors have been reported.[21,24,75,119,121] Rapid deterioration and death from hemorrhage and/or infection may be the course of the disease, with or without chemotherapy.[41,60,61,97] The survival rate for newborns with leukemia in most studies is discouragingly low. For example, only one of six newborns in the St. Jude Children's Hospital series lived for more than 1 year, and only one of eight included in the Birmingham Children's Hospital, U.K. study survived.[32,94] Of the 12 neonates with leukemia in the Rigshospitalet, Copenhagen review, the 3 included in the Children's Hospital Philadelphia study, and the 8 included in the Hospital for Sick Children, Toronto series, none survived.[19,24,47]

Across the entire pediatric age group with ALL, infants have the worst prognosis, as less than 25% of these patients survive without relapse 3 years from the time of diagnosis.[103] All three infants younger than 3 months of age with null ALL and 11q23 rearrangement in the Hospital for Sick Children, London series died.[66] Kaneko et al. reviewed the data of 34 infants with ALL from 20 different Japanese institutions; 7 were 3 months of age or younger and the longest survival time was 20 months.[65]

Recently, the outcome for infants with ANLL, as gauged by the remission rate and the

3-year survival rate, has improved considerably and appears to be almost the same as it is for older children.[71,103] However, the prognosis for newborns with AMKL and t(1;22) translocation is not as encouraging, as the three newborns included in the Pediatric Oncology Group study have died, and only two of four infants described by Chan et al. were in remission at the time of writing.[26,28]

At the present time, most agree that the newborn with leukemia should be treated cautiously and that the disease should be allowed to become established before embarking on a therapeutic regimen.[29,46,97,117] For some unexplained reason, permanent spontaneous remissions occur in the young, which is another justification for delaying treatment. With careful monitoring and supportive care, chemotherapy is almost as well tolerated in this age group as in older children (William Roberts, MD, personal communication).

REFERENCES

1. Abe R, Ryan D, Cecalupo A, et al. Cytogenetic findings in congenital leukemia: Case report and review of the literature. Cancer Genet Cytogenet 1983;9:139.
2. Allan RR, Wadsworth LD, Kalousek DK, et al. Congenital erythroleukemia: A case report with morphological, immunophenotypic and cytogenetic findings. Am J Hematol 1989;31:114.
3. Altman AJ. Cytologic diagnosis of the acute nonlymphoid leukemias. I. Morphologic, cytochemical, and ultrastructural features. Am J Pediatr Hematol Oncol 1985;7:21.
4. Altman AJ. Cytologic diagnosis of the acute nonlymphoid leukemias. II. Flow cytometry, surface markers, cytogenetics, and use of cell culture techniques. Am J Pediatr Hematol Oncol 1985;7:156.
5. Altman AJ, Schwartz AD: Malignant Diseases of Infancy, Childhood and Adolescence, 2nd ed. Philadelphia: WB Saunders, 1983.
6. Arceci RJ, Weinstein HJ. Neoplasia in the neonate and young infant. *In* Avery GB, Fletcher MA, MacDonald MG (eds): Neonatology: Pathophysiology and Management of the Newborn, 4th ed, p 1215. Philadelphia: JB Lippincott, 1994.
7. Argyle JC, Benjamin DR, Lampkin B, et al. Acute nonlymphocytic leukemias of childhood: Interobserver variability and problems in the use of the FAB classification. Cancer 1989;63:295.
8. Bader JL, Miller RM. Neurofibromatosis and childhood leukemia. J Pediatr 1978;92:925.
9. Bader JL, Miller RW. U.S. cancer incidence and mortality in the first year of life. Am J Dis Child 1979;133:157.
10. Barnett PLJ, Clark ACL, Garson OM. Acute nonlymphocytic leukemia after transient myeloproliferative disorder in a patient with Down syndrome. Med Pediatr Oncol 1990;18:347.
11. Becroft DMO, Zwi LJ. Perinatal visceral fibrosis accompanying the megakaryoblastic leukemoid reaction of Down syndrome. Pediatr Pathol 1990;10:397.
12. Benirschke K, Kaufmann P: The Pathology of the Human Placenta, 2nd ed. New York: Springer-Verlag, 1990.
13. Bennett JM, Catovsky D, Daniel M-T, et al. Proposals for the classification of acute leukemias. French-American-British (FAB) co-operative group. Br J Haematol 1976;33:451.
14. Berger R, Bernheim A, Sigaux F, et al. Acute monocytic leukemia chromosome studies. Leuk Res 1982;6:17.
15. Bernard J, Jacquillat C, Chavalet F, et al. Leucemie aigue d'une enfant de 5 mois nee d'une mere atteinte de leucemie aigue au moment de l'accouchement. Nouv Rev Fr Hematol 1964;4:140.
16. Bernard WG, Gore I, Kilby RA. Congenital leukemia. Blood 1951;6:990.
17. Bernstein R, Pinto MR, Spector I, et al. A unique 8;16 translocation in two infants with poorly differentiated monoblastic leukemia. Cancer Genet Cytogenet 1987;24:213.
18. Bevan D, Rose M, Greaves M. Leukemia of platelet precursors: Diverse features in four cases. Br J Hematol 1982;51:147.
19. Borch K, Jacobsen T, Olsen JH, et al. Neonatal cancer in Denmark 1943–1985. Pediatr Hematol Oncol 1992;9:209.
20. Brescia MA, Santora E, Sarnatora VF. Congenital leukemia. J Pediatr 1959;55:35.
21. Broadbent VA. Malignant disease in the neonate. *In* Roberton NRC (ed): Textbook of Neonatology, 2nd ed, p 879. Edinburgh: Churchill Livingstone, 1992.
22. Campbell AN, Chan HSL, O'Brien A, et al. Malignant tumours in the neonate. Arch Dis Child 1987;62:19.
23. Campbell WAB, Macafee AL. Familial congenital leukemia. Arch Dis Child 1962;37:93.
24. Cangir A, George S, Sullivan M. Unfavorable prognosis of acute leukemia in infancy. Cancer 1975;36:1973.
25. Carney LA, Kinney JS, Higgins RR, et al. X;6 translocation in a child with congenital acute lymphocytic leukemia. Cancer 1992;69:799.
26. Carroll A, Civin C, Schneider N, et al. The t(1;22)(p13;q13) is nonrandom and restricted to infants with acute megakaryoblastic leukemia: A Pediatric Oncology Group Study. Blood 1991;78:748.
27. Carroll AJ, Frankel LS, Pullen DJ, et al. Acquired cytogenetic abnormalities in blast cells of infants with acute lymphoblastic leukemia (Abstract). Blood 1986;69 (Suppl):252A.
28. Chan WC, Carroll A, Alvarado CS, et al. Acute megakaryoblastic leukemia in infants with t(1;22)(p13;q13) abnormality. Am J Clin Pathol 1992;98:214.
29. Chu J-Y, O'Connor DM, Gale GB, et al. Congenital leukemia: Two transient regressions without treatment in one patient. Pediatrics 1983;71:277.
30. Clark RH, Taylor LL, Wells RJ. Congenital juvenile chronic myelogenous leukemia: Case report and review. Pediatrics 1984;73:324.
31. Crist W, Pullen J, Boyett J, et al. Clinical and biologic features predict a poor prognosis in acute lymphoid leukemia in infants. Pediatric Oncology Group Study. Blood 1986;67:135.
32. Crom DB, Wilimas JA, Green AA, et al. Malignancy in the neonate. Med Pediatr Oncol 1989;17:101.
33. Dampier C, Chilcote RR. Acute non-lymphoid leukemia. Pediatr Ann 1983;12:293.
34. Darbyshire PJ, Smith JHF, Oakhill A, et al. Monocytic

leukemia in children: A review of eight children. Cancer 1985;56:1584.

35. Dehner LP: Neoplasms of the fetus and neonate. *In* Naeye RL, Kissane JM, Kaufman N (eds): Perinatal Diseases, International Academy of Pathology, Monograph No. 22, p 286. Baltimore: Williams and Wilkins, 1981.

36. Dinndorf PA, Reaman G. Acute lymphoblastic leukemia in infants: Evidence for B cell origin of disease by use of monoclonal antibody phenotyping. Blood 1986;68:975.

37. Djernes BW, Soukeys SW, Bove KE, et al. Congenital leukemia associated with mosaic trisomy. J Pediatr 1976;88:596.

38. Donnenfeld AE, Scott SC, Henselder-Kimmel M, et al. Prenatally diagnosed non-immune hydrops caused by congenital transient leukemia. Prenat Diagn 1994; 14:721.

39. Engel RR, Hammond D, Eitzman DV, et al. Transient congenital leukemia in 7 infants with mongolism. J Pediatr 1964;65:303.

40. Felix CA, Reaman GH, Korsmeyer SJ, et al. Immunoglobulin and T cell receptor gene configuration in acute lymphoblastic leukemia of infancy. Blood 1987; 70:536.

41. Finklestein JZ, Higgins GR, Rissman E, et al. Acute leukemia during the first year of life: Presentation, chemotherapy and clinical course. Clin Pediatr 1972; 11:236.

42. Fourcar K, Friedman K, Llewellyn A, et al. Prenatal diagnosis of transient myeloproliferative disorder via percutaneous umbilical blood sampling: Report of two cases in fetuses affected by Down's syndrome. Am J Clin Pathol 1992;97:584.

43. Fox H. Placental Metastases from fetal neoplasms. Pathology of the Placenta, Major Problems in Pathology, Vol 7, p 360. Philadelphia: WB Saunders, 1978.

44. Francis JS, Sybert VP, Benjamin DR. Congenital monocytic leukemia: Report of a case with cutaneous involvement, and review of the literature. Pediatr Dermatol 1989;6:306.

45. Fraumeni JF Jr, Miller RW. Cancer deaths in the newborn. Am J Dis Child 1969;117:186.

46. Gale GB, D'Angio GJ, Uri A, et al. Cancer in neonates: The experience at the Children's Hospital of Philadelphia. Pediatrics 1982;70:409.

47. Gale GB, Toledano SR. Congenital acute lymphocytic leukemia in a newborn with Klinefelter syndrome. Am J Pediatr Hematol Oncol 1984;6:338.

48. Garewal G, Marwaha RK, Ray R, et al. Congenital acute lymphoblastic leukemia: Report of a case with unusual immunophenotype. Am J Hematol 1993;44: 147.

49. Gilson TP, Bendon RW. Megakaryocytosis of the liver in a trisomy 21 stillbirth. Arch Pathol Lab Med 1993; 117:738.

50. Gottesfeld E, Silverman RA, Coccia PF, et al. Transient blueberry muffin appearance of a newborn with congenital monoblastic leukemia. J Am Acad Dermatol 1989;21:347.

51. Gray ES, Balch NJ, Kohler H, et al. Congenital leukemia: An unusual cause of stillbirth. Arch Dis Child 1986;61:1001.

52. Greaves MF, Sieff C, Edwards PAW. Monoclonal antiglycophorin as a probe for erythroleukemia. Blood 1983;61:64.

53. Gresik MV, Fernbach DJ. Leukemia in childhood. *In* Finegold M (ed): Pathology of Neoplasia in Children and Adolescents, Major Problems in Pathology, Vol 18, p 46. Philadelphia: WB Saunders, 1986.

54. Grier HE, Weinstein HJ. Acute myelogenous leukemia. *In* Pizzo PA, Poplack DG (eds): Principles and Practice of Pediatric Oncology, 2nd ed, p 483. Philadelphia: JB Lippincott, 1993.

55. Haahr J, Halveg AD. Congenital leukemia. Acta Paediat Scand 1971;60:720.

56. Hanada T, Ono I, Minosaki Y, et al. Translocation t(8; 16) (p11;p13) in neonatal acute monocytic leukemia. Eur J Pediatr 1991;150:323.

57. Hazani A, Barak Y, Berant M, et al. Congenital juvenile myelogenous leukemia: Therapeutic trial with interferon alpha-2. Med Pediatr Oncol 1993;21:73.

58. Heikinheimo M, Pakkala S, Juvonen E, et al. Immuno- and cytochemical characterization of congenital leukemia: A case report. Med Pediatr Oncol 1994; 22:279.

59. Hogg GR, Schmidt OA. Myelogenous leukemia in a stillborn infant. Can Med Assoc J 1958;78:421.

60. Isaacs H Jr. Congenital and neonatal malignant tumors: A 28-year experience at Children's Hospital of Los Angeles. Am J Pediatr Hematol Oncol 1987;9(2): 121.

61. Isaacs H Jr. Neoplasms in infants: A report of 265 cases. Pathol Annu 1983;18(2):165.

62. Isaacs H Jr. Perinatal (congenital and neonatal) neoplasms: A report of 110 cases. Pediatr Pathol 1985;3: 165.

63. Isaacs H Jr. Tumors of the Newborn and Infant. St. Louis: Mosby–Year Book, 1991.

64. Kalousek DK, Chan KW. Transient myeloproliferative disorder in chromosomally normal newborn infant. Med Pediatr Oncol 1987;15:38.

65. Kaneko Y, Shikano T, Maseki N, et al. Clinical characteristics of infant acute leukemia with or without 11q23 translocations. Leukemia 1988;2:672.

66. Katz F, Malcolm S, Gibbons B, et al. Cellular and molecular studies on infant null acute lymphoblastic leukemia. Blood 1988;71:1438.

67. Kelleher JF, Carbone TV. Monosomy 7 syndrome in an infant with neurofibromatosis. Am J Pediatr Hematol Oncol 1991;13:338.

68. Kojima S, Matsuyama T, Sato T, et al. Down's syndrome and acute leukemia in children: An analysis of phenotype by use of monoclonal antibodies and electron microscopic platelet peroxidase reaction. Blood 1990;76:2348.

69. Kojima S, Mimaya J, Tonouchi T, et al. Identification of myeloid origin in undifferentiated congenital leukemia. Am J Pediatr Hematol Oncol 1989;11:337.

70. Kurosawa H, Eguchi M, Sakakibara H, et al. Ultrastructural cytochemistry of congenital basophilic leukemia. Am J Pediatr Hematol Oncol 1987;9(1):27.

71. Lampkin B, Buckley J, Nesbit M, et al. Clinical and laboratory findings and responses to therapy in infants less than one year of age with acute non-lymphocytic leukemia (ANLL). Proc Am Soc Clin Oncol 1984;3:201 (C-785).

72. Lampkin BC, Peipon JJ, Price JK, et al. Spontaneous remission of presumed congenital acute nonlymphoblastic leukemia (ANLL) in a karyotypically normal neonate. Am J Pediatr Hematol Oncol 1985;7(4):346.

73. Las Heras J, Leal G, Haust MD. Congenital leukemia: Report of a case with ultrastructural study. Cancer 1986;58:2278.

74. Lazarus KH, Heerema NA, Palmer CG, et al. The myeloproliferative reaction in a child with Down's syn-

drome: Cytological and chromosomal evidence for a transient leukemia. Am J Hematol 1981;11:417.

75. Leiper AD, Chessells J. Acute lymphoblastic leukemia under 2 years. Arch Dis Child 1986;61:1007.

76. Levitt GA, Stiller CA, Chessells JM. Prognosis of Down's syndrome with acute leukaemia. Arch Dis Child 1990;65:212.

77. Lilleyman JS. Congenital monocytic leukemia. Clin Lab Haematol 1980;2:243.

78. Lin HP, Menaka H, Lim KH, Yong HS. Congenital leukemoid reaction followed by fatal leukemia. A case with Down's syndrome. Am J Dis Child 1980;134:939.

79. Ludwig W-D, Bartram CR, Harbott J, et al. Phenotypic and genotypic heterogeneity in infant acute leukemia. I. Acute lymphoblastic leukemia. Leukemia 1989;3:431.

80. MacMahon B, Levy MA. Prenatal origin of childhood leukemia: Evidence from twins. N Engl J Med 1964; 270:1082.

81. Matthay KK. Congenital malignant disorders. *In* Taeusch HW, Ballard RA, Avery ME (eds): Schaffer and Avery's Diseases of the Newborn, 6th ed, p 1025. Philadelphia: WB Saunders, 1991.

82. Miller DR. Hematologic malignancies: Leukemia and lymphoma. *In* Miller DR, Baehner RL, Miller LP (eds): Blood Diseases of Infancy and Childhood, 7th ed, p 731. St. Louis: Mosby–Year Book, 1995.

83. Miller DR, Leikin S, Albo V, et al. Prognostic factors and therapy in acute lymphoblastic leukemia of childhood: CCG-141: A report of the Children's Cancer Study Group. Cancer 1983;51:1041.

84. Miller JM, Sherrill JG, Hathaway WE. Thrombocytopenia in the myeloproliferative disorder of Down's syndrome. Pediatrics 1967;40:847.

85. Miller RW, Dalager NA. U.S. childhood cancer deaths by cell type, 1960–68. J Pediatr 1974;85:664.

86. Moir DJ, Emerson PM, Holmes-Siedel M, et al. Neonatal chronic myeloid leukemia with prolonged survival. Arch Dis Child 1983;58:64.

87. Monpoux F, Sirvent N, Sudaka I, et al. Leucemie aigue monoblastic congenitale et translocation 9;11: une observation. Pediatrie 1992;47:691.

88. Morison JE. Foetal and Neonatal Pathology, 3rd ed, p 119. New York: Appleton-Century-Crofts, 1970.

89. Nagasaka M, Maeda S, Maeda H, et al. Four cases of t(4;11) acute leukemia and its myelomonocytic nature in infants. Blood 1983;61:1174.

90. Nakagawa T, Nishida H, Arai T, et al. Hyperviscosity syndrome with transient abnormal myelopoiesis in Down syndrome. J Pediatr 1988;112:58.

91. Nathan DG, Oski FA. Hematology of Infancy and Childhood, 4th ed, Vol 2. Philadelphia: WB Saunders, 1993.

92. Nicolaides KH, Rodeck CH, Lange I, et al. Fetoscopy in the assessment of unexplained fetal hydrops. Br J Obstet Gynecol 1985;92:671.

93. Oski FA, Naiman JL. Hematologic problems in the newborn. *In* Schaffer AJ (ed): Major Problems in Clinical Pediatrics, 2nd ed, Vol 4, p 316. Philadelphia: WB Saunders, 1972.

94. Parkes SE, Muir KR, Southern L, et al. Neonatal tumours: A thirty-year population based study. Med Pediatr Oncol 1994;22:309.

95. Penchansky L, Taylor SR, Krause JR. Three infants with acute megakaryoblastic leukemia simulating metastatic tumor. Cancer 1989;64:1366.

96. Penchansky L, Wollman WR, Gartner JC, et al. Spontaneous remission of infantile acute nonlymphocytic leukemia for 11 years in a child with a normal karyotype. Cancer 1993;71:1928.

97. Pierce MI. Leukemia in the newborn infant. J Pediatr 1979;54:691.

98. Poplack DG. Acute lymphoblastic leukemia. *In* Pizzo PA, Poplack DG (eds): Principles and Practice of Pediatric Oncology, 2nd ed, p 431. Philadelphia: JB Lippincott, 1993.

99. Potter EL, Craig JM: Pathology of the Fetus and Infant, 3rd ed, p 177. Chicago: Year Book Medical Publishers, 1975.

100. Price RA. Histopathology of CNS leukemia and complications of therapy. Am J Pediatr Hematol Oncol 1979;1:21.

101. Pui C-H, Raimondi SC, Murphy SB, et al. An analysis of leukemic cell chromosomal features in infants. Blood 1987;69:1289.

102. Pullen J, Crist W, Boyett J, et al. Infants have biologically different and clinically more aggressive acute lymphocytic leukemia (ALL) than older children. Proc Am Soc Clin Oncol 1985;4:162(Abstract).

103. Reaman GH. Special considerations for the infant with cancer. *In* Pizzo PA, Poplack DG (eds): Principles and Practice of Pediatric Oncology, 2nd ed, p 303. Philadelphia: JB Lippincott, 1993.

104. Reaman G, Zeltzer P, Bleyer WA, et al. Acute lymphoblastic leukemia in infants less than one year of age: A cumulative experience of the Children's Cancer Study Group. J Clin Oncol 1985;3:1513.

105. Reimann DL, Clemmens RL, Pillsbury WA. Congenital acute leukemia: Skin nodules, a first sign. J Pediatr 1955;46:415.

106. Resnik KS, Brod BB. Leukemia cutis in congenital leukemia. Arch Dermatol 1993;129:1301.

107. Ridgway D, Beda GI, Magenis E, et al. Transient myeloproliferative disorder of the Down type in the normal newborn. Am J Dis Child 1990;144:1117.

108. Roberts W. Personal communication.

109. Rodgers R, Weiner M, Friedman AH. Ocular involvement in congenital leukemia. Am J Ophthalmol 1986; 101:730.

110. Rogers PCJ, Kalousek DK, Denegri JF, et al. Neonate with Down's syndrome and transient congenital leukemia. Am J Pediatr Hematol Oncol 1983;5:59.

111. Rosner F, Lee SL. Down's syndrome and acute leukemia: Myeloblastic or lymphoblastic? Report of 43 cases and review of the literature. Am J Med 1972;53: 203.

112. Ross JD, Moloney WC, Desforges JF. Ineffective regulation of granulopoiesis masquerading as congenital leukemia in a mongoloid child. J Pediatr 1963;63:1.

113. Sansone R, Haupt R, Strigini P, et al. Congenital leukemia: Persistent spontaneous regression in a patient with an acquired karyotype. Acta Haematol 1989;81: 48.

114. Seibel NL, Sommer A, Miser J. Transient neonatal leukemoid reactions in mosaic trisomy 21. J Pediatr 1984; 104:251.

115. Seo IS, McGuire WA, Heerema NA, et al. Congenital monoblastic leukemia cutis: A case report with chromosomal abnormality: del (10p). Am J Pediatr Hematol Oncol. 1986;8(2):158.

116. Sharief N, Kingston JE, Wright VM, et al. Acute leukemia in an infant with Marfan's syndrome: A case report. Pediatr Hematol Oncol 1991;8:323.

117. Siegel SE, Moran RG. Problems in chemotherapy of cancer in the neonate. Am J Pediat Hematol/Oncol 1981;3:287.

117a. Singer DB. The haematopoietic system. *In* Wigglesworth JS, Singer DB (eds): Textbook of Fetal and Perinatal Pathology, Vol 2, p 1283. Boston: Blackwell Scientific Publications, 1991.

118. Spier CM, Kjeldsberg CR, O'Brien R, et al. Pre-B cell acute lymphoblastic leukemia in the newborn. Blood 1984;64:1064.

119. Stark B, Umiel B, Mammon Z, et al. Leukemia of early infancy: Early B-cell lineage associated with t(4;11). Cancer 1986;58:1265.

120. Umiel T, Nadler LM, Cohen IJ, et al. Undifferentiated leukemia of infancy with t(11;17) chromosomal rearrangement: Coexpressing myeloid and B cell restricted antigens. Cancer 1987;59:1143.

121. VanEys J, Flexner JM. Transient spontaneous remission in a case of untreated congenital leukemia. Am J Dis Child 1969;118:507.

122. Voelkerding KV, Sandhaus LM, Belov L, et al. Clonal B-cell proliferation in an infant with congenital HIV infection and immune thrombocytopenia. Am J Clin Pathol 1988;90:470.

123. Warrier RP, Ravindranath Y, Inoue S, et al. Congenital leukemia: Two transient regressions without treatment in one patient. Pediatrics 1983;72:916.

124. Weinberger MM, Oleinick A. Congenital marrow dysfunction in Down's syndrome. J Pediatr 77:273,1970.

125. Weinstein HJ. Congenital leukemia and the neonatal myeloproliferative disorders associated with Down's syndrome. Clin Hematol 1978;7:147.

126. Whitfield MF, Barr DGD, O'Riordan ML. C-trisomy in a case of neonatal leukaemia. Arch Dis Child 1980; 55:551.

127. Willis RA. The Borderland of Embryology and Pathology, 2nd ed. London: Butterworths, 1962.

128. Windebank KP, Tefferi A, Smithson WA, et al. Acute megakaryocytic leukemia (M7) in children. Mayo Clin Proc 1989;64:1339.

129. Wolk JA, Stuart MJ, Davey FR, Nelson DA. Congenital and neonatal leukemia—Lymphocytic or myelocytic? Am J Dis Child 1974;128:864.

130. Wong KY, Jones MM, Srivastava AK, et al. Transient myeloproliferative disorder and acute nonlymphoblastic leukemia in Down syndrome. J Pediatr 1988; 112:18.

131. Woods WG, Rolof JF, Lukens JN. The occurrence of leukemia in patients with the Schwachman syndrome. J Pediatr 1981;99:425.

132. Yeazel MW, Buckley JD, Woods WG, et al. History of maternal fetal loss and increased risk of childhood acute leukemia at an early age: A report from the Children's Cancer Group. Cancer 1995;75:1718.

133. Zerres K, Schwanitz G, Niesen M, et al. Prenatal diagnosis of acute non-lymphoblastic leukemia in Down syndrome. Lancet 1990;335:117.

134. Zipursky A, Poon A, Doyle J. Leukemia in Down syndrome: A review. Pediatr Hematol Oncol 1992;9:139.

8

HISTIOCYTOSES

The histiocytoses represent a spectrum of conditions characterized by the infiltration and accumulation of cells of the monophagocytic system within the blood and tissues. They are a diverse group of disorders ranging from cytologically benign proliferations of mature cells to clearly malignant entities, such as acute monocytic leukemia and histiocytic lymphoma (Table 8–1). Lymphocytes may be a part of the proliferative process to a variable extent. Each of the histiocytic disorders may present with overlapping clinical and pathologic findings, making diagnosis difficult in some instances.[28,36,44,45,94,145,152,162]

Not all diseases in which histiocytic infiltrates occur are classified as histiocytoses. The infiltrates may represent a secondary process or a reaction to a condition with a known etiology. Mycobacterial infections, histoplasmosis, graft-versus-host disease, chronic granulomatous disease of childhood, the X-linked lymphoproliferative syndrome, and the lysosomal storage diseases are a few examples.[36,45,94]

ORIGIN AND FUNCTIONS OF CELLS OF THE MONOPHAGOCYTIC SYSTEM

The following discussion of the origin and functions of the cells of the monophagocytic system may be helpful in achieving a better understanding of histiocytoses. The monocyte is the precursor of the macrophage and of related phagocytic cells that comprise what was previously called the reticuloendothelial system and is now designated as the mononuclear phagocyte system. Cells of the monocytic and granulocytic series originate from a common bone marrow progenitor cell. Within the marrow, the monocyte matures through several stages from the monoblast, the promonocyte, and then the monocyte. The normal bone marrow contains 1% to 3% monocytes and their precursors.[45,94,162]

When a monocyte leaves the blood and enters the tissues, it becomes a wandering macrophage (histiocyte), subsequently undergoing further differentiation to form a variety of mononuclear phagocytic cells known by various names depending on their tissue location. For example, they become Kupffer cells in the liver, alveolar macrophages in the lung, sinus macrophages in the spleen, and Langerhans cells in the skin. Macrophages that have accumulated at a site of chronic inflammation—for example, in a tuberculous lymph node—can differentiate further into epithelioid histiocytes, or they may fuse to form multinucleated giant cells. Moreover, macrophages can divide in tissues.[45,94,162]

The properties and function of macrophages vary according to their location. Primarily, they are responsible for ingestion and killing of microorganisms. They have cytoplasmic granules composed of lysosomes, which contain hydrolytic enzymes, the antibacterial enzyme lysozyme and Fc receptors for antigen-antibody complexes. Following exposure to antigens (e.g., of an invading microorganism), T lymphocytes liberate lymphokines (soluble factors), such as interferon, which activate or assist the macrophage in disposing of the invader. Macrophages process antigen for presentation to lymphocytes in immune responses, thus initiating antibody formation. Moreover, activated macrophages secrete cytokines having important biological functions. For example, interleukin 1 plays a role in cell activation and in

Table 8–1. Histiocyte Disorders of the Fetus and Newborn

Langerhans cell histiocytosis
  Disseminated
  Focal
  Pure cutaneous histiocytosis (Hashimoto-Pritzker syndrome)
Familial erythrophagocytic lymphohistiocytosis
Infection with or without the infection-associated (reactive) hemophagocytic syndrome
  Viral
  Bacterial
  Fungal
  Parasitic
Acute monocytic leukemia
Malignant histiocytosis*
Histiocytic lymphoma*
Sinus histiocytosis with massive lymphadenopathy (Rosai-Dorfman disease)
Chronic granulomatous disease of childhood
Graft-versus-host disease
Omenn disease
X-linked lymphoproliferative syndrome (Duncan's disease)
Chédiak-Higashi syndrome (accelerated phase)
Lysosomal storage diseases (e.g., Gaucher's disease, Niemann-Pick disease, fucosidosis)
Juvenile xanthogranuloma

*Rarely occurs in the newborn.

the body's febrile reaction, whereas the tumor necrosis factor participates in host defense against tumor growth. Macrophages clear from the blood effete erythrocytes, noxious substances, and cellular debris as they pass through organs of the monophagocytic system (e.g., the liver and spleen).[45,94,162]

Based on their function, cells of the mononuclear phagocytic system are divided into two main groups: phagocytic cells (antigen processing cells) and dendritic cells (antigen presenting cells) (Table 8–2).[10,98,151,159,162]

CLASSIFICATION

The childhood histiocytoses have been classified by an international group, The Histiocyte Society,[162] into three main classes or categories according to their histopathologic characteristics (Table 8–3). Class I includes the Langerhans cell histiocytosis group, previously called histiocytosis X (Letterer-Siwe disease, Hand-Schüller-Christian syndrome, eosinophilic granuloma), self-healing histiocytosis, pure cutaneous histiocytosis, Langerhans cell granulomatosis and, "nonlipid reticuloendotheliosis." Disorders of the non-Langerhans histiocytes—namely, familial erythrophagocytic lymphohistiocytosis and the infection-associated hemophagocytic syndrome—have been designated as class II histiocytoses. Class III histiocytoses include true malignant diseases of mononuclear phagocytes: acute monocytic leukemia, malignant histiocytosis, and histiocytic lymphoma. This category represents a local or disseminated clonal proliferation of neoplastic mononuclear phagocytes (Table 8–3).[94,152,162]

Histiocytoses occurring in the newborn include Langerhans cell histiocytosis, familial erythrophagocytic lymphohistiocytosis, acute monocytic leukemia, and infection-associated hemophagocytic syndrome.[29,35,78,114,131] Malignant histiocytosis and histiocytic lymphoma are seldom described.[69,74]

LANGERHANS CELL HISTIOCYTOSIS

Langerhans cell histiocytosis is the term now applied to the older generic one, histiocytosis X, which included the clinical triad of Letterer-Siwe disease, Hand-Schüller-Christian syndrome, and eosinophilic granuloma.[57,100,127,145,162] Histologically, all three conditions are characterized by granuloma-like lesions composed of Langerhans histiocytes.[9,44–46,71,72,76,115,130] Although it behaves as a malignant disease, particularly in the young, Langerhans cell histiocytosis generally is not regarded as a true neoplasm, but instead is considered to be a

Table 8–2. Classification of the Monophagocytic Cell System Based on Function

Phagocytic Cells (Antigen-Processing Cells)	**Dendritic Cells (Antigen-Presenting Cells)**
Monocytes	Langerhans cell (skin)
Tissue macrophages	Dendritic cell (lymph node follicle)
Tingible body macrophages (lymph node follicle)	Interdigitating reticulum cell (lymph node paracortex)
Sinusoidal histiocytes	Epithelioid histiocytes

Modified from Ladisch S, Jaffe ES. The histiocytoses. *In* Pizzo PA, Poplack DG (eds): Principles and Practice of Pediatric Oncology, 2nd ed, p 617. Philadelphia: JB Lippincott, 1993. Used by permission.

Table 8–3. Histiocyte Society Classification of the Childhood Histiocytoses

---

Class I

Langerhans cell histiocytosis (formerly known as histiocytosis X—Letterer-Siwe disease, Hand-Schüller-Christian syndrome, and eosinophilic granuloma)

Pure cutaneous histiocytosis, Hashimoto-Pritzker syndrome

Class II

Familial erythrophagocytic lymphohistiocytosis

Infection-associated (reactive) hemophagocytic syndrome

Class III

Acute monocytic leukemia

Malignant histiocytosis

Histiocytic lymphoma

From Writing Group of the Histiocyte Society. Histiocytosis syndromes in children. Lancet 1987;1:208. © by The Lancet Ltd, 1987. Used by permission.

disorder of immune regulation.[22,45,94] However, a recent study questions this idea and suggests that this histiocytosis may be a neoplastic rather than a reactive process.[59]

The Langerhans cell is a member of the monophagocytic system originating from the bone marrow and migrating primarily to the skin and to other organs. It is one of three types of dendritic cells occurring in the epidermis in addition to the melanocyte and the indeterminate dendritic cell[99] (see Table 8–2). The Langerhans cell is found also in extracutaneous sites, such as the lymph nodes, thymus, oral mucosa, and vagina. Normally, it functions in the processing of antigens (e.g., those of viruses, bacteria, and tumor cells) coming into contact with the skin, and in the presentation of antigens to T lymphocytes.[16,163] In contrast to normal controls, Langerhans cell histiocytes from lesions of patients with disseminated Langerhans cell histiocytosis are unable to present alloantigens to T cells in vitro.[163]

Incidence

The Third National Cancer Survey showed that the annual incidence of Langerhans cell histiocytosis is 0.6 cases per million children younger than 15 years of age.[45,54] The male:female ratio is 2:1. Less than 50 new cases per year occur in France, according to the French Registry.[152] Disseminated Langerhans cell histiocytosis (Letterer-Siwe disease, disseminated histiocytosis X) begins before birth or within the first year of life.[121] Of 77 children with the diagnosis of Langerhans cell histiocytosis at Children's Hospital, Los Angeles, 19 (25%) were younger than 1 year of age at the time of diagnosis, and one case was congenital; this entity accounted for 19 (7%) of 265 various neoplasms and tumor-like conditions of infants.[71]

Congenital Langerhans cell histiocytosis is uncommon.[1,30,67,71,72,81,116,157] According to Dehner, 2% to 15% of children with Langerhans cell histiocytosis have manifestations in the first month of life.[35] Nezelof collected 50 examples of disseminated Langerhans cell histiocytosis over a 27-year period; 8 cases (16%) occurred in newborns.[116] Three of 127 (2.4%) were neonates in the Children's Hospital Medical Center Boston series.[57] In a later study from Children's Hospital, Los Angeles, 2 of 84 cases (2.4%) were congenital.[72] The Cincinnati Children's Hospital series, which spanned the years 1940 to 1970, had an unusually high percentage of neonatal cases, numbering 9 of the total 42 (21%).[102] Jones and colleagues collected 15 congenital examples, including 3 of their own, pointing out that skin lesions are the first manifestation from birth, that the time interval before systemic symptoms occur varies, and that there is no difference in histology between the mild and severe cases.[81]

Langerhans cell histiocytosis is not often reported in stillborns. The stillborn male infant described by Ahnquist and Holyoke had widely distributed hemorrhagic, crusted, or scaling cutaneous nodules composed of proliferating histiocytes. Similar lesions were found also in the lungs, bronchi, liver, spleen, lymph nodes, thymus, and bones at necropsy.[1]

Clinical Findings

A familial occurrence of Langerhans cell histiocytosis has been documented in both monozygotic and dizygotic twins and in sibships.[14,54,81,83] The incidence of deaths among siblings with disseminated Langerhans cell histiocytosis is significant.[54]

There is an increased frequency of congenital anomalies, particularly those involving the central nervous system, in infants with Langerhans cell histiocytosis. Patients with Langerhans cell histiocytosis who have congenital anomalies have an increased chance of developing fatal organ dysfunction during the course of their disease.[142] The findings of Glass and Miller show that most deaths occur in patients younger than 2 years of age, and their findings in five sets of siblings with the disease, including one pair of twins, suggest that the disease has prenatal origins.[54]

Disseminated Langerhans cell histiocytosis, formerly known as Letterer-Siwe disease or disseminated histiocytosis X, is the generalized form affecting primarily infants and children younger than 2 years of age. It is defined as involvement of two or more organ systems. The peak incidence of the disseminated histiocytosis is during the first 6 months of life.[13,115] The initial clinical manifestation, which already may be apparent at birth, is a seborrheic, eczematoid, and occasionally hemorrhagic rash distributed over the scalp, face, abdomen, and diaper areas (see Fig. 5–11). Subsequently, hepatosplenomegaly, lymphadenopathy, and general "failure to thrive" become evident. Hematologic studies reveal an anemia, a variable leukocytosis, abnormal clotting factors, and thrombocytopenia, all of which portend a poor prognosis.[21] Imaging studies reveal pulmonary infiltrates, which become more extensive as the disease progresses. Histiocytes are readily identified in bronchoalveolar lavage fluid with immunostaining an electron microscopy.[152] Skeletal surveys show punched-out lesions in the skull and long bones (Fig. 18–4). The diagnosis can be definitively established by a skin or lymph node biopsy.[20,36,72] Usually, the bone marrow is involved at the time of diagnosis.

Delayed umbilical cord separation is one of the ominous signs in the newborn with Langerhans cell histiocytosis.[52] The association between delayed cord separation, bacterial sepsis, and impaired neutrophil function is known.[64] Symptomatic involvement of the gastrointestinal tract occurs in disseminated Langerhans cell histiocytosis and is manifested by diarrhea and a protein-losing enteropathy. This fatal complication is described also in newborns.[18,77] According to Siegal and associates, Langerhans cell histiocytosis first appearing in the thymus is associated with a more favorable prognosis.[146] Four patients, the youngest of whom was a 2-month-old boy, presented with stridor and respiratory distress and an anterosuperior mediastinal mass detected on chest roentgenography.[146] All four patients survived after various forms of therapy.

Pathology

The gross appearance of Langerhans cell histiocytosis varies with the site and the age of the lesion. Specimens curetted from bones are soft, red, hemorrhagic, and necrotic. When visible, soft, grayish yellow to red, granuloma-like nodules, which are usually multiple, are found in the liver, spleen, and lymph nodes. Older lesions are firmer because of fibrosis and are tan-yellow instead of grayish-red owing to the presence of numerous foamy histiocytes.

The Langerhans cell has a characteristic infolded or coffee bean–shaped nucleus, small nucleolus, and eosinophilic cytoplasm (Fig. 8–1A, B, and C). Some lesions show nuclear atypia and mitotic figures, but these findings do not correlate with prognosis.[130] Extensive infiltration of histiocytes and, occasionally, eosinophils are the typical histologic findings. Histiocytic erythrophagocytosis is seldom noted.

The Langerhans cell histiocyte has distinctly different immunohistochemical and ultrastructural properties than the normal monocyte and macrophage.[10,45,61,94,135,162] The histiocytes are reactive with S-100 protein and CD1 (OKT6) surface antigen (Fig. 8–1D). CD2 and CD3 markers are positive, which is not found in normal Langerhans cell histiocytes. Reactivity with placental alkaline phosphatase, a proliferation marker Ki-S1, and a nuclear antigen Ki-67 were demonstrated by Hage et al.[59] According to these investigators, Ki-S1 and Ki-67 are indicators of neoplastic proliferation. Staining with peanut agglutinin is a useful technique for the detection of monocytes of the monophagocytic system. Langerhans cells (both normal and histiocytic cells) show a circumferential, paranuclear cytoplasmic staining, whereas diffuse cytoplasmic staining is found in other types of histiocytes.[45,126]

On ultrastructural analysis, the cytoplasm of the Langerhans histiocyte contains characteristic racket-shaped Birbeck granules, which are requisite for the diagnosis (Fig. 8–1F).[15,46,145] The significance and function of these structures is unknown. Sometimes, the granules are difficult to find, and multiple thin sections may be required. The granules are observed also in Langerhans cells, which are normally present in the epidermis but not in the intermediate dendritic cells or melanocytes.[28,99] Hashimoto and Pritzker described myelinated laminated and nonmyelinated dense bodies, in addition to Birbeck granules, in a patient with congenital self-healing Langerhans cell histiocytosis.[62,63]

Skin and bone are the tissues most often involved at the time of presentation.[106,116,127,133] In the skin, the histiocytes are situated primarily in the dermis, directly beneath the epidermal-dermal junction. Characteristically, they invade

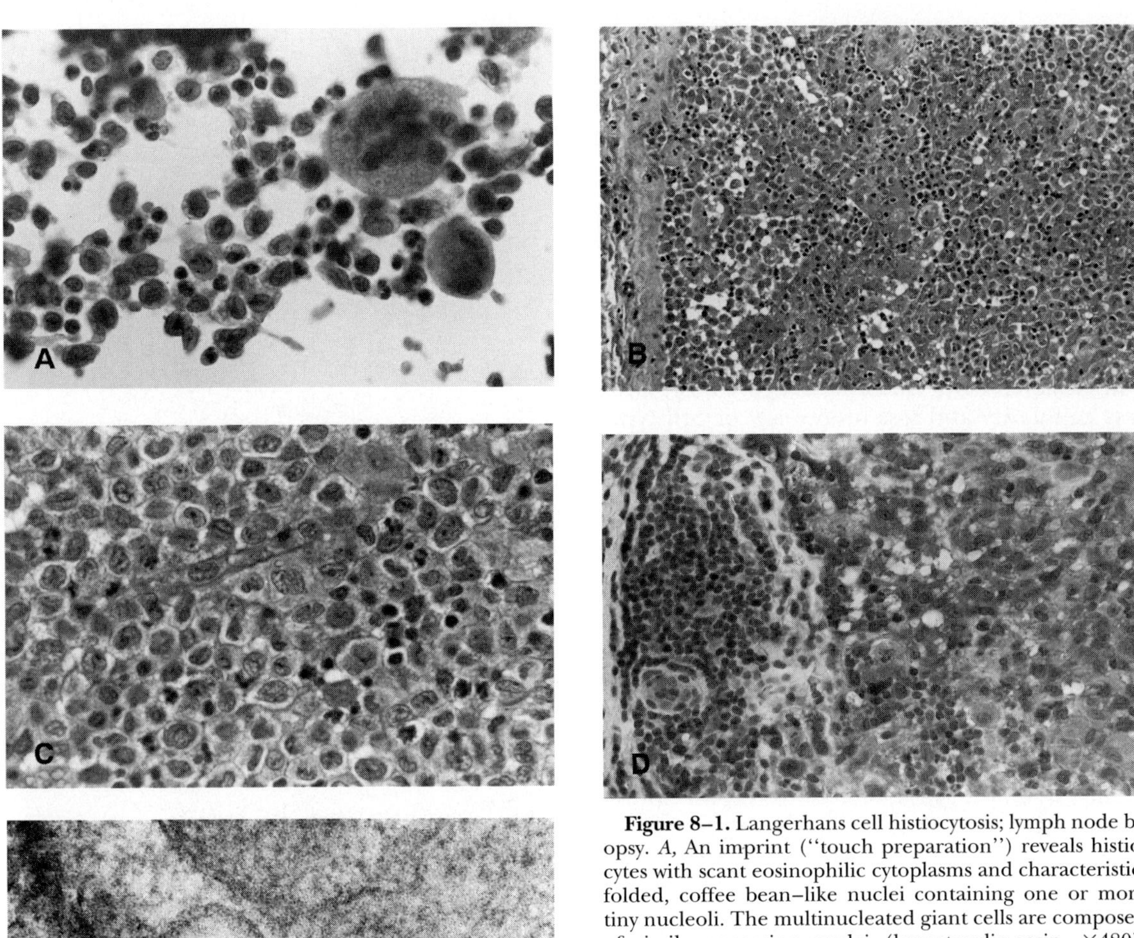

Figure 8–1. Langerhans cell histiocytosis; lymph node biopsy. *A,* An imprint (''touch preparation'') reveals histiocytes with scant eosinophilic cytoplasms and characteristic, folded, coffee bean–like nuclei containing one or more tiny nucleoli. The multinucleated giant cells are composed of similar-appearing nuclei (hematoxylin-eosin, ×480). *B,* Histiocytes are seen to be flooding the subcapsular and cortical sinusoids (hematoxylin-eosin, ×150). *C,* A higher-power view shows the histiocytes in greater detail (hematoxylin-eosin, ×480). *D,* The cytoplasms stain uniformly positive with S-100 protein (S-100, ×300). *E,* A tennis racket–shaped Birbeck granule is demonstrated by electron microscopy (×28,500). (Electron photomicrograph courtesy of Ann Peters, Children's Hospital, San Diego, CA.)

the epidermis and extend into the stratum corneum (see Fig. 5–11*B*). The differential diagnosis of cutaneous infiltrates in the newborn includes leukemia cutis, extramedullary hematopoiesis, urticaria pigmentosa (mast cell disease), metastatic rhabdomyosarcoma, and neuroblastoma (see Table 5–2).[73]

Skeletal surveys reveal lytic lesions involving the skull, ribs, pelvis, and occasionally, the long bones and vertebrae.[139] In most instances, a solitary lesion occurring in the skull or other bone is a self-limited process, even in the young, and is cured by excision and curettage (see Fig. 18–4). The lesions that are removed show granu-loma-like collections of Langerhans cell histiocytes and multinucleated giant cells, extensive necrosis with destruction of bone, eosinophilic ''abscesses,'' and variable numbers of lymphocytes and plasma cells. By contrast, older, ''end-stage,'' or healing lesions contain histiocytic foam cells that are nonreactive for S-100 protein and fibrosis and, therefore, may resemble a xanthofibroma (benign fibrous histiocytoma).

Solitary osseous lesions rarely herald the onset of soft tissue and visceral involvement and a fatal outcome. Moreover, infants with multiple bone lesions may survive.[71,106,127] Hand-Schüller-Christian syndrome is a clinical manifestation of multifocal Langerhans cell histiocytosis, involving primarily the cranial bones and adjacent structures, including the pituitary. The syndrome is very uncommon; indeed, only a few patients, usually older infants and children, actually fulfill the diagnostic criteria of exophthalmos, diabetes insipidus, and histiocytic infiltrates in membrane bone.[6] Exophthalmos results from a space-occupying histiocytic lesion in the orbit, and otitis media with drainage is the sequela of destructive infiltrates in the mastoid and petrous portion of the temporal bone. The lesions tend to be less aggressive, with less cellularity and less monotony of cell type, than in Letterer-Siwe disease, but they exhibit greater fibrosis and evidence of healing.[121] The clinical course is usually protracted, and the mortality is much less (approximately half) than that observed for the disseminated disease. The least aggressive of the three forms—eosinophilic granuloma—typically occurs in a single bone, but may be found in adolescents and adults in the skin and lungs.[6,121]

Infiltration of the pulmonary interlobular septae and alveolar spaces produces airway obstruction and, eventually, the formation of cystically dilated, emphysematous areas. Moreover, Langerhans cell histiocyte infiltration of the lungs is a significant cause of death, particularly in young infants (Fig. 8–2).[72,157] In the lymph nodes, the histiocytic infiltrate replaces and obscures the normal architecture (see Fig. 8–1). The splenic red pulp is heavily infiltrated, but the white pulp and trabeculae usually are spared. Bone marrow elements are replaced by Langerhans cell histiocytes. Granuloma-like infiltrates are found in the pancreas, gonads, liver, and salivary glands, and sometimes, in the brain and meninges.[71,72,97,121] The liver findings consist of variable degrees of periportal and sinusoidal histiocytic infiltration and fibrosis; later in the course of the disease, the lesions progress to focal biliary cirrhosis.[68,97]

A pure cutaneous form of Langerhans cell histiocytosis, also known as self-healing histiocytosis or the Hashimoto-Pritzker syndrome, is usually congenital and is associated with a good prognosis.[19,20,31,37,62,63,86,105,123,161] Surprisingly, the skin lesions, which may be extensive, undergo rapid and spontaneous regression. Ultrastructural and immunohistochemical properties of the histiocytes from patients with congenital self-healing histiocytosis are similar to both normal epidermal Langerhans cells and Langerhans histiocytosis cells.[86] Two types of histiocytes have been described, one with and one

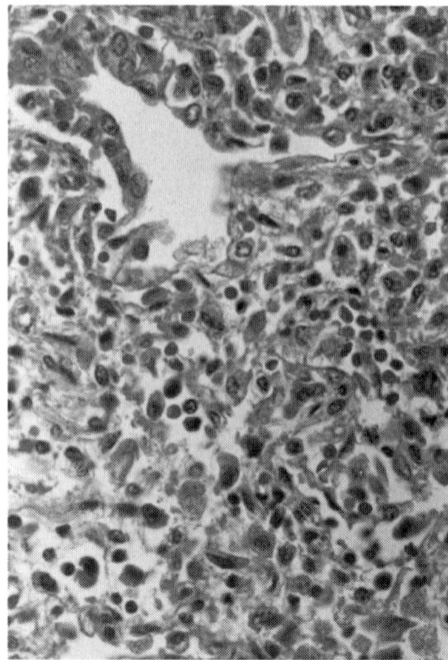

Figure 8–2. Disseminated Langerhans cell histiocytosis (Letterer-Siwe disease) involving the lung. A 5-day-old female infant with a maternal history of polyhydramnios, maculopapular rash, and severe respiratory distress. Alveoli are diffusely infiltrated by histiocytes (hematoxylin-eosin, ×380). Pulmonary involvement is an important cause of death in newborns and infants with this disease.

without Birbeck granules.[19] However, patients with self-healing histiocytosis should be monitored carefully for progression of disease.[105]

Examples of congenital "self-healing non-Langerhans cell histiocytosis" have been described, with clinical and pathologic findings practically identical to the syndrome with Langerhans histiocytes.[118,143,158] However, the histiocytes in the former react positively to Leu-M3, lysozyme, and HLA-DR, negatively to Leu-6, and variably to S-100 protein, and lack Birbeck granules by electron microscopy.

Prognosis

The clinical outcome cannot be predicted from the histologic appearance alone.[9,46,71,130] The clinical findings, particularly the age of the patient and extent of organ involvement at the time of diagnosis, are the most reliable indicators for predicting prognosis.[6,57,94,95,102,116,130,133] Lahey reports that the degree of organ dysfunction is more important than the number of organs involved.[95] Bone marrow involvement at the time of diagnosis is associated with an unfavorable outcome.[109]

Patients with disseminated Langerhans cell histiocytosis with multiple sites of involvement and organ dysfunction have a poor prognosis, with a survival rate of less than 40%.[127] Those who fall into this category are usually younger than 1 year of age and account for less than 15% of the total number of cases.[94] The overall mortality rate of children younger than 2 years of age at diagnosis is reported to be 50% to 60%, whereas that of children older than 2 years of age decreases to 15%. In an early Cincinnati Children's Hospital study (1940–1970), 7 of 9 (77%) newborns died.[102] Of 50 childhood cases of disseminated Langerhans cell histiocytosis included in the study by Nezelof et al., 8 (16%) were congenital and 50% survived.[116] In the fatal cases, death occurred between 20 days and 3.5 years of age. In a later study at the Children's Hospital of Philadelphia, 6 of 9 infants with disseminated disease died.[127]

Apparently, the form of therapy has little effect on the course of the disease and, in fact, can actually be detrimental in some instances.[22,46,57] There is no proven effective treatment; chemotherapy suppresses, but does not eradicate, the process.[46,127] Bone marrow transplantation has been attempted in some cases.[152] Because patients whose disease disappears over time usually survive even if another lesion appears later, a course of "watchful waiting" is advised before initiating potentially harmful therapeutic measures.[127]

FAMILIAL ERYTHROPHAGOCYTIC LYMPHOHISTIOCYTOSIS

In 1952, Farquhar and Claireaux reported a rapidly fatal disease in two siblings that was associated with fever, hepatosplenomegaly, and pancytopenia, which they termed "familial hemophagocytic reticulosis."[43] Ten years later, MacMahon and co-workers described two siblings with an identical disease and suggested the term "familial erythrophagocytic lymphohistiocytosis."[104] Subsequently, additional cases have appeared in the literature.[2,4,47,48,53,55,56,58,60,78–80,110,113,119,120,148,149,152,160] The German/Austrian Registry for Histiocytic Disorders reports an annual incidence of 1 per million children younger than 15 years of age.[80] The disease occurs primarily in infants and young children. Most are younger than 6 months of age at the time of diagnosis, and 10% to 15% are neonates.[53,80]

Familial hemophagocytic lymphohistiocytosis is a disorder of unknown etiology that affects the monophagocytic system. An underlying immunodeficiency has been proposed.[93] The disease has an autosomal recessive pattern of inheritance, but at least 25% of the cases are nonfamilial.[4,43,53,78,104,147] Nonspecific chromosomal abnormalities have been described in association with it.[90]

Clinical Findings

The classical presenting signs are fever, hepatosplenomegaly, and pancytopenia.[78,79] Other manifestations of this rare and usually fatal disease are irritability, anorexia, wasting, and failure to thrive. Hepatic dysfunction and bleeding diathesis are frequently present.[141,142] Typically, there is a short period of normal development and absence of symptoms after birth; however, fever or hepatomegaly may already be evident at birth.[32,38,78,79,91,92]

Stupor, or coma, and seizures with hemiplegia and cranial nerve palsies are the neurologic signs.[2,122,129] The onset of nervous system involvement heralds progression of the disease, which is reflected by an elevated cerebrospinal fluid protein level and pleocytosis.[2,4] In addition, laboratory studies reveal hypofibrinogenemia and hypertriglyceridemia.[3,44,66,78,93,94,110,162] Thrombocytopenia is accompanied by severe bleeding, and the granulocytic series may show maturational arrest.[104,147] The triad of elevated triglyceride levels, increased liver enzyme values, and low fibrinogen levels suggests the diagnosis.[79]

Frequently, the diagnosis of familial hemophagocytic lymphohistiocytosis is difficult to establish during life; it may be apparent only from postmortem findings, after which a family history of a sibling with a similar disease may be discovered.[78] In one study, 6 of 26 (23%) infants were diagnosed at necropsy.[79]

Pathology

The histopathologic hallmark of this disease is extensive lymphohistiocytic infiltration and erythrophagocytosis within the liver, spleen, lymph nodes, bone marrow, and leptomeninges (Fig. 8–3).[43,55,60,78,79,97,104,113,119,120,145] The spleen and liver are massively enlarged, up to 10 times and 2 times their normal size, respectively. Thymic involution and depletion of lymphoid tissue in lymph nodes and spleen are characteristic findings. Pulmonary infiltration is predominantly centrilobular, peribronchial,

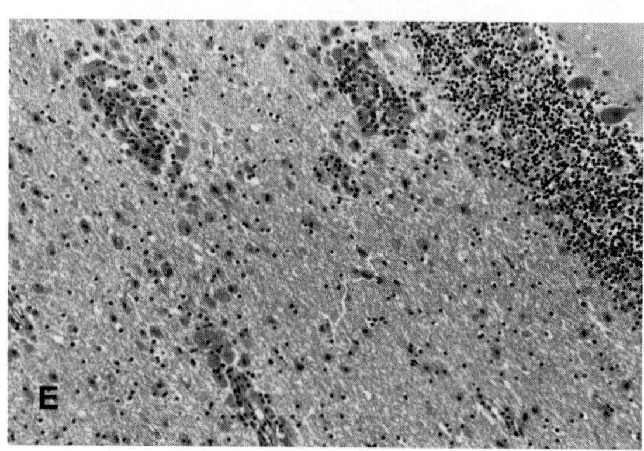

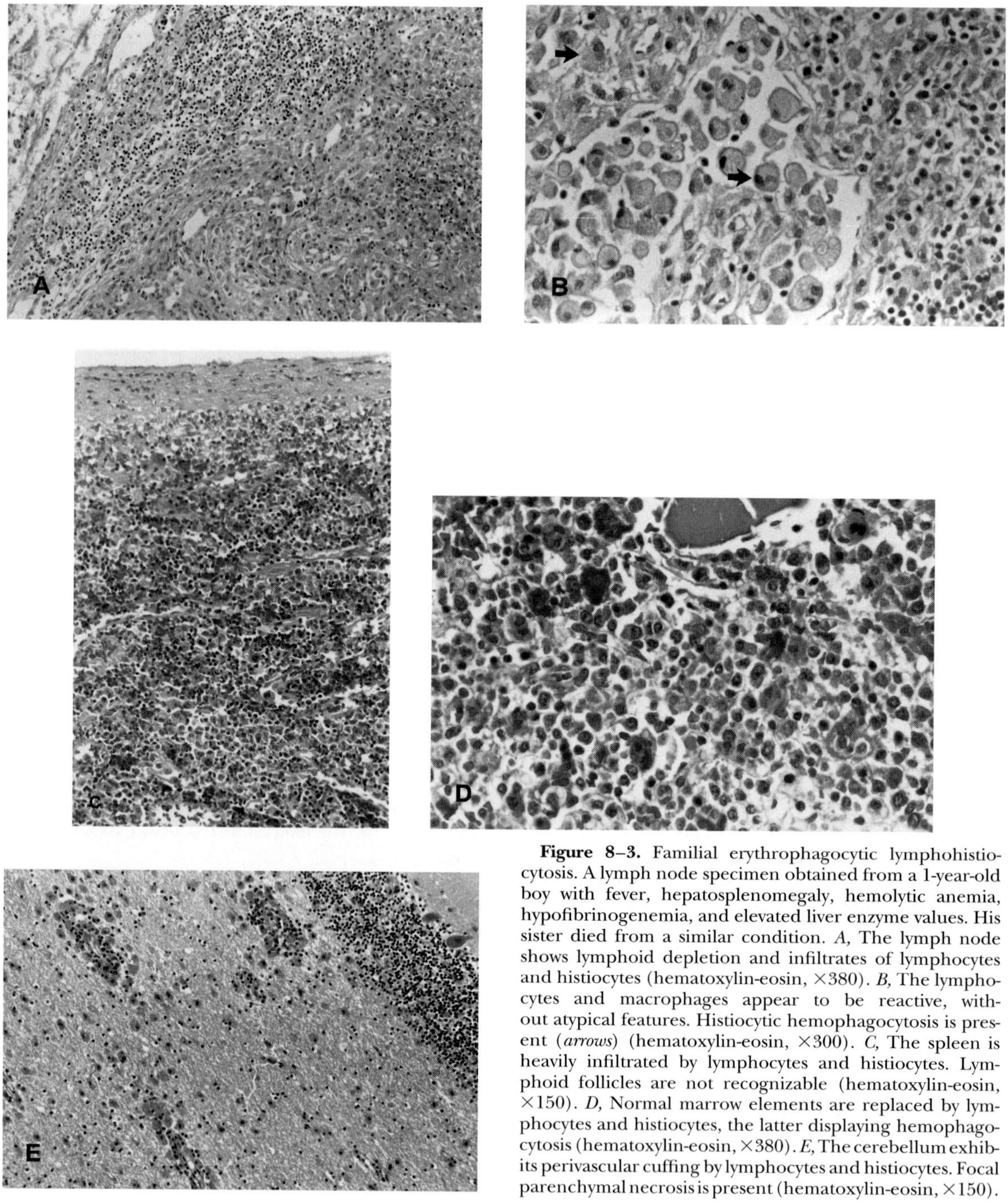

Figure 8–3. Familial erythrophagocytic lymphohistiocytosis. A lymph node specimen obtained from a 1-year-old boy with fever, hepatosplenomegaly, hemolytic anemia, hypofibrinogenemia, and elevated liver enzyme values. His sister died from a similar condition. _A,_ The lymph node shows lymphoid depletion and infiltrates of lymphocytes and histiocytes (hematoxylin-eosin, ×380). _B,_ The lymphocytes and macrophages appear to be reactive, without atypical features. Histiocytic hemophagocytosis is present (_arrows_) (hematoxylin-eosin, ×300). _C,_ The spleen is heavily infiltrated by lymphocytes and histiocytes. Lymphoid follicles are not recognizable (hematoxylin-eosin, ×150). _D,_ Normal marrow elements are replaced by lymphocytes and histiocytes, the latter displaying hemophagocytosis (hematoxylin-eosin, ×380). _E,_ The cerebellum exhibits perivascular cuffing by lymphocytes and histiocytes. Focal parenchymal necrosis is present (hematoxylin-eosin, ×150).

and perivascular in location.[97] Popper et al. described an unusual interstitial pneumonia with hemophagocytic histiocytes and lymphocytes.[120] The submucosa of the tracheal and major bronchi show extensive involvement. Many different organs are affected.[53,97,113]

The main neuropathologic finding is focal or diffuse leptomeningeal lymphohistiocytic infiltration with erythrophagocytosis.[2] The arachnoid, choroid plexus, and Virchow-Robin perivascular spaces are affected in about one third to one half of the cases.[2,53,78,97,104,113,129,141] Perivascular cuffing with extension of lymphocytes and histiocytes into the adjacent cerebral or cerebellar cortex and brain stem can also occur (Fig. 8–3*E*). Diffuse cerebral infiltration by histiocytes and multifocal necrosis are found in the most severely involved brains.[2] The severity of the central nervous system lesions seems to be related to the duration of the illness.[2] The brain is affected much more than the rest of the body in some patients.[2,122]

The histiocytes and lymphocytes within the infiltrates appear to be reactive but show no cellular atypia, abnormal mitotic activity, or other evidence of a malignant process. Histiocytic phagocytosis of erythrocytes and, sometimes, of lymphocytes and platelets is a characteristic finding. The proliferative histiocytes in familial erythrophagocytic lymphohistiocytosis have immunohistochemical and ultrastructural properties of normal, reactive histiocytes. They are positive for OKT9, OKM1, and HLA-DR, but lack the S-100 protein, T6 surface antigen, and Birbeck granules that are characteristic of Langerhans cell histiocytes.[55,60,160] Ultrastructural studies confirm the reactive nature of the histiocytes and lymphocytes and the absence of Birbeck granules.[53,160]

A diagnostic biopsy examination of an enlarged lymph node is recommended. The findings of lymphohistiocytic infiltrates, hemophagocytosis, and lymphoid depletion suggest the diagnosis.[78] However, it should be kept in mind that these findings are rather nonspecific, and hemophagocytosis is present also in a variety of other conditions, including infections, hemolytic anemia, graft-versus-host disease, and malignant histiocytosis. Lymphohistiocytic infiltrates with lymphoid depletion are found also in infection-associated hemophagocytosis, the X-linked lymphoproliferative syndrome, and the accelerated phase of Chédiak-Higashi syndrome.[17,79,124,131]

Langerhans cell histiocytosis, leukemia, nonspecific inflammation, and extramedullary hematopoiesis should be considered in the histologic differential diagnosis as well.[79]

Prognosis

Familial erythrophagocytic lymphohistiocytosis is nearly always a rapidly fatal disorder, with death occurring within 3 to 6 months of presentation. The cause of death is attributed to sepsis, bleeding, or central nervous system involvement.[47,48,53] No specific treatment has been found to improve the poor prognosis.[53,101]

Lymphohistiocytosis is a characteristic feature of the X-linked lymphoproliferative syndrome (Duncan's disease). The cause of this disease is believed to be an uncontrolled response of lymphocytes and histiocytes to infection by the Epstein-Barr virus.[97,125] Although the syndrome is present at birth, symptoms generally do not appear until later childhood. Less than 50% of the affected patients develop malignant lymphoma or fatal infectious mononucleosis.[53]

INFECTION-ASSOCIATED (REACTIVE) HEMOPHAGOCYTIC SYNDROME

Infection-associated hemophagocytic syndrome was first reported in 1979 by Risdall et al., who described a disease characterized by generalized histiocytic proliferation and hemophagocytosis associated with a systemic viral infection.[131] Cytomegalovirus, herpes simplex virus, adenovirus, and Epstein-Barr virus are the viral agents implicated.[26,34,107,131] The syndrome occurs also with other infections, such as bacterial, fungal, and parasitic infections.[5,24,84,88,111,131,154] For example, an association with congenital tuberculosis has been reported.[88] The syndrome occurs in immunocompromised and in normal individuals, but is more common in the former.[84,131] A comprehensive list of infections and the clinical, immunologic, and histopathologic findings in two infant siblings with the syndrome have been presented by Arya and colleagues.[5] Infection-associated hemophagocytic syndrome is probably the most common histiocytic disorder in the newborn, but it has been found to affect individuals of all ages, including adults.[131,144] Sometimes, the term ''reactive,'' rather than infection-associated, hemophagocytosis is used.[5]

The clinical manifestations of the infection-associated hemophagocytic syndrome are practically identical to those of the familial hemophagocytic lymphohistiocytosis, and include fever, failure to thrive, anemia, hepatosplenomegaly, and variable lymphadenomegaly.[5,94] Leukopenia, abnormal liver function tests, and a coagulopathy are the laboratory findings.[131] Bilateral pulmonary infiltrates are noted on chest roentgenograms.

Familial hemophagocytic lymphohistiocytosis is the entity that causes the greatest difficulty in the differential diagnosis.[79] In contrast to this disease, the infection-associated hemophagocytic syndrome usually is associated with under-

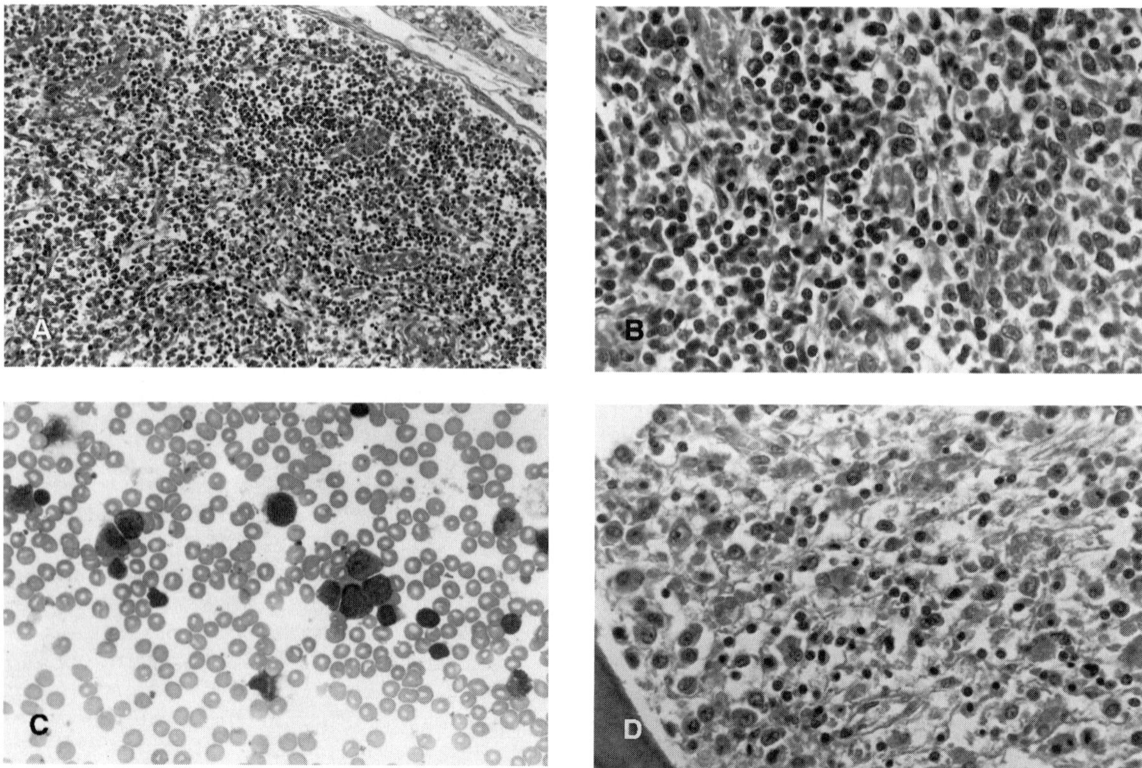

Figure 8–4. Infection-associated (reactive) hemophagocytosis. A 6-week-old female infant presented with fever, lethargy, vomiting, and diarrhea. Other findings included hepatosplenomegaly, anemia, thrombocytopenia, abnormal coagulation studies, and elevated liver enzyme values. *A,* Lymph node is replaced by lymphocytes and histiocytes (hematoxylin-eosin, ×150). *B,* The infiltrate is composed of reactive lymphocytes and histiocytes (hematoxylin-eosin, ×380). *C,* A postmortem bone marrow aspirate shows only lymphocytes and histiocytes (Wright-Giemsa, ×300). *D,* This section of rib lacks normal marrow elements. Lymphocytes and histiocytes, the latter with phagocytosed erythrocytes, comprise the cell population (hematoxylin-eosin, ×380).

lying immune deficiency (iatrogenic or otherwise), a proven infection with subsequent recovery in most instances, and usually, no family history. Some patients have been reported who were initially thought to have familial hemophagocytic lymphohistiocytosis, but in whom a viral agent was eventually recovered by tissue culture, electron microscopy, or by sensitive nucleic acid methods (e.g., hybridization with viral genome probes and polymerase chain reaction).[34,79,107] However, some researchers believe that the two diseases are essentially the same, and that the distinction between the two is superfluous.[108]

The diagnosis of infection-associated hemophagocytic syndrome is suggested by bone marrow examination. Bone marrow smears reveal prominent histiocytic hemophagocytosis (Fig. 8–4D).[26,111,131] The reactive-appearing histiocytes contain phagocytized erythrocytes and platelets. They show the cytologic, ultrastruc-

tural, and histochemical features of normal histiocytes, which is not the case in the Langerhans cell and class III malignant histiocytoses. Atypical lymphocytes (''virocytes'') and immunoblasts may be present as well. Atypical lymphocytes have large nuclei, prominent nucleoli, and a characteristic blue cytoplasm with white fluffy inclusions that give the cytoplasm a snow storm–like appearance. The peripheral blood smears exhibit varying degrees of cytopenia, with or without atypical lymphocytes. The lymph nodes and spleen are depleted of lymphoid elements, have typically ''burned-out'' germinal centers, and are infiltrated by hemophagocytic histiocytes (Fig. 8–4A).[94,111,131] Early in the disease, lymph nodes may show a florid, immunoblastic, proliferative response not unlike that observed initially in human immunodeficiency virus (HIV) infections. The liver biopsy reveals prominent portal infiltrates composed of lymphocytes, erythrophagocytic histiocytes, and sometimes, immunoblasts. If a viral or other infectious agent is found, then the diagnosis can be established with confidence.[5]

The postmortem findings in patients with infection-associated hemophagocytic syndrome have been described in the literature.[5,25–27,88,131] Reactive, benign-appearing histiocytes with erythrophagocytosis are found in the portal tracts and sinusoids of the liver, in the red pulp of the spleen, and within the leptomeninges. Focal hepatocellular necrosis is present. Interstitial pneumonia, with or without viral inclusions, constitutes the pulmonary findings. Cytomegalovirus inclusions appear in many organs of patients infected by the virus. Other infectious agents, such as acid-fast bacilli, have been identified in patients with this syndrome.[88]

At present, no specific treatment exists for infection-associated hemophagocytic syndrome.[94] In fact, it has been shown that the use of immunosuppressive therapy may be deleterious. Chemotherapy has been used when the diagnosis of infection-associated hemophagocytic syndrome was mistaken for malignant histiocytosis, monocytic leukemia, or histiocytic lymphoma, with undesirable results. Individuals presenting with symptoms of infection-associated hemophagocytic syndrome should be thoroughly investigated for evidence of a viral or other infection before therapy is begun. There are several case reports of patients with acute leukemia who died from a separate condition, considered to be a malignant histiocytosis; these patients were actually immunosuppressed following chemotherapy and subsequently developed the hemophagocytic syndrome.[27,87,131,150] Individuals with infection-associated hemophagocytic syndrome who do not have an underlying immunodeficiency and who do recover from their acute infection generally have a good prognosis.

SINUS HISTIOCYTOSIS WITH MASSIVE LYMPHADENOPATHY

The syndrome of sinus histiocytosis with massive lymphadenopathy was established as a clinicopathologic entity by Rosai and Dorfman in 1972.[134] They described a benign, chronic, massive enlargement of the cervical lymph nodes accompanied by fever, leukocytosis, and hyperglobulinemia. Since 1972, other articles on the subject have appeared.[23,42,49,50,153] The largest and most comprehensive review was presented by Fourcar, Rosai, and Dorfman, who analyzed 423 cases.[51] Less than 10 cases have been reported in the newborn and infant.[49]

The disease occurs in both children and adults, in identical twins and siblings, and is equally prevalent in blacks and in caucasians.[51] The most common presentation is cervical adenopathy, which is usually bilateral. Laboratory findings include a normochromic anemia, leukocytosis, lymphopenia, polyclonal hyperglobulinemia, and an elevated erythrocyte sedimentation rate. Approximately 10% of the patients with sinus histiocytosis with massive lymphadenopathy have an underlying immune defect, and almost 50% with this association die as a result of their immune status.[49]

Marked dilatation of lymph node sinusoids by collections of histiocytes and lymphocytes, with focal effacement of the nodal architecture, are the histologic findings. The histiocytes are benign-appearing, having abundant cytoplasm and regular nuclei. Leukocytophagocytosis (emperipolesis), whereby lymphocytes and plasma cells are phagocytized by histiocytes, is a distinguishing histologic feature that is essential for establishing the diagnosis. Reactive, vacuolated histiocytes, numerous plasma cells, and extensive fibrosis are present. The lesions are focally destructive and affect also extranodal sites, such as the nasal mucosa, salivary gland, orbit, skin, and bones.[23,42,50,51,153] The histiocytes are cytologically and immunohistochemically similar to normal histiocytes and macrophages.[42,59] In addition, placental alkaline phosphatase and S-100 protein are expressed by the histiocytes.[42,59]

Generally, patients with sinus histiocytosis with massive lymphadenopathy have a good prognosis. However, the course of the disease is often protracted, lasting 3 to 9 months, and significant morbidity and mortality can occur. Fourcar et al. analyzed the findings in 14 fatal cases, and although the cause of this syndrome remains unknown, an underlying immune defect has been suggested.[49] Treatment with cytotoxic agents and prednisone has been effective in controlling some of the complications.[153]

MALIGNANT HISTIOCYTOSES

The malignant histiocytoses are considered to be true neoplastic disorders of histiocytes. Malignant histiocytosis, acute monocytic leukemia, and histiocytic lymphoma are assigned to this group, which is classified as class III by the

Histiocyte Society (see Table 8–3).[162] Of the three, acute monocytic leukemia is the most common one in the newborn.

Malignant Histiocytosis

In 1966, Rappaport proposed the term "malignant histiocytosis" to depict a disease characterized by a disseminated, rapidly progressive, invasive process of proliferating malignant histiocytes.[128] It is a malignant disease of mononuclear phagocytes falling somewhere in the spectrum of differentiation between monocytes and monoblasts and fixed tissue histiocytes.[94] Frequently, the clinical and histologic findings of malignant histiocytosis and the other malignant histiocytoses overlap, so the distinction may be ill-defined, which accounts for the confusion in classifying these entities.[39,40,94,96,156] Malignant histiocytosis affects the whole monophagocytic system, particularly, the lymph nodes, liver, spleen, and bone marrow.[39,40,70] Skin, bone, and occasionally, the peripheral blood are additional sites of involvement.[39,75,137]

Malignant histiocytosis is a rare, nonfamilial disease that is usually found in adults. Most affected children are older than 5 years of age.[164] The clinical findings—fever, hepatosplenomegaly, lymphadenopathy, and pancytopenia—resemble those of familial erythrophagocytic lymphohistiocytosis and infection-associated hemophagocytic syndrome. Skin nodules having central ulcers representing tumor infiltrates are frequently present.

Children with this disease are the subject of only a few case reports, although malignant histiocytosis has been described in newborns and infants.[39,74,85,137] For example, the 11-month-old girl described by Di Sant'Agnese et al. had fever, a suprarenal abdominal mass, widespread metastases, and a terminal "leukemic phase."[39] The two infants depicted by Ishii et al. presented with respiratory distress, pleural effusions with malignant cells, and pulmonary infiltrates (in one).[74] The neonate reported by Schouten et al. was born with a maculopapillary rash and subsequently developed a leukemic blood pattern.[137]

Lymph node or liver biopsy is recommended to establish the diagnosis.[85,94,111] The former shows malignant histiocytes filling the sinusoids and invading the adjacent parenchyma, with effacement of the nodal architecture.[40,131] Liver biopsy reveals similar infiltrates, both in the sinusoids and portal tracts, forming nodular aggregates of histiocytes.[85] Either focal or diffuse infiltration is present in the bone marrow. The histiocytes display atypical cytologic features, in contrast to those characteristic of either familial erythrophagocytic lymphohistiocytosis or infection-associated hemophagocytic syndrome. The histiocytes have large, irregular nuclei with a reticular chromatin pattern, prominent nucleoli, and basophilic cytoplasm.[39,40,111,131] Characteristically, the histiocytes are found in all stages of maturation: malignant histiocytes, prohistiocytes, and well-differentiated histiocytes.[85,131] Erythrophagocytosis is present, but to a much lesser extent than in either of the two class II histiocytoses.

The tumor cells are reactive for nonspecific esterase, acid phosphatase, and HLA-DR antigen, but unreactive for S-100 protein and T6 surface antigen.[39,40,74,131,159] Variable reactivity is noted with lysozyme and alpha$_1$-antitrypsin.[12,40,85] An important requirement for the diagnosis is that the tumor cells lack evidence of either T- or B-cell lineage by immunophenotyping or by gene rearrangement studies.[41] Until recently, some cases thought to be malignant histiocytosis were subsequently determined to be malignant diseases of lymphoid origin, namely, Ki-1/CD30 anaplastic B- or T-cell lymphomas.[152]

Ultrastructurally, the tumor cells resemble histiocytes.[39] The noncohesive cells have irregular borders with cytoplasmic extensions and no intercellular junctions. The nuclei are large, often cleaved, and have clumped chromatin and large nucleoli. The abundant cytoplasm contains numerous lysozomes, lipid droplets, and Golgi apparatus. Birbeck granules are characteristically absent.[40]

Cytogenetic studies have been performed on several patients with malignant histiocytosis. Tumor cells display a breakpoint at 5q35 and a t(2;5)(p21 or p23;q35) translocation, which may be specific for this tumor.[12]

The mortality rate is high. Recently, however, the dismal prognosis for patients with malignant histiocytosis has improved somewhat, perhaps because of the addition of new agents to the chemotherapeutic treatment regimen.[40,94] It should be mentioned again, however, that some cases previously thought to be malignant histiocytosis were actually malignant diseases of lymphoid origin, namely, Ki-1/CD30 anaplastic B- or T-cell lymphomas.[152]

Acute Monocytic Leukemia

According to the French-American-British (FAB) classification of leukemia, the criteria for the diagnosis of acute monocytic leukemia, in addition to other findings of leukemia, are the presence of more than 30% leukemic monoblasts or more mature leukemic monocytes (FAB M5) and fewer than 20% leukemic granulocytic precursors in the bone marrow.[11] Leukemic monocytes are characteristically esterase-positive. When either malignant histiocytosis or true histiocytic lymphoma precedes bone marrow or peripheral blood involvement, leukemic conversion of these conditions, rather than monocytic leukemia, is the preferred terminology.[162]

Typically, patients with acute monocytic leukemia present with a significant leukocytosis and a high frequency of involvement of non-hematopoietic tissues, particularly, the skin and gingiva. Hepatosplenomegaly and lymphadenomegaly are found in about 50% of the cases initially (see Chapter 7, "Leukemia").[94,155]

Histiocytic Lymphoma

Histiocytic lymphoma is a malignant disease of the fixed tissue histiocyte. It occurs much less often than either acute monocytic leukemia or malignant histiocytosis.[75,94] The tumors arise from tissues of the monophagocytic system— namely, the lymph nodes and spleen—as well as from skin and bone, often presenting as a soft, greyish mass at the site of origin.

The development of terminal malignant disease, particularly lymphoma, is a known complication of inherited immunodeficiency, occurring in approximately 10% of cases.[33] B-cell lymphoproliferative disorders are the usual malignant diseases reported, but histiocytic lymphoma has been described by Hong and associates[69] as a terminal complication in an infant with Omenn disease.

Histologically, histiocytic lymphoma is composed of sheets of malignant-appearing histiocytes with large, reniform, vesicular nuclei, prominent nucleoli, and basophilic cytoplasm. Mitoses are common.[69,75,94] The tumor cells react diffusely with α-naphthol esterase, acid phosphatase, and β-glucuronidase.[94,156] The tumor cells lack evidence of T- or B-cell lineage by immunophenotyping or gene rearrangement studies.[41]

As a result of modern immunohistochemical techniques and DNA technology, most cases previously diagnosed as malignant histiocytosis or histiocytic lymphoma now probably would be classified as Ki-1 (CD30)–positive anaplastic large cell lymphoma or some other

lymphoma.[41,75,94,152] Compared to the large T- and B-cell and immunoblastic lymphomas, malignant histiocytosis and histiocytic lymphoma are extremely rare.

MISCELLANEOUS HISTIOCYTOSES

Omenn Disease

Omenn disease (Omenn's syndrome) is an uncommon, familial, immunodeficiency disorder of the lymphoid and monophagocytic systems. Eosinophilia, a widespread eczematous rash, hepatosplenomegaly, recurrent infections, and generalized lymphadenopathy with histiocytic infiltrates characterize the disease.[8,69,82,84,117,147] It occurs primarily in newborns and in infants younger than 3 months of age, and is transmitted as an autosomal recessive trait.

Severe lymphoid depletion in the presence of numerous histiocytes and eosinophils is the principal finding in the lymph nodes, spleen, and bone marrow.[8,69,82] The thymus shows practically no lymphoid elements and absence of Hassall's corpuscles. The histiocytes appear to be reactive, staining positively for esterase, acid phosphatase, S-100 protein, and OKM1 monoclonal antibody.[82,84] In addition, T6-positive histiocytes and granulocytes are found in the infiltrates. Erythrophagocytosis is not present.

The etiology of this unusual condition has not been definitively established. An immunodeficiency, with a defect primarily involving T cells, is one premise, and graft-versus-host disease associated with a primary cellular immunodeficiency is another etiologic theory.[8,69,82] With few exceptions, Omenn disease is invariably fatal by 1 year of age,[8,82,147] although recovery following bone marrow transplantation has been described.[84,152]

Chédiak-Higashi Syndrome

The cardinal features of this rare autosomal recessive disease are decreased pigmentation of the hair and eyes (partial oculocutaneous albinism), photophobia, nystagmus, frequent bacterial infections, neurologic dysfunction, and characteristically giant lysosomal granules in leukocytes and other granule-containing cells. Death often occurs from infection or from a so-called accelerated phase of the disease, usually before 7 years of age. The accelerated phase is characterized by hepatosplenomegaly,

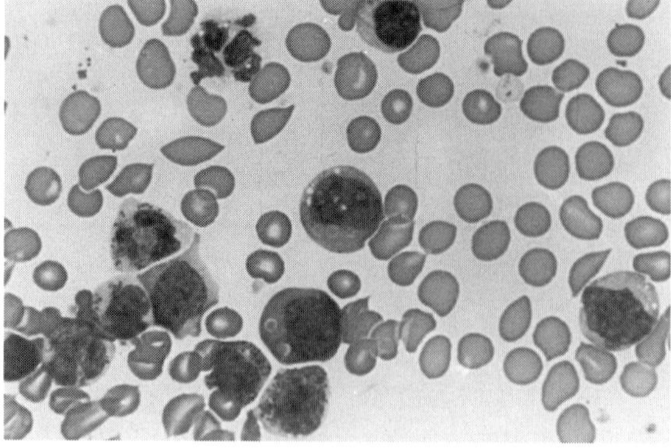

Figure 8–5. A 5-year-old girl with oculocutaneous albinism, gray hair, developmental delay, susceptibility to infection, and neutropenia. The lymphocytes contain large, eosinophilic, lysosomal inclusions diagnostic of Chédiak-Higashi syndrome. Large, irregular, cytoplasmic granules are seen in the neutrophils and other myeloid elements (Wright-Giemsa, ×750). (Courtesy of Glenn Billman, MD.)

lymphadenopathy, anemia, pancytopenia, and abnormal liver function tests. The histologic findings—namely, lymphohistiocytic infiltration with hemophagocytosis—are similar to those found in patients with the infection-associated (reactive) hemophagocytic syndrome.[7,136] Moreover, Epstein-Barr virus infection has been documented in patients with the accelerated phase of Chédiak-Higashi disease, a situation perhaps analogous to the X-linked lymphoproliferative syndrome and this virus.[89,112,136,138]

Although neonatal presentation of Chédiak-Higashi syndrome is unusual, patients may have recurrent infections beginning in the first few months of life. Nevertheless, the diagnosis can be established prenatally or at birth by finding the characteristically huge lysosomal granules within leukocytes on the peripheral blood smear or bone marrow (Fig. 8–5).[144]

Juvenile Xanthogranuloma

Juvenile xanthogranuloma may be congenital, presenting as one or more yellow nodules that range in size from 1 cm to several centimeters, particularly when the subcutaneous tissue is involved.[65,73,99,103] Microscopically, the lesion consists of histiocytes with eosinophilic or foamy cytoplasms, Touton multinucleated giant cells, and variable numbers of lymphocytes and eosinophils. The histiocytes appear to be reactive and lack Birbeck granules, S-100 pro-

tein reactivity, and the T6 surface markers that are characteristic of Langerhans cells.[56,140] The reader is referred to Chapters 4 and 5 for further discussion of this subject.

REFERENCES

1. Ahnquist G, Holyoke JB. Congenital Letterer-Siwe disease (reticuloendotheliosis) in a term stillborn infant. J Pediatr 1960;57:897.
2. Akima M, Sumi SM. Neuropathology of familial erythrophagocytic lymphohistiocytosis. Hum Pathol 1984; 15:161.
3. Ansbacher LF, Singaen BH, Hosler MW, et al. Familial erythrophagocytic lymphohistiocytosis: An association with serum lipid abnormalities. J Pediatr 1983; 102:270.
4. Arico M, Caselli D, Burgio GR. Familial hemophagocytic lymphohistiocytosis. Pediatr Hematol Oncol 1989;6:247.
5. Arya S, Hong R, Gilbert EF. Reactive hemophagocytic syndrome. Pediatr Pathol 1985;3:129.
6. Avery ME, McAfee JG, Guild HG. The course and prognosis of reticuloendotheliosis (eosinophilic granuloma, Schüller-Christian disease, Letterer-Siwe's disease). Am J Med 1957;22:636.
7. Barak Y, Nir E. Chédiak-Higashi syndrome. Am J Pediatr Hematol Oncol 1987;9:42.
8. Barth RF, Khurana SK, Vergara GG, et al. Rapidly fatal familial histiocytosis associated with eosinophilia and primary immunological deficiency. Lancet 1972;2: 503.
9. Bassett F, Nezelof C, Ferrans VJ. The histiocytoses. Pathol Annu 1983;18(2):27.
10. Beckstead JH, Wood GS, Turner RR. Histiocytosis X cells and Langerhans cells: Enzyme, histochemical and immunologic similarities. Hum Pathol 1984;15: 826.
11. Bennett JM, Catovsky D, Daniel M-T, et al. Proposals for the classification of acute leukemias. French-American-British (FAB) co-operative group. Br J Haematol 1976;33:451.
12. Benz-Lemoine E, Brizard A, Huret JL, et al. Malignant histiocytosis: A specific t(2;5) (p23;q25) translocation? Review of the literature. Blood 1988;72:1045.
13. Berry DH, Gresik MV, Humphrey GB, et al. Natural history of histiocytosis X: A pediatric oncology group study. Med Pediatr Oncol 1986;14:1.
14. Bierman HR. Apparent cure of Letterer-Siwe disease: Seventeen-year survival of identical twins with non-lipid reticuloendotheliosis. JAMA 1966;196:156.
15. Birbeck MD, Breathnach AJ, Everall JD. An electron microscopic study of basal melanocytes and high level clear cells (Langerhans cells) in vitiligo. J Invest Dermatol 1961;37:51.
16. Bjercke S, Elgo J, Braathen L, et al. Enriched epidermal Langerhans cells are potent antigen presenting cells for T cells. J Invest Dermatol 1984;83:286.
17. Blume RS, Wolf SM. The Chédiak-Higashi syndrome: Studies in four patients and a review of the literature. Medicine 1972;51:247.
18. Boccon-Gibod LA, Krichen HA, Carlier-Mercier LMB, et al. Digestive tract involvement with exudative enteropathy in Langerhans cell histiocytosis. Pediatr Pathol 1992;12:515.

19. Bonifazi E, Caputo R, Ceci A, et al. Congenital self-healing histiocytosis. Arch Dermatol 1982;118:267.

20. Broadbent VA. Malignant disease in the neonate. *In* Roberton NRC (ed): Textbook of Neonatology, 2nd ed, p 879. Edinburgh: Churchill Livingstone, 1992.

21. Broadbent V, Fadner H, Komp DM, et al. Histiocytosis syndromes in children: II. Approach to the clinical and laboratory evaluation of children with Langerhans cell histiocytosis. Med Pediatr Oncol 1989;17:492.

22. Broadbent V, Pritchard J. Histiocytosis X—Current controversies. Arch Dis Child 1985;60:605.

23. Buchino JJ, Byrd RP, Kmetz DR. Disseminated sinus histiocytosis with massive lymphadenopathy: Its pathologic aspects. Arch Pathol Lab Med 1982;106:13.

24. Campo E, Condom E, Miro MJ, et al. Tuberculosis-associated hemophagocytic syndrome. A systemic process. Cancer 1986;58:2640.

25. Chan JKC, Ng CS, Law CK, et al. Reactive hemophagocytic syndrome: A study of 7 fatal cases. Pathology 1987;19:43.

26. Chen R-L, Su I-J, Lin K-H, et al. Fulminant childhood hemophagocytic syndrome mimicking histiocytic medullary reticulosis. Am J Clin Pathol 1991;96:171.

27. Chen TK, Nesbit ME, McKenna R, et al. Histiocytic medullary reticulosis in acute lymphocytic leukemia of T cell origin. Am J Dis Child 1976;130:1262.

28. Chu T, D'Angio GJ, Favara BE, et al. Histiocytosis syndromes in children. Lancet 1987;1:208.

29. Coffin CM, Dehner LP. Congenital tumors. *In* Stocker JT, Dehner LP (eds): Pediatric Pathology, Vol 1, p 325. Philadelphia: JB Lippincott, 1992.

30. Cohen DM, Mitchell CB, Alexander JW. Letterer-Siwe disease in a newborn. Arch Pathol 1966;81:347.

31. Corbeel L, Eggermount E, Desmyter J, et al. Spontaneous healing of Langerhans cell histiocytosis (histiocytosis X). Eur J Pediatr 1988;148:32.

32. Cordier MP, Souillet G, Gilly J, et al. La lymphohistiocytose familiale. A propos de deux nouveaux cas diagnostiques au cours de la vie. Pediatrie 1981;36:291.

33. Cunningham-Rundles C, Siegel FP, Cunningham-Rundles S, et al. Incidence of cancer in 98 patients with common varied immunodeficiency. J Clin Immunol 1987;7:294.

34. Danish EH, Dahms BB, Kumar ML. Cytomegalovirus associated hemophagocytic syndrome. Pediatrics 1985;75:280.

35. Dehner LP. Neoplasms of the fetus and neonate. *In* Naeye RL, Kissane JM, Kaufman N (eds): Perinatal Diseases, International Academy of Pathology, Monograph No. 22, p 286. Baltimore: Williams and Wilkins, 1981.

36. Dehner LP. Pediatric Surgical Pathology, 2nd ed. St. Louis: CV Mosby Co, 1987.

37. Dehner LP, Bamford JT, McDonald EC. Spontaneous regression of congenital cutaneous histiocytosis X: Report of a case with discussion of nosology and pathogenesis. Pediatr Pathol 1983;1:99.

38. Devictor D, Fischer A, Marnas S, et al. Etude immunologique de la lymphohistiocytose familiale. Arch Fr Pediatr 1982;39:135.

39. Di Sant'Agnese PA, Ettinger LJ, Ryan CK, et al. Histomonocytic malignancy: A spectrum of disease in an 11-month-old infant. Cancer 1983;52:1417.

40. Ducatman BS, Wick MR, Morgan TW, et al. Malignant histiocytosis: A clinical, histologic, and immuno-histochemical study of 20 cases. Hum Pathol 1984;15:368.

41. Egeler RM, Schmitz L, Sonneveld P, et al. Malignant histiocytosis: A reassessment of cases formerly classified as histiocytic neoplasms and review of the literature. Med Pediatr Oncol 1995;25:1.

42. Eisen RN, Buckley PJ, Rosai J. Immunophenotypic characterization of sinus histiocytosis with massive lymphadenopathy (Rosai-Dorfman disease). Semin Diagn Pathol 1990;7:74.

43. Farquhar JW, Claireaux AE. Familial haemophagocytic reticulosis. Arch Dis Child 1952;27:519.

44. Favara BE. Histiocytosis syndromes and related disorders of early infancy: A pathologist's perspective. Pediatr Hematol Oncol 1989;6:213.

45. Favara BE, McCarthy RC, Mierau GW. Histiocytosis X. *In* Finegold M (ed): Pathology of Neoplasia in Children and Adolescents, p 126. Philadelphia: WB Saunders, 1986.

46. Favara BE, McCarthy RC, Mierau GW. Histiocytosis X. Hum Pathol 1983;14:663.

47. Fischer A, Cerf-Bensussan N, Blanche S, et al. Allogenic bone marrow transplantation for erythrophagocytic lymphohistiocytosis. J Pediatr 1986;108:267.

48. Fischer A, Virelizier JL, Arenzana-Seisdedos F, et al. Treatment of four patients with erythrophagocytic lymphohistiocytosis by a combination of epipodophyllotoxin, steroids, intrathecal methotrexate and cranial irradiation. Pediatrics 1985;76:263.

49. Fourcar E, Rosai J, Dorfman RF, et al. Immunologic abnormalities and their significance in sinus histiocytosis with massive lymphadenopathy. Am J Clin Pathol 1984;82:515.

50. Fourcar E, Rosai J, Dorfman RF. Sinus histiocytosis with massive lymphadenopathy: An analysis of 14 deaths occurring in a patient registry. Cancer 1984;54:1834.

51. Fourcar E, Rosai J, Dorfman R. Sinus histiocytosis with massive lymphadenopathy (Rosai-Dorfman disease): Review of the entity. Semin Diagn Pathol 1990;7:19.

52. Gannon MJ, Blayney M, Cosgrove E, et al. Histiocytosis in baby with delayed cord separation. Lancet 1987;1:507.

53. Gilbert EF, ZuRhein GM, Wester SM, et al. Familial hemophagocytic lymphohistiocytosis: Report of four cases in two families and review of the literature. Pediatr Pathol 1985;3:59.

54. Glass AG, Miller RW. U.S. mortality from Letterer-Siwe disease, 1960–1964. Pediatrics 1968;42:364.

55. Goldberg J, Nezelof C. Lymphohistiocytosis: A multifactorial syndrome of macrophagic activation. Clinicopathological study of 38 cases. Hematol Oncol 1986;4:275.

56. Gonzalez-Crussi F, Campbell RJ. Juvenile xanthogranuloma. Ultrastructural study. Arch Pathol 1970;89:65.

57. Greenberger JS, Crocker AC, Vawter G, et al. Results of treatment of 127 patients with systemic histiocytosis (Letterer-Siwe syndrome, Schüller-Christian syndrome and multiple eosinophilic granuloma). Medicine 1981;60:311.

58. Hagberg B, Hultquist G, Svennerholm L, et al. Malignant hyperlipemia in infancy. Am J Dis Child 1964;107:267.

59. Hage C, Willman CL, Favara BE, et al. Langerhans' cell histiocytosis (histiocytosis X): Immunophenotype and growth fraction. Hum Pathol 1993;24:840.

60. Hansmann ML, Rontogianni D, Janka-Schaub GE, et

al. Familial hemophagocytic lymphohistiocytosis mac-rophages showing immunohistochemical properties of activated macrophages and T-accessory cells. Pediatr Hematol Oncol 1989;6:237.

61. Harrist TJ, Bhan AK, Murphy GF, et al. Histiocytosis X: In situ characterization of cutaneous infiltrates with monoclonal antibodies. Am J Clin Pathol 1983; 79:294.

62. Hashimoto K, Griffin D, Kohsbaki M. Self-healing reticulohistiocytosis: A clinical histologic and ultrastructural study of the fourth case in the literature. Cancer 1982;49:331.

63. Hashimoto K, Pritzker MS. Electron microscopic study of reticulohistiocytoma: An unusual case of congenital self-healing reticulohistiocytosis. Arch Dermatol 1973;107:263.

64. Hayward AR, Leonard J, Wood CBS, et al. Delayed separation of the umbilical cord, widespread infections, and defective neutrophil mobility. Lancet 1979; 1:1099.

65. Helwig EB, Hackney VC. Juvenile xanthogranuloma (nevoxanthogranuloma). Am J Pathol 1954;30:625.

66. Henter J-I, Elinder G, Ost A. Diagnostic guidelines for hemophagocytic lymphohistiocytosis. Semin Oncol 1991;18:29.

67. Hertz CG, Hambrick GW Jr. Congenital Letterer-Siwe disease: A case treated with vincristine and corticosteroids. Am J Dis Child 1968;116:553.

68. Heyn RM, Hamoudi A, Newton WA Jr. Pretreatment liver biopsy in 20 children with histiocytosis X: A clinicopathologic correlation. Med Pediatr Oncol 1990; 18:110.

69. Hong R, Gilbert EF, Opitz JM. Omenn disease: Termination in lymphoma. Pediatr Pathol 1985;3:143.

70. Huhn D, Meister R. Malignant histiocytosis: Morphologic and cytochemical findings. Cancer 1978;42: 1341.

71. Isaacs H Jr. Neoplasms in infants: A report of 265 cases. Pathol Annu 1983;18(2):165.

72. Isaacs H Jr. Perinatal (congenital and neonatal) neoplasms: A report of 110 cases. Pediatr Pathol 1985;3: 165.

73. Isaacs H Jr. Tumors of the Newborn and Infant. St. Louis: Mosby–Year Book, 1991.

74. Ishii E, Hara T, Okamura J, et al. Malignant histiocytosis in infants: Surface marker analysis of malignant cells in two cases. Med Pediatr Oncol 1987;15: 102.

75. Jaffe ES. Malignant histiocytosis and true histiocytic lymphomas. *In* Jaffe ES (ed): Surgical Pathology of Lymph Nodes and Related Organs, p 381. Philadelphia: WB Saunders, 1985.

76. Jaffe R. Pathology of histiocytosis X. Perspect Pediatr Pathol 1987;9:4.

77. Jaffe R, Wollman MR, Kocoshis S, et al. Pathological cases of the month: Langerhans' cell histiocytosis with gastrointestinal involvement. Am J Dis Child 1993; 147:79.

78. Janka GE. Familial hemophagocytic lymphohistiocytosis. Eur J Pediatr 1983;140:221.

79. Janka GE. Familial hemophagocytic lymphohistiocytosis: Diagnostic problems and differential diagnosis. Pediatr Hematol Oncol 1989;6:219.

80. Janka GE. Familial hemophagocytic lymphohistiocytosis: Therapy in the German experience. Pediatr Hematol Oncol 1989;6:227.

81. Jones B, Welton WA, Gilbert EF. Congenital Letterer-Siwe disease—Report of three cases. Cutis 1967;3:750.

82. Jouan H, Le Diest F, Nezelof C. Omenn's syndrome—Pathologic arguments in favor of a graft-versus-host pathogenesis: A report of nine cases. Hum Pathol 1987;18:1101.

83. Juberg RC, Kloepfer HW, Oberman HA. Genetic determination of acute disseminated histiocytosis X (Letterer-Siwe syndrome). Pediatrics 1970;45:753.

84. Junker AK, Chan KW, Massing BG. Clinical and immune recovery from Omenn syndrome after bone marrow transplantation. J Pediatr 1989;114:596.

85. Jurco S, Starling K, Hawkins EP. Malignant histiocytosis in childhood: Morphologic considerations. Hum Pathol 1983;14:1059.

86. Kanitakis J, Zambruno G, Schmitt D, et al. Congenital self-healing histiocytosis (Hashimoto-Pritzker): An ultrastructural and immunohistochemical study. Cancer 1988;61:508.

87. Karcher DS, Head DR, Mullins JD. Malignant histiocytosis occurring in patients with acute lymphocytic leukemia. Cancer 1978;41:1967.

88. Kho LK, Goei GH, Tumbelaka WAFJ. Acute reticuloendotheliosis (Letterer-Siwe's disease) in an infant with congenital tuberculosis. Ann Paediatr 1961;197: 157.

89. Kinugara N. Epstein-Barr virus infection in Chédiak-Higashi syndrome mimicking acute lymphocytic leukemia. Am J Pediatr Hematol Oncol 1990;12:182.

90. Kletzel M, Gollin SM, Gloster ES, et al. Chromosome abnormalities in familial hemophagocytic lymphohistiocytosis. Cancer 1986;57:2153.

91. Koto A, Morecki R, Santorineou M. Congenital hemophagocytic reticulosis. Am J Clin Pathol 1976;65: 495.

92. Labbe A, Dechelotte P, Demeocq F, et al. Lymphohistiocytose familiale. Arch Fr Pediatr 1982;39:613.

93. Ladisch S, Holiman B, Poplack DG, et al. Immunodeficiency in familial erythrophagocytic lymphohistiocytosis. Lancet 1978;1:581.

94. Ladisch S, Jaffe ES. The histiocytoses. *In* Pizzo PA, Poplack DG (eds): Principles and Practice of Pediatric Oncology, 2nd ed, p 617. Philadelphia: JB Lippincott, 1993.

95. Lahey ME. Prognostic factors in histiocytosis X. Am J Pediatr Hematol Oncol 1981;3:57.

96. Lampert IA, Catovsky D, Bergier N. Malignant histiocytosis: A clinicopathological study of 12 cases. Br J Haematol 1978;40:65.

97. Landing BH. Lymphohistiocytosis in childhood: Pathologic comparison with fatal Letterer-Siwe disease (disseminated visceral histiocytosis X). Perspect Pediatr Pathol 1987;9:48.

98. Lasser A. The mononuclear phagocytic system: A review. Hum Pathol 1983;14:108.

99. Lever WF, Schaumburg-Lever G. Histopathology of the Skin, 7th ed. Philadelphia: JB Lippincott, 1990.

100. Lichtenstein L. Histiocytosis X: Integration of eosinophilic granuloma of bone, "Letterer-Siwe" and "Schüller-Christian disease" as related manifestations of a single nosologic entity. Arch Pathol 1953; 56:84.

101. Lilleyman JS. The treatment of familial erythrophagocytic lymphohistiocytosis. Cancer 1980;46:468.

102. Lucaya J. Histiocytosis X. Am J Dis Child 1971;121: 289.

103. Machin GA. The skin. *In* Wigglesworth JS, Singer DB (eds): Textbook of Fetal and Perinatal Pathology, Vol 2, p 1247. Oxford: Blackwell, 1991.

104. MacMahon HE, Bedizel M, Ellis CA. Familial erythro-

phagocytic lymphohistiocytosis. Pediatrics 1963;32:
868.

105. Marsh WI, Lew SW, Heath VC, et al. Congenital self-healing histiocytosis X. Am J Pediatr Hematol Oncol
1983;5:227.

106. Matus-Ridley M, Raney RB Jr, Thawerani H, et al. Histiocytosis X in children: Patterns of disease and results
of treatment. Med Pediatr Oncol 1983;11:99.

107. McClain K. Epstein-Barr virus DNA in lymphocytes of
patients with virus associated hemophagocytic syndrome. Am J Pediatr Hematol Oncol 1986;8:121.

108. McClain K, Gehrz R, Grierson H, et al. Virus-associated histiocytic proliferations in children: Frequent
association with Epstein-Barr virus and congenital
and acquired immunodeficiencies. Am J Pediatr
Hematol Oncol 1988;10:196.

109. McClain K, Ramsay NKC, Robison L, et al. Bone marrow involvement in histiocytosis X. Med Pediatr Oncol 1983;11:167.

110. McClure PD, Strachan P, Saunders EF. Hypofibrinogenemia and thrombocytopenia in familial hemophagocytic reticulosis. J Pediatr 1974;85:67.

111. McKenna RW, Risdall RJ, Brunning RD, et al. Virus
associated hemophagocytic syndrome. Hum Pathol
1981;12:395.

112. Merino F, Henle W, Ramirez-Duque R. Chronic active
Epstein-Barr virus infection in patients with Chédiak-Higashi syndrome. J Clin Immunol 1986;6:299.

113. Nelson P, Santamaria A, Olson RL, et al. Generalized
lymphohistiocytic infiltration. A familial disease not
previously described and different from Letterer-Siwe
disease and Chédiak-Higashi syndrome. Pediatrics
1961;27:931.

114. Nesbit ME Jr, O'Leary M, Dehner LP, Ramsay NKC.
The immune system and the histiocytosis syndromes.
Am J Pediatr Hematol Oncol 1981;3:141.

115. Nezelof C. Histiocytosis X: A histological and histogenetic study. Perspect Pediatr Pathol 1979;5:153.

116. Nezelof C, Frileux-Herbert F, Cronier-Sachot J. Disseminated histiocytosis X: Analysis of prognostic factors based on a retrospective study of 50 cases. Cancer
1979;44:1824.

117. Omenn GS. Familial reticuloendotheliosis with eosinophilia. N Engl J Med 1965;273:427.

118. Oranje AP, Vuzevski VD, de Groot R, et al. Congenital
self-healing, non-Langerhans cell histiocytosis. Eur J
Pediatr 1988;148:39.

119. Perry MC, Harrison EG, Burgert EO, et al. Familial
erythrophagocytic lymphohistiocytosis. Report of two
cases and clinicopathologic review. Cancer 1976;38:
209.

120. Popper HH, Zenz W, Mache C, et al. Familial haemophagocytic lymphohistiocytosis. A report of three
cases with unusual lung involvement. Histopathology
1994;25:439.

121. Potter EL, Craig JM. Pathology of the Fetus and Infant, 3rd ed, p 177. Chicago: Year Book Medical Publishers, 1975.

122. Price DL, Woolsey JE, Rosman NP, et al. Familial
lymphohistiocytosis of the nervous system. Arch Neurol 1971;24:270.

123. Pujol RM, Moreno A, Lopez D, et al. Childhood self-healing histiocytosis X. Pediatr Dermatol 1988;5:97.

124. Purtilo DT. Immune deficiency predisposing to
Epstein-Barr virus-induced lymphoproliferative disease: The X-linked lymphoproliferative syndrome as
a model. Adv Cancer Res 1981;34:279.

125. Purtilo DT, Yang JPS, Cassel CK, et al. X-linked recessive progressive combined variable immunodeficiency (Duncan's disease). Lancet 1975;1:935.

126. Rabkin MS, Kjeldsberg CR, Wittwer CT, et al. A comparison study of two methods of peanut agglutinin
staining with S100 immunostaining in 29 cases of histiocytosis X (Langerhans' cell histiocytosis). Arch Pathol Lab Med 1990;114:511.

127. Raney RB Jr, D'Angio GJ. Langerhans' cell histiocytosis (histiocytosis X): Experience at the Children's
Hospital of Philadelphia, 1970–1984. Med Pediatr
Oncol 1989;17:20.

128. Rappaport H. Tumors of the hematopoietic system.
In Atlas of Tumor Pathology, Section 3, Fasicle 8,
p 49. Washington, DC: Armed Forces Institute of Pathology, 1966.

129. Rettwitz W, Sauer O, Burow HM, et al. Neurological
and neuropathological findings in familial erythrophagocytic lymphohistiocytosis. Brain Dev 1983;5:
322.

130. Risdall RJ, Dehner LP, Duray P, et al. Histiocytosis X
(Langerhans histiocytosis). Prognostic role of histopathology. Arch Path Lab Med 1983;107:59.

131. Risdall RJ, McKenna RW, Nesbit ME, et al. Virus-associated hemophagocytic syndrome: A benign histiocytic proliferation distinct from malignant histiocytosis. Cancer 1979;44:993.

132. Risdall RJ, Sibley RK, McKenna RW, et al. Malignant
histiocytosis: A light and electron-microscopic and
histochemical study. Am J Surg Pathol 1980;4:439.

133. Rivera-Luna R, Martinez-Guerra G, Altamirano-Alvaraez E, et al. Langerhans cell histiocytosis: Clinical experience with 124 patients. Pediatr Dermatol
1988;5:145.

134. Rosai J, Dorfman RF. Sinus histiocytosis with massive
lymphadenopathy: A pseudolymphomatous benign
disorder: Analysis of 34 cases. Cancer 1972;30:1174.

135. Rowden G, Connelly EM, Winkleman RK. Cutaneous
histiocytosis X. The presence of S-100 protein and its
use in diagnosis. Arch Hematol 1983;119:553.

136. Rubin CM, Burke BA, McKenna RW, et al. The accelerated phase of Chédiak-Higashi syndrome: An expression of the virus-associated hemophagocytic syndrome? Cancer 1985;56:524.

137. Schouten TJ, Hustinx TWJ, Scheres JMJC, et al. Malignant histiocytosis: Clinical and cytogenetic studies in
a newborn and a child. Cancer 1983;52:1229.

138. Seibel NL, Cossman J, Magrath IT. Lymphoproliferative disorders. *In* Pizzo PA, Poplack DG (eds): Principles and Practice of Pediatric Oncology, 2nd ed, p
595. Philadelphia: JB Lippincott, 1993.

139. Senac MO Jr, Isaacs H, Gwinn JL. Primary lesions of
bone in the 1st decade of life: Retrospective survey of
biopsy results. Radiology 1986;160:491.

140. Seo S, Min KW, Mirkin LD. Juvenile xanthogranuloma: Ultrastructural and immunocytochemical studies. Arch Pathol Lab Med 1986;110:911.

141. Shapiro DN, Hutchinson RJ. Familial histiocytosis in
offspring of two pregnancies after artificial insemination. N Engl J Med 1981;304:757.

142. Sheils C, Dover GJ. Frequency of congenital anomalies in patients with histiocytosis X. Am J Hematol
1989;31:91.

143. Shimizu H, Komatsu T, Harada T, et al. An immuno-histochemical and ultrastructural study of an unusual
case of multiple non-X histiocytoma. Arch Dermatol
1988;124:1254.

144. Shurin SB. The blood and hematopoietic system. *In*
Fanaroff AA, Martin RJ (eds): Neonatal-Perinatal

Medicine: Diseases of the Fetus and Infant, 5th ed, Vol 2. St. Louis: Mosby–Year Book, 1992.

145. Sidney Farber Workshop on Histiocytoses. Pediatr Pathol 1984;2:381.

146. Siegal GP, Dehner LP, Rosai J. Histiocytosis X (Langerhans' cell granulomatosis) of the thymus: A clinicopathologic study of four childhood cases. Am J Surg Pathol 1985;9:117.

147. Singer DB. Disorders of the lymphoid tissues and the immune system. *In* Wigglesworth JS, Singer DB (eds): Textbook of Fetal and Perinatal Pathology, Vol 1. Oxford: Blackwell, 1991.

148. Soffer D, Okon E, Rosen N, et al. Familial hemophagocytic lymphohistiocytosis in Israel. Cancer 1984;54: 2423.

149. Stark B, Hershko C, Rosen N, et al. Familial hemophagocytic lymphohistiocytosis (FHLH) in Israel. 1. Description of 11 patients of Iranian-Iraqi origin and review of the literature. Cancer 1984;54:2109.

150. Starkie CM, Kenny MW, Mann JR, et al. Histiocytic medullary reticulosis following acute lymphoblastic leukemia. Cancer 1981;47:537.

151. Steinman RM, Nussenzweig MC. Dendritic cells: Features and functions. Immunol Rev 1980;53:125.

152. Stephan JL. Histiocytoses. Eur J Pediatr 1995;154:600.

153. Suarez CR, Zeller WP, Silberman S, et al. Sinus histiocytosis with massive lymphadenopathy: Remission with chemotherapy. Am J Pediatr Hematol Oncol 1983;5:235.

154. Sullivan JL, Woda BA, Herrod HG, et al. Epstein-Barr virus-associated hemophagocytic syndrome. Virological and immunopathological studies. Blood 1985;65: 1097.

155. Sultan C, Imbert M, Richard MF, et al. Pure acute monocytic leukemia. A study of 12 cases. Am J Clin Pathol 1977;68:752.

156. Turner RR, Wood GS, Beckstead JH, et al. Histiocytic malignancies: Morphologic, immunologic and enzymatic heterogeneity. Am J Surg Pathol 1984;8:485.

157. Vade A, Hayani A, Pierce KL. Congenital histiocytosis X. Pediatr Radiol 1993;23:181.

158. Valderrama E, Kahn LB, Festa R, et al. Benign isolated histiocytosis mimicking chicken pox in a neonate: Report of two cases with ultrastructural study. Pediatr Pathol 1985;3:103.

159. Vanfurth R, Taeburn JA, van Zwett TL. Characteristics of human mononuclear phagocytes. Blood 1979;54:485.

160. Wieczorek R, Greco MA, McCarthy K, et al. Familial erythrophagocytic lymphohistiocytosis: Immunophenotypic, immunohistochemical and ultra-structural demonstration of the relation to sinus histiocytes. Hum Pathol 1986;17:55.

161. Wolfson SL, Botero F, Hurwitz S, et al. Pure cutaneous histiocytosis-X. Cancer 1981;48:2236.

162. Writing Group of the Histiocyte Society. Histiocytosis syndromes in children. Lancet 1987;1:208.

163. Yu RCH, Morris JF, Pritchard J, et al. Defective alloantigen-presenting capacity of 'Langerhans cell histiocytosis cells.' Arch Dis Child 1992;67:1370.

164. Zucker JM, Caillaux JM, Vanel D, et al. Malignant histiocytosis in childhood. Clinical study and therapeutic results in 22 cases. Cancer 1980;45:2821.

BRAIN TUMORS

Brain tumors occur considerably less often in the fetus and newborn than in the older child and adolescent.[24,29,46,63,105,108,116,118,119,131,159,173,209,213,218,219,232] The peak age incidence in children is between 5 and 8 years.[91,239] Central nervous system neoplasms are the leading solid tumor in children and adolescents, surpassed only by leukemia and lymphoma in frequency.[91,239,247,248] In the fetus and neonate, brain tumors occur less often than extracranial teratomas, soft tissue tumors, neuroblastoma, and leukemia, and are responsible for 5% to 20% of the deaths secondary to neoplasms in this age group (see Table 1–1).[8,23,29,107,166]

Fetal and newborn central nervous system tumors are not entirely the same as those found in the older child and adolescent in several respects. First, the location is different. Primary intracranial tumors in the older child and adolescent are primarily infratentorial; that is, they are located within the posterior fossa (brain stem and cerebellum). By contrast, in the fetus and newborn, most occur above the tentorium (see Tables 9–1 to 9–14).[7,28,29,46,53,66,70,75,116,159,172,193,195,213,232,246] Second, the frequency of the various histologic types is not the same; for example, intracranial teratomas constitute at least one third of the total reported perinatal cases (Table 9–1).[53,159,195,232,237]

INCIDENCE

The annual incidence of brain tumors appears to vary from one decade to the next, from one institution to another, and from one part of the world to another. Neonatal intracranial tumors account for approximately 1% of those occurring during childhood.[107,232] Data from the Brain Tumor Registry in Japan show that the neonatal cases numbered 24 of 3152 (0.76%) total pediatric cases, and that the frequency of neonatal brain tumors per year in that country was estimated at 4.1.[159] The 12 neonatal brain tumors reviewed by the Children's Memorial Hospital, Chicago represented 3.3% of the 360 pediatric brain tumors diagnosed in the 9-year study.[172] A survey of 17,417 perinatal necropsies performed over a 50-year period revealed 5 brain tumors (0.03%).[234] Approximately 10% of all perinatal tumors arise from the brain, according to a comparison of 11 studies throughout the world (Table 1–1).

The number of fetuses and newborns recorded annually with intracranial lesions has increased dramatically over the past several years with the advent of ultrasonography, magnetic resonance imaging (MRI), and computerized tomography (CT), and these newer imaging techniques have significantly contributed also to earlier treatment and, thus, increased survival.[119,125,172,219,237] In the past, neurologists and neurosurgeons were reluctant to perform pneumoencephalograms in young infants because of the procedural difficulty, the inaccuracy in detecting small lesions, and the significant associated risk.

ASSOCIATION OF BRAIN TUMORS WITH HERITABLE DISORDERS AND OTHER CONDITIONS

Definite associations have been documented between brain tumors and hereditable diseases and other conditions. Neurofibromatosis type I (von Recklinghausen disease) and tuberous sclerosis are prime examples.[91,189] Generally, the tumors occurring in patients with neurofibromatosis—namely meningioma, pilocytic astro-

Table 9–1. 12 Newborn Brain Tumor Studies (170 Tumors)

Tumor	CHB	RC	HSCT	HSCL	UV	BOL	JPN	CMHC	WRAMC	KCH	CHLA	CHSD	Total (%)
Astrocytoma	3	2	3	2	1	2*	6	–	9	2	4	–	34 (20.0)
Teratoma†	2	2	–	2	1	–	8	3	12	3	–	–	33 (19.4)
Choroid plexus papilloma	3	–	–	1	–	1	1	5	3	–	5†	1	20 (11.8)
Medulloblastoma	1	2	1	3	2	–	2	1	4	–	2	–	18 (10.6)
PNET	–	–	2	–	–	–	1	1	8	–	–	3	15 (8.8)
Ependymoma‡	2	–	1	1	–	–	1	–	1	1	1	–	8 (4.5)
Meningeal tumors§	–	–	2	–	1	–	1	–	1	–	–	–	5 (2.9)
Glioblastoma	–	–	–	–	1	–	–	–	4	–	–	–	5 (2.9)
Glioma	–	1	–	2	1	–	–	1	–	–	–	–	5 (2.9)
Ganglioglioma	–	–	–	–	–	1	–	–	1	–	1	–	3 (1.7)
Craniopharyngioma	–	–	–	–	–	–	–	–	–	1	–	1	2 (1.2)
Medulloepithelioma	–	–	–	–	1	–	–	–	1	–	–	–	2 (1.2)
Miscellaneous	–	1	–	6	2	2	3	1	1	2	2	–	20 (11.8)
Total in Study	11	8	9	17	10	6	23	12	45	9	15	5	170 (100)

*A 2-month-old female infant with tuberous sclerosis and frontoparietal giant cell astrocytoma.
†Includes one choroid plexus papillary carcinoma.
‡Includes ependymoma and ependymoblastoma.
§Includes meningioma and meningeal sarcoma.
CHB = Children's Hospital Birmingham, U.K.;[166] RC = Rigshospitalet Copenhagen;[23] HSCT = Hospital for Sick Children, Toronto;[29] HSCL = Hospital for Sick Children, London;[119] UV = University of Vienna Neurological Institute;[116] BOL = Bellaria Hospital, Bologna, Italy;[70] JPN = Japan ISPN Cooperative Study;[159] CMHC = Children's Memorial Hospital, Chicago;[172] WRAMC = Walter Reed Army Medical Center, Washington, DC;[28] KCH = Kobe Children's Hospital, Japan;[195] CHLA = Children's Hospital, Los Angeles (see Table 9–2); CHSD = Children's Hospital, San Diego; PNET = primitive neuroectodermal tumor.

cytoma, ependymoma, and optic nerve glioma—do not appear in the newborn, but occur later in childhood and adolescence.[47,112,134,171,203] However, there are exceptions. The youngest patient with an optic glioma in the pediatric neurofibromatosis type I study by Shearer et al. was 5 months old; eight children had optic gliomas and two had malignant astrocytomas.[203] Similarly, the subependymal giant cell astrocytoma of tuberous sclerosis, the cerebellar hemangioblastomas and retinal tumors in patients with von Hippel-Lindau disease,[46] and medulloblastomas in the nevoid basal cell carcinoma syndrome, the Turcot intestinal polyposis syndrome, and ataxia telangiectasia usually are not apparent at birth.[91] There is an increased frequency of choroid plexus papillomas in patients with Aicardi's syndrome (seizures, mental retardation, ocular anomalies, vertebral malformations, agenesis of the corpus callosum).[3]

Brain tumors occurring in newborns with neurofibromatosis type I and tuberous sclerosis have been documented. For example, in a review of 57 cases, the Children's Memorial Hospital, Chicago group described 3 infants with neurofibromatosis and optic gliomas and 1 with a giant cell astrocytoma associated with tuberous sclerosis.[218] All four had cutaneous evidence of their phakomatosis. Occasionally, cortical tubers with bizarre, atypical neurons and

astrocytes are found in newborns with tuberous sclerosis who are undergoing surgery for craniotomy and biopsy or for postmortem examination (Table 9–2).[70,85,161,205,217] Lesions of the cerebral hemisphere, whether single or multiple, may not be discovered unless the newborn has a sizable cardiac rhabdomyoma that becomes clinically apparent or is responsible for the baby's demise.[171,205]

In a review of 200 neonatal brain tumors, Wa-

Table 9–2. Newborn Brain Tumors: Children's Hospital, Los Angeles, 1960–1991*

Tumor	Location	Number (%)
Astrocytoma	Cerebral hemisphere, thalamus, hypothalamus, optic nerve	4 (26.6)
Choroid plexus papilloma	Lateral ventricle (3 cases); 3rd ventricle (1 case)	4 (26.6)
Medulloblastoma	Cerebellum	2 (13.3)
Ependymoma	4th ventricle	1 (6.7)
Choroid plexus carcinoma	Lateral ventricle	1 (6.7)
Ganglioglioma	Frontal lobe	1 (6.7)
Cortical tuber (tuberous sclerosis)	Parietal lobe	1 (6.7)
Myxolipoma	Thalamus	1 (6.7)
Total		15 (100)

*During the same period as the study, there were seven newborns reported with intracranial vascular malformations.

kai and colleagues revealed that 23 (11.5%) had associated anomalies of various, nonspecific types.[232] Three of five fetuses with congenital brain tumors had hydrocephalus or other significant malformations.[234] In 11 newborns with intracranial teratomas reviewed by the Armed Forces Institute of Pathology, the following associated malformations were found: hydrocephalus in 5, cleft lip and palate in 2, proptosis in 2, and anencephaly in 1.[190]

An unexplained relationship exists between certain renal and liver tumors—namely, rhabdoid and Wilms' tumors—and primitive neuroectodermal tumor (PNET) of the central nervous system.[21,31,60,101] Bonnin and colleagues describe seven infants with this association, six of whom were younger than 1 year of age.[20] Chang et al. reported an example of a 14-day-old male infant with a large cerebral PNET and a solitary hepatic rhabdoid tumor discovered incidentally at necropsy.[31] They concluded from their findings that the rhabdoid tumor originated from the brain, as both PNET and rhabdoid components were found by light and electron microscopy in the brain tumor, and that the liver rhabdoid tumor was a metastasis rather than a second primary. Based on this assumption, the authors postulated that PNET and rhabdoid tumor have a common histogenesis, and that they are likely of neuroectodermal origin.

CLINICAL FINDINGS

The clinical manifestations of brain tumors in the fetus and neonate are different from those of the older child and adult.[3,63,70,112,116,117,119,122,147,159,232,239] First, there is an increased frequency of stillbirth in neonates with brain tumors (see Tables 9–6 to 9–13).[3,75,237] In the series by Wakai et al., 35 (30%) of 115 newborns were stillborn.[232] Gerlach and colleagues listed 36 cases of brain tumors in stillborns (see Table 9–4).

Macrocephaly and hydrocephalus are the main presenting signs in the fetus and neonate, which is in contrast to the older child, in whom lateralizing signs—hyperreflexia, ataxia, cranial nerve palsy, hemiparesis, and seizures—are more frequent (Table 9–3; see also Tables 9–5 through 9–13).[3] Immature development of the brain, lack of myelinization, and expansiveness of the soft cranial bones are the reasons given for the lack of lateralizing signs, particularly with cerebral and intraventricular

Table 9–3. Central Nervous System Tumors of the Perinatal Period: 736 Cases

Tumor	Group A	Group B	Number* (%)
Astrocytoma	76	58	134 (18.2)
Choroid plexus papilloma	112	7	119 (16.2)
Teratoma	80	2	82 (11.1)
Medulloblastoma	56	14	70 (9.5)
Ependymoma	38	10	48 (6.5)
Glioma, NOS	30	3	33 (4.5)
Glioblastoma	23	4	27 (3.7)
Sarcoma	20	5	25 (3.4)
Stem cell tumor	20	5	25 (3.4)
Melanoma	18	1	19 (2.6)
Lipoma	16	3	19 (2.6)
Meningioma	15	3	18 (2.4)
Craniopharyngioma	13	3	16 (2.2)
Other	68	33	101 (13.7)

*Total of groups A + B (see above). Group A includes tumors with histologic verification in the first week of life (585 cases), whereas group B includes tumors associated with symptoms within the first week of life, but with later histologic verification (151 cases).

NOS = not otherwise specified.

Abstracted from Gerlach VH, Janisch W, Schreiber D. ZNS—Tumoren der perinatalperiode. Zentralbl Allg Pathol 1982;126:23. Used by permission.

tumors.[3,173] Brain tumors in the newborn may present as intracranial hemorrhage, chronic subdural hematoma, neurologic deficits, unexplained hydrocephalus, or distortion of the cranium with bony defects.[2,28,40] The clinical manifestations may mimic those of congenital hydrocephalus, chronic subdural effusions, or cerebral palsy, making the diagnosis difficult.[116,173a]

According to Volpe,[229] the clinical findings of neonatal brain tumors can be divided into four main groups or syndromes. The first is characterized by tumors that are gigantic, producing severe macrocrania leading to cephalopelvic disproportion, dystocia, stillbirth, or premature labor associated with serious obstetrical problems. The second is characterized by a large head and bulging fontanelle secondary to hydrocephalus. The third has specific neurologic findings related to the type and site of the lesion and is typical for tumors occurring after birth in the newborn period. Seizures, noted in 14% to 25% of newborns, hemiparesis or quadriparesis, cranial nerve abnormalities, and signs of increased intracranial pressure, frequently attributable to hydrocephalus, are the findings mentioned. The fourth group is characterized by the sudden onset of intracranial hemorrhage, which occurs in 8% to 18% of neonates with brain tumors.[229]

Imaging studies show that polyhydramnios, hydrops, and hydrocephalus often accompany fetal brain tumors and, indeed, may be the initial manifestation. According to Geraghty and associates, the antenatal sonographic differential diagnosis of an intracranial mass lesion includes teratoma, astrocytoma, ependymoma, other rarer tumors, vascular malformation, and hemorrhage.[74]

Because of the remarkable ability of the skull to expand, some brain tumors grow enormously in utero, leading to a difficult delivery (dystocia) and stillbirth. Large tumors are responsible for fetal hydrops, or may require decompression of the skull to permit vaginal delivery.[16,37,40,209] Intracranial teratoma, which is the most common intracranial fetal tumor in some studies, is a prime example of such a tumor (see Fig. 9–11).[46,128,156,213,215,237] Other brain tumors detected antenatally are choroid plexus papilloma, craniopharyngioma, and astrocytoma (Tables 9–6 through 9–13).[90,128,237]

Wienk et al.[237] reviewed the clinicopathologic and sonographic findings in nine antenatal intracranial neoplasms, including two of their own, diagnosed at 31 to 40 weeks' gestation.[32,34,89,178,202,208,225,237] The review consisted of four teratomas and one each of craniopharyngioma, meningeal sarcoma, oligodendroglioma, a midline supratentorial "malignant tumor," and a lipoma of the corpus callosum. Skull decompression was required to deliver two fetuses; amniocentesis was performed in two, and two cesarean sections were performed. There was a high mortality rate—five stillbirths and three neonatal deaths—and only one survivor, the baby with the lipoma. Heckel et al. presented an example of a fetal anaplastic astrocytoma detected at 31 weeks' gestation and reviewed 19 additional brain tumors diagnosed antenatally.[90] The review included 13 teratomas and 6 astrocytomas (including 4 glioblastomas). The mortality was high in that series also, as only three survivors were reported, all of whom had astrocytomas.

Signs of increased intracranial pressure—namely, vomiting, lethargy, enlarging head size, separation of cranial sutures, and bulging fontanelles—are observed in neonates with a rapidly growing neoplasm.[119] It is possible, however, that some brain tumors are too small to produce symptoms during the perinatal period, and only become manifest when the baby is a few months older.[27]

An abnormally large head circumference is the most common physical finding observed in the neonate with a brain tumor, regardless of the histologic type; craniomegaly is the result of either hydrocephalus or the size of the tumor mass per se, or both (see Fig. 9–11).[3,28,63,67,80,107,116–118,174,209,219,232] Hydrocephalus is caused by either compression of the ventricular system or hemorrhage from the tumor.[129] The incidence of hemorrhage from neonatal brain tumors is significantly high; it occurred in 14% of the 193 symptomatic patients in the review by Wakai and colleagues,[232] and 18% of the 45 patients included in the series of Buetow and co-workers.[28] The occurrence of hemorrhage with three congenital brain tumors—astrocytoma, medulloblastoma, and cerebral PNET—was observed on imaging studies and at surgery.[2] Albert et al. suggest that rapidly changing pressure forces imposed on the baby during delivery are responsible for the hemorrhage, and that the space-occupying effect of the tumor is magnified by repeated bleeds, which accelerate the rapidly fatal outcome in some instances.[2]

In a study of 17 neonates with intracranial tumors by Jooma and colleagues, the main clinical findings in decreasing order of frequency, were macrocephaly (n = 5), seizures (n = 4), vomiting (n = 2), abnormal eye movements (n = 2), failure to thrive (n = 2), and irritability and respiratory distress (n = 1).[119] An increasing head circumference was also the most frequent finding in another study, which consisted of 4 neonates and 25 infants.[105,107] Vomiting, hydrocephalus, and bulbar paralysis were the presenting signs in the neonates with either supratentorial or infratentorial tumors.[105] Four infants with optic nerve astrocytomas had proptosis, with or without abnormal eye movements.[106]

Brain tumors occurring in the perinatal period do not always present with craniomegaly and hydrocephalus as the initial manifestations. The presenting signs and symptoms may be subtle, nonlocalizing, and, in addition, may include nuchal rigidity, paresis, rotary nystagmus, cranial nerve palsies, seizures, or general failure to thrive (see Tables 9–6 through 9–13).[7,29,61,63,66,119,219,229]

One constellation of findings that is unique to the older infant with a brain tumor is the diencephalic syndrome. Typically, infants with this condition have elfin-like facies; long, thin extremities; marked wasting in the presence of a voracious appetite; hyperalertness; and a happy disposition.[63,71,117,119] Most of these patients have a low-grade astrocytoma, usually a pilocytic type, situated in the midline in the region of the third ventricle and hypothalamus.[50,57,63,112] Increased growth hormone production by the hypothalamic-pituitary axis is believed to play a role in this rare and unusual syndrome, which is associated with a high mortality.[57,112]

With the widespread use of imaging studies, namely sonography, CT scanning, and MRI, the frequency of perinatally diagnosed brain tumors has increased considerably. Several reviews of prenatal and postnatal imaging of brain tumors have been published.[2,28,118,172,175,212] Imaging studies are most helpful in identifying and distinguishing potentially curable tumors, such as choroid plexus papillomas, from rapidly fatal ones, such as teratomas and PNETs.

DIFFERENTIAL DIAGNOSIS

Brain tumors can imitate other central nervous system conditions, such as congenital hydrocephalus, subdural hematoma, abscess, meningitis, and cerebral palsy, so the diagnosis should always be kept in mind.[173a] However, overall, neoplasms are not that common a cause of hydrocephalus in the newborn.[129] Fibrotic obstruction of the subarachnoid space or aqueduct following hemorrhage or infection occurs more frequently and is the leading cause of neonatal hydrocephalus. Other etiologies include occlusion of the aqueduct by congenital atresia or acquired gliosis and malformations, such as the Arnold-Chiari syndrome.[54] Moreover, in a normal newborn, the cerebral aqueduct is only 0.5 mm or less at its smallest diameter, which makes this structure vulnerable to injury from reactive gliosis, hemorrhage, or compression from vascular malformations and neoplasms.[65] Obstruction of the cerebral aqueduct is the most common cause of congenital hydrocephalus.

PATHOLOGY

The location and the histologic types of brain tumors of the fetus and newborn are dissimilar from those in the older child and adolescent. In most perinatal series, more than 60% of brain tumors involve regions above the tentorium cerebelli.* Intracranial teratomas account for almost one third of the total reported cases in fetuses and newborns, and astrocytoma,

____

*References: 7, 39, 52, 53, 63, 66, 70, 75, 91, 111, 112, 117–119, 125, 160, 172, 173, 195, 197, 212, 218, 232.

Table 9–4. Brain Tumors in Stillborns: 36 cases

Tumor	Number (%)
Teratoma	21 (58)
Astrocytoma	6 (16.7)
Glioma, NOS	4 (11.1)
Choroid plexus papilloma	1 (2.8)
Ependymoma	1 (2.8)
Craniopharyngioma	1 (2.8)
Mesenchymal mixed tumor	1 (2.8)
Angioblastoma	1 (2.8)

NOS = not otherwise specified.
Abstracted from Gerlach VH, Janisch W, Schreiber D. ZNS—Tumoren der perinatalperiode. Zentralbl Allg Pathol 1982;126:23. Used by permission.

medulloblastoma, ependymoma, and choroid plexus papilloma are the principal neuroepithelial tumors (see Tables 9–1 and 9–3 through 9–14).

Gerlach and associates reviewed their autopsy and surgical biopsy material and cases submitted to them for consultation, together with the world literature from 1900 to 1982, which yielded a collection of 736 perinatal brain tumors.[75] They divided the tumors into three groups: those occurring in stillborns (36 cases), those with histologic verification in the first week of life (Group A, 585 cases) and those with symptoms appearing within the first week of life with later histologic verification (Group B, 151 cases). Their data are presented in Tables 9–3 and 9–4.

Wakai and associates[232] reviewed 200 cases of congenital brain tumors, including two of their own, and recorded the distribution of the various histologic types. The results of their review are presented in Table 9–5.

The studies of Gerlach and co-workers[75] and of Wakai and colleagues[232] show that the distribution of the various types of perinatal brain tumors varies in different institutions and countries. Other conclusions that can be drawn from these findings are that astrocytoma, medulloblastoma, and choroid plexus papilloma are the major neuroglial perinatal tumors, and that teratoma is the leading non-neuroglial tumor and is responsible for the largest number of stillbirths, accounting for over one third to one half of the cases (see Table 9–4).[75,232]

In addition to light microscopy, electron microscopy and immunohistochemistry are requisite for the identification and classification of brain tumors.[10,11,19,20,91,169,192] The immunohistochemical markers specifically used for the eval-

Table 9–5. 185 Congenital Brain Tumors

Tumor	Number (%)*
Teratoma	73 (36.5)
Astrocytoma†	32 (16)
Medulloblastoma	23 (11.5)
Choroid plexus papilloma	15 (7.5)
Ependymoma	14 (7.0)
Craniopharyngioma	9 (4.5)
Meningioma	7 (3.5)
Meningeal sarcoma	7 (3.5)
Glioma, NOS	5 (2.5)

*Not all 200 brain tumors in Wakai et al.'s series are listed in this table. Rather, only 185 of the more common ones have been included for purposes of comparison. The numbers in the left column were obtained by adding the authors' groups A + B + C. The percentages in the right column are calculated on the basis of 200 cases (e.g., for teratoma 73/200 × 100 = 36.5%).

†Includes 19 astrocytomas, 7 glioblastomas, and 6 polar spongioblastomas.

Abstracted from Wakai S, Arai T, Nagai M. Congenital brain tumors. Surg Neurol 1984;21:597. Used by permission.

uation of central nervous system neoplasms are the glial fibrillary acidic protein (GFAP) and the neurofilament protein (NFP) antibodies.[10,20,192] The GFAP is helpful in distinguishing between glial and nonglial neoplasms and in identifying astrocytic elements.[10,20,192] The neurofilament proteins are intermediate filament proteins found in neurons and their processes, and are usually restricted to these cells.[10,20,192] Monoclonal antibodies directed against neuroectoderm-associated antigens include neuron-specific enolase (NSE) and the S-100 protein, which cross-reacts with many types of tissues, both neural and non-neural.[91] Despite this technical problem, neuroblastoma, medulloblastoma, and other PNETs generally show NSE positivity and are focally positive to S-100 protein. Synaptophysin is also a useful marker for identifying these neoplasms. Alpha-fetoprotein (AFP) and human chorionic gonadotropin (hCG) immunoperoxidase antibodies aid in the diagnosis of intracranial germ cell tumors, yolk sac tumor and choriocarcinoma, respectively[20] (see Chapter 2, "Germ Cell Tumors"). Electron microscopy is recommended for evaluating those brain tumors that pose a diagnostic problem.[10,11,19] Flow cytometry and Ki-67 quantitation may be useful in the prognostication of certain brain tumors (e.g., ependymomas and choroid plexus tumors) when the histologic features of malignancy are equivocal.[113] Karyotyping is increasingly becoming a useful tool in identifying certain brain tumors, as well.

CYTOGENETICS

Chromosomal abnormalities in pediatric brain tumors tend to be rather nonspecific, but nevertheless appear to be different from those found in adult brain tumors.[81,222] The most common abnormality in medulloblastoma is the total or partial loss of chromosome 17, a monosomy of i(17q), which is noted in approximately 50% of these tumors.[81,139,222] This deleted region includes the oncosuppressor gene p53. The gene most commonly amplified in medulloblastomas, as with neuroblastoma, is the N-myc oncogene. Chromosome 1 deletions (del 1q) have been described in childhood astrocytomas.[222] Cytogenetic analysis of intracranial teratomas, congenital or otherwise, show a normal 46XY or 46XX karyotype for both the patient and tumor.[139,157,185,194]

ASTROCYTOMA

Astrocytomas, the leading neuroglial tumors of infancy and childhood, are neoplasms derived from and consisting of astrocytes showing various degrees of differentiation.[13] As a group, they differ from other tumors in their gross and histologic features, as well as in their site of origin and clinical manifestations (Table 9–6). Overall, astrocytoma and intracranial teratoma occur at about the same frequency in the fetus and newborn (see Table 9–1).

In contrast to those occurring in older children and adolescents, astrocytomas of the fetus and newborn usually are found outside the cerebellum and above the tentorium cerebelli (see Table 9–6). The cerebral hemisphere is the most common primary site, where almost two thirds of the perinatal astrocytomas occur, followed by the diencephalon (thalamus, hypothalamus) and brain stem (mesencephalon, medulla, and pons) (see Table 9–6). Those arising from the cerebral hemisphere are frequently large, may involve more than one lobe, and occupy a large area of the brain. Hydrocephalus is the chief presenting finding in the fetus and newborn, regardless of the location (see Table 9–6).[209]

Newborns with hemispheric astrocytomas may present with either antenatal hydrocephalus (or macrocrania) leading to cephalopelvic disproportion and dystocia, or hydrocephalus that develops in the neonatal period. Polyhydramnios and stillbirth occur with this tumor.[4,40,69,74,75,90,182,209,232] In one series, 6 of 46

Case No.	Diagnosis	Age at Death	Location	Initial Findings	Reference
1	Astrocytoma	1 day	Basal ganglia	Hydrocephalus	Soltaire and Krigman[209]
2	Glioblastoma	After birth	Thalamus	Hydrocephalus	Soltaire and Krigman[209]
3	Astrocytoma	4 months	Midbrain	Hydrocephalus	Soltaire and Krigman[209]
4	Glioblastoma	49 days	Diencephalon	Hydrocephalus	Soltaire and Krigman[209]
5	Astrocytoma	3 days	Pons and midbrain	Hydrocephalus	Soltaire and Krigman[209]
6	Spongioblastoma	After birth	Hemisphere†	Dystocia	Soltaire and Krigman[209]
7	Spongioblastoma	Stillborn	Midbrain, pons, and medulla	Dystocia	Soltaire and Krigman[209]
8	Spongioblastoma	Stillborn	Pons	Hydrocephalus	Fuste et al.[69]
9	Astrocytoma	Stillborn	Hemisphere	Hydrocephalus	Cooperman et al.[40]
10	Desmoplastic astrocytoma	40 days	Hemisphere	Large head	Taratuto et al.[216]
11	Spongioblastoma	Stillborn	Cerebellum, pons	Hydrocephalus	Duckett and Wilson[59]
12	Astrocytoma	1 day	Hemisphere	Hemorrhage	Sandbank[196]
13	Astrocytoma	20 days	Hemisphere	Hydrocephalus, seizures, exophthalmus	Campbell et al.[29]
14	Astrocytoma‡	1 day	Hemisphere	Large head	Campbell et al.[29]
15	Astrocytoma‡	8 months	Hemisphere	Large head, strabismus	Campbell et al.[29]
16	Astrocytoma‡§	Alive	Hemisphere	Hydrocephalus	Roosen et al.[182]
17	Astrocytoma‡	8 months	Hemisphere	Hydrocephalus	Podskalny et al.[170]
18	Astrocytoma‡	After birth	Hemisphere	Large head	Osborn et al.[162]
19	Giant cell astrocytoma	Alive	Hemisphere	Tuberous sclerosis, seizures	Galassi et al.[70]
20	Astrocytoma	58 days	Roof of 3rd ventricle	Hydrocephalus	Raskind and Beigel[173]
21	Astrocytoma	3 weeks	Hemisphere	Large head	Jellinger and Sunder-Plassman[116]
22	Spongioblastoma	4 years	Optic chiasm	Ptosis, exophthalmos, cranial asymmetry	Ellams et al.[61]
23	Astrocytoma	Alive	Hemisphere	Large head	Ellams et al.[61]
24	Astrocytoma	Alive	Lateral ventricle	Vomiting	Sakamoto et al.[195]
25	Astrocytoma	3 months	Optic chiasm	Large head	Sakamoto et al.[195]
26	Astrocytoma, grade 2	Alive	Hemisphere	Hydrocephalus	Wakai et al.[232]
27	Spongioblastoma	3 days	Hemisphere	Hydrocephalus	Albert et al.[2]
28	Astrocytoma, grade 3	Alive	Hemisphere	Seizures	Albert et al.[2]
29	Astrocytoma	Alive	Hemisphere	Hemorrhage	Rothman et al.[186]
30	Astrocytoma, grade 3	18 months	Diencephalon	Large head	Jooma et al.[119]
31	Astrocytoma	3 weeks	Hypothalamus	Bulbar paralysis, dysphagia, hypotonia	Isaacs[107]
32	Astrocytoma‡	Alive	Hemisphere	Hemorrhage	Isaacs‖
33	Astrocytoma‡	Alive	Thalamus	Large head	Isaacs‖
34	Astrocytoma	LTF	Optic nerve	Proptosis	Isaacs‖
35	Astrocytoma	Alive	Hemisphere	?Hydrocephalus	Raimondi and Tomita[173]
36	Astrocytoma‡	2 months	Diencephalon, brain stem	?Hydrocephalus	Raimondi and Tomita[173]
37	Glioblastoma	20 months	Hemisphere	?Hydrocephalus	Raimondi and Tomita[173]
38	Glioblastoma	90 minutes	Hemisphere	Hydrocephalus	Sabet[193]
39	Glioblastoma§	After birth	Hemisphere	Hydrocephalus	Geraghty et al.[74]
40	Glioblastoma	43 days	Cerebellum	Large head	Itoh et al.[109]
41	Glioblastoma§	Stillborn	Hemisphere	Large head	McConachie et al.[145]
42	Glioblastoma§	20 minutes	Hemisphere	Hydramnios, hemisphere mass	Riboni et al.[177]
43	Astrocytoma‡	Stillborn§	Hemisphere	Hydrocephalus, hemisphere mass	Heckel et al.[90]
44	Glioblastoma§	1 day	Hemisphere	Hydrocephalus, large head, intracranial mass	Alvarez et al.[4]
45	Glioblastoma§	Alive	Hemisphere	Hydrocephalus, hemisphere mass	Alvarez et al.[4]
46	Astrocytoma¶	Alive	Hemisphere	Hydrocephalus, hemisphere mass	Oikawa et al.[161]

*Selected from the literature.
†Cerebral hemisphere.
‡Anaplastic astrocytoma.
§Tumor detected antenatally.
‖Refer to Table 9–2.
¶Subependymal giant cell astrocytoma associated with tuberous sclerosis.
LTF = lost to follow-up.

(13%) fetuses and newborns with astrocytoma were stillborn, and hemorrhage was the initial finding in 3 newborns (see Table 9–6).

With the advent of prenatal ultrasonography, which is practically a routine practice, fetal brain tumors are being discovered with increasing frequency. Geraghty and colleagues reported an example of a right cerebral glioblastoma detected at 33 weeks' gestation by sonography; the findings included craniomegaly and a huge, brightly echogenic mass expanding and replacing the cerebral hemisphere.[74] McConachie and co-workers and Riboni et al. reported similar examples.[145,177]

Signs of increasing intracranial pressure— namely, enlarging head size, separation of the cranial sutures, lethargy, irritability, failure to feed, and vomiting—appear in the neonatal period.[65] Sometimes seizures occur and, when present, suggest bleeding into the tumor. At this time, the cerebrospinal fluid (CSF) may be xanthochromic or contain blood.[65] Congenital astrocytoma of the brain stem is less common than hemispheric lesions and produces dysfunction of brain stem nuclei. Respiratory difficulty after birth with episodes of recurrent apnea and tremors are the clinical findings.[65] Hydrocephalus often accompanies brain stem lesions (see Table 9–6).

A newborn in the Children's Hospital, Los Angeles perinatal study with a hypothalamic astrocytoma, grade 2, was admitted to the hospital at the age of 3 weeks with bulbar paralysis, dysphagia, and hypotonia, an unusual clinical presentation for a tumor in this location. The neonate died 4 days later. The diagnosis was not established until postmortem examination.[107]

Spontaneous intracerebral hemorrhage occurs frequently with congenital astrocytoma; because of this tendency, an underlying neoplasm should be suspected when evaluating a cerebral bleed in a neonate (see Table 9–6).[2,16,46,186,196,232] Hemorrhage was the initial finding in two neonates with cerebral hemisphere lesions.[186,196] The association of an intracerebral hemorrhage secondary to a congenital cerebral artery aneurysm and an astrocytoma in the contralateral cerebral hemisphere has been described in the literature.[22]

Astrocytomas in the fetus and infant histologically range from low- to high-grade (see Table 9–6 and Figs. 9–1 and 9–2). The review of 46 perinatal astrocytomas listed in Table 9–6 shows that almost half (22 [48%]) are malignant (10 glioblastoma, 10 anaplastic, and 2

grade 3 astrocytomas). Glioblastoma multiforme occurs most often in the cerebral hemisphere as compared to the brain stem and basal ganglia (see Table 9–6).[28,59,74,109,173a,192,193,209]

The term anaplastic astrocytoma is applied to astrocytomas of intermediate grade of malignancy, roughly corresponding to grades 2 and 3. Microscopically, they display pleomorphism, hypercellularity, and to a degree, the anaplasia of glioblastoma; however, they lack the pallisading necrosis, hemorrhage, and vascular proliferation observed in the latter. Five of 17 astrocytomas reported by Asai et al.,[7] the cerebral tumors described by Roosen et al.,[182] Podskalny et al.,[170] and Osborn and colleagues,[162] and 2 of the 3 cerebral astrocytomas described by Campbell et al.[29] were diagnosed as anaplastic. Moreover, the three astrocytomas described in the Toronto neonatal study were classified as high grade.[29] Neither intracranial nor extracranial metastases were documented in the newborns with astrocytoma in any of these studies.

Although the subependymal giant cell astrocytoma associated with tuberous sclerosis is usually found in adolescents and young adults, several have been reported in neonates (see Table 9–6).[70,85,161,205,217,218] The most common sign is increased intracranial pressure produced by obstruction of the foramen of Monro.[161]

Desmoplastic cerebral astrocytoma is a form of astrocytoma that typically occurs in infants and appears to be associated with a good prognosis.[22,45,216] The desmoplastic variants are large, cystic, hemispheric tumors involving the frontal cerebral cortex and adjacent meninges, including the dura. One of the youngest infants with this form of astrocytoma was a 40-day-old girl with asymmetric macrocephaly, bulging fontanelles, the "sunset sign" (limitation of upward gaze), and cranial nerve palsies.[216]

Histologically, the desmoplastic astrocytoma consists of small clusters of astrocytes intermingled with spindle-shaped fibroblasts and a prominent collagenous stroma. Necrosis, cellular atypia, and increased mitotic activity are absent. Some tumors exhibit a storiform growth pattern. The astrocytes stain positively with GFAP and S-100 protein, and the desmoplastic stroma is reactive with vimentin.[45,138] Ultrastructural studies by de Chadarevian and associates and by Louis et al. demonstrate the presence of large amounts of external laminal material and collagen fibers between neoplastic astrocytes.[45,138] No neuronal elements are noted in the tumor.

The overall survival rate for newborns with

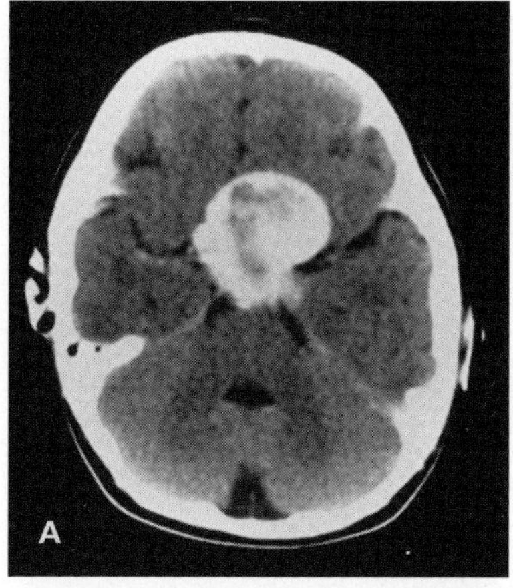

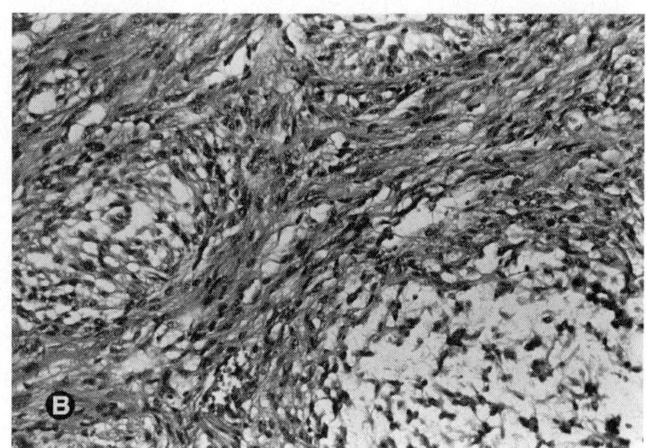

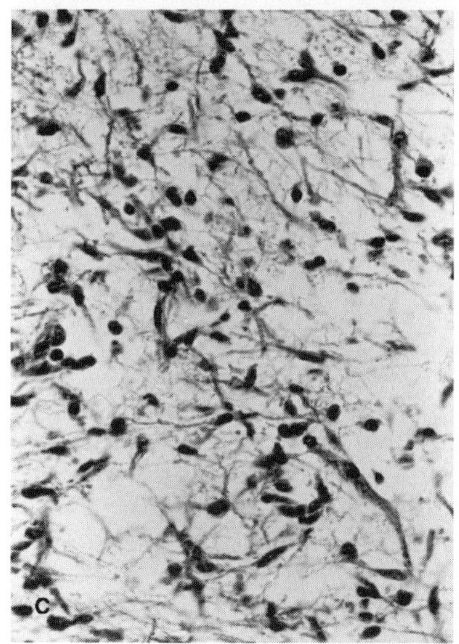

Figure 9–1. Astrocytoma. A 5-month-old girl presented with a history of intermittent vertical nystagmus. *A,* A CT scan of the head reveals a lobulated midline mass occupying the suprasellar cistern and involving the optic chiasm and left hypothalamus. *B,* A microscopic section displays a low-grade pilocytic astrocytoma with compact and microcystic areas (hematoxylin-eosin, ×300). *C,* Slender, spindle-shaped cells with elongated processes are demonstrated with the PTAH stain (PTAH, ×750). (From Isaacs H Jr. Tumors of the Newborn and Infant. St. Louis: Mosby–Year Book, 1991.)

astrocytoma remains dismal. Tables 9–6 and 9–15 show that 12 of 46 (26%) survived and 7 (15%) were stillborn. Ten of 12 survivors had cerebral hemispheric tumors. Use of chemotherapy in infants with this tumor who are younger than 3 months of age has met with limited success.[77]

PRIMITIVE NEUROECTODERMAL TUMOR

PNETs are a group of related small cell malignant tumors occurring in the central and peripheral nervous systems and soft tissues.[11,12,21,49,60,88,91,100,126,130,183] The neural crest has been proposed as the site of origin of these highly malignant neoplasms. PNETs occur primarily in the pediatric age group and are characterized by a very aggressive behavior in the central nervous system, regardless of their primary site or histologic components.

Traditionally, the term "primitive neuroectodermal" has been applied to tumors composed of undifferentiated cells (so-called fetal neuroepithelial cells) resembling germinal or matrix cells of the embryonic neural tube.[88] The term implies that the tumor cells can differentiate along either neuronal or glial cell lines. In keeping with this concept, the tumor displays a spectrum of histologic appearances varying from completely undifferentiated tumors to those showing focal or diffuse areas of neuronal and/or glial differentiation.[88] The degee of differentiation varies within areas of any given tumor and in different tumors.[126]

Characteristically, PNETs are highly aggressive, metastasizing widely within the cerebrospi-

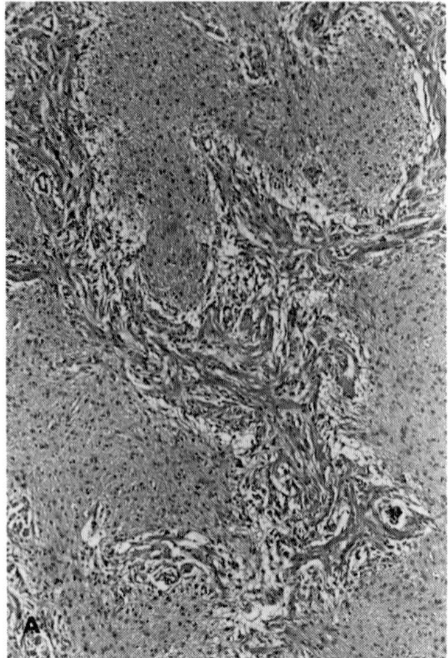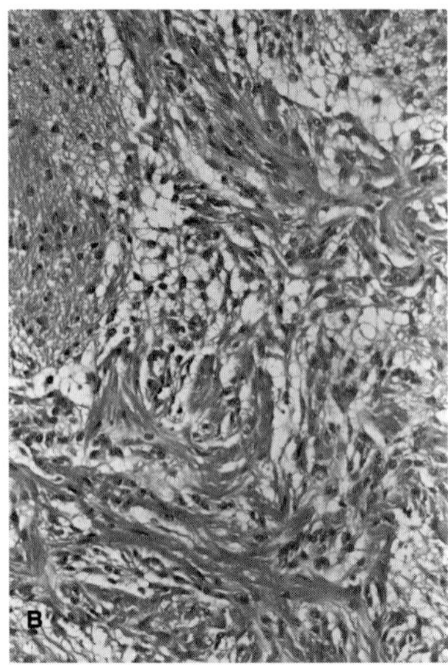

Figure 9–2. Optic glioma. A 7-month-old boy presented with seizures, facial twitching, and right eye deviation. A CT scan revealed obstructive hydrocephalus and a 3 × 4 cm suprasellar, solid and cystic mass arising from the optic chiasm, compressing the third ventricle, and producing enlargement of the right optic foramen. *A,* The cerebral cortex is infiltrated by a pilocytic astrocytoma having histologic features similar to those described in Figure 9–1 (hematoxylin-eosin, ×48). *B,* A higher-power view shows the biphasic pattern composed of compact fascicles of fibrillated, elongated, bipolar cells alternating with more loosely arranged microcystic areas (hematoxylin-eosin, ×150).

nal fluid pathways and seeding the meninges of the brain and spinal cord.[91] They occur in several locations, including (most commonly) the cerebellum, the cerebral hemispheres, pineal body, brain stem, spinal cord, olfactory nerve, and retina (Table 9–7).[11,12,126,130] Microscopically, PNETs are composed of small, often poorly differentiated, darkly staining cells. Other components, such as astrocytic, ependymal, neuronal, retinal, or melanocytic cells, may also be present, depending on the location of the tumor.[11,91,183] Mesenchymal elements— for example, skeletal muscle, fibrous tissue, cartilage, and epithelial elements—are also noted in some.

MEDULLOBLASTOMA

Medulloblastoma (so-called PNET of the cerebellum) occurs with a frequency second only to astrocytoma in older children and adolescents, and in the neonate, it is ranked fourth after intracranial teratoma, astrocytoma, and choroid plexus papilloma, again depending on the series (see Tables 9–1 to 9–3).[47,53,61,63,75,91,108,116,183,189] Most infratentorial tumors in newborns are histologically malignant, which is explained by the fact that medulloblastoma is the leading posterior fossa neoplasm in this age group.[112,117]

This malignant lesion is associated with a relatively high frequency of stillbirth, hydrocephalus, and congenital defects (see Table 9–7).[121,211] For example, cleft-palate, omphalocele, malrotation of the intestine, imperforate anus, and bladder exstrophy have been described in association with medulloblastoma.[58,158]

Medulloblastoma is a classical example of one of the neoplasms of the young that Willis designated as an "embryoma" or "embryonic tumor."[238] He defined a member of this group as "a tumor which arises during embryonic, foetal or early post-natal development from a particular organ rudiment or tissue while this is immature."[238] In the embryo, fetal neuroepithelial cells originating in the roof of the fourth ventricle migrate upward and laterally to form the external granular layer of the cerebellum, which is the proposed site of histogenesis of medulloblastoma (Fig. 9–3A).[5,11,121,192] Moreover, the medulloblastoma in a 13-week-old premature infant reported by Kadin and colleagues reinforces the idea that the tumor originates from this site.[121] The external granular layer of this patient showed areas of cellular proliferation with invasion of the adjacent molecular layer. Transitions were noted from the normal external granular layer to actual tumor formation.

Of all brain tumors in the young, familial oc-

Table 9–7. 30 Fetal and Newborn Primitive Neuroectodermal Tumors*

Case No.	Age at Death	Location	Initial Findings	Reference
1	2 months	Cerebellum†	Vomiting, large head	Campbell et al.[29]
2	11 days	Cerebellum, cerebral	Hydrocephalus, seizures	Campbell et al.[29]
3	4.5 months	Pineal	Large head, hydrocephalus	Campbell et al.[29]
4	6 hours	Cerebellum†	Hydrocephalus	Werb et al.[234]
5	7 months	Cerebellum†	Hydrocephalus	Radkowski et al.[172]
6	Alive (?)	Suprasellar	Hydrocephalus	Radkowski et al.[172]
7	3 months	Cerebellum†	Large head, seizures	Jellinger and Sunder-Plassman[116]
8	2 months	Cerebellum†	Large head, nystagmus, right hemiparesis	Jellinger and Sunder-Plassman[116]
9	Alive (4 years)	Cerebellum†	Vomiting, lethargy, hydrocephalus	Haddad et al.[84]
10	5 months	Cerebellum†‡	Hydrocephalus, hypotonia	Ehret et al.[60]
11	11 weeks	Cerebellum†	Large head	Albert et al.[2]
12	Alive	Hemisphere	Seizures, hemorrhage	Albert et al.[2]
13	After birth	Hemisphere	Hydrocephalus	Becker and Hinton[11]
14	25 days	Cerebellum†	Hydrocephalus, nystagmus, downward gaze	Taboada et al.[211]
15	7 months	Cerebellum†	Large head	Taboada et al.[211]
16	8 hours	Cerebellum†	Low APGAR scores	Amacher et al.[5]
17	2.5 months	Cerebellum†	Vomiting, head enlargement, downward gaze, opisthotonus	Papadakis et al.[164]
18	7.5 months	Cerebellum†	Vomiting, head enlargement, downward gaze, opisthotonus	Papadakis et al.[164]
19	68 days	Cerebellum†§	Hydrocephalus	Balamaric and Chau[14]
20	12 days	Cerebellum†§	Hydrocephalus	Balamaric and Chau[14]
21	3 months	Thalamus	Large head, cutaneous & cervical lymph node metastases	Yu et al.[249]
22	20 hours	Cerebellum†	Incidental necropsy finding‖	Duckett[58]
23	63 days	Cerebellum†	Vomiting, poor feeding, facial palsy	Kim et al.[123]
24	13 weeks	Cerebellum†	Large head, downward gaze	Kadin et al.[121]
25	14 days	Cerebral¶	Cephalopelvic disproportion, vomiting, irritability	Chang et al.[31]
26	Termination of pregnancy	Cerebellum	Oligohydramnios, tumor detected by antenatal sonography	Mitchell et al.[148a]
27	2 months	Cerebellum†	Vomiting, bulbar paralysis	Isaacs[107]
28	3 months	Cerebellum†	Large head, facial palsy	Isaacs#
29	2 months	Cerebral	Large head	Isaacs**
30	1.5 years	Cerebral	Hydrocephalus	Isaacs**

*Selected from the literature.
†Medulloblastoma, 20 of 29 (69%) PNETs.
‡Patient also had a renal rhabdoid tumor.
§Newborns were sisters.
‖Patient had multiple congenital anomalies (e.g., omphalocele, bladder exstrophy, imperforate anus, bifid uterus, and cleft palate).
¶Rhabdoid tumor of the liver.
#Refer to Table 9–2.
**Refer to Table 9–1.

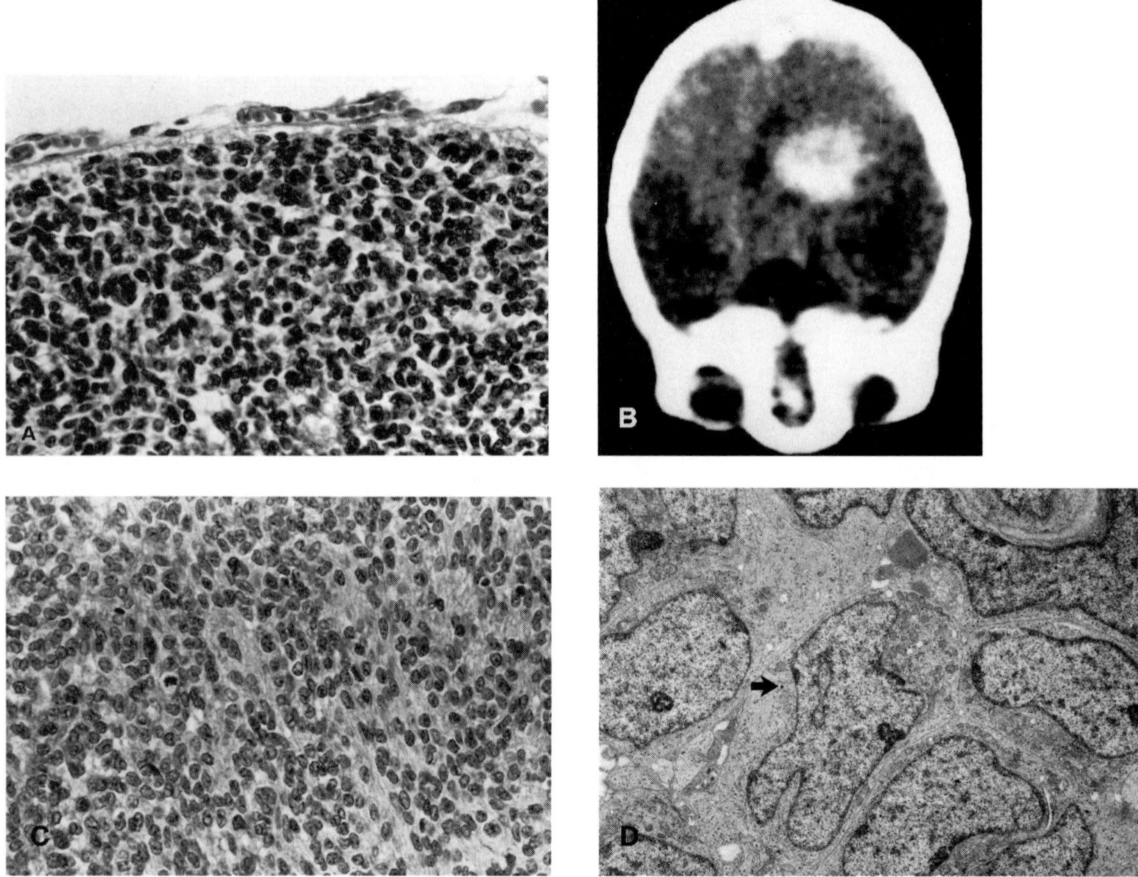

Figure 9–3. Medulloblastoma (''cerebellar PNET''). _A,_ The cerebellum of a 650-g, 10-hour-old male infant of 26 weeks' gestation shows the developing external granular layer in an immature, but otherwise normal brain (hematoxylin-eosin, ×750). Compare the cytology of this photomicrograph with that in Figure 9–3_C. B,_ A CT scan of a newborn with a several-week history of poor feeding and vomiting and terminally bulbar paresis. There is a large enhancing mass within the medial aspect of the left cerebellar hemisphere. _C,_ A photomicrograph reveals a small cell malignant tumor with a fibrillary background. Pseudorosette formation by the tumor cells is suggestive, but not well defined. Several mitotic figures are evident (hematoxylin-eosin, ×750). _D,_ The ultrastructural findings include primitive-appearing cells with irregular nuclei. The cytoplasm contains a few organelles, mostly mitochondria and scattered ribosomes. Few dense-core granules are seen (_arrow_). Microtubules are noted in some cytoplasmic processes (×9,000). (From Isaacs H Jr. Tumors of the Newborn and Infant. St. Louis: Mosby–Year Book, 1991.)

currence has been documented most often in those with medulloblastoma.[14,232] The tumor has been reported in male siblings and in two sisters with congenital tumors.[14] There is an interesting but unexplained association between medulloblastoma and rhabdoid tumor of the kidney, and it has been suggested that the neural crest is the common denominator.[21,31,60,101]

A large head and hydrocephalus are the most common findings in the fetus and newborn with a medulloblastoma (see Table 9–7).[60,65,121,148a,164] Werb et al. described a polypoid medulloblastoma measuring 1.2 cm in diameter in a fetus of 34 weeks' gestation; the tumor origi-

nated from the roof of the fourth ventricle, causing obstruction of the cerebral aqueduct and severe hydrocephalus.[234] In the neonatal period, feeding difficulty may be the initial sign, followed by lethargy, vomiting, and apnea. Other findings include nystagmus, downward gaze, opisthotonus, and seizures (see Table 9–7).[65] Hemorrhage may be the presenting finding.[2] The tumor has been detected antenatally by sonography at 30 weeks' gestation.[148a]

Medulloblastomas in the neonate arise from the midline, whereas lateral tumors are more prevalent in older individuals.[5] From the vermis of the cerebellum, the malignant process extends into the fourth ventricle and adjacent cerebellar hemispheres. Subsequently, obstructive hydrocephalus and leptomeningeal seeding along the cerebrospinal axis ensue.[11,60,121,123] At this time, cytologic examination of CSF may show tumor cells. If vascular invasion occurs, the tumor enters the blood and metastasizes— to organs outside the central nervous system in 9% to 18% of the cases—primarily to the liver, lungs, and bone marrow, and sometimes, to the lymph nodes.[143,144] Bone marrow biopsy and CSF cytologic studies are integral parts of the initial metastatic work-up before starting therapy. Occasionally, the tumor metastasizes to the cervical lymph nodes and presents as a mass in the neck, which may be mistaken clinically for lymphadenitis.[143,144] Extensive involvement of the subarachnoid space by tumor appears to be an etiologic factor associated with extraneural spread.[143]

Histologically, medulloblastomas consist of small, darkly staining cells with varying amounts of intercellular, pink-staining, fibrillar material (see Fig. 9–3C). The cells have round, oval, or carrot-shaped nuclei with coarse chromatin and small nucleoli and scant cytoplasms. Well-defined Homer-Wright pseudorosettes are present in less than 50% of the specimens.[148a] Extensive necrosis and moderate mitotic activity are typical findings.

Several other histologic forms of medulloblastoma have been described, but these are usually seen in older children. They include the nodular desmoplastic variant, medulloblastoma with glial differentiation, melanotic medulloblastoma, medullomyoblastoma, and large cell medulloblastoma.[11,33,56,79,148,201,211,250]

Desmoplasia is noted in some tumors, but apparently has no prognostic implications.[108] According to Kadin and co-workers, this histologic pattern is found when invasion of the leptomeninges occurs, and it appears to be a fibroblastic reaction to the tumor.[121] Another variation is the cerebellar PNET with a prominent desmoplastic, immature-appearing, mesenchymal stroma.[211,243] Cerebellar PNETs with glial differentiation contain several different kinds of neuroepithelial components in addition to the small, round, undifferentiated cells (e.g., astrocytoma, oligodendroglioma, and ependymoma).[250] The cerebellar tumor from a 5-month-old male infant described by Zimmer et al. had cytokeratin epithelial markers in addition to vimentin, S-100 protein, NSE, and GFAP immunoreactivity. Moreover, cytokeratin intermediate filaments were demonstrated on ultrastructural examination.[250] It is conceivable that this variant is histogenetically related to the small cell polyphenotypic tumor of the soft tissues (see Chapter 4, "Soft Tissue Tumors").

On histologic examination, the large cell variant resembles the rhabdoid tumor somewhat; that is, the cells have a large vesicular nucleus with a prominent nucleolus. However, they lack the characteristic cytoplasmic eosinophilic intermediate filament inclusions present in the latter.[79] The large cell medulloblastomas are reactive with the neuronal markers NSE and synaptophysin, as well as with vimentin. This form is associated with a particularly poor prognosis and is characterized by early CSF dissemination and death within 9 months, regardless of the mode of therapy. The youngest patient in one series of four was a 13-month-old boy.[79]

Ultrastructural studies show that medulloblastoma shares certain features with neuroblastoma.[11,108] The tumor is composed of small, primitive-appearing cells surrounded by cytoplasmic processes containing neurofilaments and neurotubules. In a few specimens, dense core granules measuring 100 nm in diameter are found, but they are seen in much smaller numbers as compared to peripheral neuroblastoma (see Fig. 9–3D). The presence of junctional complexes and cell processes containing microtubules supports the concept that the tumor is of neuroepithelial origin.[121] Some astrocytic elements may be found, but whether they are reactive or an integral part of the tumor remains unclear. The tumor cells are immunoreactive with NSE and with vimentin.[148a]

Two cases of medulloblastoma were included in the Children's Hospital, Los Angeles neonatal study (see Table 9–2).[105] Bulbar paralysis and vomiting were the initial findings in one neonate who underwent craniotomy and biopsy at 2 months of age and subsequently died on the fourth postoperative day (see Fig. 9–3). Postmortem examination revealed a mass in the cerebellar vermis that had invaded the midbrain and upper brain stem. Leptomeningeal seeding of tumor was noted over the cerebral hemispheres and pons. The second patient presented with a large head and seventh cranial nerve palsy. Liver metastases were found, in addition to the same necropsy findings as just described for the other patient.

Medulloblastomas are highly malignant neoplasms that are invariably fatal in the perinatal period. Table 9–7 shows that only 1 of 21 survived. Because there is a familial tendency for

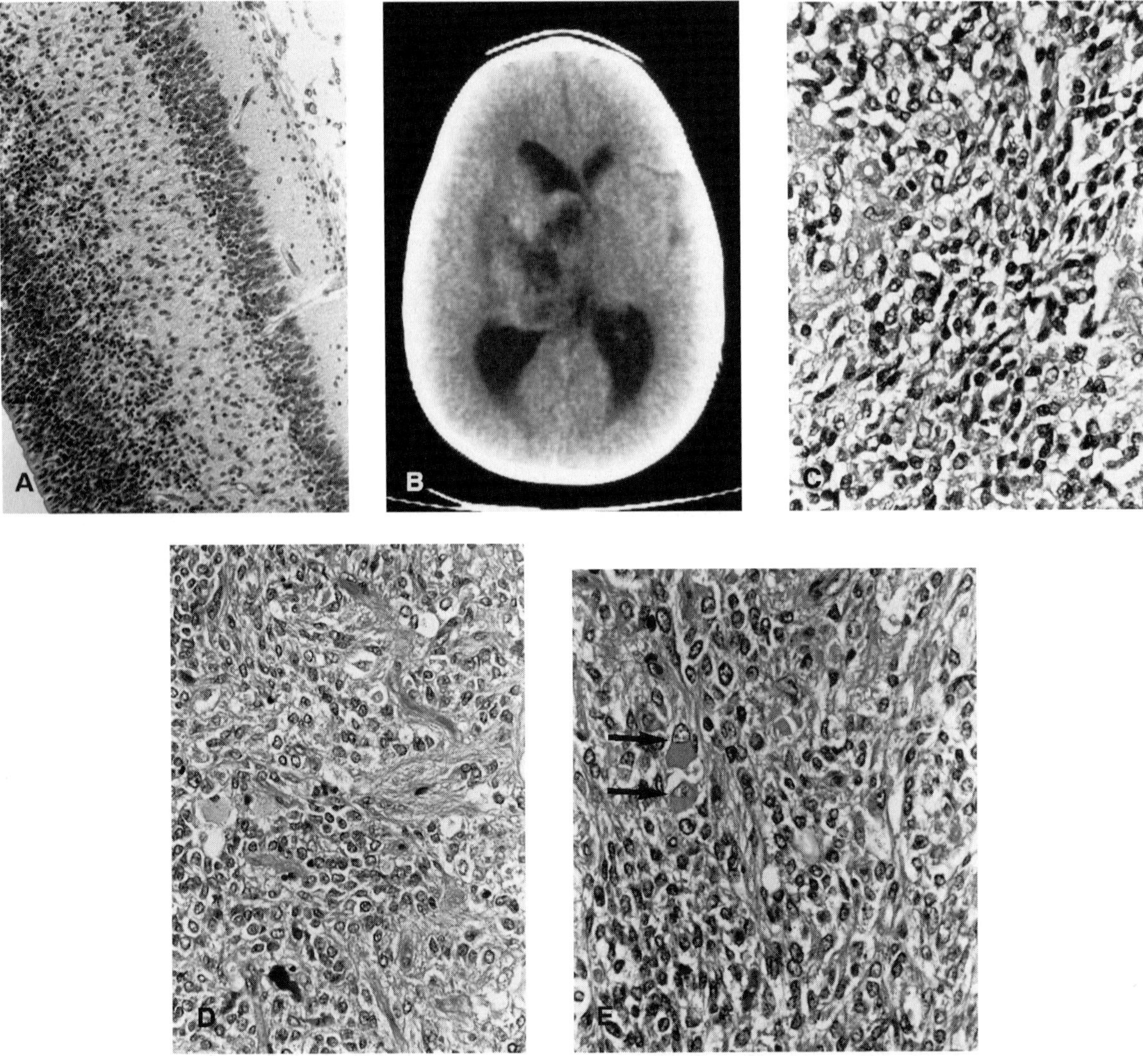

Figure 9–4. Cerebral neuroblastoma (primitive neuroectodermal tumor). *A,* Development of the cerebral hemisphere (forebrain) at an estimated 12 to 14 weeks' gestation. The wall of the cerebrum has differentiated into four layers, beginning right to left: molecular (beneath the pia-arachnoid), primordial cortical grey, intermediate, and ependymal (adjacent to the lateral ventricle). The inner part of the intermediate layer contains numerous migrating neuroblasts (hematoxylin-eosin, ×150). *B,* A CT scan of an 11-month-old boy with a history of vomiting and paresis of the left arm shows a large, heterogeneous, enhancing mass in the right frontoparietal area with irregular, low-density areas in the right basal ganglia. The lateral ventricles are dilated. *C,* The tumor consists of sheets of small, poorly differentiated, darkly staining cells (hematoxylin-eosin, ×750). *D,* An area with fibrosis (desmoplasia) and a focus of calcification (black staining material) can be seen (Masson trichrome, ×600). *E,* Foci of astrocytic differentiation are evident (*arrows*) (hematoxylin-eosin, ×750). (From Isaacs H Jr. Tumors of the Newborn and Infant. St. Louis: Mosby–Year Book, 1991.)

this tumor, accurate diagnosis is requisite so that parental counseling can be provided for future pregnancies.[65]

CEREBRAL NEUROBLASTOMA (CEREBRAL PNET)

Cerebral PNET is an uncommon, highly malignant, small cell tumor occurring primarily in young children and infants. It is characterized by early recurrence, intracranial and extracranial metastasis, and high mortality.[2,10,11,31,100,126,165] The fetal neuroepithelial cells of the subependymal plate region of the cerebrum are the proposed site of origin (Fig. 9–4A).[11,48,192]

One fourth of all cerebral PNETs occur before the age of 2 years and the tumor has been reported in stillborns.[11,48,88,192] In a study by Horten and Rubinstein, 6 of 35 affected patients were younger than 1 year of age, and the youngest was 2.5 months old.[100] The tumors were found primarily in the frontal and/or parietal lobes of the cerebral hemispheres. The frequency of this brain tumor in 12 perinatal studies was 8.8% (see Table 9–1).

Becker and Halliday described an extraordinary case of a newborn with congenital hydrocephalus who, at necropsy, was found to have a PNET that had replaced most of the cerebral hemispheres and practically the rest of the brain.[10] Yu et al. reported a similar case of a neonate who, in addition to a progressively enlarging head, had cervical lymph node and cutaneous metastases as the initial findings.[249] At necropsy, a large thalamic tumor was found which had extended into the third and fourth ventricles and had invaded the cerebellar vermis and rostral brain stem. Extensive leptomeningeal seeding had occurred. Microscopic examination showed a poorly differentiated, small cell, malignant tumor with focal astrocytic differentiation.[249]

Coexistence of cerebral PNET and rhabdoid tumor has been documented by Chang and associates.[31] The patient was a 14-day-old infant who was delivered by cesarian section because of cephalopelvic disproportion. On the second day of life, he developed jaundice, respiratory distress, irritability, and projectile vomiting. A CT scan showed a large tumor occupying most of the left cerebral hemisphere. Postmortem examination revealed, in addition to the cerebral PNET, a 2.5-cm rhabdoid tumor in the left lobe of the liver. According to the authors, the brain tumor also contained rhabdoid tumor cells, and the liver lesion was interpreted as a metastasis rather than a primary tumor.[31]

Cerebral neuroblastoma has a distinctive appearance on CT scan which may suggest the diagnosis. It appears as a large, space-occupying lesion situated in one of the cerebral hemispheres, and it consists of lobular, high- and low-density areas with extensive areas of cystic necrosis; the latter can be appreciated in the gross specimen, as well (Fig. 9–4B).[108]

Cerebral PNETs tend to be large, with extensive cystic necrosis and hemorrhage, and they occupy much of a cerebral hemisphere. The tumor is soft and friable with focal firmer gliotic or fibrotic areas.[10,31,100,249] Microscopic examination reveals a highly cellular, small cell tumor as the major component. Cerebral PNETs show areas with Homer-Wright rosettes and pink fibrillar neuropil, similar to the peripheral neuroblastoma. Focal ganglion cell differentiation, a peripheral astrocytic component, and

a prominent connective tissue (desmoplastic) stroma are additional findings (Figs. 9–4 and 9–5).[88,100,126] NSE and synaptophysin are reactive in the areas of neuronal differentiation, and the astrocytic component stains positively for S-100 protein and GFAP.[2] Ultrastructurally, the cerebral PNET cells have sparse organelles, no intercellular junctions, and occasional rosette formations.[11] There is evidence of neuronal differentiation, along with the presence of neurofilaments, dense core granules, and synaptic formations.[11]

The prognosis for the central nervous system PNET is dismal. For example, 18 patients in one series died within 2 years of diagnosis.[126] However, the newborn with the left hemispheric lesion described by Albert et al. was alive at the time of writing.[2] Few survivors have been reported (see Tables 9–7 and 9–15).

GANGLIOGLIOMA

Ganglioglioma is an infrequent central nervous system neoplasm occurring in patients of all ages, including the newborn.[10,72,87,192,207,227,241] It accounts for less than 5% and 2% of all infant and newborn brain tumors, respectively (see Table 9–1).[108] The clinical presentation is often a seizure disorder.[87,241] The cerebral hemispheres, particularly the temporal lobes, are the usual sites of origin.[207,241] The tumors vary in size, and they are well circumscribed and finely granular on cross section. Histologically, they consist of collections of mature, sometimes atypical-appearing ganglion cells and astrocytes surrounded by a network of glial fibers and gliosis (Figs. 9–6B and 9–7D). Some tumors contain microcysts and foci of calcification.[10] Wolf et al. suggest that gangliogliomas may originate from glioneuronal hamartias through neoplastic transformation of the astrocytic component.[241]

A 2-month-old infant with a ganglioglioma described by Galassi et al. presented with seizures and lethargy and was found to have a frontal lobe tumor, which was successfully excised.[70] In the Children's Hospital, Los Angeles newborn study, one ganglioglioma occurred in a 7-week-old male infant who was referred to the hospital with a markedly enlarged head, bulging tense fontanelles, and optic abnormalities (see Fig. 9–6).

The so-called desmoplastic ganglioglioma variant is a distinctive supratentorial neoplasm of infancy that typically arises from the frontal and parietal areas.[168,224] They are characterized

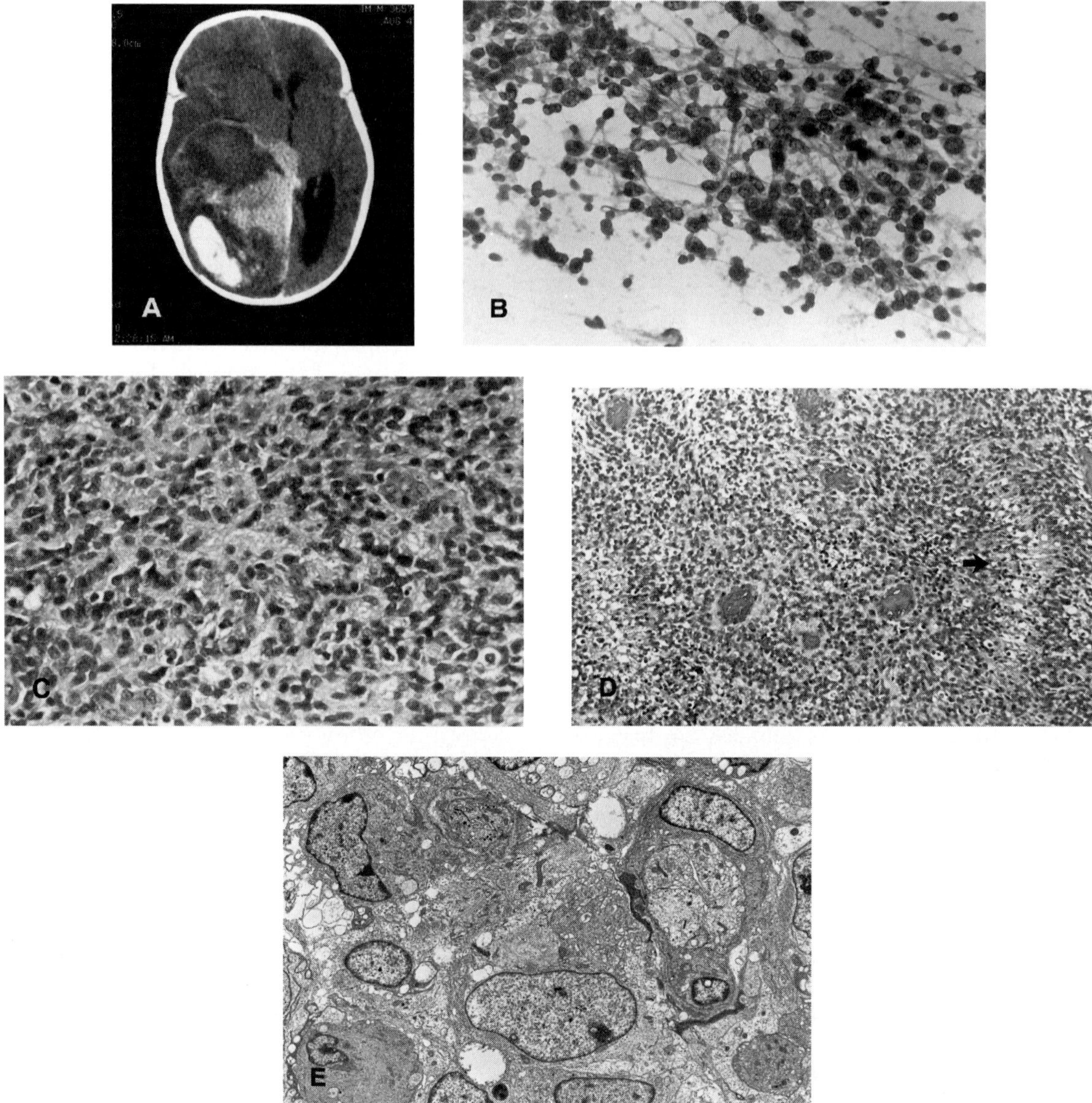

Figure 9–5. Cerebral primitive neuroectodermal tumor. *A,* A CT scan of a 6-week-old male infant with a 2-day history of vomiting and increasing lethargy. The study reveals a large, heterogeneous, enhancing mass with areas of hemorrhage and necrosis occupying much of the parieto-occipital lobes. Herniation across the midline and dilatation of the left lateral ventricle are also noted. *B,* Small, round to oval cells with delicate processes are seen on imprint cytology (hematoxylin-eosin, ×750). *C,* A section reveals a hypercellular, small cell, malignant tumor with pleomorphic nuclei and indistinct cell borders surrounded by fibrillar material. Positive immunostaining for NSE, S-100 protein, and GFAP suggest a neuroectodermal origin with glial differentiation. Cells cultured from this tumor yielded a normal male karyotype (hematoxylin-eosin, ×480). *D,* An area of pallisading necrosis is seen (*arrow*) (hematoxylin-eosin, ×150). *E,* An electron photomicrograph shows primitive-appearing cells with microfilaments. Some suggestive neurosecretory granules were found in other fields (×48,400).

by their very large size, cystic appearance, marked desmoplasia, and the presence of astrocytic and ganglionic elements. Patients with this tumor are as young as 2 months of age.[168,224] The Children's Hospital, San Diego series included a patient with this lesion who was 5 months of age at the time of presentation (see Fig. 9–7). One of the largest series was reported by VandenBerg et al.; it consisted of 11 infants, 5 of whom were 3 months of age or younger.[224] Of

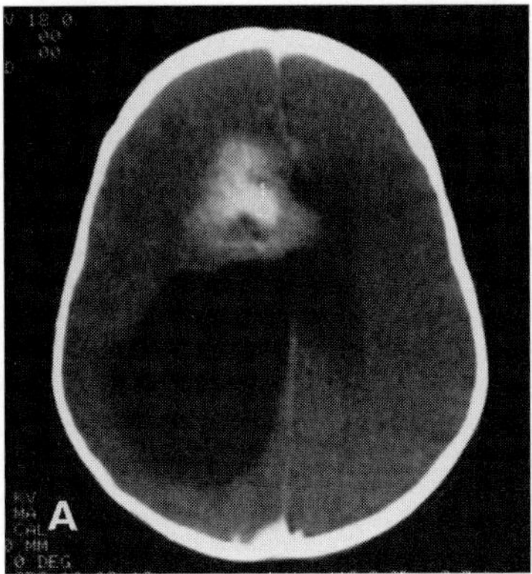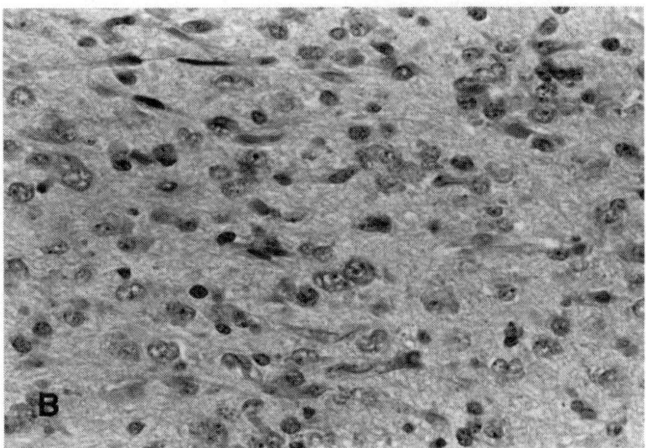

Figure 9–6. Cerebral ganglioglioma. *A,* A CT scan of a 7-week-old male infant with macrocephaly, bulging tense fontanelles, conjugate eye deviation to the right, and left homonymous hemianopsia. A large enhancing mass is seen to occupy the right frontal lobe, extending into the adjacent ventricle. Obstruction of the foramen of Monro and dilatation of the right lateral ventricle are evident. *B,* A microscopic section shows atypical-appearing ganglion cells with slightly vesicular nuclei, 1 or 2 large nucleoli, and prominent eosinophilic cytoplasms and hypertrophic astrocytes (hematoxylin-eosin, ×750). (From Isaacs H Jr. Tumors of the Newborn and Infant. St. Louis: Mosby–Year Book, 1991.)

the five newborns who survived, four underwent resection and radiation therapy, and one underwent resection only.

Histologically, the desmoplastic ganglioglioma, as the name implies, has a prominent fibrous tissue component composed of fascicles of spindle-shaped fibroblastic cells with a storiform growth pattern (Fig. 9–7*C*). Variable numbers of glial and neuronal components are present.[168,224] Schwann cells are observed in some tumors. Astrocytic cells stain positively for GFAP, and the neural component reacts with NSE and S-100 protein, but is unreactive with GFAP. The fibroblastic areas do not react with these antibodies. Moreover, focally positive macrophage antigens (Ki-M1P) are present.[168] Nuclear antigens associated with cell proliferation (Ki-67) are noted only in the astrocytic component.[241]

Electron microscopy reveals astrocytic cells containing intermediate filaments and pericellular basal lamina, as well as other cells displaying neuronal differentiation with dense core granules. The fibroblastic cells show marginated chromatin, ribosomes, intermediate filaments, and Golgi apparatus, and are surrounded by collagen reminiscent of fibrous histiocytoma.[168] Superficial cerebral astrocytomas and desmoplastic gangliogliomas are practically identical with respect to age distribution, gross and microscopic findings, and prognosis except for the presence of neuronal differentiation in the latter.[168] Similarly, patients with desmoplastic ganglioglioma have a favorable clinical outcome, provided surgical removal is complete.[168,224]

EPENDYMOMA

Ependymoma accounts for 5% to 10% of all central nervous system tumors in infants and children and is the sixth most frequently diagnosed brain tumor in the newborn (see Table 9–1).[47,91,135,189] Most perinatal ependymomas arise from the wall of the fourth ventricle.[29,127,150] Occasionally, they occur near the lateral ventricle, the usual site in adults (Table 9–8).[10,62,127,189,192]

Newborns with ependymomas present with hydrocephalus and signs of increased intracranial pressure (i.e., bulging fontanelles and split sutures); the tumors are responsible for dystocia, stillbirth, and spontaneous intracerebral hemorrhage (see Table 9–8).[62,127,150,197] Congenital familial cases have been documented only rarely (Table 9–8).[197]

Ependymomas are tumors derived from and consisting of ependymal cells originating from within or near the ependymal lining of the ventricles or central canal of the spinal cord.[91,189] The presence of cilia and blepharoplasts, demonstrated by electron microscopy and with the phosphotungstic acid hematoxylin (PTAH) stain by light microscopy, distinguish these tumors from other tumors occurring in the central nervous system. Ependymomas in the young are often classified as the cellular type

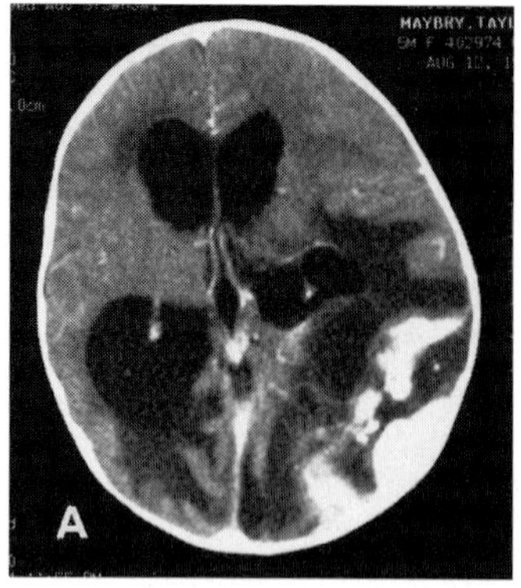
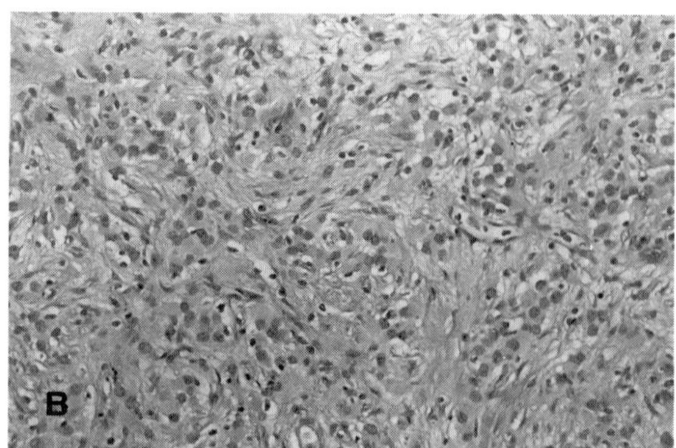
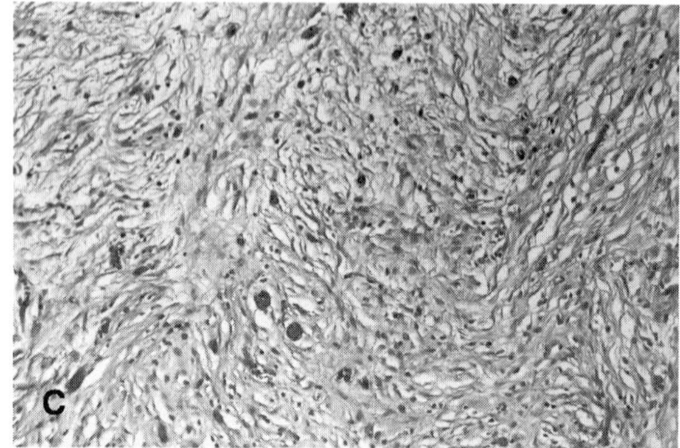
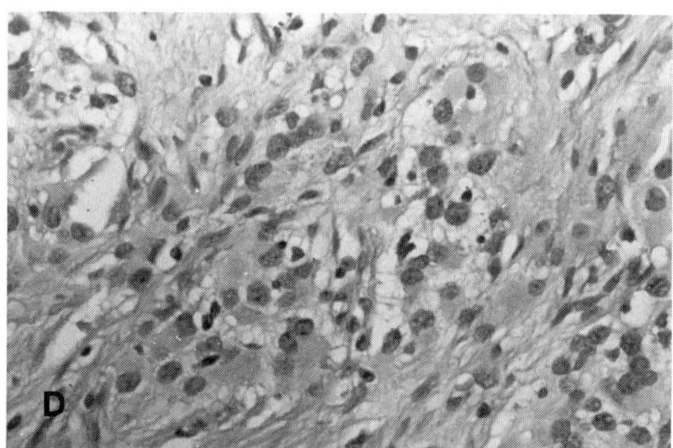
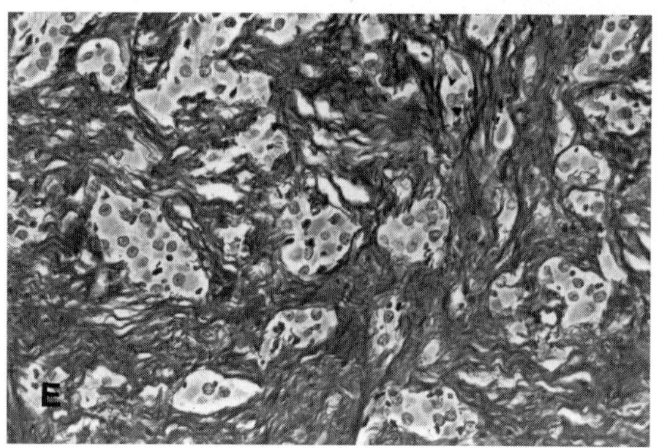

Figure 9–7. Cerebral infantile desmoplastic ganglioglioma. *A,* A CT scan of a 5-month-old girl presenting with macrocephaly and vomiting demonstrates a large, superficial, contrast-enhancing, cystic mass within the left parieto-occipital lobes that is accompanied by marked ventriculomegaly. *B,* Clusters of ganglion cells are surrounded by a fibrous tissue spindle-cell component (hematoxylin-eosin, ×120). *C,* Dense desmoplastic areas composed of spindle-shaped cells comprise most of this tumor (hematoxylin-eosin, ×120). *D,* Ganglion cells are round with slightly vesicular nuclei and prominent nucleoli (hematoxylin-eosin, ×300). *E,* Reticulin staining demonstrates collagen tissue surrounding ganglion cells (reticulin, ×150). Immunohistochemical studies revealed positive reactivity to vimentin, S-100 protein, and GFAP, and ganglion cells that were focally reactive to synaptophysin and NSE.

and consist of rather uniform, darkly staining cells with scattered ependymal perivascular rosettes (Figs. 9–8 and 9–9).[106,107] However, papillary ependymomas of the fourth ventricle occur.[35] Halos or clear zones distributed about blood vessels and surrounded by tumor cells are helpful diagnostic findings (see Fig. 9–9). Moreover, childhood ependymomas display characteristically delicate nuclear grooves or clefts on touch preparations, frozen sections, and paraffin sections stained with hematoxylin-eosin, and these, too, assist in the diagnosis.[43] Mitoses are common in these tumors.

Reyes-Mugica et al. performed histologic and DNA flow cytometry studies on 17 childhood ependymomas (the youngest patient being 1 year of age). They concluded that no statistical correlation exists between DNA index, histologic findings (necrosis, anaplasia, pleomorphism, mitotic rate, and endothelial proliferation), and outcome.[176]

The primitive, embyronic-appearing ependymoblastoma is extremely rare.[60,137,150,151,197] Few tumors fulfill the diagnostic criteria, and high-grade, anaplastic ependymomas and choroid plexus carcinomas have been misdiagnosed as ependymoblastomas. In some infant brain tumor series, malignant ependymoma was considered to be the same entity as ependymoblastoma.[127]

Table 9–8. 9 Fetal and Newborn Ependymal Tumors*

Case No.	Age at Death	Location	Initial Findings	Reference
1	14 days	4th ventricle†	Dystocia, hydrocephalus, seizures	Ehret et al.[60]
2	3 months	Lateral ventricle	Hemorrhage	Ernestus et al.[62]
3	1.5 months	4th ventricle†	Large head	Mork and Lorken[150]
4	Stillborn	Brain replaced by tumor†	Large head, dystocia hydramnios	Lorentzen and Hagerstrand[137]
5	5 weeks	4th ventricle	Hydrocephalus, vomiting	Chusid et al.[35]
6	6 months	4th ventricle‡	Hydrocephalus, vomiting	Sato et al.[198]
7	?Alive	Lateral ventricle	Large head	Sakamoto et al.[195]
8	3.5 months	4th ventricle	Hydrocephalus, vomiting	Campbell et al.[29]
9	3 months	4th ventricle	Vomiting, hydrocephalus	Isaacs§

*Selected from the literature.
†Diagnosed as ependymoblastoma.
‡Sibling died at 29 days of age with 4th ventricular glioma (?ependymoma).
§Refer to Table 9–2.

Ependymoblastoma seldom occurs in patients younger than 2 years of age. However, the tumor has been responsible for neonatal death and stillbirth (see Tables 9–4 and 9–8).[137] Ependymoblastomas, not unlike other PNETs of the central nervous system, behave in a highly malignant fashion, extensively invading adjacent structures, widely disseminating within the subarachnoid space, and seeding the brain and spinal cord with metastatic deposits.[60,137,151] The brain of a 29-week, 2.35-kg stillborn male infant described by Lorentzen and Hagerstrand was found to be replaced entirely by a thick, necrotic, yellow, and hemorrhagic

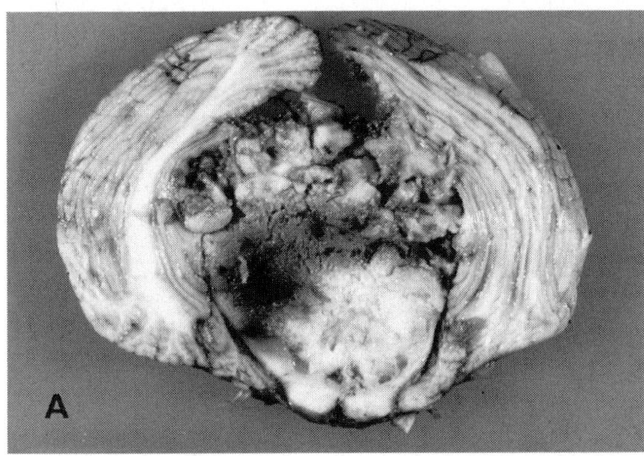

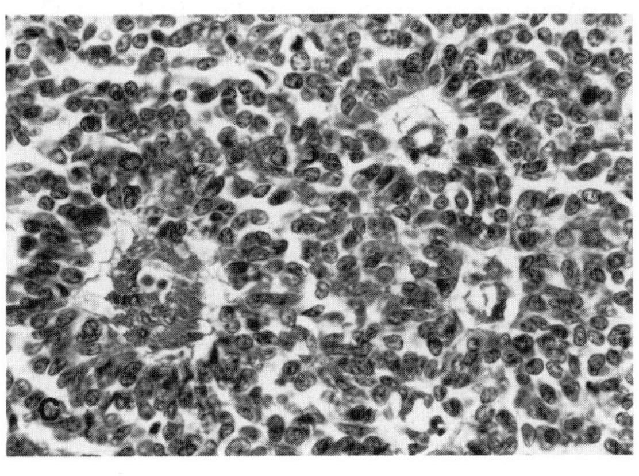

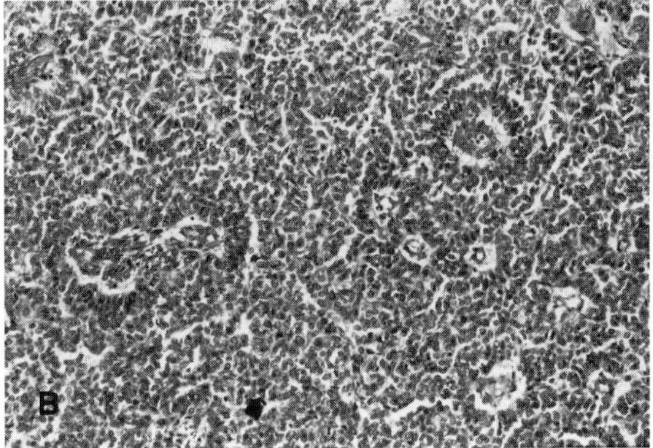

Figure 9–8. Ependymoma of the fourth ventricle. A 9-month-old boy presented with macrocephaly, vomiting, and marasmus of 5 months' duration. Imaging studies revealed severe hydrocephalus (with the mantle measuring only 1.5 cm in thickness), aqueduct stenosis, and a large, midline, cerebellar mass. *A,* This photograph depicts a 7 × 5 × 5 cm midline cerebellar tumor occupying both hemispheres and invading the mesencephalon, pons, and medulla. The immediate cause of death was a 3 × 3 cm area of recent hemorrhage within the fourth ventricle that filled the aqueduct of Sylvius. *B,* A low-power view depicts a cellular, rather uniform, small cell neoplasm forming perivascular rosettes (hematoxylin-eosin, ×64). *C,* The ependymal rosettes are seen here at higher magnification (hematoxylin-eosin, ×750). (From Isaacs H Jr. Tumors of the Newborn and Infant. St. Louis: Mosby–Year Book, 1991.)

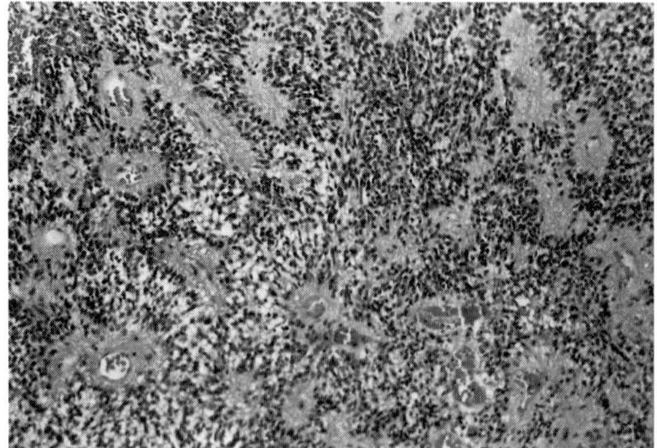

Figure 9–9. Ependymoma of the fourth ventricle showing characteristic perivascular pale zones surrounded by tumor cells (ependymal rosettes) (hematoxylin-eosin, ×300). This is a helpful diagnostic aid, particularly on frozen section. (From Isaacs H Jr. Tumors of the Newborn and Infant. St. Louis: Mosby–Year Book, 1991.)

ependymoblastoma.[137] Moreover, metastases to the spinal cord and leptomeninges were found.

Some controversy persists as to whether ependymoblastoma should be considered to be a form of malignant ependymoma or a primitive neuroectodermal tumor with ependymal differentiation.[12,48,91,151,184,192] Current opinion tends to favor the latter. Histologically, ependymoblastoma is a hypercellular tumor composed of small, uniform cells having the appearance of a "small cell malignant tumor;" in addition, it displays a high mitotic rate and characteristic, embryonic-appearing, ependymoblastic rosettes and tubules, which are requisite for diagnosis.[60,137,151,188] The ependymoblastic rosette consists of several rows of columnar cells appearing as multiple layers of nuclei situated about a central lumen lined by an internal limiting membrane with cilia.[137,151] The ependomyoblastic rosette resembles the Flexner-Wintersteiner rosette of retinoblastoma (see Fig. 10–3D). In contrast to the latter, juxtaluminal cytoplasmic blepharoplasts and cilia are present on light and electron microscopy.[44,151] Both perivascular ependymomatous rosettes, seen in the "classical" ependymoma, and ependomyoblastic rosettes are found in ependymoblastomas. The absence of pleomorphism, multinucleation, and giant cells differentiates ependymoblastoma from anaplastic (malignant) ependymoma, which occurs mostly in adults.[151]

Cruz-Sanchez et al. studied five ependymoblastomas by immunohistochemical analysis and light and electron microscopy.[44] Two patients in the study were 1 year of age or younger; both tumors occurred above the tentorium, adjacent to the lateral ventricle. The tumors stained positively for vimentin and S-100 protein, but were unreactive with cytokeratin and neurofilament antibodies. Cells were focally positive for GFAP.[44] Ultrastructurally, the tumor cells had a high nuclear:cytoplasmic ratio, few rosette formations, and small numbers of cytoplasmic organelles. In addition, junctional complexes, rudimentary cilia, basal bodies, and glial-like filaments were demonstrated.[44]

Parenthetically, some immature teratomas occurring in either intracranial or extracranial sites display a histologic pattern consisting of anastomosing cords of oval, darkly staining cells forming ependymoblastic-like rosettes (see Fig. 2–14).

Ehret et al. described a neonate with an ependymoblastoma arising from the brain stem and cerebellum, presumably from the region of the fourth ventricle, which metastasized to the hypothalamus, third and lateral ventricles, and spinal cord subarachnoid.[60] Dystocia secondary to craniomegaly and hydrocephalus was the initial antenatal finding (Table 9–8). Lorentzen and Hagerstrand reported a stillborn with an ependymoblastoma that replaced most of the brain and widely metastasized to the leptomeninges and spinal cord.[137] Hydramnios and dystocia were the initial manifestations.

An ependymoma in the Children's Hospital, Los Angeles neonatal study originated from the fourth ventricle.[107] At birth, the infant was noted to have persistent vomiting and progressively increasing head size, resulting from obstructive hydrocephalus. She had a craniotomy and biopsy performed at several weeks of age, and she expired 1 month after surgery. The biopsy showed a cellular ependymoma (see Fig. 9–9).

Newborns and infants with ependymomas and ependymoblastomas generally have a poor prognosis, and there are few survivors.[60,127,150,151,176,232] Many recur locally and progress inexorably, disseminating throughout the CSF pathways and into the peritoneal cavity via ventriculoperitoneal shunt catheters without filters.[176] One of the nine newborns listed in Table 9–8 survived.

CHOROID PLEXUS PAPILLOMA

Choroid plexus papilloma is a neoplasm composed of mature epithelial cells that line the ventricular choroid plexuses.[10,189] The incidence of choroid plexus papillomas varies in-

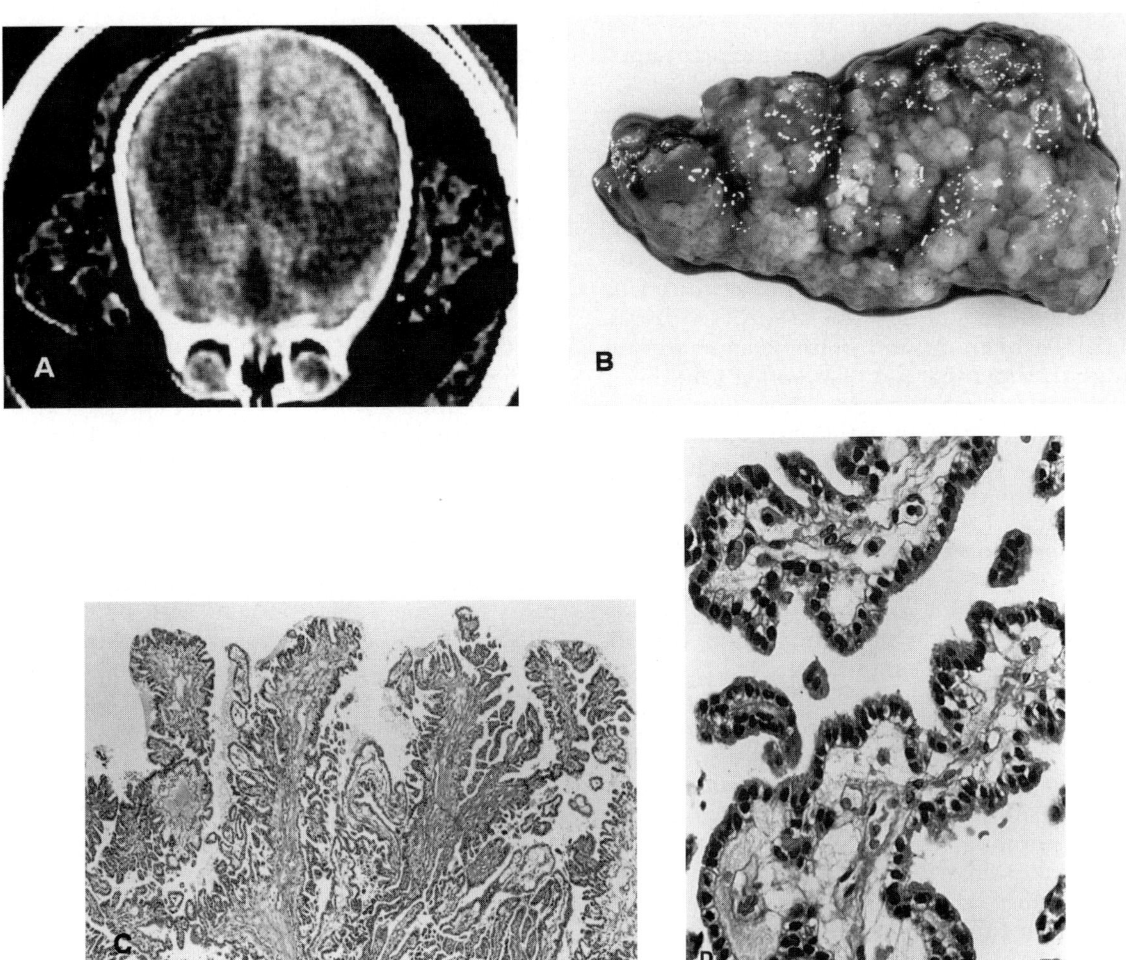

Figure 9–10. Congenital choroid plexus papilloma of the lateral ventricle. Rapidly progressive hydrocephalus, a bulging fontanelle, and vomiting were the presenting signs in this 1-month-old female infant. *A,* A CT scan shows a large, enhancing mass partially filling the left lateral ventricle, together with severe, generalized hydrocephalus. *B,* Two cauliflower-like masses, measuring 5.5 × 2.7 cm and 4.7 × 3.5 cm, were removed from the left lateral ventricle. One is depicted in the gross photograph. *C,* A low-power view shows the overall architecture and resemblance to normal choroid plexus (hematoxylin-eosin, ×48). *D,* Edematous papillary structures are lined by small cells with regular, round to oval, darkly staining nuclei (hematoxylin-eosin, ×600). (From Isaacs H Jr. Tumors of the Newborn and Infant. St. Louis: Mosby–Year Book, 1991.)

versely with age. About 50% of patients in the pediatric age group are diagnosed during the first year of life.[70,96,117,124,173a,219] Choroid plexus papillomas constitute about 12% of all neonatal brain tumors and rank third in frequency (see Table 9–1). In some series, choroid plexus papilloma is the dominant brain tumor, accounting for almost 50% of cases,[172] and they are responsible for the rapid onset of hydrocephalus in the fetus and neonate[1,25,107,159,206,219] and for stillbirth[75,116,209] (see Tables 9–3 and 9–9). An association between congenital choroid plexus papilloma and giant melanocytic nevus and Aicardi syndrome has been reported.[146,219]

Typically, the papilloma grows into the lateral ventricle, producing a large, space-occupying nodular mass that is readily observed on imaging studies (Fig. 9–10A).[107,172,175,181,212] The tumors have a predilection for the lateral ventricles, but they sometimes arise from the third and fourth ventricles (see Table 9–9).[1,133,159,167,172,197] Large quantities of CSF are produced by the tumor, resulting in marked dilatation of the entire ventricular system, which may be apparent antenatally or at birth.[108,133,181,237] Papillomas may produce a noncommunicating hydrocephalus also by obstructing the interventricular foramen of Monro.[65,167] Gertz et al. described a gigantic fetal choroid plexus papilloma that occupied most of the intracranial cavity.[76] An enlarged head was discovered by sonography at 24 weeks' gestation; because of this, the pregnancy was terminated.

The papilloma has a finely nodular, pink, cauliflower-like appearance; microscopically, the tumor displays numerous papillary formations covered by uniform, regular, cuboidal to columnar epithelial cells resembling choroid plexus (see Fig. 9–10).[142] Immunohistochemical studies, which usually are not required to establish the diagnosis, show reactivity with epithelial (cytokeratin and epithelial membrane antigen), vimentin, and glial (GFAP) markers, which reactivity is the same as for normal choroid plexus.[76] The immunocytochemical and ultrastructural features of 10 choroid plexus tumors were presented by Coffin et al.[38] Microvilli, cilia, and zonula adherens tight junctions are observed on electron microscopy.[38,78,133]

The prognosis of patients with choroid plexus papilloma is comparatively good, and is the most favorable of all newborn brain tumors (see Table 9–15). Complete surgical resection is the treatment of choice.[78,108,124,167,219] If surgery can be performed before irreversible brain damage has occurred as the result of severe hydrocephalus or hemorrhage, then a favorable outcome should be expected.[167] However, one of the puzzling, unexplained aspects of the treatment of this tumor is the persistence of hydrocephalus, along with progressive parenchymal atrophy and mental retardation, in some patients, even in those who have undergone total resection and placement of a ventriculoperitoneal shunt.[167] Nevertheless, it is important to recognize choroid plexus papilloma preoperatively because surgical removal is usually curative.

The five newborns with choroid plexus papillomas included in the Children's Memorial Hospital, Chicago series survived following surgical removal.[172,219] By contrast, an earlier series by Pascual-Castroviejo et al., consisting of six newborns who were 2 months of age or younger, reported only one survivor.[167]

Lippa et al. described a neonate with a choroid plexus papilloma that was discovered at 38 weeks' gestation during an evaluation for increased uterine size.[133] Ultrasonography revealed polyhydramnios and fetal hydrocephalus. In addition, there was an enhancing midline mass with several small cystic areas occupying most of the posterior fossa and extending well above the tentorium. At surgery, the tumor was found to involve the brain stem and cerebellum as well.[133] A neonate with a cho-

roid plexus papilloma in the Children's Hospital, Los Angeles study presented with a history of vomiting and progressive hydrocephalus since birth. A CT scan revealed a large mass, situated in the left lateral ventricle, which was removed surgically (see Fig. 9–10). The patient expired during the operation from an intracerebral hemorrhage, which is one of the serious surgical complications in such cases.[105]

CHOROID PLEXUS CARCINOMA

Fewer than one third of choroid plexus carcinomas are diagnosed in the first year of life.[78,163] In older individuals, most arise from the lateral ventricles, but in the series of Newbould et al., the fourth ventricle was the primary site in four of five newborns.[155] Other reports, however, show that the lateral ventricle is the most common site (see Table 9–9). As with papilloma, affected fetuses and newborns have hydrocephalus, which is caused by obstruction and/or hypersecretion of CSF. For example, a 1-week-old male infant described by Packer et al. had prenatal hydrocephalus, which was detected on sonography.[163] The patient survived following surgical resection.

Widespread dissemination of choroid plexus carcinoma throughout the cerebrospinal subarachnoid space is a fatal complication.[78,163] Because of this complication, CSF may contain tumor cells at the time of diagnosis; therefore, cytologic examination is an integral part of the patient's evaluation.

The diagnosis of malignant choroid plexus carcinoma rests on certain histologic criteria: infiltration into adjacent structures, hypercellularity, pleomorphic nuclei, increased mitotic activity, vascular proliferation, and necrosis.[78,155] In other words, this tumor does not closely resemble normal choroid plexus, as is the case with papilloma. Results of immunohistochemical studies are equivocal. According to one review, when testing with the carcinoembryonic antigen (CEA) is positive and testing with S-100 protein is negative, the choroid plexus tumor is probably malignant.[38] In another study, S-100 protein results were positive and CEA proved to be unreactive in a patient with choroid plexus carcinoma; however, transthyretin, carbonic anhydrase II, transferrin, and cathepsin D were uniformly reactive in all 17 carcinomas investigated.[155] These epithelial antigens are not expressed by medulloblastoma, which may resemble the anaplastic choroid plexus carcinoma.

Table 9–9. 31 Fetal and Newborn Choroid Plexus Tumors*

Case No.	Survival	Location	Initial Findings	Reference
1	+	Lateral ventricle	Hydrocephalus	Tomita et al.[219]
2	+	Lateral ventricle	Hydrocephalus	Tomita et al.[219]
3	+	Lateral ventricle	Hydrocephalus	Tomita et al.[219]
4	+	Lateral ventricle	Seizure disorder†	Tomita et al.[219]
5	+	3rd ventricle	Hydrocephalus, seizures	Knierim[124]
6	−	Lateral ventricle	Hydrocephalus, vomiting	Braunstein and Martin[25]
7	+	Lateral ventricle‡	Hydrocephalus, vomiting	Gianella-Borradori et al.[78]
8	+	Lateral ventricle§	Antenatal hydrocephalus, vomiting, lethargy	Packer et al.[163]
9	+	Lateral ventricle‖	Hydrocephalus, diffuse hypotonia, poor suck	McCune et al.[146]
10	−	Lateral ventricle	Hydrocephalus, "sunset sign"¶	Sjogren et al.[206]
11	−	4th ventricle	Increased uterine size, polyhydramnios, fetal hydrocephalus	Lippa et al.[133]
12	+	Lateral ventricle§	Hydrocephalus, vomiting	Arico et al.[6]
13	+	Lateral ventricle	Hydrocephalus	Arico et al.[6]
14	+	Lateral ventricle	Hydrocephalus, "sunset sign"	Arico et al.[6]
15	+	3rd ventricle	Hydrocephalus, "sunset sign"	Arico et al.[6]
16	+	Lateral ventricle	Large head	Radkowski et al.[172]
17	+	Lateral ventricle	Large head	Radkowski et al.[172]
18	LTF	3rd ventricle	Large head	Radkowski et al.[172]
19	+	?Lateral ventricle	Large head, eyes deviated laterally	Raskind and Beigel[173a]
20	−	Lateral ventricle	Hydrocephalus	Pascual-Castroviejo et al.[167]
21	−	Lateral ventricle§	Hydrocephalus	Pascual-Castroviejo et al.[167]
22	−	3rd ventricle	Hydrocephalus	Pascual-Castroviejo et al.[167]
23	−	4th ventricle	Hydrocephalus	Pascual-Castroviejo et al.[167]
24	−	4th ventricle	Seizures	Pascual-Castroviejo et al.[167]
25	−	4th ventricle	Hydrocephalus	Pascual-Castroviejo et al.[167]
26	−	3rd ventricle#	Large head, hydrocephalus	Adra et al.[1]
27	−	?Filled intracranial cavity	Large head**	Gertz et al.[76]
28	−	Lateral ventricle	Hydrocephalus, vomiting	Isaacs††
29	−	Lateral ventricle§	Hydrocephalus, vomiting, seizures	Isaacs††
30	+	Lateral ventricle	Large head, vomiting, downward gaze	Isaacs††
31	LTF	Lateral ventricle	Large head	Isaacs‡‡

*Selected from the literature.

†Patient presented with microphthalmia, contralateral retinal detachment, and agenesis of the corpus callosum and was diagnosed as having Aicardi's syndrome.

‡Anaplastic choroid plexus papilloma.

§Choroid plexus carcinoma: 4 of 30 (13%) of tumors; 2 survivors.

‖Newborn with a giant congenital nevus covering her back.

¶Downward deviation of the eyes.

#Detected antenatally.

**Pregnancy terminated at 24 weeks' gestation.

††Refer to Table 9–2.

‡‡Refer to Table 9–1.

+ = living; − = dead; LTF = lost to follow-up.

At times, difficulty may be encountered in distinguishing a poorly differentiated, anaplastic ependymoma from a papillary carcinoma. An example of this problem was observed by the author. The patient was a 3-month-old infant who presented with vomiting, seizures, hydrocephalus, and a bulging anterior fontanelle; the admitting diagnosis was meningitis (versus intracranial hemorrhage). The baby expired shortly after admission. A large fungating mass arising from the right lateral ventricle and replacing almost half of the adjacent cerebral hemisphere was found at necropsy. On histologic exam, the tumor was found to have features of both malignant lesions in that it was a small cell malignant tumor containing papillary structures with nuclear atypia and bizarre, multinucleated, giant cells. Immunohistochemical methods were unavailable at that time.

Total surgical resection, if it can be accomplished, offers the best chance for cure.[163] None of the five newborns in the study by Newbould

Table 9–10. 49 Fetal and Newborn Intracranial Teratomas*

Case No.	Age at Death	Location	Initial Findings	Reference
1	7 days	Brain stem	Large head	Takaku et al.[213]
2	47 days	3rd ventricle	Large head, stupor, respiratory distress	Takaku et al.[213]
3	3 weeks	Pineal region	Large head, vomiting, "sunset sign"[†]	Takaku et al.[213]
4	2 years	3rd ventricle	Large head, vomiting, dysphagia, stridor	Takaku et al.[213]
5	4 days	Hemisphere	Large head,[‡] dystocia	Wakai et al.[232]
6	Alive	3rd ventricle	Large head	Sakamoto et al.[195]
7	3 months	3rd ventricle	Large head	Sakamoto et al.[195]
8	4 months	3rd ventricle	Large head	Sakamoto et al.[195]
9	3 months	Hemisphere	Large head	Jooma et al.[119]
10	18 weeks	Hemisphere	Large head	Jooma et al.[119]
11	Stillborn	Hemisphere	Hydrocephalus,[‡] hydramnios, exophthalmos	Wienk et al.[237]
12	Stillborn	Intracranium	Hydramnios, large head	Werb et al.[234]
13	Stillborn	Intracranium	Hydramnios, large head[§]	Werb et al.[234]
14	Stillborn	Intracranium	Large head	Werb et al.[234]
15	Stillborn	Intracranium	Hydramnios[§]	Werb et al.[234]
16	2 days	3rd ventricle,[∥] both hemispheres	Large head, hydrocephalus	Radkowski et al.[172]
17	1 day	Posterior fossa[#]	Large head	Radkowski et al.[172]
18	1 day	Posterior fossa[#]	Large head	Radkowski et al.[172]
19	12 days	Left cranial fossa	Hydrocephalus[‡]	Jellinger and Sunder-Plassman[116]
20	7 days	Lateral ventricle	Large head	Whittle and Simpson[236]
21	8 months	Hemisphere, ?sella turcica	Large head, cephaloceles[§]	Whittle and Simpson[236]
22	8.5 weeks	Hemisphere	Large head, 7th nerve palsy, "sunset" sign	Hirsch[95]
23	7.5 weeks	Both hemispheres	Large head, eye deviation	Hirsch[95]
24	Stillborn	Pineal region	Large for gestation date[‡]	Lipman et al.[132]
25	At birth	Hemisphere, posterior fossa, neck	Large head, hydramnios,[‡] breech position	Lipman et al.[132]
26	At birth	Brain replaced by tumor; extension into orbit and oral cavity	Large for gestation date,[‡] hydramnios	Lipman et al.[132]
27	At birth	Brain replaced by tumor	Large for gestation, hydramnios, large head[‡]	Hoff and Mackay[99]
28	2 hours	Brain replaced by tumor	Incidental finding, large head[‡]	Crade[42]
29	At birth	Brain replaced by tumor	Large for gestation, large head[‡]	Gadwood and Reynes[69a]
30	Stillborn	Brain replaced by tumor	Hydramnios, large head[‡]	Vinters et al.[228]
31	Stillborn	Brain replaced by tumor	Incidental finding, large head[‡]	Paes et al.[163a]
32	Alive	3rd ventricle[∥]	Large head, hydrocephalus[‡]	Oi et al.[159]
33	9.5 hours	Hemispheres replaced by tumor	Hydramnios, hydrocephalus[‡]	Odell et al.[157]
34	4 days	Hemispheres replaced by tumor	Large head, "sunset sign"[†]	Odell et al.[157]
35	At birth	Hemisphere, neck, posterior fossa	Hydrocephalus, hydramnios	Rostad et al.[185]
36	At birth	Brain replaced by tumor, extension into orbit and oropharynx	Large head,[‡] hydramnios	Rostad et al.[185]
37	Stillborn	Brain replaced by tumor	Large head	Greenhouse and Neubuerger[80]
38	Stillborn	Brain replaced by tumor	Large head, dystocia	Oberman[156]
39	Stillborn	Brain replaced by tumor	Large head[‡]	Saiga et al.[194]
40	3 days	Hemispheres replaced by tumor	Large head[‡]	Nanda et al.[153]
41	Alive	Hemisphere and orbit	Orbital mass	Nanda et al.[153]

Table 9–10. 49 Fetal and Newborn Intracranial Teratomas* *Continued*

Case No.	Age at Death	Location	Initial Findings	Reference
42	35 days	Pineal body	Large for gestation date, hydramnios, hydro-cephalus‡	Dolkart et al.[55]
43	Stillborn	Brain replaced by tumor	Large head	Tamura[215]
44	Stillborn	Brain replaced by auto-lyzed tumor	Large head	Tamura[215]
45	Stillborn	Optic nerve	Hydrocephalus§	Tamura[215]
46	At birth	Brain replaced by tumor	Large for gestation date,‡§ large head, hydramnios	Weyerts[235]
47	5 days	Hemispheres replaced by tumor	Large head, hydrocepha-·lus‡	Vraa-Jensen[230]
48	Stillborn	Brain replaced by tumor	Hydramnios, hydrocepha-lus, intracranial mass‡	DiGiovanni and Sheikh[51]
49	Stillborn	Cerebral hemispheres re-placed by tumor	Hydramnios, hydroceph-alus	Washburne et al.[232a]

*Selected from the literature.
†Downward deviation of the eyes.
‡Detected antenatally.
§Associated malformations included atrial and ventricular septal defects (case 13); cleft lip and bilateral cleft palate (case 15); cleft lip and palate, hypertelorism, coloboma, and proptosis plus embryonal carcinoma recurrence (case 21); ear deformity, absence of auditory canal, cup-like defect of the right eye (case 45); and pulmonary and adrenal hypoplasia (case 46).
‖Diagnosed as malignant.
#Invaded and displaced the cerebellum and brain stem.

et al. survived, and only 2 of the 4 newborns listed in Tables 9–9 and 9–15 survived. The use of chemotherapy in patients with choroid plexus carcinoma is currently of unproven benefit, but has produced some encouraging results in older individuals.[6,78,163]

INTRACRANIAL TERATOMA

Teratoma is the major intracranial germ cell tumor occurring in the first year of life and is the leading neonatal brain tumor in several series (Tables 9–1, 9–4, and 9–5).[28,116,159,190,209,213,215,232,234,237] It accounted for one third of the 24 neonatal brain tumors in the Japanese cooperative study reported by Oi et al.[159] Four of five newborns with brain tumors described by Takaku et al. had teratomas.[213] Of 54 pediatric intracranial germ cell tumors analyzed by Rueda-Pedraza et al., 11 (20%) occurred in infants younger than 3 months of age, and almost 50% were stillborn.[190] Intracranial teratoma accounted for 2 of 7 (28.6%) of the total number of neonatal brain tumors in the Children's Hospital of Philadelphia series.[153] The tumor is associated with a high perinatal mortality rate (see Table 9–15).

Perinatal intracranial teratomas consist of mature and immature tissues of various types, but lack germinoma or other malignant germ cell tumor components. They arise from midline supratentorial locations, such as the pineal body and third ventricular and suprasellar regions, and occasionally, other sites, such as the cerebral hemisphere and brain stem (see Table 9–10).[116,157,189,190,199,209,213] In almost 50% of affected fetuses and newborns, the teratoma reaches gigantic proportions, effacing the brain so that the exact site of origin cannot be determined (see Table 9–10 and Fig. 9–11).[132,232,232a] For example, a teratoma in the series of Rueda-Pedraza et al. measured 16 × 12 cm and was both craniopharyngeal and intraoral in location.[190] Moreover, the two tumors mentioned by Odell et al. measured 15 cm in diameter and replaced most of the brain.[157,190] According to Nanda and co-workers, perinatal intracranial teratomas can be divided into three main groups: massive tumors replacing the intracranial contents, smaller tumors causing hydrocephalus, and tumors with extension into the orbit or neck.[153]

Until recently, most intracranial teratomas were diagnosed at postmortem examination. Now, however, increasing numbers are being detected in utero or in the neonatal period using modern imaging techniques (see Table 9–10 and Fig. 9–11A).[42,51,55,99,132,154,157,160,178,185,222,230,235,237] Table 9–10 shows that 19 of 49 (40%) of perinatal tumors culled from the literature were diagnosed antenatally. Some are found in-

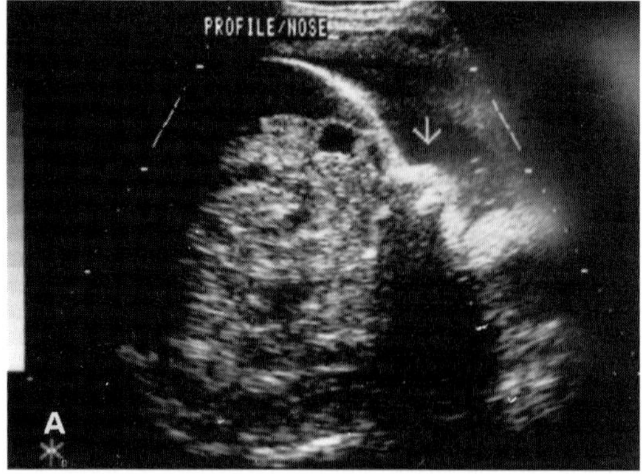

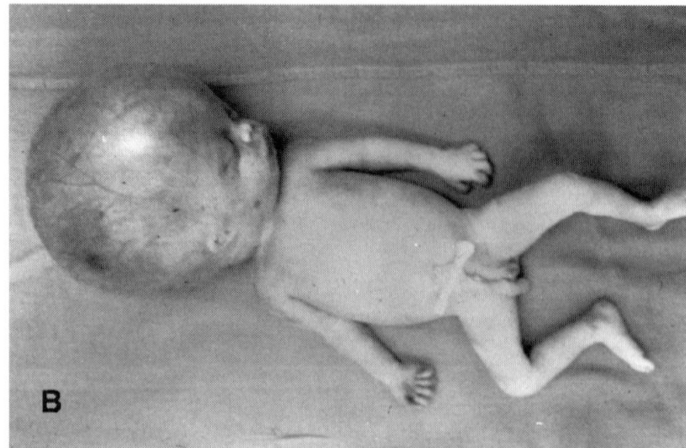

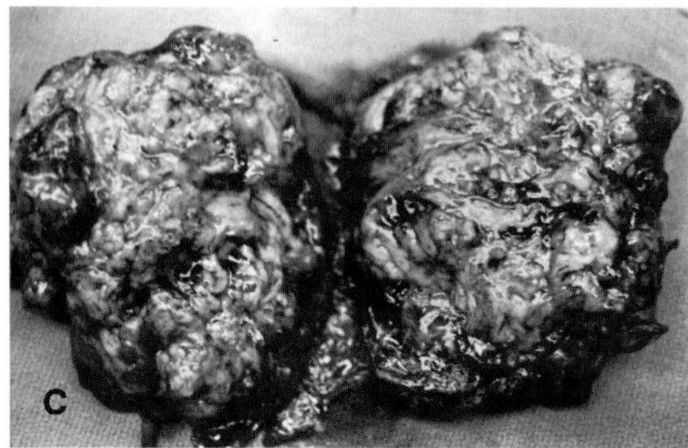

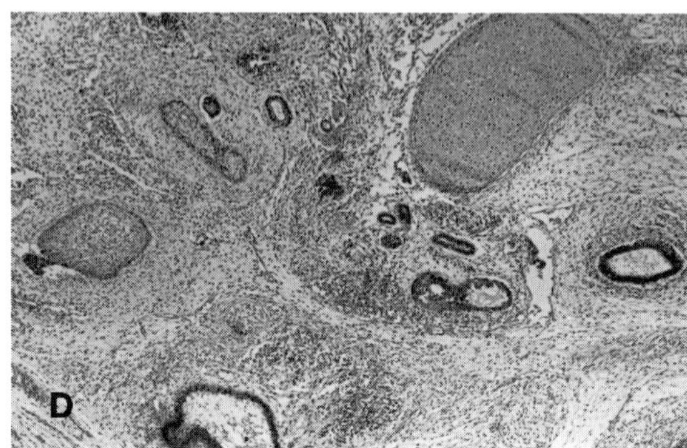

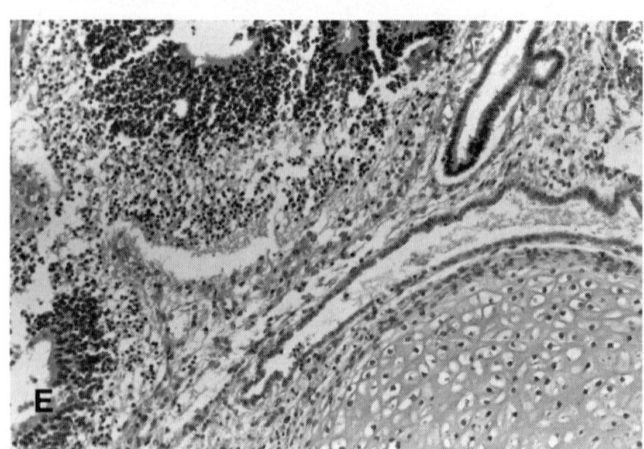

Figure 9–11. Intracranial teratoma. *A,* An ultrasonogram was performed at 31 weeks' gestation. The coronal view displays a large cystic and solid mass filling the cranial vault. The arrow is pointed at the nose. The forehead is the curved structure above the arrow and the mouth and chin are below it. (Courtesy of Val Catanzarite, MD.) *B,* The macrocephalic infant at birth. *C,* The intracranial contents consist of a variety of cystic and solid tissues; there was no recognizable brain. *D,* A photomicrograph reveals cartilage, squamous and respiratory epithelium, and immature neuroglial elements (hematoxylin-eosin, ×48). *E,* The immature neuroglial elements, epithelium, and cartilage at higher magnification (hematoxylin-eosin, ×150). (*B–E:* Courtesy of Arturo Mendoza, MD.) (From Weyerts LK, Catanzarite V, Jones MC, et al. Prenatal diagnosis of a giant intracranial teratoma associated with pulmonary hypoplasia. J Med Genet 1993;30:880. Used by permission of the BMJ Publishing Group.)

cidentally on "routine" prenatal ultrasonography, whereas others are detected during evaluation for a sudden onset of large uterine size in otherwise normal pregnancies.[132,175,235] The rapid growth in maternal girth results from the accompanying hydramnios, which is found in 50% of the cases. Cephalopelvic disproportion occurs as early as the second trimester.[132]

The sonographic findings consist of cranial enlargement and distortion of the normal cerebral architecture by an intracranial mass of mixed densities that contain solid and cystic areas, with or without foci of calcification (see Fig. 9–11*A*).[28,119,132,172,232]

Intracranial teratomas can cause stillbirth and perinatal death.[75,157,160,175,194,215,230,232a,234,237] Fetal death occurs because the teratoma effaces the brain or the enlarged head prevents passage through the maternal birth canal, causing dystocia.[215] Sometimes, the cranium ruptures during delivery, with extrusion of the cranial contents. The review by Gerlach and associates showed that, of all perinatal brain tumors, teratoma was the one most responsible for stillbirth, accounting for 58% of the cases (see Table 9–4).[75] Almost one third of the patients with this tumor who are listed in Table 9–10 were stillborn. Naudin Ten Cate et al. described an intracranial teratoma containing six distinct dysmorphic fetuses which occurred in a hydrocephalic stillborn female fetus.[154] The tumor was detected by antenatal sonography at 30 weeks' gestation. The authors pointed out that a clear distinction between fetus in fetu and teratoma may be an artificial one.

Hydrocephalus occurs in association with intracranial teratomas, and it may be the initial finding. Serial prenatal sonograms demonstrate the onset of hydrocephalus prior to the detection of a massive teratoma.[153,157,185,228] This observation suggests that early obstruction to the flow of CSF by the midline location of the lesion is followed by effacement of the brain by continued tumor growth.[95,153,157] The pineal region, quadrigeminal plate, or the walls of the third ventricle are the main sites of origin.[153,157,238] In neonates with small teratomas, the midline location of the tumor compresses or obstructs the cerebral aqueduct, producing hydrocephalus during the first week of life.[65,157] As mentioned earlier, because of the size of the tumor and resulting distortion of the intracranial architecture, the exact site of origin may be impossible to determine.

In their review of 25 newborns with intracranial teratoma prior to 1960, Greenhouse and Neubuerger divided the cases into three main groups with characteristic clinicopathologic findings.[80] Group I consisted of 11 stillborns: 7 whose brain had been totally replaced by the teratoma and 2 others who had large tumors with obstructive hydrocephalus. The neonates in group 2 were born alive with hydrocephalus and with tumors of intermediate size; their survival ranged from 1/2 hour to 9 weeks. Group 3 comprised 9 neonates who were born healthy but subsequently developed hydrocephalus within 2 days to 3 months after birth. This last group had the smallest tumors, but nevertheless, only 1 patient in this group survived 9 months.

Nine of 12 intracranial teratomas reviewed by Soltaire and Krigman were located in the cerebral hemispheres.[209] Some tumors may be enormous and may erode through the skull into the orbit or extend into the neck.[153,185] Tamura et al. described three stillborn fetuses with teratoma.[215] One occurred in a fetus measuring 29.5 cm crown-heel; the tumor had replaced the brain and filled the cranial cavity. Another

had a teratoma attached to the optic nerve, as well as malformations involving the ear, auditory canal, and orbit, with a cup-like excavation of the ipsilateral eye.[215] Oberman presented a striking example of a massive intracranial teratoma that essentially replaced the entire brain and caused dystocia and stillbirth.[156] Odell et al. reported two similar tumors causing perinatal death.[157] Other examples of enormous perinatal intracranial teratomas effacing most of the brain have been reported (see Table 9–10).[228,230,235]

Cytogenetic data show that intracranial teratomas, as well as extracranial teratomas, have the same karyotype as their host (i.e., 46XX or 46XY).[157,185,194] Saiga et al. described a stillborn with an intracranial teratoma who had a normal DNA histogram; the amniotic fluid had very high values of AFP, CEA, carbohydrate (CA19-9), and cancer 125 antigens.[194]

Typically, intracranial teratomas are large and cystic, with solid areas.[157,234] Calcification, teeth, bone, and cartilage may be present. These tumors have a gross appearance that is identical to that of extracranial teratomas (see Chapter 2, "Germ Cell Tumors"). Frequently, the tumor grows aggressively, effacing the intracranial contents to the extent that the normal architecture of the brain is ill-defined or absent (see Table 9–10 and Fig. 9–11C).[132,237] Histologically, the teratomas consist of both mature tissues from all three germ layers and immature neuroglial elements, which is characteristic for teratomas occurring in various sites in this age group (Fig. 9–11D).[64,153,157,185,194,234] The 11 perinatal intracranial tumors included in the Armed Forces Institute of Pathology series were composed of both mature and immature neuroglial tissues without malignant germ cell tumor elements.[190] The same histologic findings have been reported by other investigators, as well.[156,157,209,215] The two intracranial teratomas depicted by Odell et al.[157] contained mostly immature neuroepithelial tissues, which has been reported before.[157,184,185,230]

The immunohistochemical and ultrastructural features of intracranial germ cell tumors have been discussed by Felix and Becker,[64] Saiga et al.,[194] and Vance et al.,[223] all of whom concur that the findings are essentially the same as those observed for extracranial teratomas. Very infrequently, malignant germ cell tumor components occur in perinatal intracranial teratomas.[236] Immature neuroglial tissues, generally found in intracranial teratomas, have been misinterpreted as malignant lesions, such as ependymoma, neuroblastoma, or medulloblastoma. However, a newborn described by Whittle and Simpson had what was first diagnosed as a benign teratoma; this recurred as embryonal carcinoma 8 months after the initial surgery.[236]

Despite recent advances in diagnosis and therapy, fetal and neonatal intracranial teratomas remain a potentially fatal condition (see Table 9–15).[119,132,157,232,236]

CHORIOCARCINOMA

Choriocarcinoma is a malignant germ cell neoplasm that occurs either in association with an intracranial teratoma or as the result of a placental primary tumor metastatic to the brain.[46,122,240] Primary intracranial choriocarcinoma has not been reported in the newborn.[30,204] Nevertheless, this malignant lesion may present in the neonate or infant as a distinctive syndrome characterized by widespread metastases, bleeding tendencies, and elevated hCG levels. The increased hCG levels result from a placental primary tumor that has invaded the chorionic villous vessels, entered the umbilical vein, and become disseminated throughout the fetal circulation.[240] Chandra et al. analyzed 10 cases of choriocarcinoma in infancy.[30] Their patient, a 1-month-old male infant, died from a massive intracranial hemorrhage secondary to metastatic choriocarcinoma to the brain that presumably originated from the placenta. This case was unique in that the metastatic tumor was confined to the brain. Moreover, in their review, no examples of primary intracranial choriocarcinoma occurring in the perinatal period were found.

CRANIOPHARYNGIOMA

Although craniopharyngioma is a relatively common tumor of childhood, accounting for approximately 10% of intracranial neoplasms, it seldom occurs in the fetus and newborn, in which group it constitutes only 1% of the perinatal brain tumors (see Table 9–1).[45,73,103,133, 245]

Because of their epithelial morphology and location, which is intimately related to the pituitary gland, craniopharyngiomas are thought to arise from Rathke's pouch, an ectodermal diverticulum or upgrowth developing from the roof of the mouth (stomodeum) at about 24 days' gestation.[10] In the region of the sella turcica, Rathke's pouch comes into contact with the infundibulum, the future posterior pituitary, arising as a downgrowth from the floor of the forebrain at about the sixth week.[149] The anterior lobe of the pituitary (adenohypophysis) develops from the anterior wall of Rathke's pouch. The anlage of the adenohypophysis consists of glandular formations composed of pseudostratified columnar epithelia, which are hormonally active at about the ninth week.[245] The ectoderm of the stomodeum further differentiates into the oral mucosa squamous epithelium and the enamel-forming organ of the tooth bud.

Craniopharyngiomas grow by expansion superiorly into the optic chiasm and into the floor of the third ventricle and posteriorly into the posterior fossa.[10] Macrocephaly, resulting from either hydrocephalus and/or the size of the tumor, is the most frequent clinical presentation in the fetus and newborn (Table 9–11).[9,103,110,208,210,221,245] Stillbirth secondary to craniopharyngioma has been reported (see Tables 9–4 and 9–11).[75,233,245]

Imaging studies reveal peripherally located transonic areas or a large, heterogeneous, calcified, cystic mass in the suprasellar region of a fetus or neonate.[92,103,208,237] In addition, the third and lateral ventricles may show signs of obstruction manifested by hydrocephalus.

Perinatal craniopharyngiomas vary in size, but generally tend to be large, occupying much of the cranial volume.[103] One of the smallest ones recorded was only 3 cm in diameter; perhaps one of the largest was 12 cm in greatest dimension.[140,208] The latter tumor, described by Snyder et al., was an enormous, central, calcified, lobulated, solid and cystic mass that had replaced most of the brain. Neither the cortical mantle nor the ventricular system was identifiable.

Craniopharyngiomas are characterized histologically by solid and cystic areas, both squamous and adamantinomatoid patterns, keratin pearl formation, and foci of calcification (Fig. 9–12).[103,208,233] When the tumor invades brain tissue, it provokes a marked reactive gliosis with Rosenthal fiber formation.[10,233]

Yamada et al. described a fetal craniopharyngioma with unique gross and histologic features.[245] At 23 weeks' gestation, a large intracranial mass was detected incidentally on routine antenatal sonography. Induction of labor produced a 1480-g, stillborn male infant with macrocephaly. At necropsy, a large, sponge-like tumor with multiple small cysts

Table 9–11. 14 Fetal and Newborn Craniopharyngiomas*

Case No.	Age at Death	Location	Initial Findings	Reference
1	3 months	3rd ventricle	Large head	Sakamoto et al.[195]
2	48 days	Sella turcica, 3rd ventricle	Large head, bilateral subdural hematoma	Gass[73]
3	?Alive	Suprasellar region	Large head, seizures, jaundice	Majd et al.[140]
4	Alive	Suprasellar region	Large head, incidental sonographic finding†	Hurst et al.[103]
5	3 months	Suprasellar region‡	Large head, hydrocephalus	Iyer[110]
6	39 days	Suprasellar region	Large head	Sobin[208a]
7	2.5 months	Suprasellar region	Large head,§ hydrocephalus, downward gaze	Tabbador et al.[210]
8	Stillborn	Suprasellar region	Large head,† hydrocephalus	Weber and Mori[233]
9	4 days	Suprasellar region	Large head†	Helmke et al.[92]
10	8 hours	Suprasellar region	Large head	Ueyama et al.[221]
11	3 days	Suprasellar region	Large for gestation date,† hydramnios, large head	Snyder et al.[208]
12	8 weeks	Suprasellar region	Hydramnios, hydrocephalus†	Bailey et al.[9]
13	Stillborn	Suprasellar region	Intracranial mass†	Yamada et al.[245]
14	Alive	Suprasellar region	Upward gaze, nystagmus	Isaacs‖

*Selected from the literature.
†Detected antenatally.
‡Diagnosed at necropsy.
§Bilateral rudimentary sixth fingers.
‖Refer to Table 9–1.

filled with gelatinous material and hemorrhage was seen to have replaced the hypothalamus, thalamus, and corpus callosum, and was attached to the sella. The ventricles were markedly dilated, leaving only a thin rim of recognizable cerebral mantle. The tumor had a histologic appearance reminiscent of developing stomodeum (Rathke's pouch) in the embryo, forming squamous cells, enamel organ (ameloblasts), tooth buds, and anterior pituitary, primordial, pseudostratified, columnar epithelium. Transitions between the various types of epithelia were noted. Residual anterior pituitary tissue was present about the periphery, suggesting that the tumor originated from the gland anlage. Moreover, the primordial adenohypophysial epithelium was immunoreactive for chromogranin A and six different anterior pituitary hormones.[245] The squamous epithelial cells were cytokeratin-positive. The term "em-

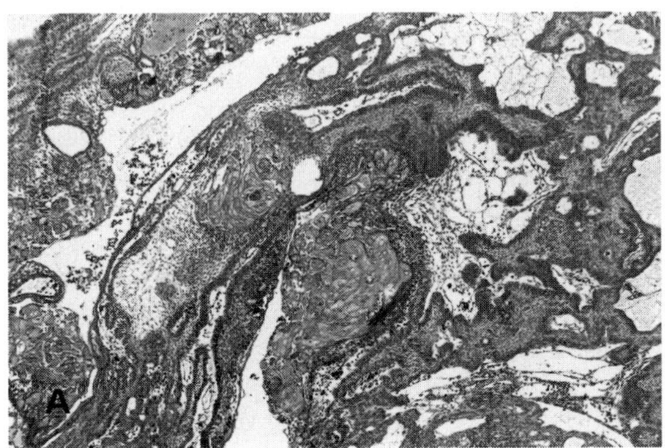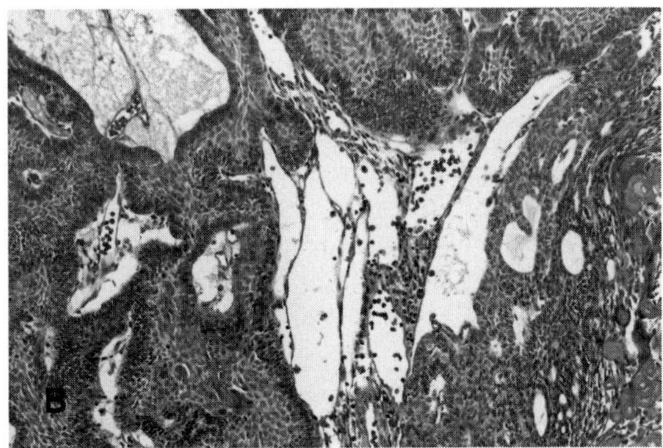

Figure 9–12. Craniopharyngioma. A 3-month-old female infant presented with upward gaze nystagmus and a suprasellar mass (with enhancement) detected on CT scan. *A,* The tumor consists of epithelial cells forming compact masses or lining cysts (hematoxylin-eosin, ×48). *B,* Nests of epithelial cells are surrounded by a layer of columnar "basal" cells separated by a myxoid stroma consisting of stellate cells ("adamantinomatous" pattern). Clusters of keratin pearls are seen on the right side of the photomicrograph (hematoxylin-eosin, ×120).

Table 9–12. 13 Miscellaneous Fetal and Newborn Central Nervous System Tumors*

Case No.	Age at Death	Diagnosis	Location	Initial Findings	Reference
1	3 months	Rhabdoid tumor	Cerebellum	Large head, irritability	Biggs et al.[18]
2	5 months	Rhabdoid tumor	Hemisphere	?Large head	Briner et al.[26]
3	3 years	Rhabdoid tumor	Hemispheres	Large head, hydran-encephaly	Velasco et al.[226]
4	9 months	Medulloepithelioma	Hemisphere	Large head, vomiting, paresis	Jellinger[115]
5	8 months	Medulloepithelioma	Midbrain	Large head, seizures	Treip[220]
6	5 days	Hamartoma	Hypothalamus	Respiratory distress	Sakamoto et al.[195]
7	?Alive	Hamartoma	Hypothalamus	Seizures	Guibaud et al.[82]
8	6 weeks	Hemangioblastoma	Spinal cord	Spinal cord section syndrome	Roig et al.[180]
9	Alive	Hemangioblastoma	Hemisphere	Large head, "sunset" sign	Richmond and Schmidt[179]
10	8 months	Pineoblastoma	Pineal	Large head, irritability, hydrocephalus	Lilue et al.[130]
11	5 months	Pineoblastoma	Pineal	Large head, hydrocephalus	Lilue et al.[130]
12	Stillborn	Oligodendroglioma†	Hemisphere	Hydramnios, large head, hydrocephalus	Wienk et al.[237]
13	2 months	Oligodendroglioma	Hemisphere	Large head, hydrocephalus	Ellams et al.[61]

*Selected from the literature.
†Detected prenatally.

bryonal craniopharyngioma,'' applied by Yamada et al. for this tumor, seems to be an appropriate designation.

Generally, the prognosis for craniopharyngioma is unfavorable. Tables 9–11 and 9–15 show that, of 14 newborns with this tumor, only 3 (21%) survived and 2 were stillborn.

RHABDOID TUMOR

Rhabdoid tumor is a highly malignant neoplasm that occurs also in the central nervous system and has been described in the newborn: two tumors arising from the cerebrum, three from the cerebellum, and one from the fourth ventricle (Table 9–12).[17,18,26,41,226] The three rhabdoid tumors reported by the Philadelphia Children's Hospital group had a monosomy 22 defect.[17] This malignant lesion occurs solely as a primary neoplasm of the brain or concomitantly with rhabdoid tumor of the kidney or liver.[21,31]

Rhabdoid tumor is described in association with hydranencephaly.[226] In the bizarre case depicted by Velasco et al., the tumor was responsible for massive destruction of the cerebral hemispheres with secondary hydranencephaly.[226] The cerebral cortex and white matter were replaced by membranous sacs infiltrated by tumor and filled with viscous CSF. Despite this, the patient had an unbelievably long survival of 3 years.

Generally, the biological behavior of a central nervous system rhabdoid tumor is not unlike that of the primitive neuroectodermal tumor, and is characterized by aggressive growth locally, early metastases through the CSF pathways, seeding of the leptomeninges, invasion of the adjacent brain and spinal cord, and a rapidly fatal course.[17,18,26,41] Hematogenous spread from the central nervous system has not been documented.[226]

On histologic examination, the tumors are similar to those found in the kidney, soft tissues, and other sites, consisting of cells with an eosinophilic cytoplasm, a characteristic round vesicular nucleus with a large nucleous, and paranuclear cytoplasmic bodies composed of intermediate filaments. The light microscopic findings are so distinctive that, in most instances, the diagnosis is suggested from the hematoxylin-eosin staining of sections. The immunohistochemical and ultrastructural features of the intracranial rhabdoid tumor have been discussed by Biggs et al. and by Cossu et al.[18,41] (See Chapter 4, "Soft Tissue Tumors.") Immunohistochemical analysis reveals that the neoplasms react with cytokeratin and with vimentin, but are unreactive with muscle markers. Histogenesis remains an enigma. It is conceivable that some neonatal brain tumors formerly diagnosed as "sarcoma" could possibly have been rhabdoid tumors.

Central nervous system rhabdoid tumors are refractory to radiation therapy and chemotherapy, and patients experience a rapidly fatal, progressively declining, clinical course. The three cases reported by Biegel et al. and the one described by Briner et al. died within 5 months of diagnosis (see Table 9–12).[17,26]

MEDULLOEPITHELIOMA

Medulloepithelioma is an unusual multipotential "embryonal tumor" or "embryoma" recapitulating the primitive medullary epithelium of the medullary plate and neural tube. It forms papillary and tubular structures composed of pseudostratified columnar cells.[10,11,116,200,220] The primitive ventricular matrix cell is thought by Rubinstein to be the cytogenetic origin of the tumor.[187] The tumor displays divergent differentiation ranging from embryonal to mature neuroepithelial cell types. In addition to the neural tube–like epithelium just described, foci of astrocytic, oligodendroglial, and ependymal elements, as well as neuroblasts and mature ganglion cells, are present in varying proportions.

The cerebral medulloepithelioma is a neoplasm of early childhood (average age of 2 years), and congenital cases have been reported (Table 9–12).[28,115,116,200,243] In the Children's Hospital of Philadelphia series, it represented only 1% of the primary brain tumors.[243] The youngest patient in their series of seven children was 6 months of age and had a primary tumor involving the fourth ventricle. The periventricular region of the cerebrum is a common site, but the tumor can occur in almost any location in the brain and spinal cord.[200]

The infant with medulloepithelioma reported by Jellinger and Sunder-Plassmann had a clinical history of a rapidly enlarging head since birth, followed by vomiting and paresis of the left arm at the age of 8 months and opisthotonus at the time of death.[116] At necropsy, a large tumor found in the right parieto-occipital region extended to the dilated lateral ventricles and compressed the aqueduct of Sylvius. Histologically, the tumor consisted of tubular and papillary structures, with columnar epithelium forming ependymal rosettes, neural tube–like

formations, and poorly differentiated neuroblastoma–like areas.

Medulloepitheliomas are highly malignant neoplasms that extensively invade structures locally, metastasizing through the CSF pathways. They are invariably associated with a fatal outcome.

MENINGEAL TUMORS

In the fetus and newborn, the meninges are the source of a variety of benign and malignant tumors, including meningioma, sarcoma, and melanoma.[152] The meningeal neoplasms arise from primitive mesenchymal cells that surround the neural tube and form the dura.[65] Examples are described in the newborn[15,116,136,152,159] and fetus[225] (Table 9–13). Most perinatal meningeal tumors show histologic features of malignancy. Table 9–13 shows that 9 of 12 are sarcomas. Leptomeningeal melanomatosis and malignant melanoma are associated with congenital giant melanocytic nevi, which are discussed in greater detail in Chapter 5, "Tumors and Tumor-Like Conditions of the Skin."

Meningiomas in the young are distinctly different from those found in older age groups.[15] They occur most often in male patients. They are more frequently convex (supratentorial) rather than infratentorial in location, and the distribution of the histologic types is not the same. Fibroblastic and angioblastic meningiomas are among the most common.[15,93,136] The former are characterized on histologic examination by a uniform, spindle cell tumor resembling fibromatosis, whereas in the latter, whorls of small, spindle-shaped cells with oval nuclei are seen to surround the capillaries. Some tumors attain a large size; for example, a fibroblastic meningioma removed from a 5-month-old male infant weighed 600 g.[136]

Meningeal sarcoma presents as an intracranial mass, an occipital protuberance mimicking an encephalocele, or as a spinal cord compression syndrome.[65,98,116,252] These tumors can occur both above and below the tentorium (see Table 9–13). The major signs of meningeal sarcoma in the perinatal period are macrocephaly, hydrocephalus, a tense fontanelle, and cranial asymmetry.[93] In addition, vomiting, seizures, and diffuse spasticity may occur (see Table 9–13).

Two main histologic types of meningeal sarcoma are found in the perinatal period: "sarcoma" and myxofibrosarcoma (see Table 9–

Table 9–13. 12 Fetal and Newborn Meningeal Tumors*

Case No.	Age at Death	Diagnosis	Location	Initial Findings	Reference
1	Alive	Angiomatous meningioma	Supratentorial and infratentorial and orbital	Exophthalmos, seizures	Benli et al.[15]
2	Stillborn	Fibromatous meningioma	Middle fossa	Stillborn	Soltaire and Krigman[209]
3	15 days	Sarcoma	Brain stem, cerebellum	Bulbar syndrome	Jellinger and Sunder-Plassman[116]
4	3 months	Sarcoma	Hemisphere	Large head, spastic quadriparesis	Ellams et al.[61]
5	15 months	Myxofibrosarcoma	Posterior fossa	Occipital mass, vomiting	Campbell et al.[29]
6	Alive	Myxofibrosarcoma	Hemisphere	Frontoparietal mass	Campbell et al.[29]
7	15 months	Sarcoma	Occipital	Fontanelle mass	Nakamura and Becker[152]
8	3 years	Sarcoma	Parieto-occipital	Fontanelle mass	Nakamura and Becker[152]
9	Stillborn	Sarcoma†	Middle cranial fossa	Large-for-date uterus, large head	van Vliet et al.[225]
10	14 months	Myxofibrosarcoma	Occipital	Occipital swelling	Hockley et al.[98]
11	Alive	Myxofibroma	Occipital	Occipital scalp mass	Hockley et al.[98]
12	28 days	Sarcoma	Spinal cord	Respiratory distress, flaccid paralysis of upper extremities	Zwartverwer[252]

*Selected from the literature.
†Detected antenatally.

13).[152] Both are composed of small, spindle-shaped cells, but myxofibrosarcoma, as the name implies, has a prominent pale grey–staining myxoid background. Mitotic activity is brisk, but nuclear atypia varies. The pleomorphic sarcoma, hemangiopericytoma, and fibrous histiocytoma occur more commonly in older individuals.[152] The perinatal sarcomas arise from the dura and tend to grow extradurally, eroding through the cranium and attaining a large size outside the skull forming a visibly large scalp mass.[65,98] For example, one of the newborns described by Hockley et al. had a large, asymmetric scalp mass at birth, which gave the infant's head an odd configuration.[98]

In a survey from the Hospital for Sick Children, Toronto, 1.8% of all intracranial tumors of childhood were meningeal in origin (as compared to 14% in adults).[152] Of 17 patients with meningeal sarcoma, 2 were younger than 4 months of age. The tumors in both of these patients presented as rapidly growing fontanelle masses that protruded through the fontanelle and eroded through the adjacent cranium. The bulk of the tumors were extradural but attached to the dura, and infiltrated the venous sinuses.[152] Both tumors were diagnosed as myxofibrosarcoma, and on microscopic examination, they consisted of stellate or spindle-shaped cells with oval nuclei surrounded by a

loose myxoid stroma, which stained positively with Hale's colloidal iron and alcian blue stains. Moderate mitotic activity, foci of necrosis, and mild to moderate pleomorphism were among the findings. Ultrastructurally, the tumor cells were found to have elongated cytoplasms with irregular borders, rough endoplasmic reticulum, glycogen deposits, vacuoles, and clusters of intermediate filaments. Immunostaining for S-100 protein, GFAP, and muramidase was nonreactive.

van Vliet et al. reported an example of a meningeal sarcoma detected by sonography at 32 weeks' gestation.[225] Progressive, asymmetric hydrocephalus and a space-occupying lesion in the middle cranial fossa were the sonographic findings. Postmortem examination of the hydrocephalic stillborn revealed a large middle cranial fossa tumor invading adjacent brain.[225]

A spinal cord meningeal sarcoma occurred in a 12-day-old female neonate who developed respiratory distress and flaccid paralysis of the arms shortly after birth.[252] At necropsy, the sarcoma partially surrounded the spinal cord from the mid-thoracic area to the foramen magnum. The brain per se was not involved. The neonate described by Jellinger and Sunder-Plassmann developed a bulbar syndrome shortly after birth that was manifested by areflexia, extremities in flexion, and respiratory distress.[116] At necropsy, a 65-g posterior fossa sarcoma measuring 5 × 4 cm was found in the cerebellar hemispheres, fourth ventricle, and caudal brain stem. In addition, there was tumor spread along the leptomeninges. A rapidly enlarging occipital mass was the presentation in two newborns with fatal meningeal myxofibrosarcomas reported by Becker and Halliday.[10] Initially, the tumors were hypocellular with low mitotic activity, but subsequently, the neoplasm began to grow at a rapid rate and eventually showed histologic evidence of frank malignancy. The authors cited six similar cases from the literature.[10]

Surgery is the treatment of choice for meningeal tumors. The prognosis is favorable for the meningioma, provided that the tumor can be completely excised in older individuals; however, Table 9–13 shows that, for both benign and malignant lesions, the survival is only 25% (3 of 12) in the perinatal period. Moreover, one of the survivors had a meningeal sarcoma.[15,136]

HYPOTHALAMIC TUMORS

The hypothalamus is the site of certain distinctive tumors in the young that are associated with unusual syndromes and malformations. The hypothalamic hamartoblastoma is part of a complex congenital malformation syndrome characterized by absence of the pituitary, abnormal facies, short limb dwarfism with postaxial polydactyly, anorectal atresia, renal and pulmonary anomalies, and hypogenitalism.[36,68,83,86,102,104] Some patients have hypopituitarism and hypoadrenalism. This fortunately rare but fatal condition has been called congenital hypothalamic hamartoblastoma, or the Pallister-Hall syndrome. More than 50% of the infants with this tumor die within the first week of life, and the remainder die within 4 months.[36,83,102,104]

The hamartoblastoma may be an unexpected finding at necropsy in a newborn with multiple congenital anomalies.[102] The tumor arises from the hypothalamus and ranges in size from 1 cm to 2.5 cm in diameter.[36,102,104] The larger lesions are observed on the inferior surface of the cerebrum, extending from the optic chiasm to the interpeduncular fossa.[36,104] The tumor may invade the pituitary stalk.[104] Microscopically, hamartoblastoma consists of small, dark, uniform cells resembling primitive, undifferentiated germinal cells.[104] The embryonic hypothalamic plate is the proposed site of origin. A constella-

Table 9–14. Brain Lesions Observed in the Pallister-Hall Syndrome

Hypothalamic hamartoblastoma
Short or absent olfactory tracts
Leptomeningeal cyst
Holoprosencephaly
Absent corpus callosum
Polymicrogyria
Dandy-Walker cyst*
Heterotopic nodules
Encephalocele

*Cystic malformation of the fourth ventricle with partial or complete absence of the cerebellar vermis.

From Finnigan DP, Clarren SK, Haas JE. Extending the Pallister-Hall syndrome to include other central nervous system malformations. Am J Med Genet 1991;40:439. Reprinted by permission of Wiley-Liss, Inc., a subsidiary of John Wiley & Sons, Inc.

tion of central nervous system lesions occur in association with the Pallister-Hall syndrome (Table 9–14).[68]

Hypothalamic hamartomas are more mature-appearing on histologic examination than hamartoblastomas, and are associated with precocious puberty or seizures, which may be evident at birth.[82,97,120,195,251] Guibaud et al. described a female newborn with a hamartoma measuring 5 cm in diameter that was detected on MRI studies and confirmed by biopsy.[82] The infant presented with seizures during the first week of life, but without signs of increased intracranial pressure. Sakamoto et al. reported a 5-day-old male infant with an extensive hypothalamic hamartoma who had respiratory distress at birth and survived 1 day following surgery.[195]

The hamartoma is small in size, ranging from 0.5 to 2 cm in diameter, and arises from the posterior hypothalamus between the tuber cinereum and the mamillary bodies, bulging into the interpeduncular fossa.[97] Ultrastructurally, the hamartoma shows neurons with dense core granules and blood vessels with fenestrated endothelium and double basement membranes, features similar to those cells observed in the normal hypothalamus.[251] The mechanisms causing the precocious puberty in these patients are poorly understood.

VASCULAR MALFORMATIONS OF THE BRAIN

Cyanosis and congestive heart failure are the manifestations of large, intracranial, arteriovenous malformations, making it easy to confuse these with congenital heart disease.[107] Dur-

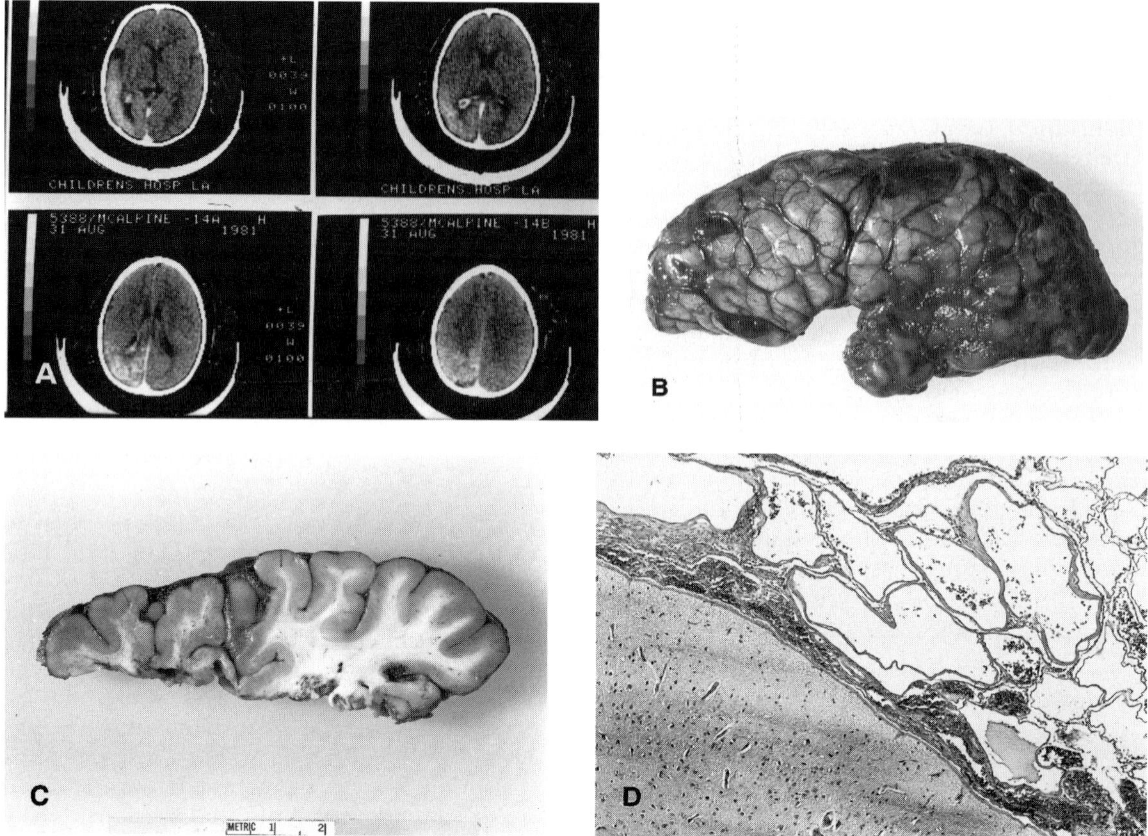

Figure 9–13. Sturge-Weber disease. *A,* A CT scan of a 1-year-old boy who presented with a port wine stain hemangioma distributed over the left side of the face, forehead, and parietal area and intractable seizures. Left cerebral atrophy and focal calcifications are present. *B,* The external surface of the left cerebral hemisphere displays thickening and discoloration of the leptomeninges secondary to multiple hemangiomas situated over the temporal, parietal, and occipital areas. *C,* The cut surface of the cerebral hemisphere shows diffuse involvement of the leptomeninges and a focal lesion in the cortical grey and white matter. *D,* A microscopic section of the temporal lobe depicts a leptomeningeal hemangioma composed of numerous, thin-walled vessels lined by a single layer of flattened endothelium and separated by variable amounts of loose connective tissue. The adjacent gray and white matter show gliosis and focal neuronal necrosis (hematoxylin-eosin, ×120). (From Isaacs H Jr. Tumors of the Newborn and Infant. St. Louis: Mosby–Year Book, 1991.)

ing the 1958–1982 Children's Hospital, Los Angeles perinatal study, five cases were reported of newborns with large intracerebral arteriovenous malformations accompanied by cyanosis and congestive heart failure.[107,108] Because of the clinical presentation in three of the five infants, a presumptive diagnosis of congenital heart disease was made. However, cranial bruits in the other two suggested an arteriovenous malformation. All five newborns died within 3 days after birth. Postmortem findings revealed anastomoses or fistulae between the cerebral or meningeal arteries and the cerebral veins, sagittal sinus, or vein of Galen. The adjacent brain showed variable amounts of hemorrhage, necrosis, or calcification. The hearts of these neonates were considerably enlarged and

dilated, with right ventricular hypertrophy, suggesting high-output heart failure resulting from the large intracranial arteriovenous shunt. At the time of this study, another infant with Sturge-Weber syndrome (flat facial hemangiomata, meningeal hemangiomata with seizures) was reported to have intractable seizures and a port wine stain hemangioma distributed over the left side of the face, forehead, and parietal area. CT scans revealed left cerebral atrophy and focal calcifications in the left parietal area, which were confirmed on gross and microscopic examination of the hemispherectomy specimen (Fig. 9–13). Diffuse hemangiomatosis of the leptomeninges, with focal involvement of gray and white matter of the temporal and occipital lobes, were also found.

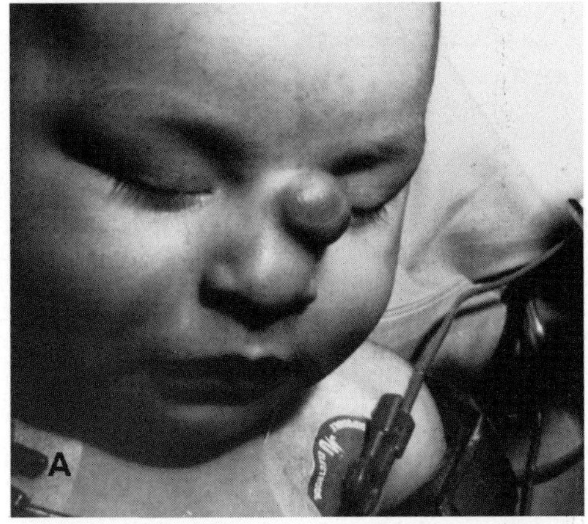

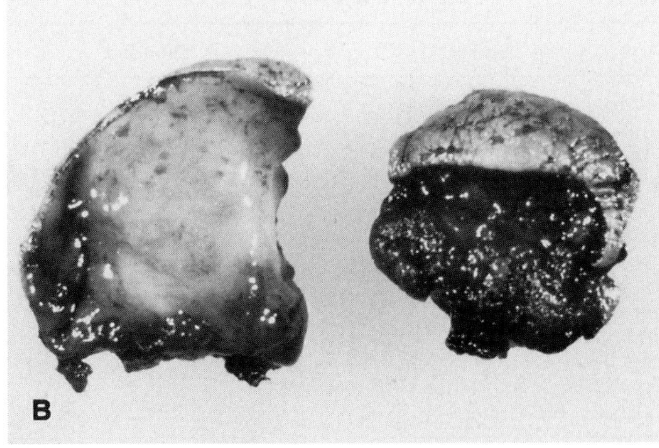

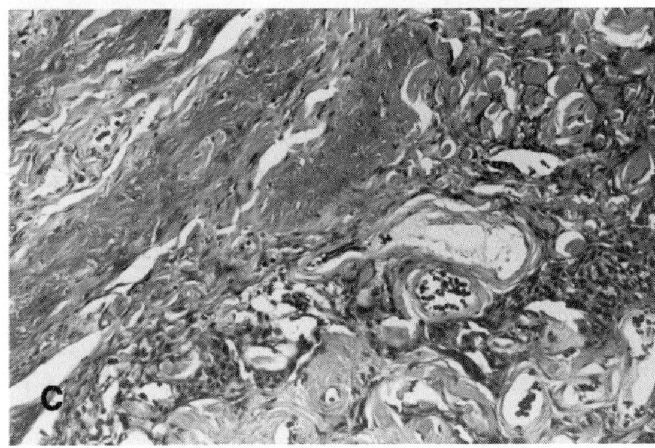

Figure 9–14. Nasal encephalocele ("nasal glioma"). *A,* A newborn with a firm, round nodule situated on the bridge of the nose. A CT scan of the head did not reveal a communication with the brain. *B,* The nasal mass has a firm, fibrous-appearing cut surface. *C,* The lesion consists of dense fibrous connective tissue containing glial elements, pictured on the left of the photomicrograph, and meninges (small, dark, round cells) pictured on the right (trichrome, ×120).

MISCELLANEOUS NEOPLASMS

Herzog et al. reported the findings in six cases of intracranial hemangiopericytomas in children, five of which occurred in newborns.[94] The tumors were situated near the surface of the brain on the convexity or parasagittal region. The authors concluded that infantile intracranial hemangiopericytomas generally have a good prognosis, similar to that of those arising in the soft tissues (see Chapter 4, "Soft Tissue Tumors"). Histologically, they are highly cellular, consisting of cells with irregular or oval nuclei surrounding thin-walled blood vessels. Many mitoses and pleomorphic and hyperchromatic nuclei are present. The tumor cells react with vimentin, and the vessel endothelial cells react with factor VIII–related antigen. Reticulin staining shows reticulin fibers around individual cells. Although the tumors can recur after incomplete excision, spontaneous regression has been documented in some instances.[94] Surgical excision is the treatment of choice.

Two examples of congenital hemangioblastoma have been described, one arising from the left cerebral hemisphere and manifesting as craniomegaly and the "sunset sign," and the other arising from the spinal cord with signs of spinal cord section syndrome.[179,180] Examples of other brain tumors rarely reported in the perinatal period include oligodendroglioma[141] (although no photomicrograph was shown), lipoma of the corpus callosum associated with Goldenhar syndrome,[114] myxolipoma of the thalamus in a newborn with Down syndrome,[107] and a cerebellar neuroepithelial tumor with "multiple divergent differentiation."[199]

Nasal encephalocele ("nasal glioma") arises from a bony defect in the midline between the nasal and the frontal bone, and may have an intracranial connection.[171] The lesion may present either extranasally as a firm mass (Fig. 9–14A) or intranasally, in which case it may be mistaken for a nasal polyp.[147] Microscopically, it consists of neuroglial elements, which are GFAP-positive, meningeal remnants (in some cases), fibrous connective tissue, and rarely, brain tissue (see Fig. 9–14). The differential diagnosis includes hemangioma, dermoid cyst, and nasal polyp.

Table 9–15. Survival Rates for 204 Fetal and Newborn Brain Tumors*

Tumor	Number	Living/Dead	LTF	% Survival
Teratoma	49	3/46		6
Astrocytoma	46	12/34		26
Choroid plexus tumors†	31	16/13	2	52
Primitive neuroectodermal tumors‡	30	3/27		10
Craniopharyngioma	14	3/11		21
Meningeal tumors	12	3/9		25
Ependymoma‖	9	1/8		11
Rhabdoid tumor	3	0/3		0
Medulloepithelioma	2	0/2		0
Pineoblastoma	2	0/2		0
Oligodendroglioma	2	0/2		0
Hypothalamic hamartoma	2	1/1		50
Hemangioblastoma	2	1/1		50
Total	204	43/159		21¶

*Compiled from Tables 9–6 through 9–13.
†Includes 4 papillary carcinomas (2 of 4 survivors).
‡Includes 20 medulloblastomas (1 of 20 survivors).
§Includes 9 sarcomas (2 survivors) and 3 meningiomas (2 survivors).
‖Includes 3 ependymoblastomas (no survivors).
¶Overall survival rate: 43/204 × 100 = 21%.
LTF = lost to follow-up.

PROGNOSIS

Generally, fetuses and newborns with brain tumors have a poor outcome (Tables 9–15).[23,29,107,119,166,229] The overall survival rate has improved somewhat, however, with newer imaging and neurosurgical techniques. Survival figures and neurologic deficits are variable and are related to the age of the patient and the size, location, and histologic type of the tumor. For example, patients with choroid tumors (52% survival) and astrocytomas (26% survival) have a relatively better prognosis compared to those with intracranial teratomas (6% survival) and primitive neuroectodermal tumors (10% survival) (see Table 9–15). Moreover, the gestational age at the time of diagnosis is significant in that usually, there are no survivors when the tumor is found before 30 weeks' gestation.[4,90]

Surgery remains the treatment of choice. Nevertheless, the prognosis for neonates with brain tumors remains dismal, with a high operative and case mortality being reported for example (20% and 75%, respectively, according to Albright,[3] and 35% and 82%, respectively, according to Jooma and co-workers.[119] In the Hospital for Sick Children, London neonatal study, all but 2 of 17 patients died.[119] One survivor had a vascular malformation, and the other was a child with an optic glioma who became blind and retarded at 4 years of age. Of 12 patients in the Children's Memorial Hospital, Chicago series, 5 died within 1 day to 8 months after diagnosis.[172] Only the five patients with choroid plexus papilloma survived. Of nine newborns included in The Hospital for Sick Children, Toronto study, one lived. None of the four patients included in the Children's Hospital, Los Angeles series survived.[29,105]

The Birmingham Children's Hospital, U.K., reported a 7% survival rate; 1 of 14 patients who lived had a choroid plexus papilloma.[166] None of the 14 neonates with various brain tumors who were included in the Danish study survived.[23] In the Japanese Cooperative Study reported by Oi and colleagues, the mortality within 4 months was 48% for neonates and 77.6% for infants.[159] Again, the outcome in these studies was related to the location of the tumor and the histologic features of the tumors.

Although there is a relatively high operative mortality, surgery remains the treatment of choice. Operations are not, however, indicated for neonates with enormous tumors that replace most of the brain.[3] Radiotherapy in the newborn and infant is not recommended because of the deleterious effects of this form of treatment on the immature, developing brain.[119,174] Radiation therapy is also contraindicated in patients younger than 2 years of age. The use of chemotherapy in this age group is controversial;[52,53] however, some authors advocate radical resection whenever possible, followed by chemotherapy, for malignant tumors (e.g., PNETs and astrocytomas).[84]

REFERENCES

1. Adra AM, Mejides AA, Salman FA, et al. Prenatal sonographic diagnosis of a third ventricle choroid plexus papilloma. Prenatal Diagn 1994;14:865.
2. Albert FK, Gaedicke G, Wenzel D, et al. Congenital brain tumors: Diagnostic and therapeutic approach with a report of 3 cases. Zentralbl Neurochir 1989;50:101.
3. Albright AL. Brain tumors in neonates, infants and toddlers. Contemp Neurosurg 1985;7:1.
4. Alvarez M, Chitkara U, Lynch L, et al. Prenatal diagnosis of fetal brain tumors. Fetal Ther 1987;2:203.
5. Amacher AL, Torres QU, Rittenhouse S. Congenital medulloblastoma: An inquiry into origins. Child's Nerv Syst 1986;2:262.
6. Arico M, Raiteri E, Bossi G, et al. Choroid plexus carcinoma: Report of one case with favorable response to treatment. Med Pediatr Oncol 1994;22:274.
7. Asai A, Hoffman HJ, Hendrick EB, et al. Primary intracranial neoplasms in the first year of life. Child's Nerv Syst 1989;5:230.
8. Bader JL, Miller RW. U.S. Cancer incidence and mortality in the first year of life. Am J Dis Child 1979;133:157.
9. Bailey W, Freidenberg GR, James HE, et al. Prenatal diagnosis of a craniopharyngioma using ultrasonography and magnetic resonance imaging. Prenatal Diagn 1990;10:623.
10. Becker LE, Halliday WC. Central nervous system tumors of childhood. Perspect Pediatr Pathol 1987;10:86.
11. Becker LE, Hinton D. Primitive neuroectodermal tumors of the central nervous system. Hum Pathol 1983;14:538.
12. Becker LE, Hinton D. Primitive neuroepithelial tumors of the central nervous system. *In* Finegold M (ed): Pathology of Neoplasia in Children and Adolescents, Major Problems in Pathology, Vol 18, p 397. Philadelphia: WB Saunders, 1986.
13. Becker LE, Yates AJ. Astrocytic tumors in children. *In* Finegold M (ed): Pathology of Neoplasia in Children and Adolescents, Major Problems in Pathology, Vol 18, p 373. Philadelphia: WB Saunders, 1986.
14. Belamaric J, Chau AS. Medulloblastoma in newborn sisters—Report of two cases. J Neurosurg 1968;30:76.
15. Benli K, Cataltepe O, Oge HJ, et al. Giant congenital meningioma in a newborn. Child's Nerv Syst 1990;6:462.
16. Berry PJ. Congenital tumours. *In* Keeling JW (ed): Fetal and Neonatal Pathology, 2nd ed, p 273. Berlin: Springer-Verlag, 1993.
17. Biegel JA, Rorke LB, Packer RJ, et al. Monosomy 22 in rhabdoid or atypical tumors of the brain. J Neurosurg 1990;73:710.
18. Biggs PJ, Garen PD, Powers JM, et al. Malignant rhabdoid tumor of the central nervous system. Hum Pathol 1987;18:332.
19. Boesel CP, Suhan JP, Bradel EJ. Ultrastructure of primitive neuroectodermal neoplasms of the central nervous system. Cancer 1978;42:194.
20. Bonnin JM, Rubinstein LJ. Immunohistochemistry of central nervous system tumors. J Neurosurg 1984;60:1121.
21. Bonnin JM, Rubenstein LJ, Palmer NF, et al. The association of embryonal tumors originating in the kidney and in the brain: A report of seven cases. Cancer 1984;54:2137.
22. Boop FA, Chadduck WM, Sawyer J, et al. Congenital aneurysmal hemorrhage and astrocytoma in an infant. Pediatr Neurosurg 1991–92;17:44.
23. Borch K, Jacobsen T, Olsen JH, et al. Neonatal cancer in Denmark 1943–1985. Pediatr Hematol Oncol 1992;9:209.
24. Branch CE, Dyken PR. Choroid plexus papilloma and infantile spasms. Ann Neurol 1979;5:302.
25. Braunstein H, Martin F Jr. Congenital papilloma of choroid plexus: Report of a case, with observations on pathogenesis of associated hydrocephalus. Arch Neurol Psychol 1952;68:475.
26. Briner J, Bannwart F, Kleihues P, et al. Malignant small cell tumor of the brain with intermediate filaments—A case of a primary cerebral rhabdoid tumor. Pediatr Pathol 1985;3:117.
27. Broadbent VA. Malignant disease in the neonate. *In* Roberton NRC (ed): Textbook of Neonatology, 2nd ed, p 879. Edinburgh: Churchill Livingstone, 1992.
28. Buetow PC, Smimiotopoulos JG, Done S. Congenital brain tumors: A review of 45 cases. Am J Neuroradiol 1990;11:793.
29. Campbell AN, Chan HSL, O'Brien A, et al. Malignant tumours in the neonate. Arch Dis Child 1987;62:19.
30. Chandra SA, Gilbert EF, Viseskul C, et al. Neonatal intracranial choriocarcinoma. Arch Pathol Lab Med 1990;114:1079.
31. Chang C, Ramirez N, Sakr WA. Primitive neuroectodermal tumor of the brain associated with malignant rhabdoid tumor of the liver: A histologic, immunohistochemical and electron microscopic study. Pediatr Pathol 1989;9:307.
32. Chervanak FA, Isaacson G, Touloukian R, et al. Diagnosis and management of fetal teratomas. Obstet Gynecol 1985;66:666.
33. Chowdhury C, Roy S, Mahapatra AK, et al. Medullomyoblastoma. A teratoma. Cancer 1985;55:1495.
34. Christensen RA, Pinckney LE, Higgins S, et al. Sonographic diagnosis of lipoma of corpus callosum. J Ultrasound Med 1987;6:449.
35. Chusid JG, de Gutierrez-Mahoney CG, Garvey TQ. Ependymoma of the cerebellopontine angle in an infant. Neurology 1956;6:152.
36. Clarren SK, Alvord EC Jr, Hall JG. Congenital hypothalamic hamartoblastoma, hypopituitarism, imperforate anus, and postaxial polydactyly—A new syndrome? Part II. Neuropathological considerations. Am J Med Genet 1980;7:75.
37. Coffin CM, Dehner LP. Congenital tumors. *In* Stocker JT, Dehner LP (eds): Pediatric Pathology, Vol 1, p 325. Philadelphia: JB Lippincott, 1992.
38. Coffin CM, Wick MR, Braun JT, et al. Choroid plexus neoplasms: Clinicopathologic and immunohistochemical studies. Am J Surg Pathol 1986;10:394.
39. Colangelo M, Buonaguro A, Ambrosio A. Intracranial tumors in early infancy: Under one year of age. J Neurosurg Sci 1980;24:27.
40. Cooperman E, Marshall KG, Haust D. Congenital astrocytoma. Can Med Assoc J 1967;97:1406.
41. Cossu A, Massarelli G, Manetto V, et al. Rhabdoid tumors of the central nervous system: Report of three

cases with immunocytochemical and ultrastructural findings. Virchows Arch [A] 1993;422:81.

42. Crade M. Ultrasonic demonstration in utero of an intracranial teratoma. JAMA 1982;247:1173.

43. Craver RD, McGarry P. Delicate longitudinal nuclear grooves in childhood ependymomas. Arch Pathol Lab Med 1994;118:919.

44. Cruz-Sanchez FF, Haustein J, Rossi ML, et al. Ependymoblastoma: A histological, immunohistological and ultrastructural study of five cases. Histopathology 1988;12:17.

45. de Chadarevian J-P, Pattisapu JV, Faerber EN. Desmoplastic cerebral astrocytoma of infancy: Light microscopy, immunocytochemistry and ultrastructure. Cancer 1990;66:173.

46. Dehner LP. Neoplasms of the fetus and neonate. In Naeye RL, Kissane JM, Kaufman N (eds): Perinatal Diseases, International Academy of Pathology, Monograph No. 22, p 286. Baltimore: Williams and Wilkins, 1981.

47. Dehner LP. Pediatric Surgical Pathology, 2nd ed. St. Louis: CV Mosby, 1987.

48. Dehner LP. Peripheral and central primitive neuroectodermal tumors. Arch Pathol Lab Med 1986;110:997.

49. Dehner LP. Primitive neuroectodermal tumors of the central nervous system in childhood. Retrospective and overview. Med Pediatr Oncol 1981;1:227.

50. De Sousa AL, Kalsbeck JE, Mealey J Jr, et al. Diencephalic syndrome and its relation to opticochiasmatic glioma: Review of twelve cases. Neurosurgery 1979;4:207.

51. DiGiovanni LM, Sheikh Z. Prenatal diagnosis, clinical significance and management of fetal intracranial teratoma: A case report and literature review. Am J Perinatol 1994;6:420.

52. Di Rocco C. Intracerebral tumors in the first year of life. Pediatr Neurosurg 1990–91;16:99.

53. Di Rocco C, Iannelli, Ceddia A. Intracranial tumors of the first year of life: A cooperative survey of the 1986–1987 Education Committee of the ISPN. Child's Nerv Syst 1991;7:150.

54. Dohrmann GJ, Farwell JR, Flannery JT. Ependymomas and ependymoblastomas in children. J Neurosurg 1976;45:273.

55. Dolkart LA, Balcom RJ, Eisinger G. Intracranial teratoma: Prolonged neonatal survival after prenatal diagnosis. Am J Obstet Gynecol 1990;162:768.

56. Dolman CL. Melanotic medulloblastoma. Acta Neuropathol 1988;76:528.

57. Drop SLS, Guyda HJ, Colle E. Inappropriate growth hormone release in the diencephalic syndrome of childhood: Case report and 4 year endocrinology follow-up. Clin Endocrinol 1980;13:181.

58. Duckett S, Claireaux AE, Pearse AGE. Histoenzymatic study of fetal medulloblastoma associated with congenital malformations. Neurology 1966;16:283.

59. Duckett S, Wilson RR. Fetal spongioblastoma. J Neuropathol Exper Neurol 1964;23:560.

60. Ehret M, Jacobi G, Hey A, et al. Embryonal brain neoplasms in the neonatal period and early infancy. Clin Neuropathol 1987;6:218.

61. Ellams ID, Neuhauser G, Agnoli AL. Congenital intracranial neoplasms. Childs Nerv Syst 1986;2:165.

62. Ernestus R-I, Schroder R, Klug N. Spontaneous intracerebral hemorrhage from an unsuspected ependymoma in early infancy. Child's Nerv Syst 1992;8:357.

63. Farwell JR, Dohrman GJ, Flannery J. Intracranial neoplasms in infants. Arch Neurol 1978;35:533.

64. Felix I, Becker LE. Intracranial germ cell tumors in children: An immunohistochemical and electron microscopic study. Pediatr Neurosurg 1990–1991;16:156.

65. Fenichel GM. Hydrocephalus and congenital tumors. In Fenichel GM (ed): Neonatal Neurology, 3rd ed, p 211. London: Churchill Livingstone, 1990.

66. Fessard C. Cerebral tumors in infancy: 66 clinico-anatomical case studies. Am J Dis Child 1968;115:302.

67. Finck FM, Antin R. Intracranial teratoma of newborn. Am J Dis Child 1965;109:439.

68. Finnigan DP, Clarren SK, Haas JE. Extending the Pallister-Hall syndrome to include other central nervous system malformations. Am J Med Genet 1991;40:395.

69. Fuste FG, Snyder DE, Price A. Congenital spongioblastoma of the pons. Am J Clin Pathol 1967;47:790.

69a. Gadwood KA, Reynes CJ. Intracranial teratoma. Illinois Med J 1983;164:196.

70. Galassi E, Gonado U, Cavallo M, et al. Intracranial tumors during the first year of life. Child's Nerv Syst 1989;5:288.

71. Gareis FJ, Johnson JA. Inanition in infants associated with diencephalic neoplasms. Am J Dis Child 1965;109:349.

72. Garrido E, Becker LF, Hoffman HJ. Gangliogliomas in children: A clinicopathologic study. Child's Brain 1978;4:339.

73. Gass HH. Large calcified craniopharyngioma and bilateral subdural hematomata present at birth. Survey of neonatal brain tumors. J Neurosurg 1956;13:514.

74. Geraghty AV, Knott PD, Hanna HM. Prenatal diagnosis of fetal glioblastoma multiforme. Prenatal Diagn 1989;9:613.

75. Gerlach VH, Janisch W, Schreiber D. ZNS—Tumoren der perinatalperiode. Zentralbl Allg Pathol 1982;126:23.

76. Gertz HJ, Unger M, Lobeck H, et al. Histological and immunocytochemical findings in a case of fetal choroid plexus papilloma. Zentralbl Allg Pathol 1990;136:719.

77. Geyer JR, Finlay JL, Boyett JM, et al. Survival of infants with malignant astrocytomas. A report from the Children's Cancer Group. Cancer 1995;75:1045.

78. Gianella-Borradori A, Zeltzer PM, Bodey B, et al. Choroid plexus tumors in childhood: Response to chemotherapy, and immunophenotypic profile using a panel of monoclonal antibodies. Cancer 1992;69:809.

79. Giangaspero F, Rigobello L, Badiali M, et al. Large-cell medulloblastomas: A distinct variant with highly aggressive behavior. Am J Surg Pathol 1991;16:687.

80. Greenhouse AH, Neubuerger KT. Intracranial teratoma of the newborn. Arch Neurol 1960;3:718.

81. Griffin CA, Hawkins AL, Packer RJ, et al. Chromosome abnormalities in pediatric brain tumors. Cancer Res 1988;48:175.

82. Guibaud L, Rode V, Saint-Pierre, et al. Giant hypothalamic hamartoma: An unusual neonatal tumor. Pediatr Radiol 1995;25:17.

83. Haas JE, Clarren SK, Beckwith JB, et al. Hypothalamic hamartoblastoma, hypoendocrinism and hypomelia: A new syndrome? Lab Invest 1980;42:172.

84. Haddad SF, Menezes AH, Bell WE, et al. Brain tumors occurring before 1 year of age: A retrospective review of 22 cases in an 11 year period (1977–1987). Neurosurgery 1991;29:8.

85. Hahn JS, Bejar R, Gladson C. Neonatal subependymal giant cell astrocytoma associated with tuberose sclerosis: MRI, CT and ultrasound correlation. Neurology 1991;41:124.

86. Hall JG, Pallister PD, Clarren SK, et al. Congenital hypothalamic hamartoblastoma, hypopituitarism, imperforate anus, and postaxial polydactyly—A new syndrome? Part I. Clinical, causal, and pathogenetic considerations. Am J Med Genet 1980;7:47.

87. Hall WA, Yunis EJ, Albright AL. Anaplastic ganglioglioma in an infant: Case report and review of the literature. Neurosurgery 1986;19:1016.

88. Hart MN, Earle KM. Primitive neuroectodermal tumors of the brain in children. Cancer 1973;32:890.

89. Hecht F, Grix A Jr, Hecht BK, et al. Direct prenatal chromosome diagnosis of a malignancy. Cancer Genet Cytogenet 1984;11:107.

90. Heckel S, Favre R, Gasser B, et al. Prenatal diagnosis of a congenital astrocytoma: A case report and literature review. Ultrasound Obstet Gynecol 1995;5:63.

91. Heideman RJ, Packer RJ, Albright LA, et al. Tumors of the central nervous system. *In* Pizzo PA, Poplack GP (eds): Principles and Practice of Pediatric Oncology, 2nd ed, p 633. Philadelphia: JB Lippincott, 1993.

92. Helmke K, Hausdorf G, Moehrs D, et al. CCT and sonographic findings in congenital craniopharyngioma. Neuroradiology 1984;26:523.

93. Herz DA, Shapiro K, Shulman K. Intracranial meningiomas of infancy, childhood and adolescence: Review of the literature and addition of 9 case reports. Child's Brain 1980;7:43.

94. Herzog CE, Leeds NE, Bruner JM, et al. Intracranial hemangiopericytomas in children. Pediatr Neurosurg 1995;22:274.

95. Hirsch LF, Rorke LB, Schmidek HH. The unusual cause of relapsing hydrocephalus: Congenital intracranial teratoma. Arch Neurol 1977;34:505.

96. Ho DM, Wong T-T, Liu H-C. Choroid plexus tumors in childhood: Histopathologic study and clinicopathological correlation. Child's Nerv Syst 1991;7:437.

97. Hochman HI, Judge DM, Reichlin S. Precocious puberty and hypothalamic hamartoma. Pediatrics 1981;67:236.

98. Hockley AD, Hoffman HJ, Hendrick EB. Occipital mesenchymal tumors of infancy: Report of three cases. J Neurosurg 1977;46:239.

99. Hoff NR, Mackay IM. Prenatal ultrasound diagnosis of intracranial teratoma. J Clin Ultrasound 1980;8:247.

100. Horten BC, Rubinstein LJ. Primary cerebral neuroblastoma: A clinicopathological study of 35 cases. Brain 1976;99:735.

101. Howat AJ, Gonzales MF, Waters KD, et al. Primitive neuroectodermal tumour of the central nervous system associated with a malignant rhabdoid tumour of the kidney: Report of a case. Histopathology 1986;10:643.

102. Huff DS, Fernandes M. Two cases of congenital hypothalamic hamartoblastoma, polydactyly and other congenital anomalies (Pallister-Hall syndrome) (Letter). N Engl J Med 1982;306:430.

103. Hurst RW, McIlhenny J, Park TS, et al. Neonatal craniopharyngioma: CT and ultrasonographic features. J Comput Assist Tomogr 1988;12:858.

104. Iafolla K, Fratkin JD, Spiegel PK, et al. Case report and delineation of the congenital hypothalamic hamartoblastoma syndrome (Pallister-Hall syndrome). Am J Med Genet 1989;33:489.

105. Isaacs H Jr. Congenital and neonatal malignant tumors: A 28-year experience at Children's Hospital of Los Angeles. Am J Pediatr Hematol/Oncol 1987;9(2):121.

106. Isaacs H Jr. Neoplasms in infants: A report of 265 cases. Pathol Annu 1983;18(2):165.

107. Isaacs H Jr. Perinatal (congenital and neonatal) neoplasms: A report of 110 cases. Pediatr Pathol 1985;3:165.

108. Isaacs H Jr. Tumors of the Newborn and Infant. St. Louis: Mosby–Year Book, 1991.

109. Itoh Y, Kowada M, Mineura K, et al. Congenital glioblastoma of the cerebellum with cytofluorometric deoxyribonucleic acid analysis. Surg Neurol 1987;27:163.

110. Iyer CGS. Case of an adamantinoma present at birth. J Neurosurg 1952;9:221.

111. Janisch W. Zur epidemiologie der primaren Geschwulste des zentralnervensystems im ersten lebensjahr. Arch Geschwulstforsch 1985;55:489.

112. Janisch W, Schreiber D, Martin H, Gerlach H. Primare intrakranielle tumoren als todesursache bei feten und sauglingen. Zentralbl Allg Pathol 1984;192(2):75.

113. Jay V, Parkinson D, Becker L, et al. Cell kinetic analysis in pediatric brain and spinal tumors: A study of 117 cases with Ki-67 quantitation and flow cytometry. Pediatr Pathol 1994;14:253.

114. Jeanty P, Zaleski W, Fleischer AC. Perinatal sonographic diagnosis of lipoma of the corpus callosum in a fetus with Goldenhar syndrome. Am J Perinatol 1991;8:89.

115. Jellinger K. Cerebral medulloepithelioma. Acta Neuropathol 1972;22:95.

116. Jellinger K, Sunder-Plassman M. Connatal intracranial tumors. Neuropaediatrics 1973;4:46.

117. Jooma R, Hayward RD, Grant DN. Intracranial neoplasms during the first year of life: Analysis of one hundred consecutive cases. Neurosurgery 1984;14:31.

118. Jooma R, Kendall BE. Intracranial tumors in the first year of life. Neuroradiology 1982;23:267.

119. Jooma R, Kendall B, Hayward R. Intracranial tumors in neonates: A report of seventeen cases. Surg Neurol 1984;21:165.

120. Judge DM, Kulin HE, Page R, et al. Hypothalamic hamartoma: A source of luteinizing-hormone-releasing factor in precocious puberty. N Engl J Med 1977;296:7.

121. Kadin ME, Rubinstein LJ, Nelson JS. Neonatal cerebellar medulloblastoma originating from the fetal external granular layer. Neuropathol Exp Neurol 1970;29:593.

122. Kelly DL Jr, Kushner J, McLean WT. Neonatal intracranial choriocarcinoma. J Neurosurg 1971;35:465.

123. Kim JH, Duncan C, Manuelides EE. Congenital cerebellar medulloblastoma. Surg Neurol 1985;23:75.

124. Knierim DS. Choroid plexus tumors in infants. Pediatr Neurosurg 1990–91;16:276.

125. Kobayashi T, Kayama T, Yoshimoto T. Brain tumor in infancy: Comparative study of before and after CT scan era. Pediatr Neurosurg 1990–91;16:99.

126. Kosnik EJ, Boesel CP, Bay J, et al. Primitive neuroectodermal tumors of the central nervous system in children. J Neurosurg 1978;48:741.

127. Kudo H, Oi S, Tamaki N, et al. Ependymoma diagnosed in the first year of life in Japan in collaboration with the International Society for Pediatric Neurosurgery. Child's Nerv Syst 1990;6:375.

128. Kurjak A, Zalud I, Jurkovic Z, et al. Ultrasound diagnosis and evaluation of fetal tumors. J Perinatol Med 1989;17:173.

129. Laurence KM. Hydrocephalus and malformations of the central nervous system. _In_ Keeling JW (ed): Fetal and Neonatal Pathology, 2nd ed, p 541. London: Springer-Verlag, 1993.

130. Lilue RE, Jequier S, O'Gorman AM. Congenital pineoblastoma in the newborn: Ultrasound evaluation. Radiology 1985;154:363.

131. Lin SR, Lee KF, O'Hara AE. Congenital astrocytomas: The roentgenographic manifestations. Am J Roentgenol Radium Ther Nucl Med 1972;115:78.

132. Lipman SP, Pretorius DH, Rumack CM, et al. Fetal intracranial teratoma: US diagnosis of 3 cases and a review of the literature. Radiology 1985;157:491.

133. Lippa C, Abroms IF, Davidson R, et al. Congenital choroid plexus papilloma of the fourth ventricle. J Child Neurol 1989;4:127.

134. Listernick R, Charrow J, Greenwald M. Emergence of optic pathway gliomas in children with neurofibromatosis type 1 after normal neuroimaging results. J Pediatr 1992;121:584.

135. Liu HM, Boggs J, Kidd J. Ependymomas of childhood. I. Histological survey and clinicopathological correlation. Child's Brain 1976;2:92.

136. Lopez MJ, Olivares JL, Ramos F, et al. Giant meningioma in a 5-month-old infant. Child's Nerv Syst 1988; 4:112.

137. Lorentzen M, Hagerstrand I. Congenital ependymoblastoma. Acta Neuropathol (Berl) 1980;49:71.

138. Louis DN, Von Deimling A, Dickersin GR, et al. Desmoplastic cerebral astrocytomas of infancy: A histopathologic, immunohistochemical, ultrastructural and molecular genetic study. Hum Pathol 1992;23: 1402.

139. Magee JF, McFadden DE, Pantzar JT. Congenital tumors. _In_ Dimmick JE, Kalousek DK (eds): Developmental Pathology of the Embryo and Fetus, p 235. Philadelphia: JB Lippincott, 1992.

140. Majd M, Farkas J, LoPresti JM, et al. A large calcified craniopharyngioma in the newborn. Radiology 1971; 99:399.

141. Marwaha RK, Joss CV. A rare congenital intracranial tumor. Med Pediatr Oncol 1994;22:348.

142. Matsushima T. Choroid plexus papillomas and human choroid plexus: A light and electron microscopic study. J Neurosurg 1983;59:1084.

143. McComb JG, Davis RL, Isaacs H Jr. Extraneural metastatic medulloblastoma in childhood. Neurosurgery 1981;9:548.

144. McComb JG, Davis RL, Isaacs H Jr, et al. Medulloblastoma presenting as neck tumors in 2 infants. Ann Neurol 1980;7:113.

145. McConachie NS, Twinning P, Lamb MP. Case report: Antenatal diagnosis of congenital glioblastoma. Clin Radiol 1991;44:121.

146. McCune AB, Cohen BA, Gartner JC. Congenital choroid plexus papilloma and giant nevomelanocytic nevus: Report of a case. J Am Acad Dermatol 1990;22: 849.

147. Menkes JH. Miscellaneous neurologic disorders presenting in the newborn. _In_ Taeusch HW, Ballard RA, Avery ME (eds): Schaffer and Avery's Diseases of the Newborn, 6th ed, p 456. Philadelphia: WB Saunders, 1991.

148. Misugi K, Liss L. Medulloblastoma with cross-striated muscle: A fine structural study. Cancer 1970;25: 1279.

148a. Mitchell D, Rojiani AM, Richards D, et al. Congenital CNS primitive neuroectodermal tumor: Case report

and review of the literature. Pediatr Pathol Lab Med 1995;15:949.

149. Moore KL. The Developing Human: Clinically Oriented Embryology, 5th ed. Philadelphia: WB Saunders, 1993.

150. Mork SJ, Loken AC. Ependymoma. A follow up study of 101 cases. Cancer 1977;40:907.

151. Mork SJ, Rubinstein LJ. Ependymoblastoma: A reappraisal of a rare embryonal tumor. Cancer 1985;55: 1536.

152. Nakamura Y, Becker LE. Meningeal tumors of infancy and children. Pediatr Pathol 1985;3:341.

153. Nanda A, Schut L, Sutton LN. Congenital forms of intracranial teratoma. Child's Nerv Syst 1991;7:112.

154. Naudin Ten Cate L, Vermeij-Keers C, Smit DA, et al. Intracranial teratoma with multiple fetuses: Pre- and post-natal appearance. Hum Pathol 1995;26:804.

155. Newbould MJ, Kelsey AM, Arango JC, et al. The choroid plexus carcinomas of childhood: Histopathology, immunohistochemistry and clinicopathological correlations. Histopathology 1995;26:137.

156. Oberman B. Intracranial teratoma replacing brain. Arch Neurol 1964;11:423.

157. Odell JM, Allen JK, Badura RJ, et al. Massive congenital teratoma: A report of two cases. Pediatr Pathol 1987;7:333.

158. Ogasawara H, Inagawa T, Yamamoto M, et al. Medulloblastoma in infancy associated with omphalocele, malrotation of the intestine, and exstrophy of the bladder. Child's Nerv Syst 1988;4:108.

159. Oi S, Kokunai T, Matsumoto S. Congenital brain tumors in Japan (ISPN Cooperative Study): Specific clinical features in neonates. Child's Nerv Syst 1990; 6:86.

160. Oi S, Tamaki N, Kondo T, et al. Massive congenital intracranial teratoma diagnosed in utero. Child's Nerv Syst 1990;6:459.

161. Oikawa S, Sakamoto K, Kobayashi N. A neonatal huge subependymal giant cell astrocytoma: Case report. Neurosurgery 1994;35:748.

162. Osborn RA, McGahan JP, Dublin AB. Sonographic appearance of congenital malignant astrocytoma. Am J Neuroradiol 1984;5:814.

163. Packer RJ, Perilongo G, Johnson D, et al. Choroid plexus carcinoma of childhood. Cancer 1992;69:580.

163a. Paes BS, DeSa DJ, Hunter JD, et al. Benign intracranial teratoma—prenatal diagnosis influencing early delivery. Am J Obstet Gynecol 1982;143:600.

164. Papadakis N, Millan J, Grady DF, et al. Medulloblastoma of the neonatal period and early infancy. J Neurosurg 1971;34:88.

165. Parker JC Jr, Mortara RH, Mcloskey JJ. Biological behavior of the primitive neuroectodermal tumors: Significant supratentorial childhood gliomas. Surg Neurol 1975;4:383.

166. Parkes SE, Muir KR, Southern L, et al. Neonatal Tumours: A thirty-year population based study. Med Pediatr Oncol 1994;22:309.

167. Pascual-Castroviejo I, Villarejo F, Perez-Higueras A, et al. Childhood choroid plexus neoplasms: A study of 14 cases less than 2 years old. Eur J Pediatr 1983;140:51.

168. Paulus W, Schlote W, Perentes E, et al. Desmoplastic supratentorial neuroepithelial tumours of infancy. Histopathology 1992;21:43.

169. Perentes E, Rubinstein LJ. Recent applications of immuno-peroxidase histochemistry in human neuro-oncology: An update. Arch Pathol Lab Med 1987;111: 796.

170. Podskalny GD, Haller JS, Emrich JF, et al. Report of congenital anaplastic astrocytoma discovered in a newborn. J Child Neurol 1993;8:389.

171. Potter EL, Craig JM. Pathology of the Fetus and Infant, 3rd ed, p 177. Chicago: Year Book Medical Publishers, 1975.

172. Radkowski MA, Naidich TP, Tomita T, et al. Neonatal brain tumors: CT and MR findings. J Comput Assist Tomogr 1988;12:10.

173. Raimondi AJ, Tomita T. Brain tumors during the first year of life. Child's Brain 1983;10:193.

173a. Raskind R, Beigel F. Brain tumors in early infancy— probably congenital in origin. J Pediatr 1961;65:727.

174. Reaman GH. Special considerations for the infant with cancer. In Pizzo PA, Poplack DG (eds): Principles and Practice of Pediatric Oncology, 2nd ed, p 303. Philadelphia: JB Lippincott, 1993.

175. Reece EA. Fetal neoplasm. In Reece EA, Hobbins JC, Mahoney MJ, Petrie RH (eds): Medicine of the Fetus and Mother, p 617. Philadelphia: JB Lippincott, 1992.

176. Reyes-Mugica M, Chou PM, Myint MM, et al. Ependymomas in children: Histologic and DNA-flow cytometric study. Pediatr Pathol 1994;14:453.

177. Riboni G, De Simoni M, Leopardi O, et al. Ultrasound appearance of a glioblastoma in a 33-week fetus in utero. J Clin Ultrasound 1985;13:345.

178. Richards SR. Ultrasonic diagnosis of intracranial teratoma in utero. A case report and literature review. J Reprod Med 1987;32:73.

179. Richmond BK, Schmidt JH. Congenital cystic supratentorial hemangioblastoma. J Neurosurg 1995;82:113.

180. Roig M, Ballesca M, Navarro C, et al. Congenital spinal cord haemangioblastoma: Another cause of spinal cord section syndrome in the newborn. J Neurol Neurosurg Psychiatry 1988;51:1091.

181. Romero R, Oilu G, Jeanty P, Ghidini A, Hobbins JC. Prenatal Diagnosis of Congenital Anomalies, p 34. Norwalk: Appleton & Lange, 1988.

182. Roosen N, Deckert MD, Nikolas N, et al. Congenital anaplastic astrocytoma with favorable prognosis: Case report. J Neurosurg 1988;69:604.

183. Rorke LB. The cerebellar medulloblastoma and its relationship to primitive neuroectodermal tumors. J Neuropathol Exp Neurol 1983;42:1.

184. Rorke LB, Gilles FH, Davis RL, et al. Revision of the World Health Organization classification of brain tumors for childhood brain tumors. Cancer 1985;56:1869.

185. Rostad S, Kleinschmidt-DeMasters BK, Manchester DK. Two massive congenital intracranial immature teratomas with neck extension. Teratology 1985;32:163.

186. Rothman SM, Nelson JS, DeVivo DC, et al. Congenital astrocytoma presenting with intracerebral hematoma. J Neurosurg 1979;51:237.

187. Rubinstein LJ. Cytogenesis and differentiation of primitive central neuroepithelial tumors. J Neuropathol Exp Neurol 1972;31:7.

188. Rubinstein LJ. The definition of the ependymoblastoma. Arch Pathol 1970;90:35.

189. Rubinstein LJ. Tumors of the Central Nervous System, Atlas of Tumor Pathology, Second Series, Fascicle 6. Washington, DC: Armed Forces Institute of Pathology, 1972.

190. Rueda-Pedraza ME, Heifetz SA, Sesterhenn IA, et al. Primary intracranial germ cell tumors in the first two decades of life. Perspect Pediatr Pathol 1987;10:160.

191. Russell AA. A diencephalic syndrome of emaciation in infancy and childhood. Arch Dis Child 1951;26:274.

192. Russell DS, Rubinstein LJ. Pathology of Tumours of the Nervous System, 5th ed. Baltimore: Williams & Wilkins, 1989.

193. Sabet LM. Congenital glioblastoma multiforme associated with congestive heart failure. Arch Pathol Lab Med 1982;106:31.

194. Saiga T, Osasa H, Hatayama H, et al. The origin of extragonadal teratoma: Case report of an immature teratoma occurring in a prenatal brain. Pediatr Pathol 1991;11:759.

195. Sakamoto K, Kobayashi N, Ohtsubo H, et al. Intracranial tumors in the first year of life. Child's Nerv Syst 1986;2:126.

196. Sandbank U. Congenital astrocytoma. J Pathol Bacteriol 1962;84:226.

197. Sato O, Tamura A, Sano K. Brain tumors in early infants. Child's Brain 1975;1:121.

198. Sato T, Shimoda A, Takahashi T, et al. Congenital anaplastic ependymoma: A case report of familial glioma. Child's Brain 1984;11:342.

199. Sato T, Shimoda A, Takahashi T, et al. Congenital cerebellar neuroepithelial tumor with multiple divergent differentiations. Acta Neuropathol (Berl) 1980;50:143.

200. Scheithauer BW, Rubinstein LJ. Cerebral medulloepithelioma: Report of a case with multiple divergent neuroepithelial differentiation. Child's Brain 1979;5:62.

201. Schiffer D, Giordana MT, Pezzotta S, et al. Medullomyoblastoma: Report of two cases. Child's Nerv Syst 1992;8:268.

202. Shawker TH, Schwartz RM. Ultrasound appearance of a malignant brain tumor. J Clin Ultrasound 1983;11:35.

203. Shearer P, Parham D, Kovnar E, et al. Neurofibromatosis type I and malignancy: Review of 32 pediatric cases treated at a single institution. Med Pediatr Oncol 1994;22:78.

204. Shitara T, Oshima Y, Yugami S, et al. Choriocarcinoma in children. Am J Pediatr Hematol/Oncol 1993;15:268.

205. Simopoulos AP, Breslow A. Tuberous sclerosis in the newborn. Am J Dis Child 1966;111:313.

206. Sjogren I, Grotte G, Olding L. Choroid plexus papilloma and infantile hydrocephalus. Acta Paediatr 1964;53:182.

207. Smith NM, Carli MM, Hanieh A, et al. Gangliogliomas in childhood. Child's Nerv Syst 1992;8:258.

208. Snyder JR, Lustig-Gillman I, Milio L, et al. Antenatal ultrasound diagnosis of an intracranial neoplasm (craniopharyngioma). J Clin Ultrasound 1986;14:304.

208a. Sobin LH. Multiple congenital neoplasms. Arch Pathol 1963;76:602.

209. Soltaire GB, Krigman MR. Congenital intracranial neoplasm. A case report and review of the literature. J Neuropathol Exp Neurol 1964;23:280.

210. Tabaddor K, Shulman K, Dal Canto MC. Neonatal craniopharyngioma. Am J Dis Child 1974;128:381.

211. Taboada D, Froufe A, Alonso A, et al. Congenital medulloblastoma. Report of two cases. Pediatr Radiol 1980;9:5.

212. Tadmor R, Harwood-Nash DCF, Savoiardo M, et al. Brain tumors in the first two years of life: CT diagnosis. Am J Neuroradiol 1980;1:411.

213. Takaku A, Kodama N, Ohara H, et al. Brain tumors in newborn babies. Child's Brain 1978;4:365.

214. Tamura A, Sano K. Brain tumors in early infants. Child's Brain 1975;1:121.

215. Tamura H. Intracranial teratoma in fetal life and infancy. Obstet Gynecol 1966;27:134.

216. Taratuto AL, Monges J, Lylyk P, et al. Superficial cerebral astrocytoma attached to dura: Report of six cases in infants. Cancer 1984;54:2505.

217. Tien RD, Hesselink JR, Duberg A. Rare subependymal giant-cell astrocytoma in a neonate with tuberous sclerosis. Am J Neuroradiol 1990;11:1251.

218. Tomita T, McLone DG. Brain tumors during the first twenty-four months of life. Neurosurgery 1985;17:913.

219. Tomita T, McLone DG, Flannery AM. Choroid plexus papillomas of neonates, infants and children. Pediatr Neurosci 1988;14:23.

220. Treip CS. A congenital medulloepithelioma of the midbrain. J Pathol Bacteriol 1957;74:357.

221. Ueyama Y, Kuratsuji T, Lee JY, et al. Congenital giant craniopharyngioma. Acta Pathol Jpn 1985;35:1273.

222. Vagner-Capodano AM, Gentet GC, Gambarelli D, et al. Cytogenetic studies in 45 pediatric brain tumors. Pediatr Hematol Oncol 1992;9:223.

223. Vance RP, Geisinger KR, Randall MB, et al. Immature neural elements in immature teratomas: An immunohistochemical and ultrastructural study. Am J Clin Pathol 1988;90:397.

224. VandenBerg SR, May EE, Rubinstein LJ, et al. Desmoplastic supratentorial neuroepithelial tumors with divergent differentiation potential ("desmoplastic infantile gangliogliomas"): Report of 11 cases of a distinctive embryonal tumor with favorable prognosis. J Neurosurg 1987;66:58.

225. van Vliet MAT, Bravenboer B, Kock HCLV, et al. Congenital meningeal sarcoma—A case report. J Perinat Med 1983;11:249.

226. Velasco ME, Brown JA, Kini J, et al. Primary congenital rhabdoid tumor of the brain with neoplastic hydranencephaly. Child's Nerv Syst 1993;9:185.

227. Ventureyra E, Herder S, Mallya BK, et al. Temporal lobe gangliomas in children. Child's Nerv Syst 1986;2:63.

228. Vinters HV, Murphy J, Wittmann B, et al. Intracranial teratoma: Antenatal diagnosis at 31 weeks' gestation by ultrasound. Acta Neuropathol (Berl) 1982;58:233.

229. Volpe JJ. Brain tumors and vein malformations. _In_ Volpe JJ: Neurology of the Newborn, 3rd ed, p 795. Philadelphia: WB Saunders, 1995.

230. Vraa-Jensen J. Massive congenital intracranial teratoma. Acta Neuropathol 1974;30:271.

231. Wagner JA, Douglas LH, Slager UT. Dystocia caused by fetal intracranial teratoma. Report of a case. Obstet Gynecol 1954;4:647.

232. Wakai S, Arai T, Nagai M. Congenital brain tumors. Surg Neurol 1984;21:597.

232a. Washburne JF, Magann EF, Chauhan SP, et al. Massive congenital intracranial teratoma with skull rupture at delivery. Am J Obstet Gynecol 1995;173:226.

233. Weber F, Mori Y. Craniopharyngioma congenital geant. Helv Paediatr Acta 1976;31:261.

234. Werb P, Scurry J, Ostor A, et al. Survey of congenital tumors in perinatal necropsies. Pathology 1992;24:247.

235. Weyerts LK, Catanzarite V, Jones MC, et al. Prenatal diagnosis of a giant intracranial teratoma associated with pulmonary hypoplasia. J Med Genet 1993;30:880.

236. Whittle JR, Simpson DA. Surgical treatment of neonatal intracranial teratomas. Surg Neurol 1981;15:268.

237. Wienk MATP, van Geijn HP, Copray FJA, et al. Prenatal diagnosis of fetal tumors by ultrasonography. Obstet Gynecol Surv 1990;45:639.

238. Willis RA. The Borderland of Embryology and Pathology, 2nd ed. London: Butterworths, 1962.

239. Wilson CB. Diagnosis and surgical treatment of childhood brain tumors. Cancer 1975;35:950.

240. Witzleben CL, Bruninga G. Infantile choriocarcinoma: A characteristic syndrome. J Pediatr 1968;73:374.

241. Wolf HK, Muller MB, Spanle M, et al. Ganglioglioma: A detailed histopathological and immunohistochemical analysis of 61 cases. Acta Neuropathol 1994;88:166.

242. Yachnis A, Lang B, Zimmerman RA, et al. CNS medulloepithelioma in children: A clinicopathologic study. Pediatr Neurosurg 1990–91;16:100.

243. Yachnis AT, Rorke LB, Biegel JA, et al. Desmoplastic primitive neuroectodermal tumor with divergent differentiation. Broadening the spectrum of desmoplastic infantile neuroepithelial tumors. Am J Surg Pathol 1992;16:998.

244. Yagishita S, Itoh Y, Chiba Y, et al. Cerebral neuroblastoma. Virchows Arch [A] 1978;381:1.

245. Yamada H, Haratake J, Narasaki T, et al. Embryonal craniopharyngioma. Cancer 1995;75:2971.

246. Yates AJ, Becker LE, Sachs LA. Brain tumors in childhood. Child's Brain 1979;5:31.

247. Young JL, Heiss HW, Silverberg E, et al. Cancer Incidence, Survival and Mortality for Children Under 15 Years of Age. Atlanta: American Cancer Society, 1978.

248. Young JL, Miller RW. Incidence of malignant tumors in U.S. children. J Pediatr 1975;86:254.

249. Yu I-T, Ho DM, Wong T-T, et al. Congenital cerebral primitive neuroectodermal tumor with astrocytic differentiation and extracranial metastases. Child's Nerv Syst 1990;6:179.

250. Zimmer C, Figols J, Patt S, et al. Cytokeratin expression in congenital multipotential primitive neuroectodermal tumor. Child's Nerv Syst 1991;7:405.

251. Zuniga OF, Tanner SM, Wild WO, et al. Hamartoma of CNS associated with precocious puberty. Am J Dis Child 1983;137:127.

252. Zwartverwer FL, Kaplan AM, Hart MC, et al. Meningeal sarcoma of the spinal cord in a newborn. Arch Neurol 1978;35:844.

10

TUMORS OF THE EYE

RETINOBLASTOMA

Retinoblastoma is the principal intraocular neoplasm of infancy and childhood, originating from the retina of one or both eyes as a single mass or multifocal tumors. Although it is relatively uncommon in the pediatric age group overall as compared to other neoplasms, it is responsible for significant morbidity and mortality during the first year of life.[3,5,21,37,38,61] The neoplasm occurs in both the fetus and newborn (Tables 10–1 through 10–3; see Fig. 10–3).[3,13,39,51,63]

Incidence

The frequency of retinoblastoma varies considerably with different ethnic groups, both in the United States and elsewhere in the world.[29] The average annual incidence rate given for the United States is in the range of 1 in 18,000 to 1 in 30,000 live births,[61,64] and the average age at diagnosis is 13 months.

Retinoblastoma was the second most common malignant neonatal tumor, accounting for 17 of 102 cases (17%), following neuroblastoma in the Hospital for Sick Children, Toronto study reported by Campbell et al.[13] Of the 148 pediatric retinoblastomas in that institution, it represented 11.5% of the total. Thirteen neonates had bilateral disease, whereas four had unilateral tumors. The initial finding in these 13 patients was leukokoria, strabismus, or heterochromia iridis, in that order; tumors were found in four neonates during eye examinations performed because of a positive family history. The patients were treated with enucleation or irradiation or both. Thirteen (76.5%)

are long-term survivors without evidence of second malignant lesions.[13]

Of 51 neonatal tumors reviewed at the Royal Hospital for Sick Children, Glasgow, 3 (5.9%) were retinoblastomas.[17] Two with a positive family history had bilateral disease. All three patients survived following a combination of enucleation, irradiation, and photocoagulation. The St. Jude Children's Hospital review in 1989 revealed 34 neonatal tumors, of which 3 (8.8%) were retinoblastomas; these accounted for 2.3% of the total 132 retinoblastomas in that institution.[16] All three patients survived following various therapies. Two of 76 (2.6%) neonatal malignant tumors in the Danish cancer study were identified as retinoblastoma.[9] Both of these patients underwent enucleation; one died of a second malignant tumor (osteosarcoma) and the other from an unrelated cause. In the Institut Gustave-Roussy review, retinoblastoma accounted for 1 of 88 (1.1%) of the total number of pediatric ocular malignant lesions, and 1 of 75 (1.3%) of the neonatal malignant tumors.[72] The infant survived after enucleation.

The Children's Hospital of Birmingham, U.K. reported 170 cases of neonatal tumors, 14 (8.2%) of which were diagnosed as retinoblastoma.[63] Eleven of the 14 were bilateral and 3 were unilateral. A positive family history was documented in five patients with bilateral disease and in two with unilateral tumors. Enucleation of one eye was performed in all neonates with bilateral tumors, followed by irradiation to the other eye; two subsequently required a second enucleation. Chemotherapy was administered to two patients, one as the primary treatment, the other when the tumor recurred. The treatment of the unilateral cases consisted of

Table 10–1. Four Newborn Retinoblastomas, Children's Hospital, Los Angeles, 1962–1990

Case No., Sex (Year)	FH	Initial Findings	Location	Group*	Optic Nerve Involvement	Therapy	Outcome
1 M (1962)	–	Leukokoria	O.D.	1	–	Enucleation	Alive
2 F (1984)	+	Leukokoria, bilateral; proptosis and retinal detachment, O.S.	Bilateral	5	–	Enucleation, O.S.; RT and CT, O.D.	Alive
3 F (1986)	–	Leukokoria, O.D.	Bilateral	5	–	Enucleation, bilateral; CT; photocoagulation; cryotherapy, O.S.	Died Age 4 yr.
4 F (1989)	–	Leukokoria, O.S.†	Bilateral	5	–	Enucleation, O.S.; cryotherapy, O.D.	Alive

*According to the Ellsworth staging system (see Table 10–4).[24]
†13q-syndrome.
FH = family history; O.D. = right eye; O.S. = left eye; RT = radiation therapy; CT = chemotherapy.
Clinical data courtesy of Linn Murphree, MD.

Table 10–2. Clinical Presentation of 71 Infants Younger than 3 Months of Age with Retinoblastoma

Finding	No. of Patients
Family history	21
Leukokoria	41
Strabismus	3
Miscellaneous*	6

*Miscellaneous findings included anisocoria, heterochromia, tearing, swelling, proptosis, cataract, nystagmus, and perforation of the globe.

Data abstracted from Abramson DH, Notterman RB, Ellsworth RM, et al. Retinoblastoma treated in infants in the first six months of life. Arch Ophthalmol 1983;101:1362.

enucleation alone in two patients and radiation therapy only in one patient. Six patients with bilateral retinoblastomas died, all of whom had evidence of further tumor. Three developed "trilateral retinoblastoma;" that is, an additional tumor appeared in the pineal region several years after the diagnosis of bilateral retinal tumors. Two others developed second malignant lesions, an orbital osteosarcoma and a sarcoma of the maxilla, several years after diagnosis. The remaining patients survived.[63]

Parkes et al. concluded from their study that the incidence of retinoblastoma in the neonatal period is influenced by the recognition of a family history of the disease. Half the patients in their series had a known family history. Survival is related also to the risk of second malig-nant lesions; 3 of 11 children with bilateral tumors died of second malignant lesions.[63]

Cytogenetics

Cytogenetic and clinical studies in patients with retinoblastoma, and their families have paved the way for a better understanding of the carcinogenesis of this tumor and other childhood tumors in general.[15,26,45,46,60,61] The retinoblastoma gene, a suppressor gene, is situated at the 13q14 chromosome locus, and deletions or mutations of both gene copies at this site are believed to be responsible for the formation of tumors.[23,26–28,60] The two alleles normally found at the 13q14 locus provide double protection against carcinogenesis.[61] This observation seems to apply not only to retinoblastoma, but also to other childhood tumors, such

Table 10–3. Distribution of Reese-Ellsworth-Stage Tumors in 123 Eyes from 73 Infants Younger than 3 Months of Age with Retinoblastoma

Group (Stage)	No. of Eyes (%)
I	35 (28.5)
II	16 (13.0)
III	18 (14.6)
IV	7 (5.7)
V	45 (36.6)
Advanced	2 (1.6)
	123 (100)

Data abstracted from Abramson DH, Notterman RB, Ellsworth RM, et al. Retinoblastoma treated in infants in the first six months of life. Arch Ophthalmol 1983;101:1362.

as neuroblastoma, Wilms' tumor, and osteosarcoma.[61]

Genetic factors should be taken into consideration, both in the diagnosis and in the treatment of individuals and their families with retinoblastoma.[61] This tumor can be classified into two main categories: hereditary and nonhereditary ("sporadic"). The nonhereditary form, resulting from two somatic mutations, comprises 60% of the cases, whereas the hereditary form, resulting from one germinal mutation and one somatic mutation, accounts for the remainder.[30,61] Only 5% to 6% of hereditary cases have a family history of either unilateral or bilateral tumors. Unilateral disease is present in roughly 60% of children with retinoblastoma, and bilateral tumors are seen in about 40%; the bilateral cases are usually hereditary. In the neonate and infant, bilateral disease is by far more prevalent, being seen in almost 70%.[1] Bilateral retinoblastoma is a dominant trait; patients are heterozygous for chromosome 13 deletion, and the genotype (Rb+/rb−) is transmitted to approximately 50% of their offspring.[61] Because so many retinal cells are at risk, 1 of 3 cells in each eye will undergo a second sporadic tumorigenic inactivation mutation, resulting in loss of all tumor suppression and the appearance of a tumor.[61]

Clinical Findings

The clinical manifestations depend upon when the tumor is discovered, which is usually by a parent or by an examining physician. Generally, the diagnosis of bilateral retinoblastoma is established during the first year of life, with unilateral disease being discovered most often during the second year.[21,61] An inherited predisposition to retinoblastoma in bilateral cases shortens the time period to the appearance of tumor. Leukokoria, or white pupillary reflex, is the chief early sign, being noted in more than 50% of affected newborns (see Tables 10–1 and 10–2; Fig. 10–1).[3] Funduscopic examination at this time reveals one or more yellow-white, creamy, rather smooth-shaped lesions on the retina. Strabismus is the presenting sign in less than 10% of cases (see Table 10–2).[3] Infrequent clinical findings in newborns with retinoblastoma include anisocoria, heterochromia, cataract, swelling, nystagmus, and retinal detachment.[3,61] When the optic nerve is involved by tumor, rubeosis iridis (the formation of blood vessels and fibrosis on the surface of the

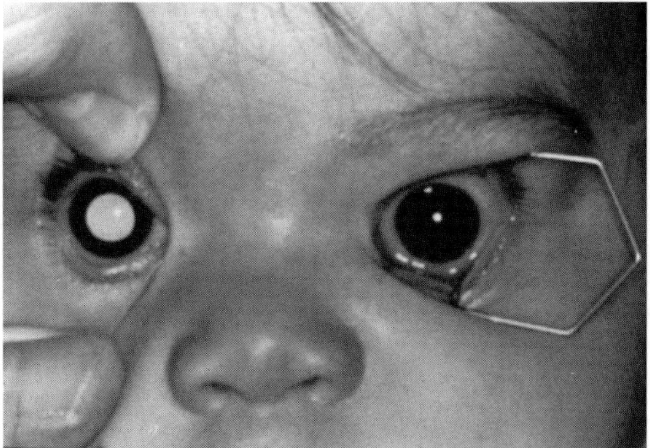

Figure 10–1. Leukokoria (white pupillary reflex) is the most common finding in the newborn and infant with retinoblastoma. The photograph depicts a 9-month-old girl with leukokoria of the right eye, which was noted by her mother 2 weeks prior to diagnosis. (Courtesy of Linn Murphree, MD, and Ben Szirth.) (From Isaacs H Jr. Tumors of the Newborn and Infant. St. Louis: Mosby–Year Book, 1991.)

iris) is observed.[61] With advanced disease, later findings include proptosis, perforation of the globe, and blindness. When metastases occur outside the globe, the patient eventually develops a large, disfiguring, orbital mass, with or without adjacent bone and paranasal sinus invasion (see Fig. 10-4*C*). Irritability, vomiting, seizures, and coma are ominous signs of central nervous system metastases.

Abramson et al. concluded from their study of infants younger than 6 months of age that, because of their young age, the diagnosis of retinoblastoma does not preclude the discovery of advanced disease on initial examination (see Table 10–3).[61] Table 10–3 shows that more than one third of the newborns had group V retinoblastoma. Moreover, the stage V disease in one newborn was so far advanced that there was spontaneous perforation of the globe.

Retinoblastoma is diagnosed in utero by ultrasonography.[51] Maat-Kievit et al. described a large mass arising from the right eye of a fetus of 21 weeks' gestation. The mother was referred for ultrasound examination because of a large-for-date uterus. At necropsy, the tumor measured 8 × 7 cm, weighed 165 g, and effaced the normal anatomy of the orbit, facial bones, mouth, palate, and jaw. Part of the tumor extended into the middle cranial fossa. Ultrasonography suggests the diagnosis when prenatal DNA diagnosis (13q deletion) is not possible.[51]

Less than 5% of children with retinoblastoma have the 13q (del) syndrome, which, in addition to the chromosomal defect, is characterized by a variety of abnormalities, including microcephaly, mental retardation, hypotonia, imperforate anus, malformed digits, and growth failure.[81] Riccardi et al. described a newborn male with the 13q-syndrome who had bilateral retinoblastomas and multiple congenital defects, including a broad nasal bridge, synophrys, large mouth, micrognathia, cryptorchidism, hypotonia, and craniomegaly.[69] At birth, a large, centrolateral retinoblastoma was found in the left eye, which was enucleated, and a small one was found in the right eye. The infant failed to thrive, developed another tumor in the right eye, as well as congestive heart failure, and died at 111 days of age. In addition to the retinoblastoma of the right eye, at necropsy, the heart showed bilateral myocardial and septal hypertrophy and subaortic stenosis.

Diagnosis

Other than funduscopic examination, which often suggests the diagnosis, imaging studies can also assist in establishing diagnosis.[21,61] The finding of one or more retinal masses with calcifications on computed tomography (CT) is pathognomonic for the tumor in most instances. Magnetic resonance imaging (MRI) confirms the CT findings (Fig. 10–3*A* and *B*). Cerebrospinal fluid (CSF) cytology and bone marrow biopsy, together with imaging studies, are requisite for establishing the presence of metastases.[61]

N-myc amplification is noted in tumors removed from patients with advanced stages of retinoblastoma; this is also observed in stage III and IV neuroblastomas.[33,40] Both the enzyme esterase D and the retinoblastoma genes are situated at the same chromosomal locus, 13q14.[27,28,61] Decreased amounts of this enzyme indicate a deletion at this locus. Therefore, determination of esterase D levels is a useful method for detection of prenatal and postnatal patients who are at risk.[23]

Differential Diagnosis

According to Murphree and Munier, retinoblastoma can imitate other conditions involving the eye, particularly hemorrhage and inflammation.[61] Examples include hypopyon (pus in the anterior chamber), orbital cellulitis (painful red eye), and hyphema (hemorrhage into the anterior chamber). Coat's disease (vascular malformation or hemangioma of the retina with retinal detachment) and persistent hyperplastic primary vitreous (partial covering of the retina by a fibrovascular membrane or plaque) are the diseases most easily mistaken for retinoblastoma.[61] Toxoplasmosis, *Toxocara canis* infection, and other forms of severe uveitis have been confused with this tumor.[21] Retinal astrocytoma can mimic this malignant lesion; the astrocytoma would be more likely in a child with tuberous sclerosis.[78]

Spontaneous Regression

Spontaneous regression has been documented in infants and children with retinoblastoma, as with neuroblastoma. The process in patients with retinoblastoma is heralded clinically by inflammation of the involved eye; microscopic changes include hemorrhage, necrosis, lymphocytic infiltrates, and vascular changes, resulting in retinal gliosis of varying degrees, phthisis bulbi (shrinkage, fibrosis, and disorganization of the eye), or even a normal eye.[43] The exact incidence and the cause of spontaneous regression are unknown, but it occurs most often in patients with bilateral disease.[31,43,74,76] Shuangshoti and co-workers reported one example of regression of retinoblastoma that occurred in a 1-month-old male infant who had an enlarged left eye with leukokoria; these signs disappeared spontaneously, leaving the eye blind.[76] At 2 years of age, a similar event occurred in the right eye, which was subsequently enucleated and shown to have tumor.

According to Abramson et al., spontaneous regression occurs in two different settings: (1) in patients with phthisis bulbi, in whom retinoblastoma is often suspected, and (2) in retinoblastoma-like lesions in the fundus of parents of children with retinoblastoma.[3] The family depicted by Gangwar et al. is an example of both instances—namely, bilateral spontaneous regression with phthisis bulbi in a parent (the father) and retinoblastoma in the daughter.[31] The father had leukokoria in the right eye in early infancy, followed by inflammation and phthisis bulbi. When a white reflex and tumor was discovered in the daughter's left eye at 1 month of age, enucleation was performed and the diagnosis of retinoblastoma (well differentiated) was confirmed. In addition to the phthisical right eye, the father had chalky white retinal

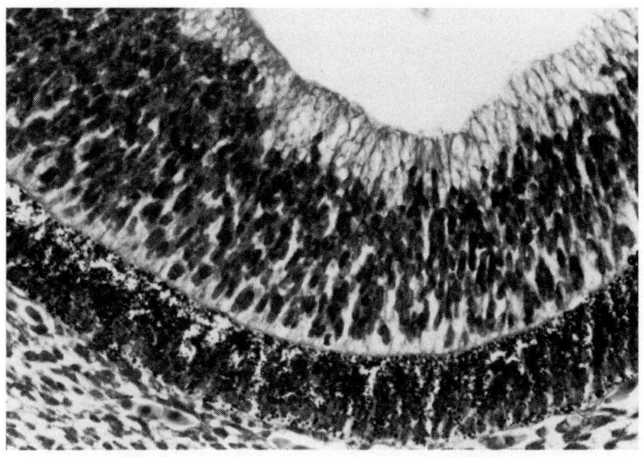

Figure 10–2. Developing retina from a fetus of 8 to 10 weeks' estimated gestation. The external layer of the optic cup contains retinal pigment, whereas the inner layer contains the sensory (neural) retina. At this stage, the neural retina consists of four zones: proliferative (next to the pigment layer), external neuroblastic, transient fiber, and internal neuroblastic zone (hematoxylin-eosin, ×750). (From Isaacs H Jr. Tumors of the Newborn and Infant. St. Louis: Mosby–Year Book, 1991.)

deposits that were consistent with regressed tumor detected on fundoscopic examination.[31]

Garner suggests that some spontaneously regressed retinoblastomas actually represent a benign variant known as retinocytoma (retinoma).[32] Margo et al. reported the pathologic findings (based on light microscopic, ultrastructural, and immunohistochemical analysis) in six retinocytomas occurring in five children treated by enucleation alone.[56] The youngest patient at the time of enucleation was 26 months old, and the oldest was 5 years of age. Histologically, the tumor is composed of differentiated retinal cells with numerous fleurettes but without necrosis or mitotic activity.[56] Occasionally, calcification is present. It is proposed that retinocytomas represent yet another manifestation of the retinoblastoma gene, but with the same genetic implications of a retinoblastoma.[1,8,30,56,61]

Pathology

Light microscopic and ultrastructural findings support the concept that retinoblastoma resembles and probably originates from the retinal precursor cells of photoreceptor cells. (Figs. 10–2 and 10–3D).[61,66,67,70,76,77] During embryonic life, the retina develops from the primitive neuroectoderm lining the optic vesicle, which is an evagination of the neural tube.[59,76]

This neuroepithelium is capable of differentiating into both neuronal and neuroglial elements (see Fig. 10–2).

Retinoblastoma arises from the retina of one or both eyes as a single mass or as multifocal lesions. The involved eye on cross section shows a well-defined, soft, gray-white mass containing tiny white flecks of calcification situated in the retina (see Fig. 10–3C).[35,61,70,74] When there are multifocal primary lesions or foci of vitreous seeding, they appear as white nodules or plaques on the retina or choroid. Large and mostly necrotic tumors tend to be less well demarcated, and sometimes have the appearance of thick white paste within the vitreous cavity. Retinal detachment is found in both the endophytic and exophytic lesions, particularly in advanced disease, but it may be seen earlier in the former, where the tumor grows toward the choroid from the retina. Most retinoblastomas are exophytic; that is, they grow anteriorly into the vitreous from the retina (see Fig. 10–3C). The rare diffuse infiltrating form is characterized by diffuse infiltration of both the retina and choroid by tumor without a well-defined mass.[19,35] Choroidal invasion per se is not always an unfavorable prognostic sign, but it is frequently seen when the optic nerve is involved.[61,68]

The three findings associated with an unfavorable outcome are (1) optic nerve invasion beyond the lamina cribosa, (2) choroidal involvement, and (3) orbital extension.[2,18,47,53,68,74]

Careful examination and taking proper microscopic sections of the optic nerve are crucial in the evaluation of a retinoblastoma specimen. The presence or absence of tumor at the line of resection determines the outcome. When the tumor invades the nerve for a distance of 10 mm or more, it will inevitably enter the subarachnoid space, leading to fatal dissemination of tumor cells into the CSF with seeding of the leptomeninges at the base of the brain and spinal cord (Fig. 10–4). In approximately 40% of cases, choroidal vessels are invaded by tumor cells, which then enter the circulation and metastasize, primarily to the bone marrow, lymph nodes, and liver.[70] In advanced disease with extensive involvement of the eye, the tumor eventually perforates the globe and invades the orbital soft tissues and bone, forming a large, disfiguring mass (Fig. 10–4C).[40]

Retinoblastoma is a prime example of one of the small blue cell tumors of infancy and childhood; therefore, it belongs in the category of primitive neuroectodermal tumor (PNET). It

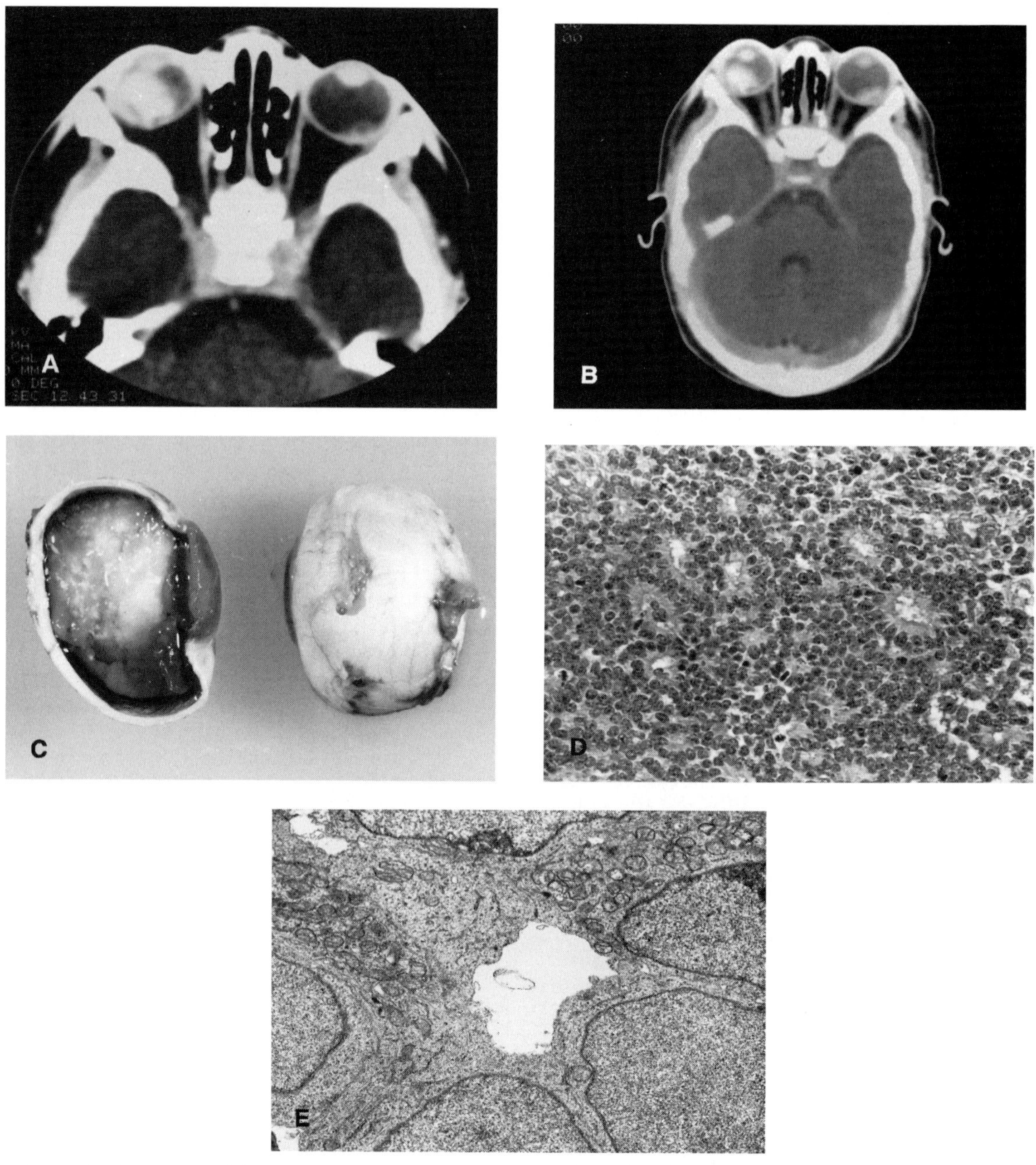

Figure 10–3. Congenital bilateral retinoblastoma in a 1½-month-old female infant with leukokoria of the right eye. *A,* A CT scan reveals tumors in both eyes. *B,* MRI confirms the diagnosis of bilateral tumors of the eye. *C,* The globe of the right eye is bisected, revealing a gray-white tumor mass measuring 11 × 13 mm, filling most of the vitreous cavity, and containing white flecks of calcification. The stub of the optic nerve is situated on the posterior external surface of the globe on the right. Microscopic examination revealed that the optic nerve was not involved. At the time of enucleation, the left eye was noted to have a 12 × 12 disc diameter lesion in the posterior pole and four additional smaller ones. *D,* The tumor is a differentiated retinoblastoma composed of small, round cells with scant cytoplasms and round to oval nuclei with a fine peppery chromatin pattern containing one or two small nucleoli. Several Flexner-Wintersteiner rosettes are evident (hematoxylin-eosin, ×750). *E,* An electron photomicrograph of a Flexner-Wintersteiner rosette shows a clear space in the center surrounded by four poorly differentiated tumor cells. Clusters of mitochondria and scattered microtubules are present in the cytoplasm. In the left lower corner of the photograph, there is a primitive cell junction (×18,900). (*E:* Courtesy of Darkin Chan.) (From Isaacs H Jr. Tumors of the Newborn and Infant. St. Louis: Mosby–Year Book, 1991.)

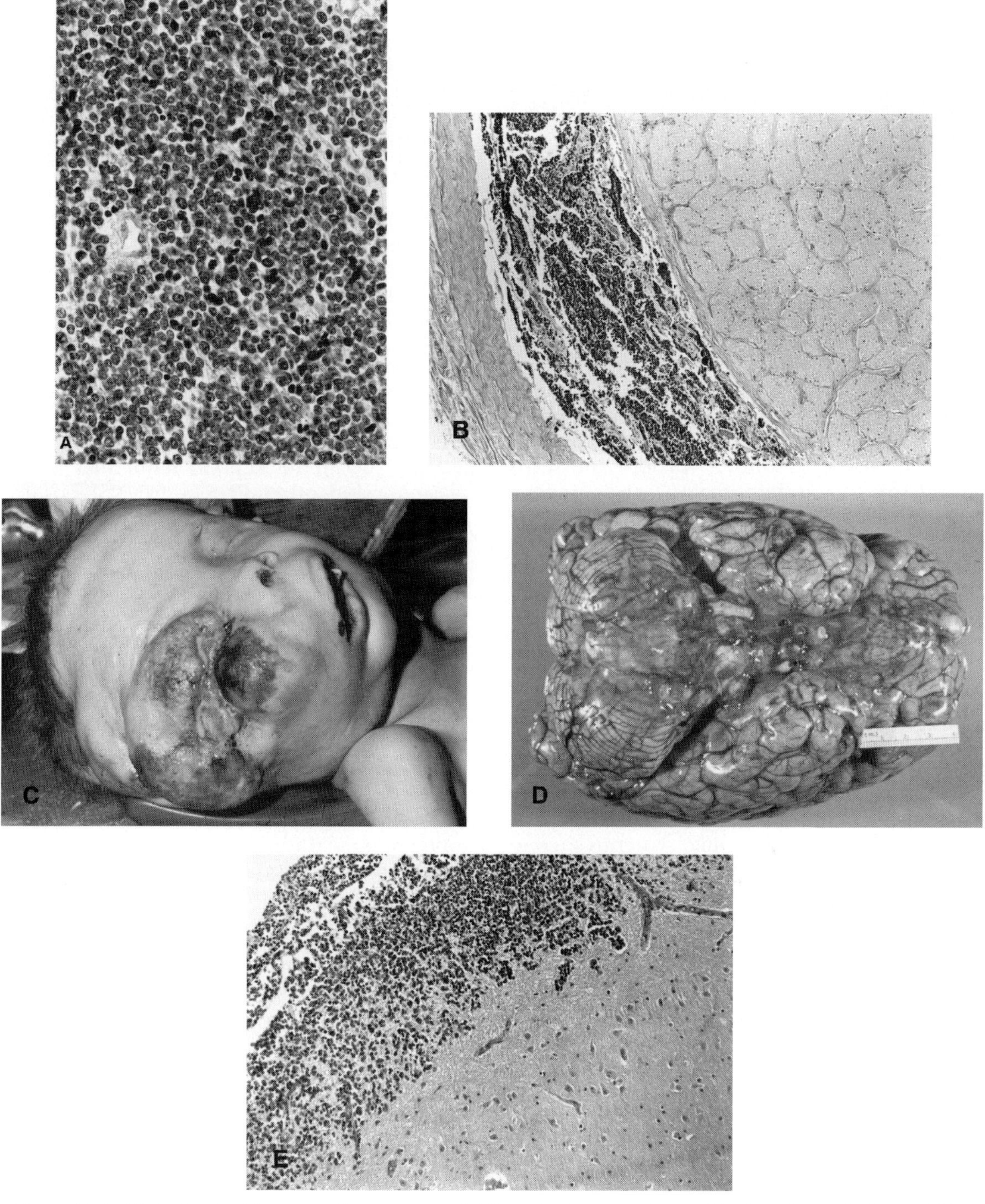

Figure 10–4. Bilateral retinoblastoma with metastases. *A,* The retinoblastoma detected in the left eye of a 1-year-old boy with bilateral disease has the appearance of a poorly differentiated, small cell, malignant tumor. Essentially no photoreceptor cell differentiation is apparent (hematoxylin-eosin, ×750). *B,* This section of the optic nerve shows subarachnoid tumor spread (hematoxylin-eosin, ×120). *C,* At postmortem examination, the patient was found to have a fungating mass protruding from the right orbit and involving the right maxilla and frontal bone. The tumor had spread inferiorly to the right maxilla and medially and posteriorly to the nasal cavity and pharynx, obstructing these structures. It had also invaded the right orbital plate, extended into the floor of the anterior and middle cranial fossae, and involved the base of the brain. *D,* The leptomeninges of the inferior and medial frontal and temporal lobes and cerebellar hemispheres are seen to be infiltrated by tumor. The cranial nerves, mesencephalon, pons, and medulla (the cut surface) are encased by metastases. *E,* The leptomeninges and adjacent insular cerebral cortex are seen to be invaded by tumor cells (hematoxylin-eosin, ×240). (From Isaacs H Jr. Tumors of the Newborn and Infant. St. Louis: Mosby–Year Book, 1991.)

shares certain histologic and biologic features in common with other PNETs, such as neuroblastoma and medulloblastoma, which presumably are also of neural crest origin.[30,74] The main difference between retinoblastoma and other members of this group is that the more differentiated retinoblastomas display neuronal or photoreceptor cell differentiation in the form of Flexner-Wintersteiner rosettes and fleurettes. Once outside the globe, the tumor's aggressive behavior is typical of all the PNETs of the central nervous system (see Chapter 9, "Brain Tumors").

Histologically, retinoblastoma is a hypercellular neoplasm consisting of sheets of small, round to oval, primitive-looking cells with a hyperchromatic, basophilic nucleus and scant cytoplasm. Cytodifferentiation, the amount varying with each specimen, is manifested by the formation of Homer-Wright rosettes, composed of a ring of tumor cells distributed about a central area containing pink fibrillar material, and the distinctive Flexner-Wintersteiner rosettes, consisting of a single layer of cells situated about a well-defined inner circular membrane with a clear zone in the center (see Fig. 10–3D). Most tumors contain Homer-Wright rosettes, but only the Flexner-Wintersteiner rosette is considered to be pathognomonic because it is related to photoreceptor cells and is present in about 50% of retinoblastoma specimens.[18,30,67,70,76,77] Fleurette-like structures, composed of clusters of cells having a "fleur-de-lis" arrangement, and representing further cytodifferentiation, are observed occasionally.[70,74,76,77] Fleurettes are present in retinocytomas.[56] On electron microscopy, the cells forming the Flexner-Wintersteiner rosettes show, at their luminal borders, clusters of mitochondria, zonula adherens–like cell junctions, and characteristic cilia.

Other histologic features include extensive necrosis and calcification and numerous mitoses. Although little or no recognizable stroma is present, a prominent vascular network coursing through the tumor with more viable cells forms sheaths about small vessels. The necrosis and calcification may be so extensive that a diagnosis will not be able to be established with certainty on the basis of histologic findings alone.

Riccardi et al. performed light and electron microscopic studies on an eye removed from a newborn with the 13q-syndrome and retinoblastoma.[69] They found that the tumor had essentially the same ultrastructural features as those described before for the non-(del) 13q-

syndrome patients.[67] However, in addition, areas sampled from portions of the eye not involved by tumor showed a "widespread retinal developmental defect, which they thought was related to the (del)13q" anomaly.[69]

Immunoperoxidase studies performed on both retinoblastoma specimens and on human retina show certain features in common, further supporting the proposed histogenesis of this tumor.[22,30,55,58] For example, neuron-specific enolase (NSE) is the neuronal marker that is positive in tumor cells forming the Flexner-Wintersteiner rosettes and in human retina neurons. NSE staining may be helpful in establishing the diagnosis in the bone marrow when there is a question of metastatic disease. However, it should be kept in mind that neuroblastoma and other PNETs are NSE-positive, and this procedure will not distinguish between the two. In addition to the neuronal components just depicted, Shuangshoti et al. demonstrated the presence of neuroglial elements using both morphologic criteria and immunoperoxidase labeling (NSE and glial fibrillary acidic protein [GFAP]).[76] According to their findings, neoplastic ependymal cells were found in all tumors, and astrocytes, oligodendrocytes, and glioblastoma were found to a lesser degree.

Carbajal described the results of a necropsy study performed on 12 patients with retinoblastoma, demonstrating that the principle routes of spread were the CSF in 9, the bone marrow in 7, orbit-to-orbit spread through the meninges in 6, and the liver in 6.[14] The routes of metastases were classified as to whether they were intracranial (9 of 12) or extracranial (3 of 12). It is significant that all children in the study had optic nerve involvement and that, of the seven with choroid involvement, all but one had distant metastases. Every patient with orbital recurrence died. In a similar postmortem study, Merriam found distant metastases in 9 of 17 patients and intracranial spread in 8.[57] The findings of these investigators further confirm the observation that once retinoblastoma escapes from the eye, there is essentially no survival (see Fig. 10–4).

Treatment

Patients with retinoblastoma are treated by a variety of modalities, depending on whether one or both eyes are affected, the extent of tumor involvement, and whether or not there are metastases present at the time of diagno-

Table 10–4. Criteria for Staging
of Retinoblastoma

___

Group I (Very Favorable)
  A. Solitary tumor, less than 4 disc diameters in size, at or behind the equator
  B. Multiple tumors, none greater than 4 disc diameters in size, all at or behind the equator

Group II (Favorable)
  A. Solitary lesion, 4 to 10 disc diameters in size, at or behind the equator
  B. Multiple tumors, 4 to 10 disc diameters in size, behind the equator

Group III (Doubtful)
  A. Any lesion anterior to the equator
  B. Solitary tumors larger than 10 disc diameters and behind the equator

Group IV (Unfavorable)
  A. Multiple tumors, some larger than 10 disc diameters
  B. Any lesion extending anterior to the ora serrata retinae

Group V (Very Unfavorable)
  A. Massive tumors involving more than half the retina
  B. Vitreous seeding

___

From Ellsworth, RM. The practical management of retinoblastoma. Trans Am Ophthalmol Soc 1969;67:462. Used by permission.

sis.[2,21,61,75] Traditionally, the primary treatment of the disease is enucleation. Other forms of therapy used currently include external beam radiotherapy, photocoagulation, cryotherapy, and chemotherapy in metastatic disease. When the tumor is confined to one eye, in most instances, there is a high probability of cure following enucleation alone. However, according to Murphree and Munier, if the lesion is small, every attempt should be made to salvage the vision in the affected eye(s) by using a treatment modality other than enucleation initially.[61] As a discussion of specific treatment measures is beyond the scope of this book, the reader is referred elsewhere for discussions on the therapy of retinoblastoma.[2,3,21,61,75]

Prognosis

The extent of the tumor, or stage of the disease at the time of diagnosis, is the most important factor with regard to the salvage of the eye(s) and prognosis (see Table 10–4).[3,21,24,61,75] Left untreated, the mortality from retinoblastoma approaches 100%, but in pediatric centers in which radiation therapy, chemotherapy, and other treatment modalities are available, there is a long-term survival rate of greater than 90%. The prognosis is guarded for patients with massive tumors involving more than half the globe and for those with vitreous seeding (Ellseworth group V). A family history of retinoblastoma leads to earlier recognition of the disease and, therefore, increases the likelihood of salvaging the eye(s); however, there appears to be no difference in prognosis between those with a family history and those without.[61] Nevertheless, all children of parents with a family history of this tumor should be examined by an ophthalmologist immediately after birth in order to detect and treat this malignant disease as early as possible.[75]

In a study of 158 children with retinoblastomas diagnosed in the first 6 months of life, Abramson et al. concluded that a young age at the time of diagnosis (mean age of 3.6 months) did not necessarily guarantee that the tumor(s) would be found at an early stage.[61] Indeed, more than one third were classified as group V (see Table 10–3).[61] All 10 (6%) who developed metastases died. Second malignant lesions occurred in 12 (8%) patients, 11 of whom had bilateral tumors. Although most were diagnosed with advanced disease, the 7.4-year survival of 85% was surprisingly high, as it is greater than the overall survival estimated by Jensen and Miller[82] for both unilateral and bilateral cases in the United States.

The survival rate in patients of all ages who were diagnosed as having retinoblastoma and who were treated at Children's Hospital, Los Angeles over the past 25 years is surprisingly good. Of the 200 or so cases, there were only 6 (roughly 3%) known deaths (Linn Murphree, MD, personal communication). There were no instances of trilateral tumors.

It should be emphasized again that the most significant findings that determine the likelihood of survival are optic nerve involvement, particularly at the line of resection, and extraorbital spread.[61,74] At the present time, a definite relationship between tumor cytodifferentiation and prognosis has not been confirmed.[61] When distant metastases occur, or when there is local extension outside the eye, the mortality rate approaches 100%, regardless of the form of therapy.[3,61] The length of survival after diagnosis of metastatic retinoblastoma ranges from 6 months to 1 year.[61]

Trilateral Retinoblastoma

The association of bilateral retinoblastoma with retinoblastoma in the pineal region was termed "trilateral retinoblastoma" in 1980 by Bader and colleagues.[4,6] Retinoblastomas arise from the photoreceptor cells of both eyes and from vestigial photoreceptor cells of the pineal. In lower vertebrates, the pineal serves as the primary photoreceptor, in some animals, acting as a "third eye."[42] Pineoblastomas unassociated with retinoblastomas occasionally display photoreceptor differentiation.[34,42] The midline intracranial tumors usually occur in the pineal region, but occasionally, they are found in the suprasellar and parasellar regions.[20,36,42,65,83] Of 13 patients included in the study by De Potter and associates, the intracranial tumor had a pineal location in 10 and a parasellar location in 3.[20] Extraocular extension or local invasion into the central nervous system from the ocular retinoblastoma or from distant metastases has not been documented in the trilateral syndrome.[4,42,65] It is conceivable that some cases of trilateral retinoblastoma were not recognized in the past because the midline intracranial malignant lesion was interpreted as an intracranial metastasis of retinoblastoma.[65]

The histology of unilateral, bilateral, and pineal retinoblastomas from the same patient may be essentially the same, with or without photoreceptor differentiation.[42] On the other hand, trilateral lesions may have the appearance of an undifferentiated small blue cell tumor.

This ultimately lethal triad is uncommon. Of 245 consecutive children with retinoblastoma in one study, 7 (3%) developed a pineal retinoblastoma.[65] In another study of 32 trilateral cases, a positive family history was noted in 68%, as was an earlier age of presentation of retinoblastoma (7 months) compared to classic bilateral retinoblastoma (15 months).[36] The mean survival time from diagnosis of trilateral disease to death was 6.6 months, and all patients died with spinal metastases.

Holladay et al. found that treatment prolonged survival: survival was 1.3 months with no treatment, as compared to 9.7 months with therapy.[36] Of the 13 patients included in the study by De Potter and associates, there was only one survivor (7.7%) at 30 months post therapy.[20] None of the three patients in the series of Johnson et al. survived.[42]

One of the earliest ages at which pineal retinoblastoma was detected in a patient after the diagnosis of bilateral tumors was 6 months. Kingston and co-workers described a 2-month-old female infant with bilateral retinoblastomas and a positive family history who developed a pineal tumor 4 months later.[44] However, this is not the typical clinical course. After a quiescent period of 1 to several years, tumor in the pineal region is heralded by signs and symptoms of increased intracranial pressure, namely, lethargy, irritability, ataxia, vomiting, hydrocephalus, and papilledema.[36] In De Potter and colleagues' review of 13 patients with trilateral disease, 7 (55%) were asymptomatic, and the intracranial tumor was found on routine brain imaging studies.[20] For this reason, patients should be screened for an intracranial lesion at the time of diagnosis of bilateral retinoblastoma, and ophthalmologists recommend additional imaging studies at appropriate intervals until at least 4 years of age (Linn Murphree, MD, personal communication).[20,44,65,83] Rarely, the symptoms of the intracranial tumor precede those of the ocular lesion(s).[61] Although very uncommon, Kingston and colleagues suggest that the associated pineal malignant lesion is one of the most frequent causes of death in children with bilateral retinoblastoma.[44]

Second Malignant Lesions

The high incidence of second malignant tumors in patients with retinoblastoma, particularly those with bilateral disease, is well known.[3,21,61] Sarcomas of various types, mostly osteosarcoma, are the usual second malignant lesions. Intraorbital rhabdoid tumor following bilateral retinoblastoma has been reported.[26,79] Walford and co-workers described a 2-month-old male infant who was apparently cured following enucleation of the left eye and irradiation of the fellow eye; the patient developed exophthalmos 27 months after the first presentation.[79] Further investigation revealed a rhabdoid tumor arising within the right orbit which eroded through the sphenoid bone into the middle cranial fossa.

It is estimated that approximately 50% of the patients with bilateral retinoblastoma eventually die, from either retinoblastoma or from a second malignant lesion, within 32 years after the diagnosis of the original tumor.[3,21,61]

MEDULLOEPITHELIOMA

Medulloepithelioma is a neoplasm that is thought to arise from the medullary epithelium lining the optic cup, which begins in early embryonic life as an outpouching of the neural tube. Broughton and Zimmerman consider the medulloepithelioma to be a neoplasm of non-pigmented ciliary epithelium.[11] It occurs most often in the ciliary body and/or iris, and occasionally, in the optic nerve or retina. One of the youngest patients with this tumor was a 6-month-old infant described in the Armed Forces Institute of Pathology's series of 56 cases.[11] The main initial clinical findings identified in that study were a cyst or mass in the iris, anterior chamber, or ciliary body, and glaucoma.

On histologic examination, the tumor is composed of sheets and cords of small, blue, neuroblast-like cells (''medullary epithelium'') forming tubular structures and cyst formations.[11,12,80] The net-like appearance formed by anastomosing cords of medullary epithelium is termed the diktyomatous pattern (from the Greek word ''dikty,'' meaning net). When heterotopic tissues (e.g., skeletal muscle, cartilage, or neuroglial tissue) are present, the tumor is classified as a teratoid medulloepithelioma.[11]

During the 33 years of the Children's Hospital, Los Angeles study (see Table 10–1), there were approximately 200 retinoblastomas, 4 of which occurred in newborns. During the same time period, two teratoid medulloepitheliomas were diagnosed in older children who survived disease-free following enucleation as the only therapy.

Medulloepitheliomas are usually slow-growing lesions, and are associated with a favorable outcome, provided they are localized to the eye and completely excised. However, the tumors are potentially fatal when they perforate the globe and extend into the orbit. Death results from intracranial metastases. Therefore, the most important prognostic factor is the presence or absence of orbital invasion.[11,12,80]

ASTROCYTIC TUMORS OF THE RETINA

Retinal tumors or hamartomas of astrocytic origin occur in association with tuberous sclerosis and neurofibromatosis, in 54% and 14% of the patients, respectively.[62,78] In addition, they are observed in the retinas of children who do not have either one of these phakomatoses. Early, the lesion presents as a small, flat, transparent, retinal thickening; later in childhood and adulthood, it appears as a raised, nodular, and calcified whitish mass within the retina or optic disc. Funduscopically, these tumors may resemble a retinoblastoma. The astrocytic lesions, presumably originating from the nerve fiber and ganglion cell layers, grow slowly in childhood, are confined to the eye, and do not invade the sclera. Histologic findings include spindle-shaped astrocytes separated by glial fibrils with foci of calcification. Giant astrocytes are seen in the tumors (hamartomas) of patients with tuberous sclerosis.[78] Replacement of the retina by tumor or recurrent vitreous hemorrhage results in blindness.[62]

JUVENILE XANTHOGRANULOMA

Juvenile xanthogranuloma is regarded as a benign disorder of histiocytes that is typically manifested in the newborn or infant as one or more yellow to reddish-brown cutaneous nodules measuring less than 1 cm in diameter. Most occur on the head and neck and extremities and spontaneously regress within 2 years or less after diagnosis.[19,25,48] Rarely, cutaneous xanthogranulomas are associated with similar lesions in other sites, such as the eye, lung, or deep soft tissues (see Chapter 5, ''Tumors and Tumor-Like Conditions of the Skin'').[19,25,48]

Xanthogranulomas occur not only in the conjunctiva and orbit, but, more importantly from the perspective of ophthalmologists, also in the iris and ciliary body.[35,73] The clinical presentation of spontaneous unilateral hyphema (hemorrhage within the anterior chamber), yellow nodules in the iris, and secondary glaucoma should suggest the diagnosis and prompt a search for skin lesions for biopsy examination.[35,73] However, skin nodules are not always present when there is eye involvement. Sanders reviewed 20 cases of intraocular xanthogranuloma, 5 of which occurred in infants younger than 3 months of age.[73] Four of the five patients had associated skin lesions, five had hyphema, and four had glaucoma.

Histologically, the iris shows nodular infiltration by large histiocytes with eosinophilic cytoplasms and regular, round, oval or reniform nuclei; in addition, smaller numbers of multinucleated Touton giant cells and eosinophils are noted. The intraocular microscopic findings are basically similar to those observed in the skin, except there is less lipid vacuolization in the former. The histiocytes exfoliate into the anterior and posterior chambers, filling the chamber angles and intratrabecular spaces. The blockage that results is responsible for the secondary glaucoma. Neovascularization is a prominent feature, and rupture of the thin-walled vessels accounts for the hyphema.[35,73]

MALIGNANT MELANOMA

Malignant melanoma is a neoplasm derived from melanocytes which, during embryonic life, migrate from the neural crest into various tissues, such as skin, mucous membranes, meninges, and eye. Cases of malignant melanoma have been reported in the fetus and newborn.[10,41,52] As in older children and adults, the skin is the most common site, particularly those arising from giant melanocytic nevi (see Chapter 5, "Tumors and Tumor-Like Conditions of the Skin"). Two known cases of intraocular malignant melanoma have been reported to have occurred at birth.[10] One, depicted by Broadway et al., was a female infant born with a large, darkly pigmented ocular tumor measuring 5.2 × 4 cm and weighing 45-g, multiple melanocytic nevi, and neoplastic hepatomegaly.[10] A CT scan revealed a large neoplasm replacing the left eye and invading the orbit, cavernous sinus, and anterior wall of the middle cranial fossa, but sparing the dura and brain. Following enucleation, the infant received chemotherapy and, surprisingly enough, was living and well 2 years and 10 months after treatment. On macroscopic examination, the melanoma was found to have replaced most of the eye, and there were no recognizable ocular structures. Histologically, the tumor was hypercellular, consisting of round, epithelioid, and spindle-shaped cells with round or oval vesicular nuclei. There was a high mitotic rate. The cytoplasm contained abundant pigment, which was demonstrated ultrastructurally in melanosomes. Tumor cells were immunoreactive with S-100 protein, NSE, and vimentin, but unreactive with cytokeratin and GFAP. Biopsy of a representative skin lesion showed a benign, congenital, melanocytic nevus. However, a liver biopsy taken at 1 week of age revealed metastatic malignant melanoma.

Another neonate with an intraocular melanoma was described by Magee and colleagues.[52] The tumor presumably arose from the uveal tract, filled the globe, and invaded the orbit and adjacent structures. Histologically, it consisted of plump, eosinophilic cells arranged in nests with centrally placed cells containing melanin. The infant was well at the time of writing,

a few months after enucleation. There were no placental or other metastases.

Jensen and associates reported a 7-month-old male infant with the dysplastic nevus syndrome who, at the age of 3 months, had a large vitreous hemorrhage and subluxation of the lens, leading to phthisis bulbi.[41] At the age of 7.5 months, the right eye was enucleated and showed a large, pigmented, hemorrhagic lesion filling the vitreous cavity. The tumor arising from the choroid extended from the posterior lens capsule to the optic nerve, sparing the optic nerve per se and the sclera, but effacing the retina. The light and electron microscopic appearance of the lesion was similar to the tumor described by Broadway et al.[10] The patient was living and well at 25 months of age.

It appears that congenital ocular melanoma, even with metastases, may have a better prognosis than its adult counterpart. However, this tenuous assumption is based only on a few cases.

NEUROFIBROMATOSIS

Neurofibromatosis is one of the phakomatoses, a generalized systemic disease that affects the skin, eyes, and central nervous system. Tuberous sclerosis, Sturge-Weber disease, and von Hippel-Lindau disease are other examples. Less than 50% of infants with neurofibromatosis exhibit physical signs at birth, such as multiple café-au-lait spots, plexiform neurofibromas, and hamartomas of the ocular structures. The condition may involve the entire uveal tract, including the iris, ciliary body, and choroid. When affected, the choroid shows generalized thickening owing to the presence of spindle-shaped Schwann cells, in addition to ganglion cells, nerve fibers, ovoid bodies, and melanocytes (Fig. 10–5A).[76a] Plexiform neurofibroma of the eyelid is associated with a high incidence of congenital glaucoma. Although Lisch nodules, which are focal collections of melanocytic cells situated on the anterior border of the iris, are the most common intraocular abnormality seen in adults, they are rarely found in children younger than 5 years of age.[76a]

ORBITAL TUMORS

Rhabdomyosarcoma occurs in the lid and orbit of the newborn (Fig. 10–6).[38] Teratoma, rhabdoid tumor, neurofibroma, and poly-

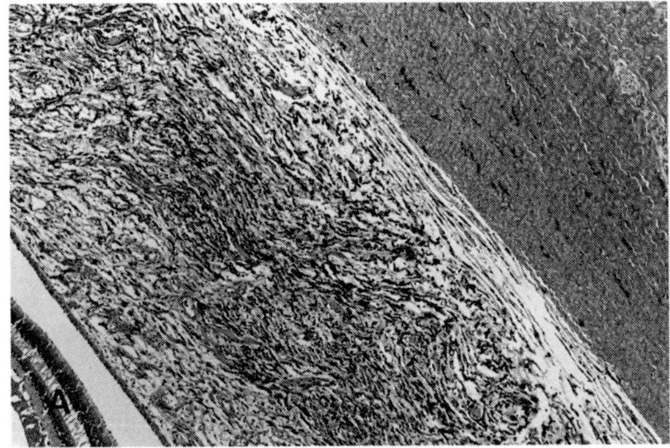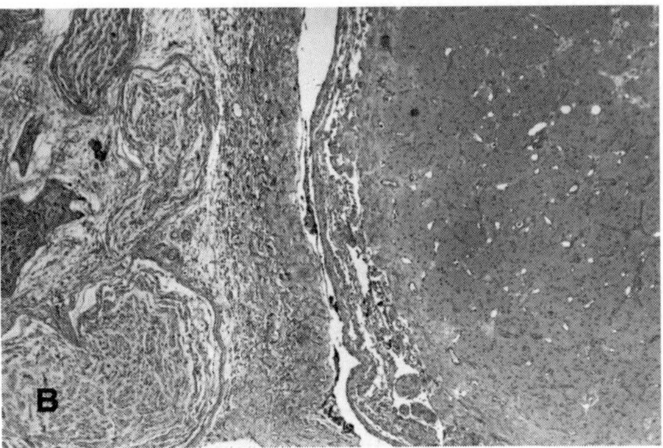

Figure 10–5. Neurofibromatosis of the eye and optic nerve. A 21-month-old boy had neurofibromatosis and glaucoma. *A,* A section was obtained of sclera, ciliary body, and retina. The ciliary body is diffusely thickened by collections of melanocytes, spindle-shaped Schwann cells, and fibrocytes. The sclera contains a nerve with a plexiform neurofibroma (*upper right corner*) (hematoxylin-eosin, ×120). *B,* The meninges are thickened. Adjacent to the optic nerve is a plexiform neurofibroma (hematoxylin-eosin, ×36). (Courtesy of Glenn Billman, MD.)

phenotypic tumor are examples of other tumors involving these structures.[7,17,49,50,54,71,76a]

Orbital teratoma is found at birth, presenting with proptosis and exophthalmus.[7,49,54] The tumor is detected on prenatal sonography.[54] The teratoma is characterized by moderately rapid growth, extensive enlargement of the bony orbit, transillumination of part or all of the tumor, and usually, an associated normally developed eye.[7] Occasionally, it involves the intracranial cavity or is part of an intracranial teratoma with secondary orbital involvement.[7,54] Orbital teratomas contain mature tissues and immature neuroglial elements and, sometimes, unique, embryonic-appearing, optic cup-like structures (see Fig. 2–16).[54]

Rootman and co-workers described a 6-week-old male infant with progressive proptosis noted at 1 week of age.[71] A CT scan revealed a large, enhancing, retrobulbar mass that was examined at biopsy and diagnosed as a malignant rhabdoid tumor. Following excision of most of the mass, radiation therapy, and chemotherapy, the child was alive 2 years after treatment. The tumor cells consisted of a large, round to oval, vesicular nucleus, a prominent nucleolus, and characteristic cytoplasmic eosinophilic bodies that were noted on ultrastructural examination as packets of intermediate filaments. Immunohistochemically, the tumor was reactive with both epithelial membrane antigen and vimentin, but unreactive with cytokeratin, leukocyte common antigen, myoglobin, and desmin.[71]

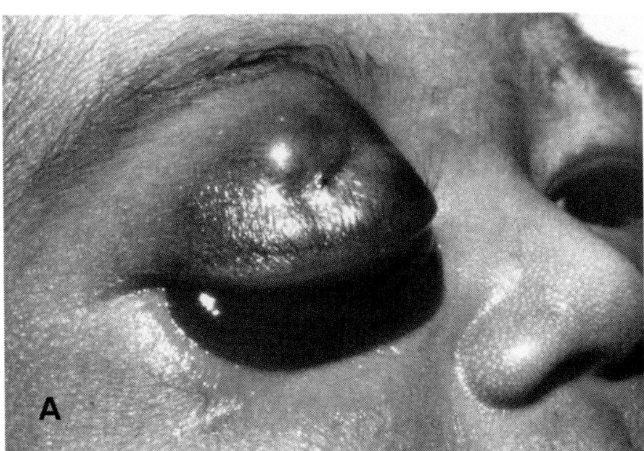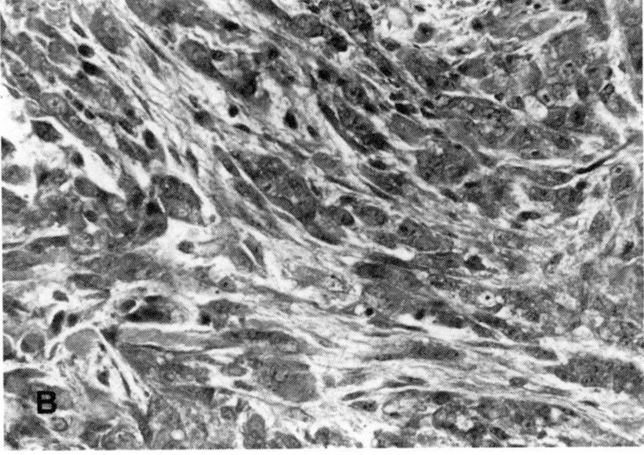

Figure 10–6. Rhabdomyosarcoma of the eyelid. A 6-day-old male infant presented with a mass on the right upper eyelid which was excised. *A,* A picture of the patient shortly after birth shows the eyelid tumor and the underlying hemorrhagic, chemotic conjunctiva. *B,* This is a photomicrograph of a right preauricular lymph node metastasis removed 9 days after the initial surgery. Large, spindle-shaped cells consistent with rhabdomyoblasts are present (hematoxylin-eosin, ×600). (From Isaacs H Jr. Tumors of the Newborn and Infant. St. Louis: Mosby–Year Book, 1991.)

A giant, congenital, orbitocranial, polyphenotypic, small cell tumor was reported by Lyon et al.[50] The infant died as the result of local extension despite orbital exenteration and chemotherapy.

REFERENCES

1. Abramson DH. Retinoma, retinocytoma, and the retinoblastoma gene (Editorial). Arch Ophthalmol 1983; 101:1517.
2. Abramson DH, Ellsworth RM, Tretter P, et al. Treatment of bilateral groups I through III retinoblastoma with bilateral radiation. Arch Ophthalmol 1981;99: 1761.
3. Abramson DH, Notterman RB, Ellsworth RM, et al. Retinoblastoma treated in infants in the first six months of life. Arch Ophthalmol 1983;101:1362.
4. Bader JL, Meadows AT, Zimmerman LE, et al. Bilateral retinoblastoma with ectopic intracranial retinoblastoma: Trilateral retinoblastoma. Cancer Genet Cytogenet 1982;5:203.
5. Bader JL, Miller RW. U.S. cancer incidence and mortality in the first year of life. Am J Dis Child 1979;133: 157.
6. Bader JL, Miller RW, Meadows AT, et al. Trilateral retinoblastoma. Lancet 1980;2:582.
7. Berlin JA, Rich LS, Hahn JF. Congenital orbital teratoma. Child's Brain 1983;10:208.
8. Boniuk M, Zimmerman LE. Spontaneous regression of a retinoblastoma. Int Ophthalmol Clin 1962;2:525.
9. Borch K, Jacobsen T, Olsen JH, et al. Neonatal cancer in Denmark 1943–1985. Pediatr Hematol Oncol 1992; 9:209.
10. Broadway D, Lang S, Harper J, et al. Congenital malignant melanoma of the eye. Cancer 1991;67:2642.
11. Broughton WL, Zimmerman LE. A clinicopathologic study of 56 cases of intraocular medulloepitheliomas. Am J Ophthalmol 1978;85:407.
12. Brownstein S, Barsoum-Homsy M, Conway VH, et al. Nonteratoid medulloepithelioma of the ciliary body. Ophthalmology 1984;91:1118.
13. Campbell AN, Chan HSL, O'Brien A, et al. Malignant tumours in the neonate. Arch Dis Child 1987;62:19.
14. Carbajal UM. Metastases in retinoblastoma. Am J Ophthalmol 1959;48:47.
15. Cowell JK, Hungerford J, et al. A chromosomal breakpoint that separates the esterase D and retinoblastoma predisposition loci in a patient with del (13)(q14q31). Cancer Genet Cytogenet 1987;27:27.
16. Crom DB, Wilimas JA, Green AA, et al. Malignancy in the neonate. Med Pediatr Oncol 1989;17:101.
17. Davis CF, Carachi R, Young DG. Neonatal tumors: Glasgow 1966–86. Arch Dis Child 1988;63:1075.
18. Dehner LP: Neoplasms of the fetus and neonate. In Naeye RL, Kissane JM, Kaufman N (eds): Perinatal Diseases, International Academy of Pathology, Monograph No. 22, p 286. Baltimore: Williams and Wilkins, 1981.
19. Dehner LP. Pediatric Surgical Pathology, 2nd ed. St. Louis: CV Mosby, 1987.
20. De Potter P, Shields CL, Shields JA. Clinical variations of trilateral retinoblastoma: A report of 13 cases. J Pediatr Ophthalmol Strab 1994;31:26.
21. Donaldson SS, Egbert PR, Lee W-H. Retinoblastoma. In Pizzo PA, Poplack DG (eds): Principles and Practice of Pediatric Oncology, 2nd ed, p 683. Philadelphia: JB Lippincott, 1993.
22. Donoso LA, Shields CL, Lee EY. Immunohistochemistry of retinoblastoma. A review. Ophthalmic Pediatr Genet 1989;10:3.
23. Dryja TP, Cavenee W, White R, et al. Homozygosity of chromosome 13 in retinoblastoma. N Engl J Med 1984; 310:550.
24. Ellsworth RM. The practical management of retinoblastoma. Trans Am Ophthalmol Soc 1969;67:462.
25. Enzinger FM, Weiss SW: Soft Tissue Tumors, 3rd ed. St. Louis: CV Mosby, 1995.
26. Friend SH, Bernards R, Rogelj S, et al. A human DNA segment with properties of the gene that predisposes to retinoblastoma and osteosarcoma. Nature 1986;323: 643.
27. Friend SH, Dryja TP, Weinberg RA. Oncogenes and tumor suppressing genes. N Engl J Med 1988;318:618.
28. Fung Y-KT, Murphree AL, T'Ang A, et al. Structural evidence for the authenticity of the human retinoblastoma gene. Science 1987;236:1657.
29. Gaitan-Yanguas, M. Retinoblastoma: Analyses of 235 cases. Int J Radiol Oncol Biol Phys 1978;4:359.
30. Gallie BL, Hinton D. Retinoblastoma: A prototype childhood malignancy. In Finegold M (ed): Pathology of Neoplasia in Children and Adolescents, Major Problems in Pathology, Vol 18, p 419. Philadelphia: WB Saunders, 1986.
31. Gangwar DN, Jain MSIS, Gupta A, et al. Bilateral spontaneous regression of retinoblastoma with dominant transmission. Ann Ophthalmol 1982;14:479.
32. Garner A. Retinoblastoma (Commentary). Histopathology 1989;15:113.
33. Gilbert F, Potluri VR, et al. Retinoblastoma, chromosome abnormalities and oncogene expression. Ophthalmol Paediatr Genet 1987;8:3.
34. Herrick MK, Rubinstein LJ. The cytological differentiating potential of pineal parenchymal neoplasms (true pinealomas). A clinicopathological study of 28 tumours. Brain 1979;102:289.
35. Hogan MJ, Zimmerman LE. Ophthalmic Pathology: An Atlas and Textbook, 2nd ed, pp 449 & 516. Philadelphia: WB Saunders, 1962.
36. Holladay DA, Holladay A, Montebello JF, et al. Clinical presentation, treatment and outcome of trilateral retinoblastoma. Cancer 1991;67:710.
37. Isaacs H Jr. Congenital and neonatal malignant tumors: A 28-year experience at Children's Hospital of Los Angeles. Am J Pediatr Hematol/Oncol 1987;9:121.
38. Isaacs H Jr. Neoplasms in infants: A report of 265 cases. Pathol Annu 1983;18(2):165.
39. Isaacs H Jr. Perinatal (congenital and neonatal) neoplasms: A report of 110 cases. Pediatr Pathol 1985;3: 165.
40. Isaacs H Jr: Tumors of the Newborn and Infant: St. Louis: Mosby–Year Book, 1991.
41. Jensen OA, Movin M, Muller J. Malignant melanoma of the choroid in an infant with the dysplastic naevus syndrome. Acta Ophthalmol 1987;65:91.
42. Johnson DL, Chandra R, Fisher WS, et al. Trilateral retinoblastoma: Ocular and pineal retinoblastoma. J Neurosurg 1985;63:367.
43. Khoudadoust AA, Roozitalab HM, Smith RE, et al. Spontaneous regression of retinoblastoma. Surv Ophthalmol 1977;21:467.
44. Kingston JE, Plowman PN, Hungerford JL. Ectopic in-

tracranial retinoblastoma in childhood. Br J Ophthalmol 1985;69:742.

45. Knudson AG Jr. Hereditary cancer, oncogenes, and antioncogenes. Cancer Res 1985;45:1437.

46. Knudson AG Jr. Retinoblastoma: A prototypic hereditary neoplasm. Semin Oncol 1978;5:57.

47. Kobrin J, Blodi F. Prognosis in retinoblastoma. Influence of histopathologic characteristics. J Pediatr Ophthalmol Strab 1978;15:278.

48. Lever WF, Schaumburg-Lever G: Histopathology of the Skin, 7th ed. Philadelphia: JB Lippincott, 1990.

49. Levin ML, Leone CR, Kincaid MC. Congenital orbital teratomas. Am J Ophthalmol 1986;102:476.

50. Lyon DB, Dortzbach RK, Gilbert-Barness E. Polyphenotypic small-cell orbitocranial tumor. Arch Ophthalmol 1993;111:1402.

51. Maat-Kievit JA, Oepkes D, Hartwig NG, et al. A large retinoblastoma detected in a fetus at 21 weeks' gestation. Prenatal Diagn 1993;13:377.

52. Magee JF, McFadden DE, Pantzar JT. Congenital tumors. *In* Dimmick JE, Kalousek DK (eds): Developmental Pathology of the Embryo and Fetus, p 235. Philadelphia: JB Lippincott, 1992.

53. Magramm I, Abramson DH, Ellsworth RM. Optic nerve involvement in retinoblastoma. Ophthalmology 1989; 96:217.

54. Mamalis N, Garland PE, Argyle JC, et al. Congenital orbital teratoma: A review and report of two cases. Surv Ophthalmol 1985;30:41.

55. Marangos PJ, Polak JM, Pearse AGE. Neurone specific enolase. A probe for neurones and neuroendocrine cells. Trends Neurosci 1982;5:193.

56. Margo C, Hidayat A, Kopelman J, et al. Retinocytoma: A benign variant of retinoblastoma. Arch Ophthalmol 1983;101:1519.

57. Merriam GR. Retinoblastoma: Analysis of 17 autopsies. Arch Ophthalmol 1950;44:71.

58. Molnar ML, Stefansson K, Marton LS, et al. Immunohistochemistry of retinoblastoma in humans. Am J Ophthalmol 1984;97:301.

59. Moore KL: The Developing Human—Clinically Oriented Embryology, 5th ed. Philadelphia: WB Saunders, 1993.

60. Murphree AL, Benedict WF. Retinoblastoma: Clues to human oncogenesis. Science 1984;223:1028.

61. Murphree AL, Munier FL. Retinoblastoma. *In* Ryan S (ed): Retina, 2nd ed, Vol 1, p 571. St Louis: CV Mosby, 1994.

62. Nicholson DH, Green WR: Ocular tumors in children. *In* Nelson LB, Kalhoun JH, Harley RD (eds): Pediatric Ophthalmology, 3rd ed, p 382. Philadelphia: WB Saunders, 1991.

63. Parkes SE, Muir KR, Southern L, et al. Neonatal tumours: A thirty-year population based study. Med Pediatr Oncol 1994;22:309.

64. Pendergrass TW, Davis S. Incidence of retinoblastoma in the United States. Arch Ophthalmol 1980;98:1204.

65. Pesin SR, Shields JA. Seven cases of trilateral retinoblastoma. Am J Ophthalmol 1989;107:121.

66. Popoff N, Ellsworth RM. The fine structure of nuclear alterations in retinoblastoma and in human developing retina: In vivo and in vitro observations. J Ultrastruc Res 1969;29:535.

67. Popoff NA, Ellsworth RM. The fine structure of retinoblastoma. In vivo and in vitro observations. Lab Invest 1971;25:389.

68. Redler LD, Ellsworth RM. Prognostic importance of choroidal invasion in retinoblastoma. Arch Ophthalmol 1973;90:294.

69. Riccardi VM, Hittner HM, Francke U, et al. Partial triplication and deletion of 13q: Study of a family presenting with bilateral retinoblastomas. Clin Genet 1979;15: 332.

70. Rootman J, Carruthers JDA, Miller RR. Retinoblastoma. Perspect Pediatr Pathol 1987;10:208.

71. Rootman J, Damji KF, Dimmick JE. Malignant rhabdoid tumor of the orbit. Ophthalmology 1989;96:1650.

72. Rubie H, Baunin C, Guitard J, et al. Tumeurs neonatales malignes. Rev Prat (Paris) 1993;43(17):2208.

73. Sanders TE. Intraocular juvenile xantho-granuloma (nevoxantho-endothelioma): A survey of twenty cases. Am J Ophthalmol 1962;53:455.

74. Sang DN, Albert DM. Retinoblastoma: Clinical and histopathologic features. Hum Pathol 1982;13:133.

75. Shields JA, Shields CL. Current management of retinoblastoma. Mayo Clin Proc 1994;69:50.

76. Shuangshoti S, Chaiwun B, Kasantikul V. A study of 39 retinoblastomas with particular reference to morphology, cellular differentiation and tumor origin. Histopathology 1989;15:113.

76a. Spencer WH: Ophthalmic Pathology: An Atlas and Textbook, 3rd ed, Vol 3, p 1382. Philadelphia: WB Saunders, 1986.

77. Ts'o, M, Zimmerman LE, Fine BS. The nature of retinoblastoma. I. Photoreceptor differentiation: A clinical and histopathologic study; II. Photoreceptor differentiation: An electron microscopic study. Am J Ophthalmol 1970;69:339.

78. Ulbright TM, Fulling KH, Helveston EM. Astrocytic tumors of the retina: Differentiation of sporadic tumors from phakomatosis-associated tumors. Arch Pathol Lab Med 1984;108:160.

79. Walford N, Deferrai R, Slater RM. Intraorbital rhabdoid tumour following bilateral retinoblastoma. Histopathology 1992;20:170.

80. Wilson DJ, Green WR. Miscellaneous uveal tumors. *In* Ryan S (ed): Retina, 2nd ed, Vol 1, p 864. St Louis: CV Mosby, 1994.

81. Wilson MG, Melnyk J, Towner JW. Retinoblastoma and deletion D (14) syndrome. J Med Genet 1969;6:322.

82. Young JL, Heiss HW, Silverberg E, et al. Cancer incidence, survival and mortality for children under 15 years of age. Am Cancer Soc 1978.

83. Zimmerman LE. Trilateral retinoblastoma. *In* Blodi FC (ed): Retinoblastoma, p 185. New York: Churchill Livingstone, 1985.

RENAL TUMORS

11

Although tumors of the kidney are uncommon in the fetus and neonate, non-neoplastic conditions are far more prevalent, with hydronephrosis and renal cystic disease accounting for more than 40% of all abdominal masses in this age group (Figs. 11–1 through 11–4).[91,94,96,112] Approximately 5% of perinatal tumors arise from the kidney (see Table 1–1).[7,20,94,125] Mesoblastic nephroma is the most common renal neoplasm, followed in order of frequency by Wilms' tumor, rhabdoid tumor, and clear cell sarcoma (see Tables 11–4 through 11–6).[27,34,43,49,51,55,87,125,130,187] The typical clinical presentation is an abdominal mass, but sometimes renal tumors can present with hematuria or manifestations of metastases (e.g., hydrocephalus secondary to brain involvement[29,126] and neck masses secondary to metastasis to the cervical lymph nodes.[92] Moreover, mesoblastic nephroma and rhabdoid tumors have been detected in utero by sonography,[1,35,42,64,69] and the former has been described in stillborn infants.[4,77,125,196]

Other unique clinical findings are noted in the perinatal period. There is a high incidence of polyhydramnios when the diagnosis is congenital mesoblastic nephroma. Moreover, hypercalcemia occurs with congenital mesoblastic nephroma and rhabdoid tumor of the kidney.[14,98,162,163,190]

The association of renal tumors and separate, concomitant, primary brain tumors has been reported, as mentioned previously. Bonnin and his colleagues[29] described seven patients—six with rhabdoid tumors and 1 with Wilms' tumor—who developed brain tumors, four of which were primitive neuroectodermal tumors[29] (see Table 11–6 and Chapter 9, ''Brain Tumors'').

The author's proposed classification for newborn renal tumors is presented in Table 11–1. A list of distinguishing gross and microscopic features is included in Table 11–2.

EMBRYOLOGY

Before continuing a discussion of renal tumors, it is appropriate at this time to discuss briefly the embryologic development of the kidney, as this has some bearing on the understanding of the histogenesis and histology of these neoplasms.

In the 5-week embryo, the genitourinary system develops from a longitudinal mass of mesoderm situated on each side of the aorta, called the nephrogenic cord.[137] The kidneys and ureters are derived from two structures in the caudal end of the nephrogenic cord called the metanephric blastema and ureteric bud. The metanephric blastema forms the nephrons and interstitium of the kidney, whereas the ureteric bud forms the ureter, pelvis, calyces, and collecting tubules (Fig. 11–5).[137]

Because Wilms' tumors are believed to arise from the metanephric blastema,[26,202] it would seem likely that they would display a wide variety of histologic appearances. Indeed, they vary considerably in morphology, ranging from diffusely cellular, undifferentiated-appearing blastemal proliferations, to heterogeneous neoplasms consisting of differentiating nephrons and heterotopic tissues, such as skeletal muscle and cartilage.[202] Moreover, the congenital mesoblastic nephroma, composed of fibroblastic and myofibroblastic elements, probably arises from interstitial mesenchyme derived from the metanephric blastema.[26]

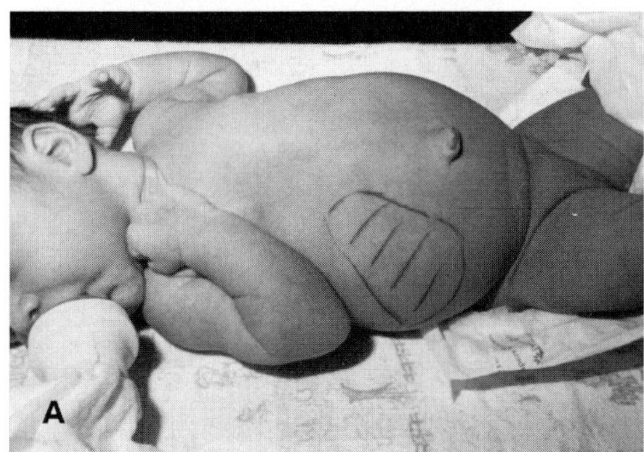

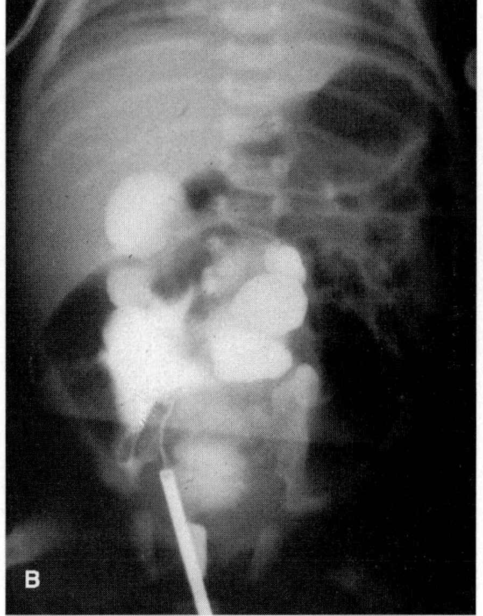

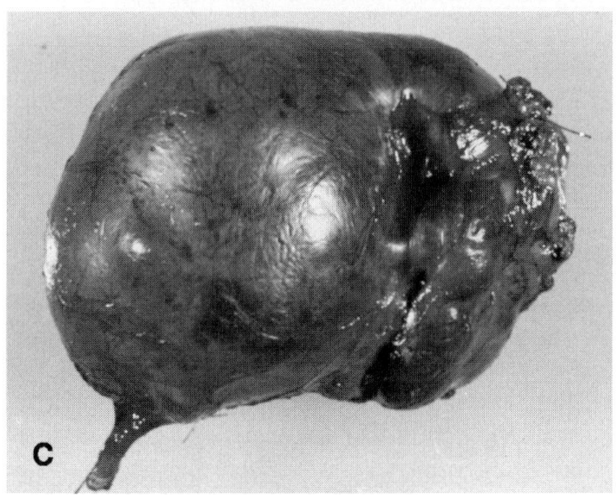

Figure 11–1. Hydronephrosis presenting as an abdominal mass. *A,* A 1-week-old female infant presented with an abdominal mass. *B,* A retrograde pyelogram revealed a dilated renal pelvis outlined by injected contrast medium. *C,* The dilated pelvis and stub of ureter are situated on the left side of the kidney. A ureteropelvic junction obstruction (stenosis) was demonstrated, and was presumably the cause of the hydronephrosis. (From Isaacs H Jr. Tumors of the Newborn and Infant. St. Louis: Mosby–Year Book, 1991.)

More than 20 years ago, Potter proposed that Wilms' tumor resulted from interference with the normal maturation of metanephric blastema.[152] According to her, primitive nephrogenic tissue normally differentiates into the metanephric blastema, which forms nephrons and interstitial connective tissue stroma. Abnormal proliferation of the metanephric blastema may result in either epithelial and/or stromal tumors, which are found almost exclusively in young infants.[152]

CONGENITAL MESOBLASTIC NEPHROMA

Congenital mesoblastic nephroma (CMN) (fetal renal hamartoma) is a benign mesenchymal tumor of the kidney composed of spindle-shaped cells.[27,200] It is the leading renal tumor of the fetus and the newborn, and is surpassed in frequency only by Wilms' tumor during the first year of life overall.* In 1967, CMN was clearly distinguished from Wilms' tumor by Bolande and co-workers[27] and by Wigger,[200] who emphasized the importance of its benign clinical behavior. A decade later, Bolande reviewed 48 cases of CMN, including 8 of his own cases, confirming its benign behavior and suggesting that CMN arises from the metanephric blastema and thus is histogenetically related to Wilms' tumor.[26] Moreover, he pointed out that CMN-like areas are noted in Wilms' tumors,

---

*References: 20, 21, 24–27, 37, 49, 51, 55, 66, 75, 87, 93, 94, 117, 145, 159, 166, 172, 192, 196, 200, 204.

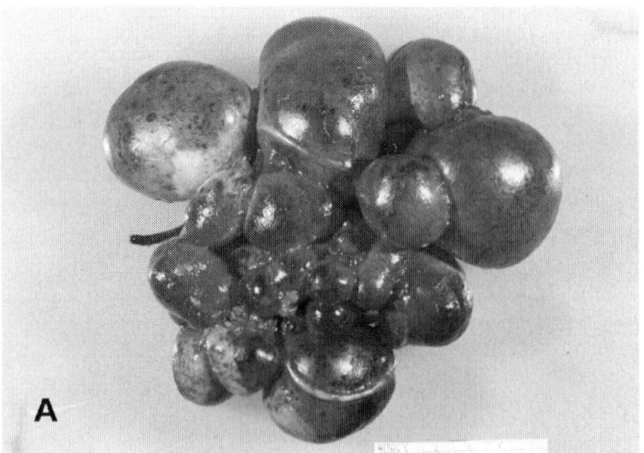 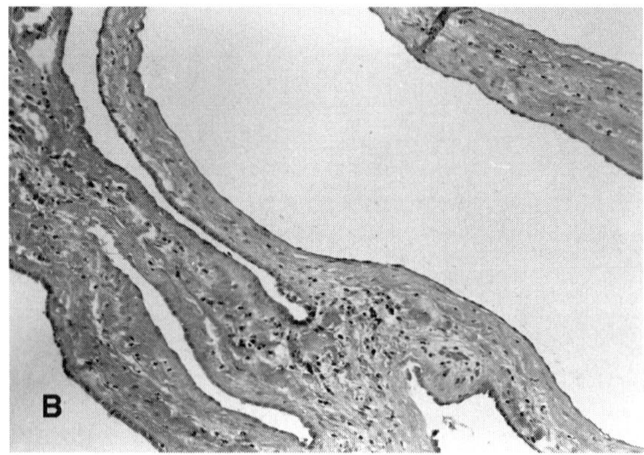

Figure 11–2. Multicystic kidney. The patient was an infant with an abdominal mass. *A,* The entire left kidney has been replaced by multiple cysts of various sizes that are filled with clear, straw-colored fluid that resemble a bunch of grapes. The specimen weighed 368 g and measured 13 × 9 × 5 cm. An atretic ureter is attached to the cystic kidney on the left. *B,* The cysts are lined by cuboidal and flattened epithelial cells. In one section, a small area of recognizable renal parenchyma was found on microscopic examination (not shown here) (hematoxylin-eosin, ×120). Compare this photograph with Figure 11–16*B* and note the close resemblance between the two. Potter and Craig believe that the two conditions are related[152] (see earlier discussion). (From Isaacs H Jr. Tumors of the Newborn and Infant. St. Louis: Mosby–Year Book, 1991.)

and that nephroblastoma-like foci are present in CMNs. Occasionally, CMN is observed in patients with hemihypertrophy and the Beckwith-Wiedemann syndrome, further supporting a histogenetic relationship to Wilms' tumor.[203]

One of the largest reviews of CMN prior to 1982 was by Yazaki et al.,[204] who analyzed 78 and 12 cases of CMN in the English and Japanese literature, respectively. Their review emphasized the benign behavior of CMN and the necessity for accurate diagnosis to prevent overtreatment.

Typically, patients with CMN present with an abdominal mass, which may be discovered on antenatal sonography or by physical examination of the neonate (Fig. 11–6).[9,20,26,27] The clinical findings that should alert the physician to the possibility of this diagnosis are a maternal history of hydramnios, prematurity in the infant, and a renal mass. Hematuria may be the initial manifestation.[89] Fetal hydrops, hypercalcemia, hypertension, increased renin production, congestive heart failure secondary to arteriovenous shunting, and stillbirth have also been described in association with this tumor.[21,26,35,77,89,104,108,117,127,143,186,196,205]

Of particular note is the high incidence of polyhydramnios in mothers of fetuses with CMN and of prematurity in the newborn.[21,26,55,117,143,204] Polyhydramnios, the accumulation of more than 2 L of amniotic fluid, occurs in approximately 1 in 1000 pregnancies, and in 71% of pregnancies associated with

CMN.[21] CMN is the most common renal tumor associated with excessive urine production in the perinatal period.[143] Of the neonates with CMN who were reviewed by Yazaki et al., more than two thirds for whom birth weight was recorded weighed less than 3000 g.[204]

Hypercalcemia is attributed to the secretion of parathormone or prostaglandins.[98,162,163,190] Elevated calcium levels have no prognostic significance per se, but they can be used as a tumor marker in some patients.[98] The 2-month-old female infant with CMN reported by Vido and colleagues had elevated levels of both blood calcium and urinary prostaglandins.[190] These values returned to normal after the tumor was removed. Prostaglandin production by the tumor was considered to be the cause of the hypercalcemia.

Tsuchida et al. reviewed five patients with CMN, elevated renin production, and hypertension, including one of their own.[186] Their patient was a 39-day-old male infant with a left flank mass and hypertension. Both the plasma renin activity and plasma renin concentration were elevated prior to surgery, but returned to normal values after the tumor was removed. Renin immunoperoxidase reactivity was found in the juxtaglomerular apparatus adjacent to glomeruli entrapped by tumor, but not in the CMN per se. Compared to the reported cases of Wilms' tumor, renin production in CMN is considerably higher.[186]

CMN can be detected by antenatal sonogra-

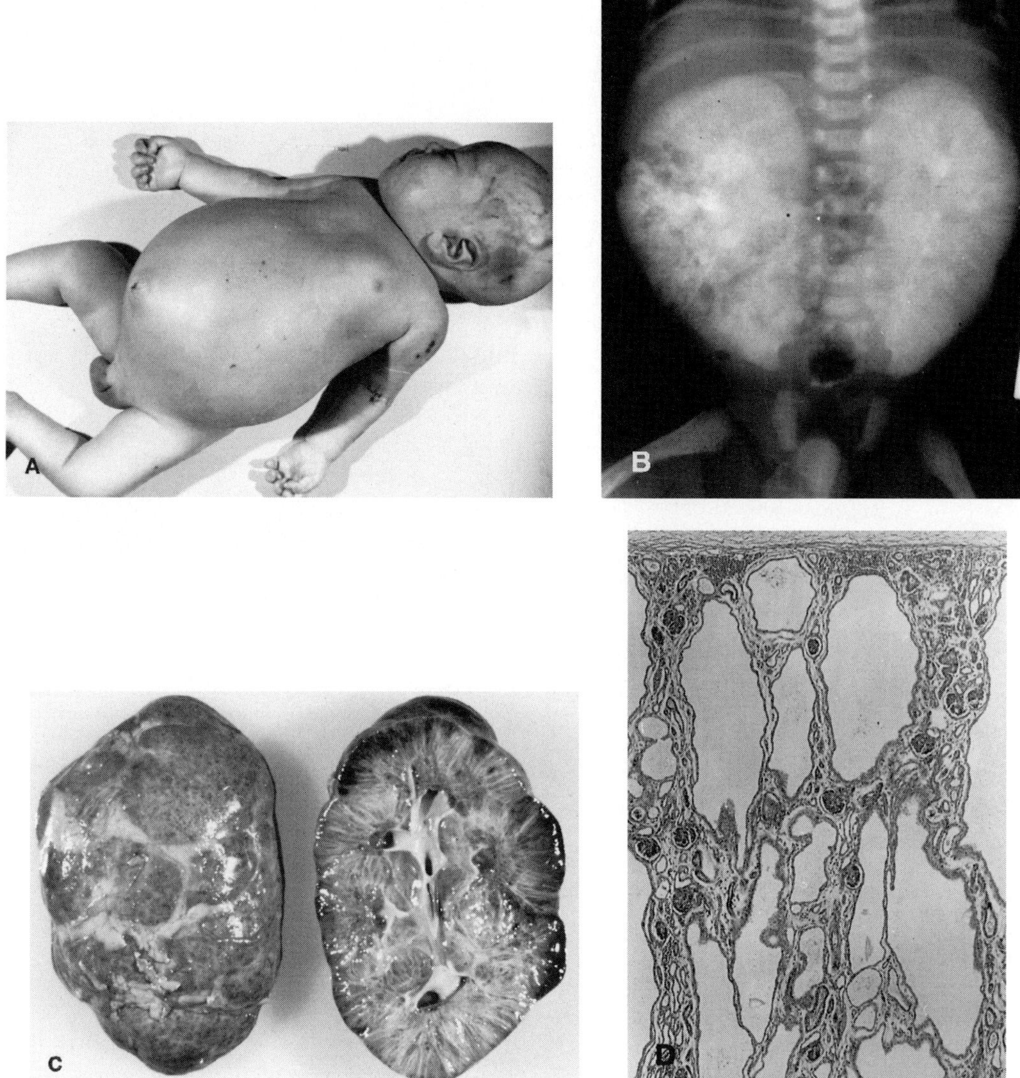

Figure 11–3. Infantile polycystic disease of the kidney and liver (autosomal recessive). *A,* A 3-month-old male infant with bilateral flank masses noted at birth subsequently died of renal failure and *Escherichia coli* sepsis. The abdomen is distended by markedly enlarged kidneys and liver. *B,* An intravenous pyelogram reveals bilateral renomegaly and cystically dilated tubules filled with dye. *C,* Radially arranged, fusiform cysts are situated in the cortex and medulla. The blackened cortical areas represent foci of acute pyelonephritis due to *E. coli. D,* Cystically dilated collecting ducts are evident (hematoxylin-eosin, ×48).

phy; practically all of the affected fetuses were in the third trimester.[1,35,64,69,127,134,143,185,199] Moreover, CMN is the renal tumor most often found on antenatal imaging studies. As mentioned earlier, polyhydramnios and preterm labor occur with increased frequency in mothers whose infants have CMN. Mothers of affected fetuses are initially examined because of either a discrepancy between uterine size and gestational dates or polyhydramnios.[21,64,134,143] The tumor

can be diagnosed prenatally with sonography because of its characteristic sonographic appearance, which is different from that of Wilms' tumor.[5,37,64] The sonographic findings consist of a large, unilateral, renal lesion, measuring 4 to 8 cm, with nodular densities or diffuse renal enlargement (Fig. 11–7A).[64] The CMN is predominantly solid, but sometimes cystic areas are present, particularly in the cellular variants.[41,171] No well-defined capsule is

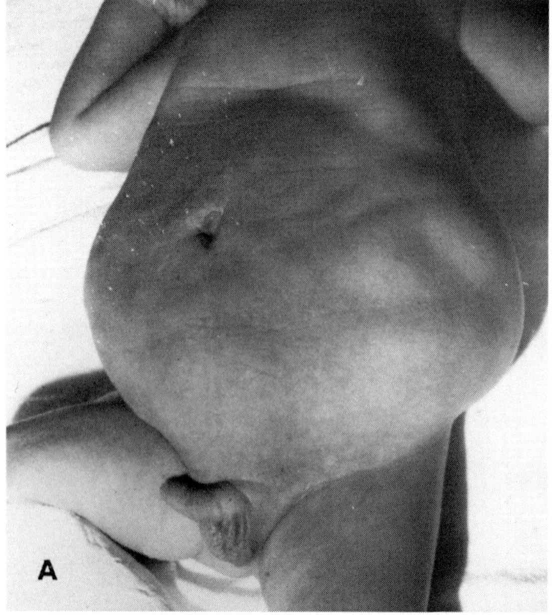

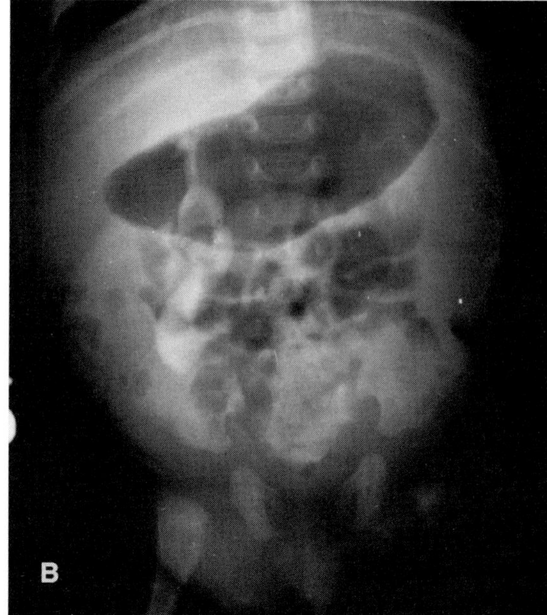

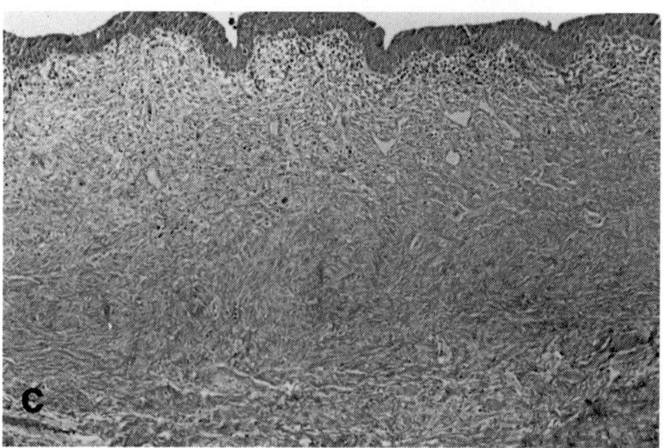

Figure 11–4. Prune belly syndrome (megacystis, megaureter, and absence of abdominal musculature). *A,* An infant presented with a distended, scaphoid, "doughy" abdomen and bilateral undescended testes. *B,* An intravenous pyelogram depicts a markedly dilated ureter and enlarged urinary bladder. (Courtesy of Melvin O. Senac, Jr., MD, Department of Radiology, Children's Hospital, San Diego, CA.) *C,* A portion of megaureter from a 1-year-old boy with prune belly syndrome shows intramural fibrosis and markedly decreased smooth muscle. Skeletal muscle was not found in a full-thickness biopsy specimen from the abdominal wall (hematoxylin-eosin, ×48).

noted, which is in direct contrast to Wilms' tumor. Chan et al. describe a characteristic sonographic finding, not seen in Wilms' tumor, consisting of a concentric, echogenic, and echopoor ring pattern—the so-called "ring sign."[37]

Occasionally, CMNs are responsible for stillbirth. Werb et al. described two such cases, one with hydrocephalus, Arnold-Chiari malformation, and a thoracolumbar meningomyelocele.[196] The second stillborn infant was delivered because of rapid-onset polyhydramnios; a renal tumor measuring 8 × 6 cm was found at necropsy. The association between CMN and nonimmunologic hydrops fetalis, in addition to polyhydramnios, was noted by Gray.[77] According to this author, massive hemorrhage into the tumor and retroperitoneum, producing circulatory problems and anemia, were contributing factors. Angulo et al. reported an additional example of hydrops fetalis and CMN in a stillborn.[4] The abdominal mass in the fetus may be so large as to produce dystocia or rupture.[26,134]

Generally, the diagnosis of CMN is suggested by its distinctive gross appearance, which is different from that of Wilms' tumor, clear cell sarcoma, rhabdoid tumor, and multilocular cyst. CMN occupies half or more of the involved kidney, and cut sections reveal an unencapsulated, bulging mass having a whorled pattern similar to that of a uterine leiomyoma (see Fig. 11–6*B* and 11–7*C*).[11,26,27,94,96,159] Unlike the renal neoplasms described later in this chapter, CMN characteristically has finger-like projections which extend into the adjacent renal parenchyma. The perinatal tumors vary considerably in size and weight, ranging from 5 to 14 cm and 38 to 550 g.[26,169]

Table 11–1. Classification of Fetal and Newborn Renal Tumors

Congenital mesoblastic nephroma
   Classic mesoblastic nephroma
   Cellular mesoblastic nephroma
Wilms' tumor
   Classic triphasic
   Blastemal
   Epithelial (monomorphous)
   Fetal rhabdomyomatous
   Wilms' tumor with anaplasia*
Nephroblastomatosis complex
Cystic renal tumors
   Cystic nephroma (multilocular cyst)*
   Cystic partially differentiated nephroblastoma
   Cystic Wilms' tumor
Rhabdoid tumor of kidney
Clear cell sarcoma of kidney
Ossifying renal tumor of infancy
Renal cell carcinoma*
Clear cell "tumor"

*Usually does not occur in newborns.
Modified from Isaacs H Jr. Tumors of the Newborn and Infant. St. Louis: Mosby–Year Book, 1991.

Although unusual, extension of CMN into the renal vein, vena cava, or extrarenal soft tissues, and cystic variants does occur.[14,21,107,149,207] Two newborns with CMNs presented with gross hematuria and a flank mass, and had hemorrhagic cysts within their tumors.[41] Rare cases of bilateral CMN have been documented.[26] There have also been single case reports of CMNs occurring in solitary and in horseshoe kidneys.[9,140]

Microscopically, CMN displays a proliferation of uniform, spindle-shaped cells, demonstrated by electron microscopy to be myofibroblasts and fibroblasts.[169] These infiltrate the renal parenchyma, appearing to push aside the glomeruli and tubules rather than to invade them (see Fig. 11–7D and E).[26,55,149,169] Mitotic figures and small islands of cartilage are noted in some instances. Vimentin and actin staining both yield positive results, but the lesion is unreactive to desmin or the desmin is sometimes focally expressed.[35,149] Ultrastructural, immunohistochemical, and karyotypic findings suggest that CMN shares certain histologic and cytogenetic features with infantile fibromatosis and other myofibroblastic tumors of childhood (see Chapters 4, "Soft Tissue Tumors," and Chapter 16, "Cardiac Tumors").[149]

Pettinato et al.[149] and Barrantes et al.[9] performed flow cytometric studies on CMNs with classical, cellular, and mixed histology. They found that the classical form generally has a diploid DNA content whereas the cellular and mixed tumors have either diploid or aneuploid DNA ploidy. Both groups of investigators inferred that flow cytometry is not particularly helpful in selecting patients who need further treatment or in predicting outcome.

Molecular studies were performed on two classical CMNs by Tomlinson et al.[185] and on a classical CMN and a cellular CMN metastasis by Afshan et al.[1] Northern and Southern blot analyses revealed a high level of expression of insulin-like growth factor (IGF-2) in both CMN and Wilms' tumor, but no reactivity of N-myc oncogene or Wilms' tumor supressor gene (WT1) in the CMN.[1,185] Moreover, loss of heterozygosity of 3p, 11p13, or 11p15 was not demonstrated in the CMN, in contrast to the Wilms' tumor samples. Subsequently, karyotypic analysis of CMN detected antenatally by Carpenter et al. showed certain features in common with leiomyoma.[35] They found a trisomy 11 and breakpoints in the q13–15 region of chromosome 12, which are observed also in leiomyomas. A subsequent report by this group showed that trisomy 11 is associated with the cellular histologic variant of CMN (Fig. 11–8F).[133] The authors noted that trisomy 11 is found also in congenital fibrosarcoma, which, on microscopic examination, resembles cellular CMN.

Cellular Mesoblastic Nephroma

Cellular mesoblastic nephroma is a variant of CMN distinguished from the latter by the presence of increased cellularity, nuclear atypia, and numerous mitotic figures.[10,11,18,37,58,103,104,107,193,207] The series of Chan et al., consisting of 17 patients, showed that cellular CMN is noted after 1 month of age and as late as 18 months of age, as compared to classical (typical) CMN, which is usually detected in patients younger than 1 week of age.[37]

The gross appearance of cellular CMN differs from the classical CMN in that it has a softer, more cystic, and sometimes hemorrhagic-appearing cut surface (Fig. 11–8B).[37] The cellular tumor also appears to be more circumscribed, without the interdigitating periphery seen in classical CMN. Gigantic cystic cellular CMNs weighing as much as 1300 g have been described in older infants.[107]

It is conceivable that, in the past, some examples of the cellular variant were called fibrosarcoma or sarcoma of the kidney because of their ominous microscopic appearance, which is characterized by the presence of increased mi-

Table 11–2. Renal Tumors and Tumor-Like Conditions of the Fetus and Newborn:
Distinguishing Features

Tumor	Gross Findings	Histopathologic Findings
Mesoblastic Nephroma		
Classic	Nonencapsulated, noncircumscribed, light tan, with finger-like projections, resembles leiomyoma	Monomorphous, uniform, spindle-shaped cells surrounding normal parenchymal elements; rare mitoses Vim +, Act + EM: spindle cells with features of fibroblasts and myofibroblasts
Cellular	Encapsulated, pale gray, circumscribed, cystic, gelatinous	Monomorphous, spindle-shaped cells; hypercellular; mitoses; slight nuclear atypia Vim +, Act ± EM: primitive, spindle-shaped cells with features of fibroblasts and myofibroblasts
Wilms' Tumor	Encapsulated, well circumscribed, light tan-gray, soft, cystic, necrotic, hemorrhagic	*Epithelial:* primitive tubules and glomeruli; scant stroma *Blastemal:* small, round to oval cells; many mitoses *Triphasic:* epithelial, blastemal, mesenchymal elements (e.g., skeletal muscle, fibroblasts) *Fetal rhabdomyomatous:* triphasic histology with 40% skeletal muscle **Anaplasia:* bizarre, mulberry-like giant cells; huge mitoses
Nephroblastomatosis Complex		
Nephrogenic Rests		
Perilobar (PLNR)†‡	Small, tan-gray nodules present beneath the capsule; may be visible depending on their size	Nodules of small, dark, embryonic-appearing tubules and glomeruli resembling the nephrogenic zone of the developing kidney
Intralobar (ILNR)	Small, tan-gray nodules present in the cortex or medulla; may be visible depending on their size	Nodules of small, dark, embryonic-appearing tubules and glomeruli resembling the developing kidney
Nephroblastomatosis		
Perilobar (PLNR)	Tan-gray nodules present beneath the capsule; kidney may be diffusely enlarged with irregular, nodular, capsular surfaces	Nodules of small, dark, embryonic-appearing tubules and glomeruli resembling the nephrogenic zone of the developing kidney
Intralobar (ILNR)	Tan-gray nodules present in the cortex or medulla; kidney may be diffusely enlarged	Nodules of small, dark, embryonic-appearing tubules and glomeruli resembling the developing kidney
Combined (PLNR + ILNR)	Tan-gray confluent nodules present beneath the capsule and in the cortex and medulla; kidneys diffusely enlarged	Nodules of small, dark, embryonic-appearing tubules, glomeruli, and blastema resembling the developing kidney
Universal (PANLOBAR)	Hyperlobulated, cerebriform appearance; no recognizable cortex or medulla; kidney diffusely enlarged	Diffuse, hyperplastic-appearing tubules, glomeruli, and blastema occupying the cortex and medulla; tubulointerstitial dysplasia
Multilocular Cyst of Kidney (Cystic Nephroma)	Multilocular cysts with thin fibrous septa containing clear fluid; does not communicate with renal pelvis	Regular, low, cuboidal, epithelium-lined cysts; no metanephric elements in cyst walls; no atypia; no mitoses
Cystic, Partially Differentiated Nephroblastoma	Multilocular cysts with thin fibrous septa containing clear fluid; does not communicate with renal pelvis	Regular, low, cuboidal, epithelium-lined cysts; immature or mature metanephric elements and skeletal muscle in cyst walls

Table 11–2. Renal Tumors and Tumor-Like Conditions of the Fetus and Newborn:
Distinguishing Features *Continued*

Tumor	Gross Findings	Histopathologic Findings
Cystic Wilms' Tumor	Multilocular cyst with a nodule of Wilms' tumor, the latter containing a multilocular cyst	Regular, low, cuboidal, or atypical epithelium-lined cysts; Wilms' tumor histopathology (as described earlier)
Rhabdoid Tumor of Kidney	Encapsulated, tan-gray, well-circumscribed, large areas of cystic necrosis, hemorrhage	Monomorphous population of polygonal cells with abundant eosinophilic cytoplasm; vesicular nucleus with single big nucleolus EM: globular cytoplasmic body consisting of intermediate filaments Vim +, Cytok +, Des −, Act −
Clear Cell Sarcoma of Kidney	Encapsulated, well circumscribed, hemorrhagic and cystic	Monomorphous population of round to oval cells with watery, clear cytoplasm; vesicular nucleus, fine chromatin, and tiny nucleolus; few mitoses; rows of cells separated by delicate fibrous septa; pallisading and vascular patterns Vim +, NSE −, Cytok −, Desm −, Act − EM: primitive small cells with sparse organelles and fluffy intracellular and extracellular deposits
Ossifying Renal Tumor of Infancy	Calcified mass projecting into dilated calyx	Osteoid trabeculae surrounded by osteoblasts and spindle-shaped cells related to nephrogenic rests

*"Unfavorable histology" associated with a poor prognosis; anaplasia has not been described in the newborn.
†Found in association with bilateral Wilms' tumor and congenital anomalies.
‡According to the Beckwith classification, "this condition also includes entities such as metanephric hamartoma and tubular adenoma."
Vim = vimentin; Act = actin; Cytok = cytokeratin; Des = desmin; NSE = neuron-specific enolase; EM = electron microscopy.
Modified from Isaacs H Jr. Congenital malignant tumors. *In* Reed GB, Claireaux AE, Bain AD (eds): Diseases of the Fetus and Newborn: Pathology, Radiology and Genetics, p 131. London: Chapman Hall, 1989. Used by permission; and from Isaacs H Jr. Tumors of the Newborn and Infant. St. Louis: Mosby–Year Book, 1991.

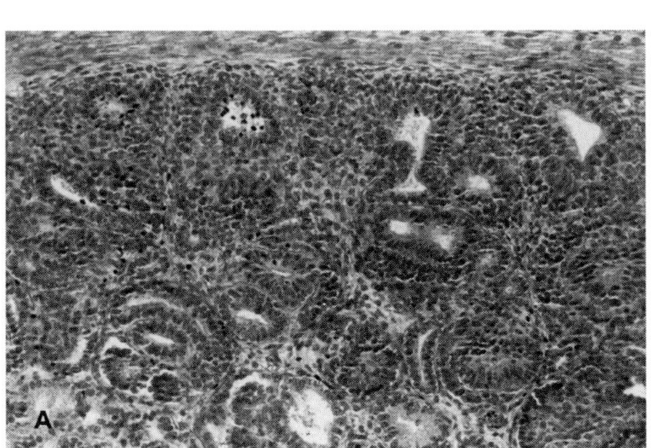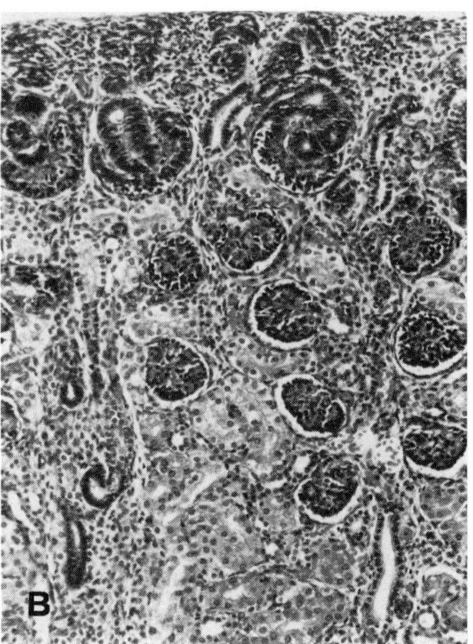

Figure 11–5. Development of the kidney. *A,* Glomeruli and tubules are beginning to form in the cellular metanephric blastema of the nephrogenic zone (hematoxylin-eosin, ×60). (This specimen was taken from an embryo of estimated 10 to 12 weeks' gestation.) *B,* At the top of the photograph, there is a row of immature glomeruli and tubules arising from the metanephric blastema. Three or four layers of definitive glomeruli are evident beneath. Nephrogenic zone in a 650-g fetus (hematoxylin-eosin, ×200). (*B:* From Isaacs H Jr. Tumors of the Newborn and Infant. St. Louis: Mosby–Year Book, 1991.)

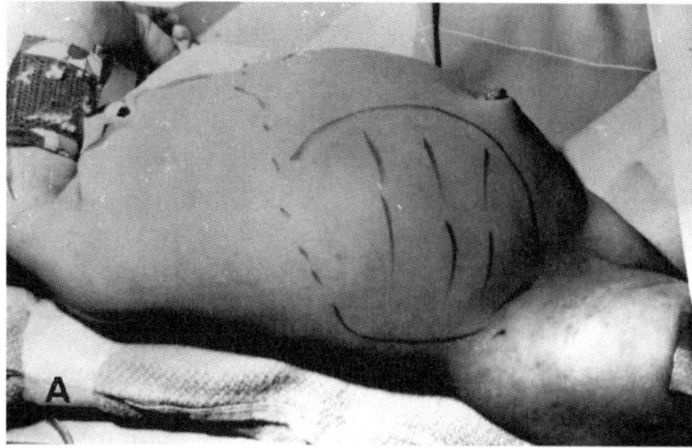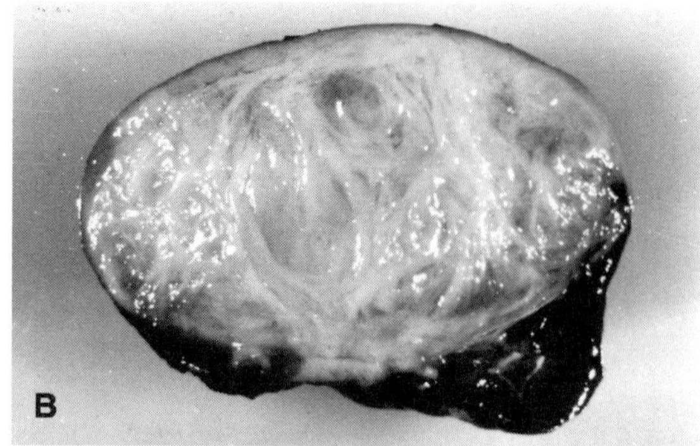

Figure 11–6. Congenital mesoblastic nephroma. *A,* A 1-week-old female infant with an abdominal mass (the most common finding) and a maternal history of polyhydramnios. *B,* The tumor, which weighed 94 g and measured 8 × 5 cm, is seen to have replaced the lower two thirds of the kidney. It has a light tan-yellow, whorled appearance. It is nonencapsulated, and small, finger-like projections extend into the adjacent hemorrhagic kidney. (From Isaacs H Jr. Neoplasms in infants: A report of 265 cases. Pathol Annu 1983;18(2):165. Used by permission.)

totic activity, hypercellularity, and nuclear atypia. Haas and colleagues suggest that CMN represents a spectrum of lesions ranging from classical CMN at the benign end, cellular CMN somewhere in the middle, and clear cell sarcoma of the kidney at the malignant end.[81] From their study of 16 cases of CMN, Pettinato et al. concluded that the classic (conventional) and cellular (atypical) forms of CMN are histogenetically related, as there were three tumors with combined (mixed) histologic patterns, all of which occurred in infants younger than 4 months of age.[149] Moreover, as was described in the report of Haas and co-workers, Pettinato et al. also noted clear cell sarcoma–like areas in classical, cellular, and mixed CMNs. Nevertheless, they found no correlation between the histologic features and prognosis.[81,149]

Ultrastructural studies performed on conventional and cellular CMNs reveal that the spindle-shaped cells have both fibroblastic and myofibroblastic features (Fig. 11–8*E*).[58,149,169] The cells contain peripheral bundles of thin filaments with focal, dense body formations and prominent, rough-surfaced, endoplasmic reticulum profiles. Zonula adherens–type cell junctions, lipid droplets, pinocytotic vesicles, and interstitial collagen bundles are additional findings. However, the cellular CMNs are characterized by smaller cells, with a higher nuclear:cytoplasmic ratio and fewer organelles; thus, they have a more primitive or immature appearance than the classical form (see Fig. 11–8*E*). Shen and Yunis described the cellular tumor cells as "mesenchymal, fibroblast-like."[169] Tumor cells of both the classical and cellular CMNs are reactive with vimentin, but

only one third of the cellular CMNs express actin, according to Pettinato et al.[149]

The cellular variant is found in almost one third of infants with CMN who are younger than 3 months of age, a fact that apparently has no prognostic significance in this younger age group, *provided the lesion is completely removed.* However, in older children, the chances of recurrence or metastases, although small, are comparatively increased.[11,76] Pulmonary metastases were noted in two infants, ages 4 and 7 months, who recovered following irradiation and chemotherapy.[74,179] Brain metastasis was documented in an 8-month-old male infant who had a cellular CMN detected by antenatal sonography, who had undergone nephrectomy at birth, and who had an abdominal recurrence at the age of 3 months.[1]

It is important to recognize CMN because it can be cured by surgical resection alone, provided it is *completely* excised.[10,25–27,37,51,76,89,93,149,159,166,172,204] Occasionally, inappropriately aggressive therapy has been prescribed.[89] Recurrences and metastases have, however, been documented in 6.7% of the cases of CMN by the National Wilms' Tumor Study. In the series of Gormley et al., 7 of 38 patients with cellular CMN had recurrences and/or pulmonary metastases, and 3 of the 7 died; the other 31 patients survived.[76] The authors suggest that tumor at the surgical margins, not the histologic findings, appears to be the only statistically significant factor that predicts recurrence.[76] Another case, reported by Heidelberger et al., involved a male infant who had a renal mass detected on prenatal ultrasound and who underwent nephrectomy at 10 days of age.[84] Histo-

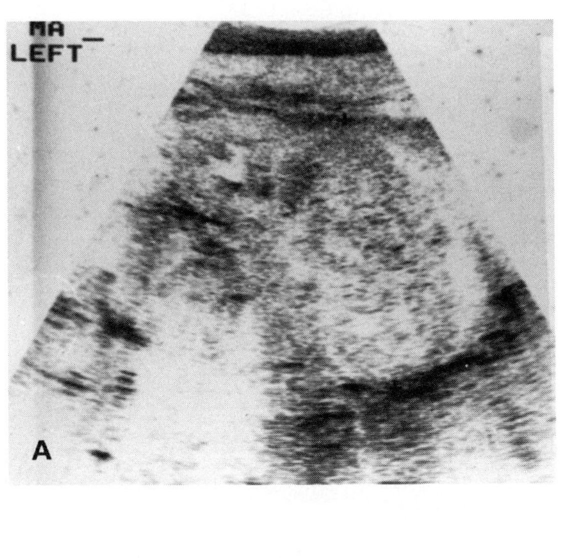

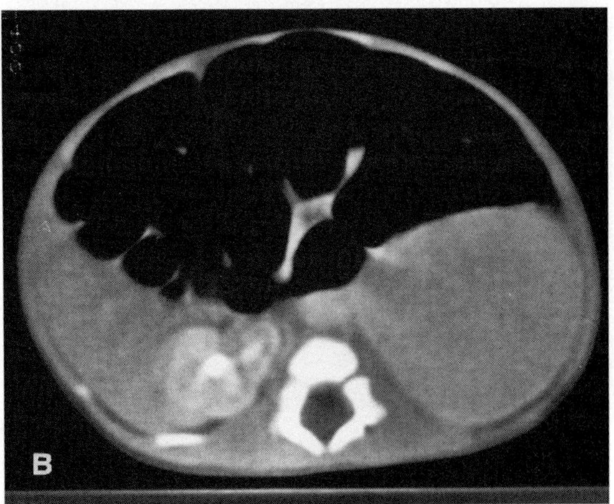

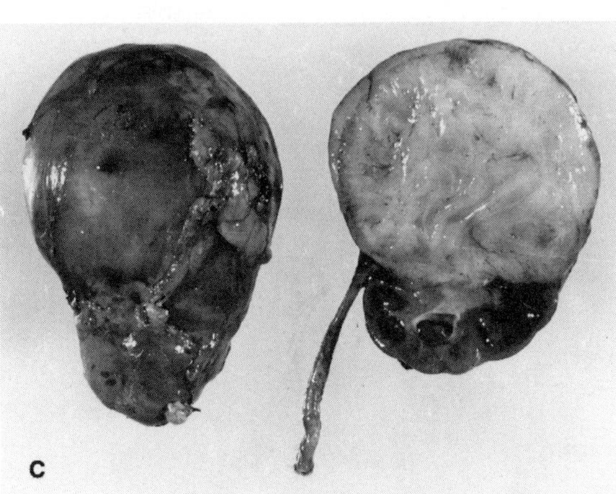

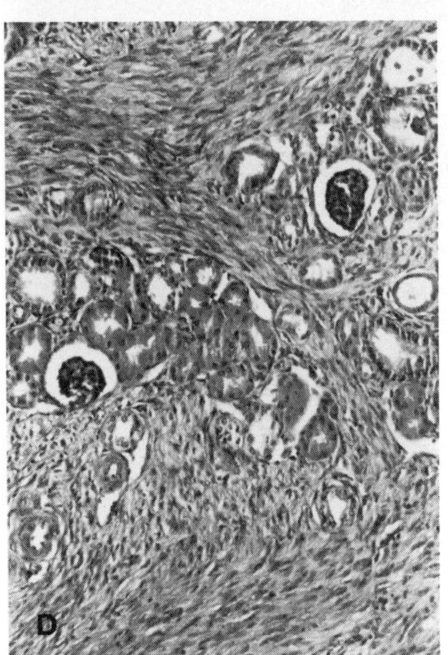

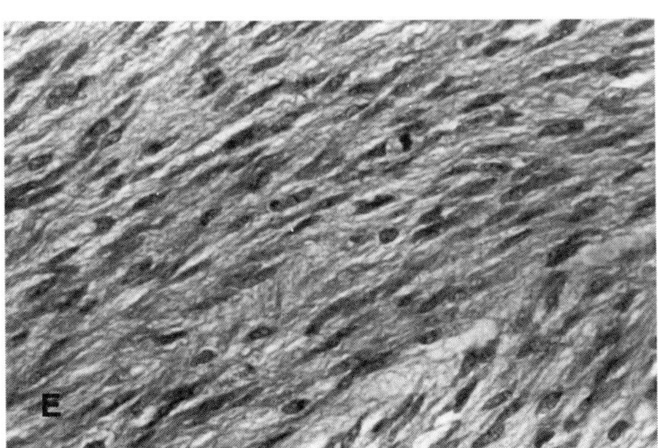

Figure 11–7. Congenital mesoblastic nephroma. *A,* A sonogram of a 5-day-old male infant demonstrates a left flank mass, which was noted at birth. *B,* A CT scan confirms the sonographic findings. *C,* The tumor, which weighed 50 g and measured 5 × 5 cm, has a whorled appearance not unlike that of a uterine leiomyoma and involves the pelvis and calyces. *D,* Regular, spindle-shaped cells are seen to encircle tubules and glomeruli (hematoxylin-eosin, ×300). *E,* The tumor cells are elongated and spindle-shaped, with regular oval to fusiform nuclei. Mitoses are seldom noted (hematoxylin-eosin, ×380). (From Isaacs H Jr. Tumors of the Newborn and Infant. St. Louis: Mosby–Year Book, 1991.)

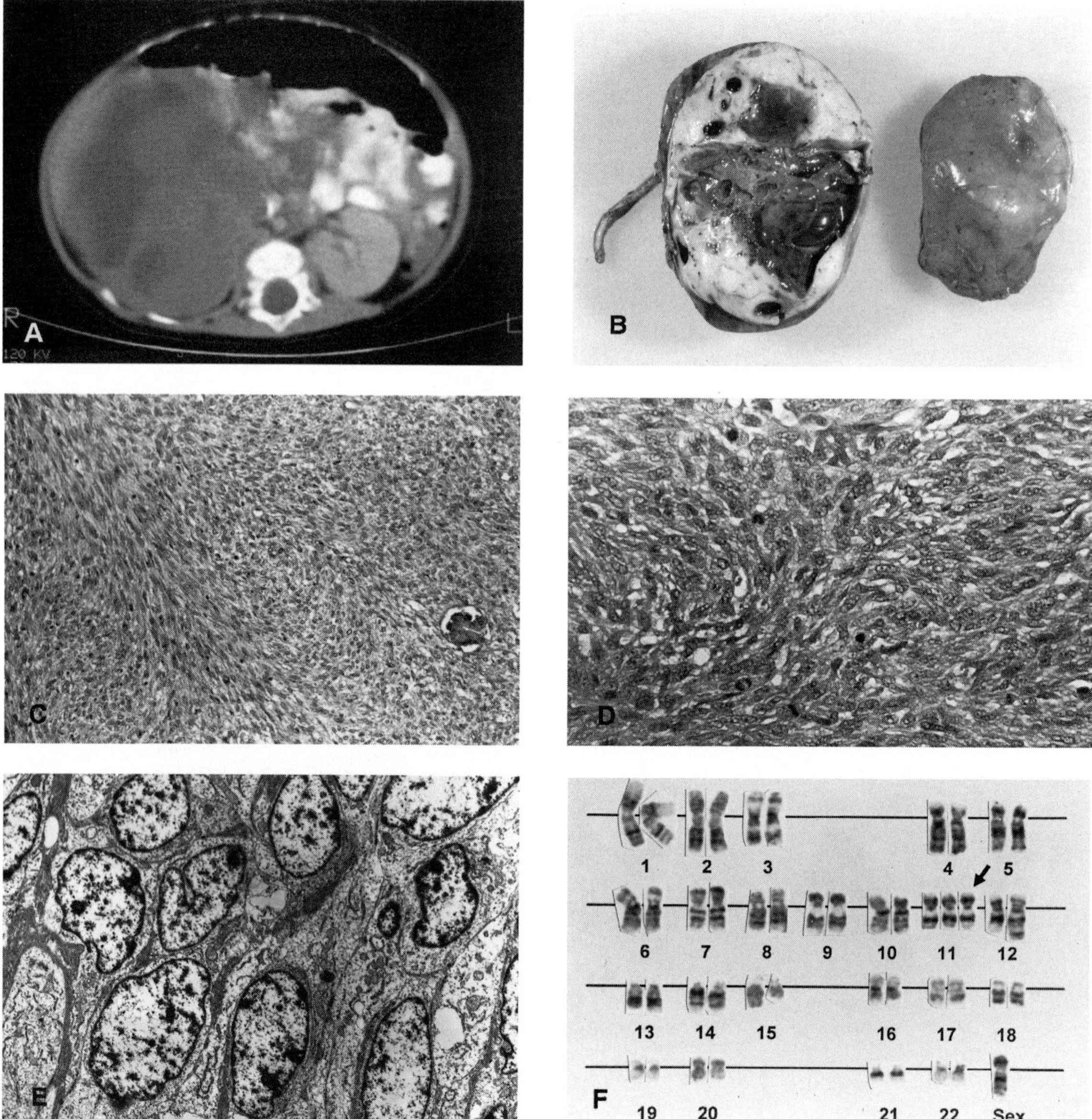

Figure 11–8. Cellular congenital mesoblastic nephroma. *A,* A CT scan of a 4-month-old female infant with an abdominal mass reveals a large right renal lesion composed of both solid and cystic elements. *B,* The right kidney weighed 254 g and measured 10 × 8 cm. Most of the kidney is seen to have been replaced by a soft, light tan-gray tumor with a prominent cystic component. In contrast to the congenital mesoblastic nephroma described in Figure 11–6*B,* this tumor is encapsulated, circumscribed, and cystic. *C,* Spindle-shaped cells with plump, oval or fusiform nuclei are separated by a slightly vacuolated fibrillary stroma. It displays an interdigitating (herringbone) growth pattern. *D,* The tumor is more cellular than the "classic" mesoblastic nephroma described in Figure 10–7*E* and *F,* and the mitotic activity is greater (hematoxylin-eosin, ×300). *E,* An electron photomicrograph reveals spindle cells with features consistent with fibroblasts. (Cytoplasmic fibrillar material is present ×8300.) (Courtesy of Ann Peters, Children's Hospital, San Diego, CA.) *F,* A karyotype reveals a trisomy 11, which has previously been described in association with this tumor.[133] (Courtesy of James Mascarello, PhD, Department of Genetics, Children's Hospital, San Diego, CA.) (*A–C:* From Isaacs H Jr. Tumors of the Newborn and Infant. St. Louis: Mosby–Year Book, 1991.)

Table 11–3. Wilms' Tumor Clinicopathologic Staging

Stage I	Tumor confined to the kidney and totally resected
Stage II	Tumor extending beyond the kidney (i.e., capsular invasion) but completely resected. Tumor thrombi in vessels outside the kidney. Presurgical biopsy and local tumor spillage are also included in this stage.
Stage III	Residual tumor confined to the abdomen. Positive intra-abdominal lymph nodes, whatever the site. Gross or microscopic lines of resection are positive. Gross tumor spillage and peritoneal implants. Tumor is unresectable because vital structures are involved.
Stage IV	Hematogenous metastases to distant organs
Stage V	Bilateral Wilms' tumors

From Green DM, D'Angio GJ, Beckwith JB, et al. Wilms' tumor (nephroblastoma, renal embryoma). *In* Pizzo PA, Poplack DG (eds): Principles and Practice of Pediatric Oncology, 2nd ed, p 713. Philadelphia: JB Lippincott, 1993. Used by permission.

logic examination revealed a CMN with both classical and focal cellular patterns. There was extension of the tumor into the perirenal fat. Seven months later, a fatal brain metastasis was discovered which had the morphologic characteristics of cellular CMN.

A more positive outlook was presented by The International Society of Pediatric Oncology (SIOP). Although the study group reported that 50% of the cellular CMNs had ruptured or infiltrated the renal pelvis or perirenal tissue at the time of surgery,[166] surprisingly, all but two patients (who died postoperatively) survived. In the series of Barrantes et al., 10 of 13 infants with CMN were younger than 3 months of age, and all but 2 lived.[9] One newborn died from surgical complications and the other from progressive local disease. Both had the classical pattern of CMN and were classified as having stage II disease (Table 11–3).[9] The National Wilms' Tumor Study reported by Howell et al. in 1982 showed an impressive survival rate of 98%; 49 of 50 patients with CMN survived after surgery, which was the sole treatment, and the one fatality was attributable to sepsis.[89] Even more impressive was the study by Chan et al., in which all 17 patients, 9 with typical CMN and 8 with cellular CMN, survived following nephrectomy as the main treatment.[37] Thus, nephrectomy is the treatment of choice, and adjuvant chemotherapy is recommended only if the lesion ruptures during surgery or if the surgical margins

contain tumor in an infant older than 3 months of age.[37,76] In patients with initially inoperable, advanced disease, biopsy is recommended to establish the diagnosis, followed by chemotherapy and nephrectomy.

WILMS' TUMOR

Less than 2% of all Wilms' tumors are diagnosed in the first 3 months of life.[7,11,90,160,164] Of a total of 6832 patients enrolled in the National Wilms' Tumor Study from 1969 to 1993, 11 (0.16%) were neonates.[160] Although Wilms' tumor is the major renal neoplasm of childhood, the classic form, characterized by triphasic histologic features, is not as common in the newborn as in older children.[20,43,96] The so-called infantile congeners of Wilms' tumor, a term coined by Bolande to describe renal lesions resembling Wilms' tumor in early infancy, occur more often.[25,60] This group includes CMN, nephroblastomatosis complex, and monomorphic epithelial Wilms' tumor (see Table 11–1).[12,20,26,27,43,55,90,125,187]

Of the 36 infant renal neoplasms in the Children's Hospital, Los Angeles study, 24 were classified as Wilms' tumor, none of which was diagnosed in a newborn.[96] The youngest in this series with the diagnosis of Wilms' tumor was 4 months old. The youngest with this diagnosis in the study by Ugarte and colleagues of 11 infants with renal tumors was 6 months of age.[187] By contrast, all four malignant renal tumors reported in The Hospital for Sick Children, Toronto neonatal study were diagnosed as Wilms' tumor.[34]

Wilms' tumors, particularly the well-differentiated ones, appear to recapitulate or imitate histologically the embryologic development of the kidney. For this reason, the synonym nephroblastoma and the class name embryoma were applied to this tumor by Willis more than 30 years ago.[202] Currently, however, the term nephroblastoma is not recommended, and should not be used in the same context as a Wilms' tumor, because it creates confusion with the nephroblastomatosis group of renal lesions (see Tables 11–1 and 11–2).

Congenital Malformations and Syndromes Associated with Wilms' Tumor

Wilms' tumor is found in association with certain congenital defects and malformation syndromes. In 1964, Miller and colleagues reported the excessive occurrence of Wilms' tumor with a variety of congenital defects, including aniridia, hemihypertrophy, and genitourinary anomalies.[136] Meadows and co-workers reported similar findings in a later study.[135] Of 3442 patients enrolled in the National Wilms' Tumor Study, 252 (7%) had congenital malformations consisting mainly of hemihypertrophy, hypospadias, and cryptorchidism.[78] The incidence of congenital anomalies was 13% (33/248) in the Institut Gustave-Roussy study.[119] Urogenital defects were the most common defects (7%), and hemihypertrophy, aniridia, and microcephaly each accounted for 2% of the cases. Spina bifida and other vertebral defects have also been known to occur.[105] Bilateral tumors, aniridia, and hypospadias are conditions associated with early presentation.[146] The combination of Wilms' tumor, hypospadias, and cryptorchidism has been reported in infant twins.[28] Newborns with any of these associated conditions should be screened carefully and monitored for Wilms' tumor.[47]

Other associations with Wilms' tumor have been described, including Beckwith-Wiedemann syndrome (omphalocele, macroglossia, visceromegaly, and gigantism); WAGR syndrome (Wilms' tumor, aniridia, mental retardation, and genitourinary abnormalities); 11p deletion syndrome; Denys-Drash syndrome (ambiguous genitalia, nephritis, and Wilms' tumor); Perlman syndrome (fetal gigantism, renal hamartomas, and nephroblastomatosis with Wilms' tumor); the VATER association (vertebral malformations, anal atresia, tracheoesophageal fistula, limb dysplasias, and renal anomalies); Prader-Willi syndrome (obesity, short stature, hypogonadism, mental retardation), and Bloom syndrome (growth failure, sun-sensitive facial telangiectasia, and defective immunity).[11,20,25,32,33,45,71,78,97,128,144,147,148,156,157,164,168,175,177] In two of the four cases of neonatal Wilms' tumor depicted by Campell et al., the mothers were diagnosed as having renal and colon carcinoma, respectively.[34]

Gallo and Chemes reported that the youngest patient with Wilms' tumor and terminal renal failure in a series of eight children with the Denys-Drash syndrome was 7 months old.[61] The onset of nephrotic syndrome preceded the Wilms' tumor, which was found at necropsy, by 1.5 months. In the study by Jadresic et al., three of seven children with this syndrome had bilateral tumors, and all neoplasms showed favorable histologic features.[97]

The familial occurrence of Wilms' tumors is not as uncommon as originally thought. Of 3442 patients enrolled in the National Wilms' Tumor Study, 42 (1.2%) had one or more family members affected by the neoplasm.[13] Perlman et al. described a syndrome in siblings consisting of fetal gigantism, unusual facies, hypertrophy and hyperplasia of the islets of Langerhans, bilateral renal hamartomas, and nephroblastomatosis with Wilms' tumor in one sibling.[148] The absence of macroglossia, omphalocele, and adrenocortical cytomegaly distinguishes this syndrome from the Beckwith-Wiedemann syndrome.[148]

Cytogenetics

Karyotypic analyses performed on Wilms' tumors show a deletion in the short arm of chromosome 11, del 11p13.[67,113,120,158,168] The studies demonstrate chromosome 11 deletions both in the leukocytes and in the tumor, a fact that is useful in identifying individuals and families at risk for developing this malignant tumor and in confirming an equivocal histologic diagnosis. For instance, some poorly differentiated blastemal Wilms' tumors and cellular mesoblastic nephromas may present a diagnostic problem. Koufos et al. identified another locus—11p15.5—which occurs both in Wilms' tumor and in patients with the Beckwith-Wiedemann syndrome, but which is not observed in the WAGR syndrome.[113] As in neuroblastoma, retinoblastoma, hepatoblastoma, medulloblastoma, and human fetal kidney, Wilms' tumor expresses the N-myc oncogene.[141]

Giangiacomo et al. described a male neonate with bilateral Wilms' tumors, B-C chromosomal translocation, and multiple congenital anomalies, including Potter's facies, undescended testes, broad spade-like hands, polydactyly, talipes equinovarus, and webbing of the toes.[68] Exploratory laparotomy performed in this patient at 3 weeks of age revealed a large, unresectable tumor occupying the pelvocaliceal collecting system of the left kidney. The right kidney contained a similar, smaller mass. Histologically, the Wilms' tumors showed mostly epithelial elements, with lesser amounts of blastemal elements (considered to be a "favorable histology"). The infant died at 5 weeks of age.

Pathology

In many respects, the morphologic features of perinatal Wilms' tumor are similar to those

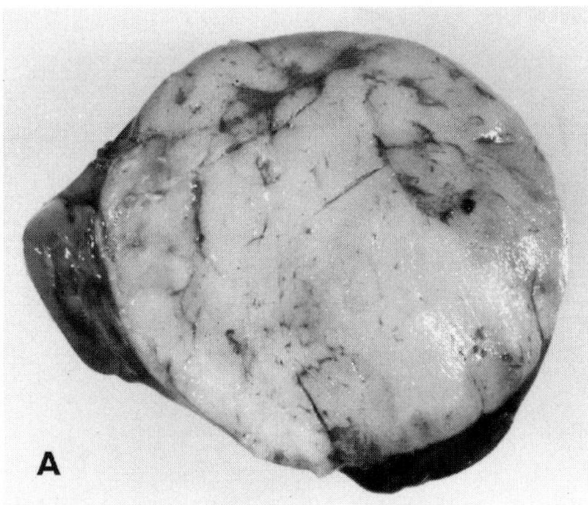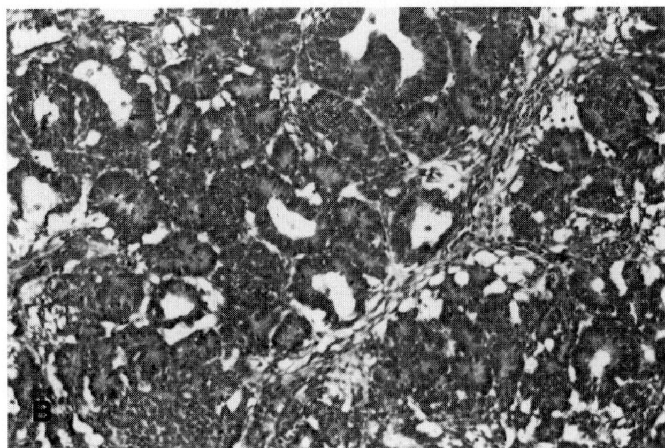

Figure 11–9. Wilms' tumor. *A,* A renal tumor, weighing 170 g and measuring 8 × 6.5 cm, was completely resected from a 4-month-old male infant who presented with an abdominal mass. The cut surface has a white, pasty appearance. *B,* The tumor displayed a predominantly epithelial growth pattern consisting of small, darkly staining cells forming tubules and rosettes. A round nest of blastemal cells is seen near the lower left hand corner (hematoxylin-eosin, ×150).

in older children (Figs. 11–9 through 11–14). The weight of neonatal tumors ranges from 30 to 500 g.[160] Macroscopically, the cut surface is pale tan to light gray, with or without areas of necrosis or cyst formation. The tumor is encapsulated and well circumscribed. Rupture of the capsule with spillage and/or extension of tumor through the capsule can occur, particularly in the larger specimens. Renal vein invasion is noted in less than 25% of the specimens examined.

Practically all neonatal Wilms' tumors have a "favorable histology," as defined by the National Wilms' Tumor Study (Table 11–4).[13,14,160] The monomorphic epithelial tumors, which account for more than 50% of the Wilms' tumors in this age group, are composed predominantly of epithelial tubular elements (see Fig. 11–9). Moreover, the more differentiated neoplasms resemble developing kidney, and may be indistinguishable from nephroblastomatosis.

Differentiated monomorphic epithelial Wilms' tumors appear to be associated with a better prognosis than the triphasic tumors, which consist of epithelial elements with varying degrees of differentiation; small, spindle-shaped blastemal cells; and interstitial fibroblastic or myoblastic stromal cells (see Fig. 11–12).[25,38] According to Bolande, well-differentiated tubular adenoma, multiloculated cystic nephroma, and polycystic Wilms' tumor should all be classified as monomorphic epithelial Wilms' tumor.[25] Chatten's study of 95 Wilms' tumors revealed that the differentiated epithelial neoplasms correlated with a better outcome

than those in which there was little or no epithelial differentiation.[38] Moreover, she found that Wilms' tumors in the young tend to have a more organized histologic pattern and a better prognosis than those that occur in older patients.[38]

Blastemal Wilms' tumors, which consist of small, round to spindle-shaped cells with high mitotic activity, are less common than either the epithelial or the triphasic tumors (see Fig. 11–13). Other histologic patterns of Wilms' tumor have also been noted, particularly in the first year of life. Fetal rhabdomyomatous nephroblastomas (tumors with a prominent skeletal muscle component) and botryoid tumors of the renal pelvis, which show a triphasic pattern with or without skeletal muscle differentiation, are examples of histologic variants (see Fig. 11–14).[72,126,130,187,195,201] Rhabdomyogenic differentiation in a Wilms' tumor removed from a 2-month-old male infant was documented by Gonzalez-Crussi and colleagues.[72] The tumor presented as a well-circumscribed, multiloculated, cystic mass consisting of 20% muscle and 40% blastema. Because blastemal elements were noted within the cyst walls, the lesion was categorized as a cystic, partially differentiated Wilms' tumor.[72] In a review of 20 fetal rhabdomyomatous nephroblastomas by Wigger, the youngest patient was 6 months of age.[201] Reinberg et al. described a 5-month-old female infant with the VATER association and a Wilms' tumor arising from the pelvis and having a botryoid appearance.[156] In addition to the triphasic histology, neoplastic papillary projections

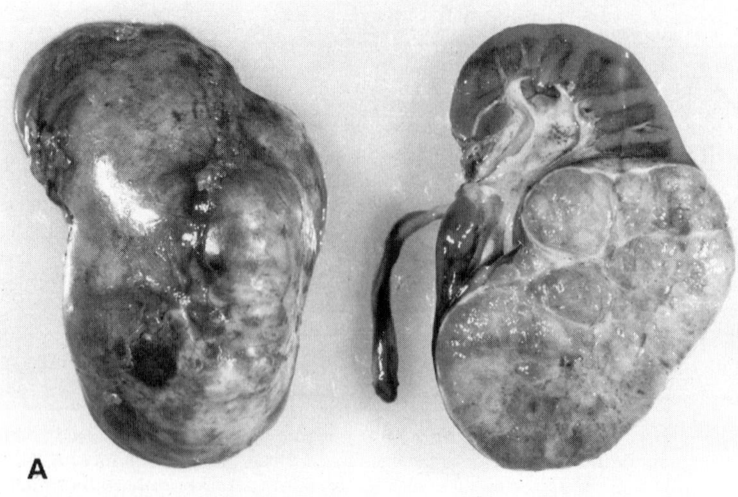

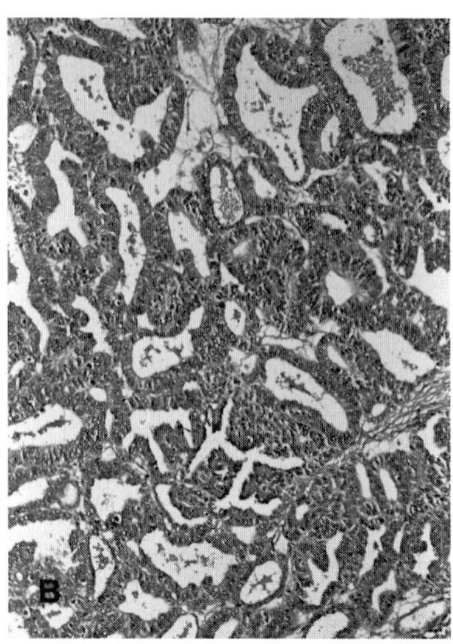

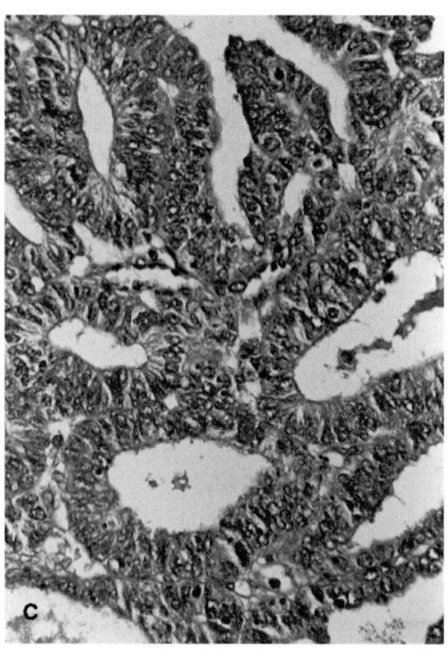

Figure 11–10. Wilms' tumor. *A,* A renal tumor, weighing 250 g and measuring 9 × 5.5 cm, was excised from an 11-month-old male infant with an abdominal mass. The cut surface of the kidney on the right shows a bulging, lobulated, encapsulated, and well-circumscribed neoplasm with a pale, slimy, translucent appearance. *B,* A low-power view reveals predominantly epithelial tubular elements with very little stroma in between the tubules (hematoxylin-eosin, ×240). *C,* At a higher magnification, back-to-back tubular formations, composed of vacuolated columnar cells with variably shaped nuclei and moderate mitotic activity, can be seen (hematoxylin-eosin, ×600). (From Isaacs H Jr. Tumors of the Newborn and Infant. St. Louis: Mosby–Year Book, 1991.)

within the renal pelvis were lined by metaplastic intesinal epithelium. Parenthetically, this type of epithelium is observed in lesions of cloacal origin (e.g., bladder exstrophy), in which the interior mucosal lining is exposed to the surface of the body.[152] Kurtz reported a 3-month-old male infant with Wilms' tumor having a prominent granular cell tumor component.[116] The infant had a favorable outcome. The prognosis of these microscopic variants is essentially the same as the triphasic Wilms' tumor with "favorable histology."

Anaplastic features—that is, the presence of large, mulberry-like cells with hyperchromatic nuclei and multipolar mitotic figures—are associated with an adverse prognosis and occur almost exclusively in older children.[13,17,174]

Treatment

The main treatment of the newborn with Wilms' tumor is resection of the primary tumor, if this can be accomplished. Based on the review of Ritchey et al., it is recommended that neonates with stage I tumors weighing less than 550 g should be observed, without adjuvant chemotherapy (Table 11–3). In addition, they should be monitored closely, using imaging studies, at appropriate intervals until 2 years of age.[160] Those infants who receive chemotherapy should have a 50% dose reduction. The treatment of patients with bilateral Wilms' tumor should be managed in such a way as to conserve as much noninvolved renal parenchyma as possible (i.e., performing focal resection,

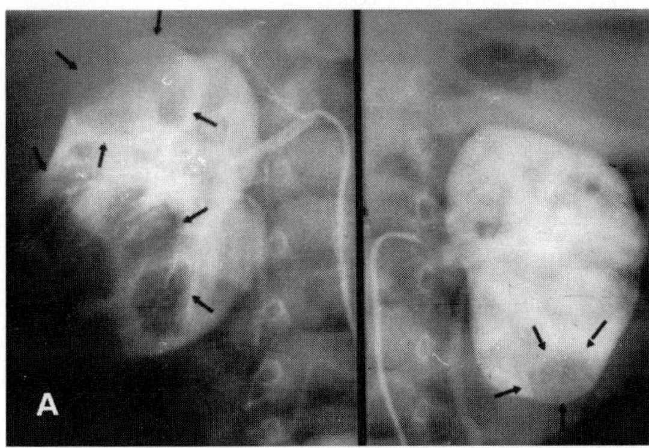

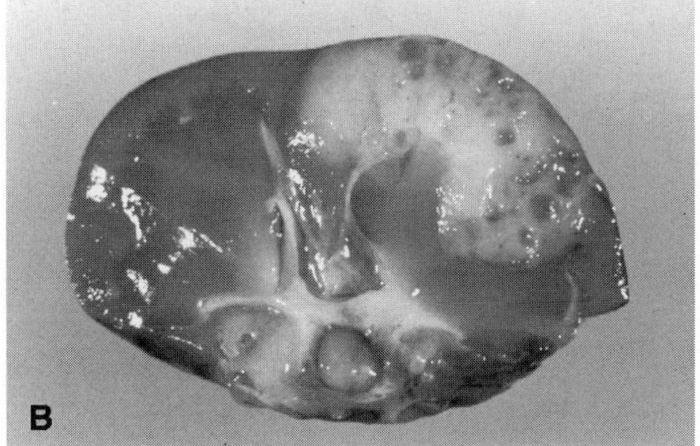

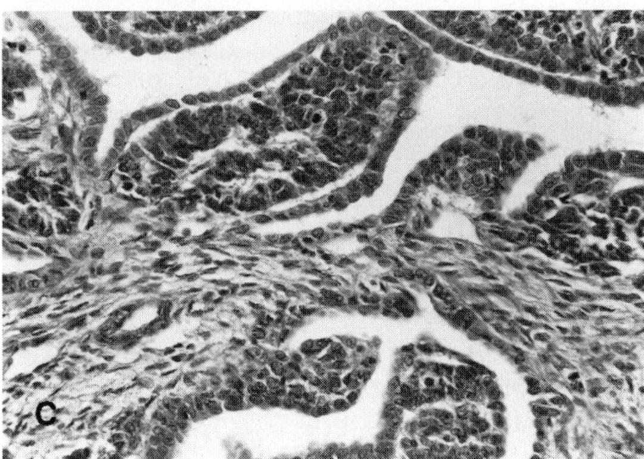

Figure 11–11. Bilateral Wilms' tumor. A 1-year-old boy with congenital anomalies associated with this malignant lesion. The clinical presentation of hypospadias, bilateral undescended testes, and aniridia prompted an investigation of the patient for the possibility of Wilms' tumor. *A,* An arteriogram demonstrates two large masses in the right kidney and a smaller one in the left. The lesions are outlined by arrows. The patient underwent a total right nephrectomy (as this kidney was more involved) and a partial left nephrectomy. *B,* The 2 × 1 cm tumor nodule situated beneath the capsule of the lower pole of the left kidney has a light tan-grey, cystic, gelatinous appearance which was similar to the gross appearance of the two larger tumors in the right kidney. *C,* All three tumors displayed the same histologic appearance, with both triphasic and epithelial patterns. Polypoid epithelial components, consisting of papillary formations, are lined by single rows of cuboidal cells and nests of more atypical-appearing epithelial cells beneath (hematoxylin-eosin, ×600). (From Isaacs H Jr. Tumors of the Newborn and Infant. St. Louis: Mosby–Year Book, 1991.)

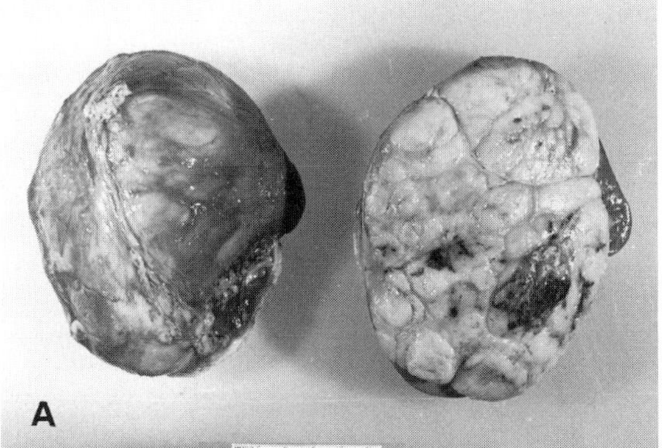

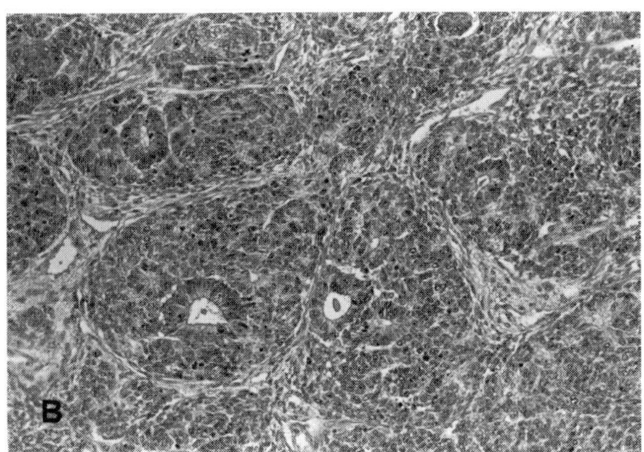

Figure 11–12. Wilms' tumor. *A,* The kidney (658 g, 13 × 11 × 9 cm) from a 1-year-old boy is seen to have been replaced by a soft, tan-gray, lobular neoplasm that is encapsulated and well circumscribed. Areas of hemorrhagic necrosis are evident. *B,* The tumor has blastemal, tubular, and fibrous connective tissue components (hematoxylin-eosin, ×300). The so-called triphasic histologic pattern is the most common one seen in Wilms' tumors in children overall, whereas the epithelial histologic pattern occurs more frequently in newborns. Notice how the spindle-shaped stromal cells blend imperceptibly with the small, round, more darkly-staining blastemal cells. This microscopic feature is helpful when attempting to establish the diagnosis, for example, on the basis of frozen section. (From Isaacs H Jr. Tumors of the Newborn and Infant. St. Louis: Mosby–Year Book, 1991.)

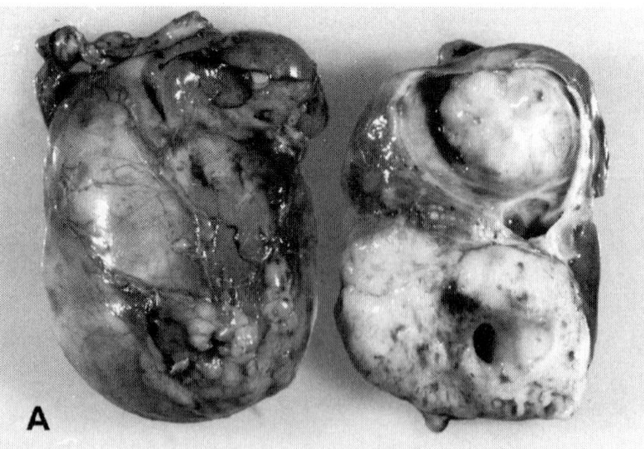 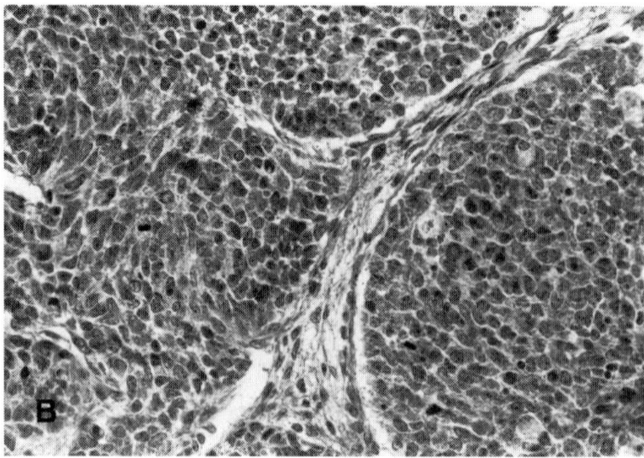

Figure 11–13. Wilms' tumor. *A*, A 192-g, solid and cystic neoplasm measuring 9.5 × 7 cm was removed from a 4-month-old female infant who presented with an abdominal mass. *B*, Lobules of small, round to oval, blastemal cells with a high nuclear:cytoplasmic ratio are separated by delicate fibrovascular septa (hematoxylin-eosin, ×300). The blastemal pattern can have the appearance of a small cell malignant tumor.

rather than nephrectomy, if feasible, in order to preserve renal function) (see Fig. 11–11).[96]

Prognosis

Most Wilms' tumors in the newborn and infant are classified as stage I or II, which probably accounts for the favorable prognosis in this age group.[78,130,160] Table 11–5 shows that stages I and II account for 83% of the neonatal Wilms' tumors culled from the literature. The inci-

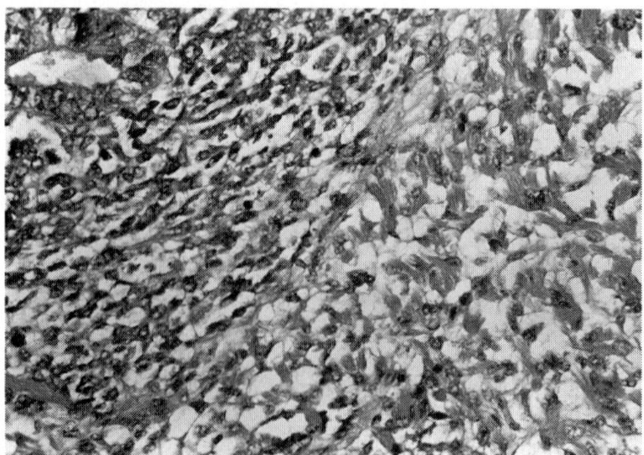

Figure 11–14. Wilms' tumor with a predominant skeletal muscle component (''fetal rhabdomyomatous'' Wilms' tumor). Rhabdomyoblasts with cytoplasmic cross-striations (right side of the field) are bordered by blastemal cells and an embryonic tubule formation in the left upper corner. This renal tumor (845 g, 15 × 11 cm) was removed from a 10-month-old boy. The renal pelvis was extensively involved. This histologic pattern is unusual in the newborn (hematoxylin-eosin, ×600). (From Isaacs H Jr. Tumors of the Newborn and Infant. St. Louis: Mosby–Year Book, 1991.)

dence of bilateral tumors (stage V) ranges from 8% to 50%, depending on the study.[11,130,174] Of the 30 newborn Wilms' tumors listed in Table 11–5, 3 (10%) were bilateral. As compared to patients with unilateral lesions, patients with bilateral tumors tend to be younger at diagnosis and have an increased frequency of congenital malformations and nephrogenic rests.[78]

The Hospital for Sick Children, Toronto study reported by Campbell et al., revealed four newborns with Wilms' tumor, accounting for 1.4% of the total number of Wilms' tumors and 4% of all neonatal tumors at that institution.[34] Two patients had bilateral tumors, which were manifested at birth as bilateral abdominal masses. One patient with bilateral tumors died of pulmonary hyaline membrane disease 11 hours after birth. The other survived following a total unilateral nephrectomy, a partial resection on the contralateral side, irradiation, and chemotherapy. Two additional neonates with unilateral tumors presented with an abdominal mass and hematuria, respectively. All four of these newborns had Wilms' tumors of favorable histology. Three of the four neonates survived (see Table 11–4).[34]

Of 3340 patients with various renal tumors enrolled in the National Wilms' Tumor Study, 27 (0.8%) were younger than 30 days of age; of the 27, 19 had mesoblastic nephroma, 3 had Wilms' tumor, 1 had rhabdoid tumor, and 4 had non-neoplastic conditions.[60] Two of the neonates with Wilms' tumors had stage I disease and one had stage II disease. All three of these patients had favorable histologic findings, and all survived. The Wilms' tumor in the patient with stage II disease contained areas suggestive

Table 11–4. 30 Newborn Wilms' Tumors*

Case No.	Age at Death	Initial Findings	Treatment	Comments	Reference(s)
1	Alive	Abdominal mass	S	Stage I, FH	Rubie et al.[164]
2	21 yr†	?Abdominal mass	S, RT	Stage IIA, FH	Crom et al.[46a]
3	Alive	?Abdominal mass	S, CT, RT	Stage IIIB, FH	Crom et al.[46a]
4	11 hr‡	Abdominal masses, bilateral	–	Stage V, FH	Campbell et al.[34]
5	Alive	Abdominal masses, bilateral	Left total, right partial nephrectomy; CT, RT	Stage V, FH	Campbell et al.[34]
6	Alive	Abdominal mass	S	Stage I, FH	Campbell et al.[34]
7	Alive	Hematuria	S	Stage I, FH	Campbell et al.[34]
8	Alive	Abdominal mass	S	Stage I, FH§	Kurtz[116]
9	9 days	Bilateral flank masses‖	Biopsy	Stage V, FH	Giangiacomo et al.[67,68]
10	8 days	Abdominal mass	S	Stage IV; metastases to the periaortic lymph nodes	Giangiacomo and Kissane[67]
11	4 days	Hydramnios, bilateral renal enlargement	–	Left Wilms' tumor, FH; nephroblastomatosis, right;¶ ?stage I	Perlman et al.[148]
12	Alive	?Abdominal mass	S	Partially differentiated cystic Wilms' tumor, FH; stage I	Gonzalez-Crussi and Baum[72]
13	Alive	Abdominal mass	S	Stage I, FH (epithelial)	Hrabovsky et al.,[90] Ritchey et al.[160]
14	Alive	Abdominal mass	S	Stage I, FH (epithelial)	Hrabovsky et al.,[90] Ritchey et al.[160]
15	Alive	Abdominal mass	S, CT	Stage II, FH (epithelial)	Hrabovsky et al.,[90] Ritchey et al.[160]
16	Alive	?Abdominal mass	S§?	Stage I?, FH (triphasic)	Marsden and Lawler[130]
17	Alive	?Abdominal mass	S§?	Stage I?, FH (epithelial)	Marsden and Lawler[130]
18	Alive	Abdominal mass	S, CT	Stage I, ?FH	Gale et al.[60a]
19	Alive	Abdominal mass#	S, CT	Stage II, FH	Andrews;[3a] Ritchey et al.[160]
20	Alive	UTS screen	S, CT	Stage I, FH, B-W	Ritchey et al.[160]
21	Alive	Abdominal mass	S	Stage I, FH	Ritchey et al.[160]
22	Alive	Prenatal UTS	S	Stage I, FH	Ritchey et al.[160]
23	Alive	Abdominal mass	S, CT, RT	Stage II, FH	Ritchey et al.[160]
24	Alive	Prenatal UTS	S, CT	Stage I, FH	Ritchey et al.[160]
25	Alive	Abdominal mass	S, CT	Stage I, FH	Ritchey et al.[160]
26	Alive	Abdominal mass	S, CT	Stage I, FH	Ritchey et al.[160]
27	Alive	Abdominal mass	S, CT	Stage I, FH	Ritchey et al.[160]
28	Alive	Abdominal mass	S, CT	Stage I, FH	Ritchey et al.[160]
29	Alive	Abdominal mass	S	Stage I, FH	Ritchey et al.[160]
30	16 mo	Prenatal UTS	S, CT	Stage I, FH	Ritchey et al.[160]

*Selected from the literature.

†Died of an unrelated cause.

‡Pulmonary hyaline membrane disease.

§With a prominent granular cell tumor component.

‖Multiple congenital anomalies: Potter facies; undescended testes; broad, spade-like hands; polydactyly; talipes equinovarus; webbing of the toes; B-C chromosomal translocation.

¶Perlman syndrome.

CT = chemotherapy; FH = favorable histology; RT = radiation therapy; S = surgery; UTS = ultrasonography; B-W = Beckwith-Wiedemann syndrome.

#Extrarenal Wilms' tumor in the sacrococcygeal area possibly associated with an immature teratoma.

of mesoblastic nephroma, which could conceivably represent evolution of a Wilms' tumor from a mesoblastic nephroma (or vice versa).[60] Included in the study of infant renal tumors by Marsden and Lawler were 21 Wilms' tumors,[130] two of which occurred in 2-month-old infants. One of these tumors displayed a classical (tri-phasic) pattern, whereas the other showed an epithelial pattern; both patients survived.

As reported by Ritchey et al.,[160] one of the largest neonatal Wilms' tumor reviews is derived from the archives of the National Wilms' Tumor Study, the Pediatric Oncology Group, and the Children's Cancer Study Group. This

Table 11–5. 30 Neonatal Wilms' Tumors:
Stage (Group) Versus Survival*

Stage (Group)†	Number (%)‡	Survival (%)
I	21 (70.0)	19 (90)
II	4 (13.4)	3 (75)
III	1 (3.3)	1 (100)
IV	1 (3.3)	0
V (Bilateral)	3 (10.0)	2 (67)
	30 (100)	25 (83)§

*Data compiled from Table 11–4.
†See Table 11–3 for staging of Wilms' tumors.
‡All tumors were determined to have "favorable histology."
§Overall survival: 25/30 × 100 = 83%.

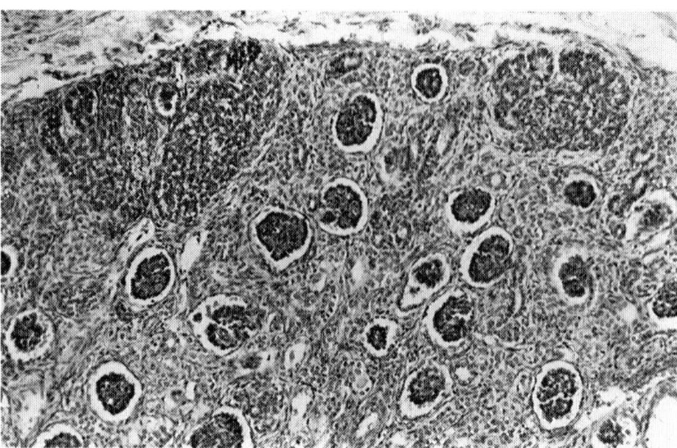

Figure 11–15. Nephrogenic rests. Well-circumscribed nodules of darkly staining blastemal cells are situated beneath the renal capsule at the top of the photomicrograph (perilobar nephrogenic rests). Early tubule and glomerulus formation is evident. This was an incidental postmortem microscopic finding in both kidneys of a 3-week-old, 1984-g, female patient of 35 weeks' gestation with the Pierre-Robin syndrome and terminal bronchopneumonia. In addition, malformations of the genitourinary tract, including a hypoplastic right kidney with a double collecting system and hydronephrosis, were found (hematoxylin-eosin, ×240). (From Isaacs H Jr. Tumors of the Newborn and Infant. St. Louis: Mosby–Year Book, 1991.)

study included 15 patients (see Table 11–4). Three tumors were detected by antenatal sonography, and 1 was diagnosed by postnatal sonography. Most of the tumors (12) were classified as stage I, and three were assigned to stage II. All of the tumors had a favorable histologic picture. There was a high frequency of nephrogenic rests—in 8 of 15 renal tumors (4 perilobar and 4 intralobar nephrogenic rests)—which is higher than expected for unilateral Wilms' tumor. All newborns were treated with nephrectomy. Postoperative chemotherapy was administered to 10, and one received radiation therapy. Fourteen of 15 (93%) survived, which is about the same survival rate as for childhood Wilms' tumor overall. One patient died of progressive disease.[160]

According to the results of the National Wilms' Tumor Study, most histologic forms of Wilms' tumor, including the fetal rhabdomyomatous and the monomorphic epithelial types, are associated with a favorable outcome.[11] There is a relatively high cure rate—greater than 90%—for patients younger than 2 years of age.[11,13] One plausible explanation for this is that most neonatal Wilms' tumors are classified as being low-stage lesions, mainly stages I and II, and are probably detected relatively early on physical examination (see Tables 11–4 and 11–5). Another possible explanation is that anaplastic Wilms' tumor is seen in only 2% of patients younger than 2 years of age and rarely, if at all, in the newborn. The favorable prognosis for Wilms' tumor in the young has been confirmed in several studies. As indicated in Table 11–5, 25 of 30 tumors (83%) were categorized as stage I or II. Nineteen of 21 (90%) newborns diagnosed as having stage I disease with favorable histology survived, which is less than the

overall survival rate for children reported by the National Wilms' Tumor Study for that stage (96.5%). However, looking just at the results of the review of Ritchey et al., 14 of 15 (93%) neonates with stage I Wilms' tumor survived, which is closer to the 96.5% figure. However, Table 11–5 shows an 83% overall survival rate for 30 newborns with Wilms' tumor, stages I through V, and this figure is much lower than the 92.4% 2-year survival for children of all ages reported by the Third National Wilms' Tumor Study.[47] Owing to the rarity of this tumor in the newborn and the small number of cases reported, it is impossible to obtain statistically significant survival data at this time.

NEPHROBLASTOMATOSIS COMPLEX (NEPHROGENIC RESTS AND NEPHROBLASTOMATOSIS)

Nephrogenic rests and nephroblastomatosis are terms used to designate a group of renal lesions resembling the metanephric blastema (nephrogenic zone) of the developing kidney (see Figs. 11–5 and 11–15).[11,12,20,25,30,31,46,50,78] Nephrogenesis normally ceases at 34 to 36 weeks' gestation, and persistence of nephrogenic rests beyond this time period is considered abnormal.[46,180] Nephrogenic rests, nephroblastomatosis, and Wilms' tumor appear to be different lesions belonging to the same disease spectrum.[60,161] Indeed, the progression of nephrogenic rests to nephroblastomatosis, and eventually to Wilms' tumor, has been documented.[114,180]

Nephrogenic rests and nephroblastomatosis may be single, multiple, or bilateral in distribution, and may be grossly or microscopically visible, depending on their size. Beckwith and associates have devised an elaborate classification scheme for this group.[16] Nephrogenic rests consist of two main types: perilobar (PLNR) and intralobar (ILNR), whereas nephroblastomatosis is categorized according to four main types: perilobar (PLNR only), intralobar (ILNR only), combined (PLNR and ILNR), and universal (panlobar).[12,16] PLNR is the most frequent form, occurring at the lobar (cortical) surface (see Fig. 11–15); ILNR is less common and may be found anywhere in the cortex or medulla. Panlobar (universal) nephroblastomatosis is the rarest form of all and usually is fatal.[20,88] In these specimens, there is no recognizable renal cortex or medulla on microscopic examination.

Hou and Holman reported an example of panlobar nephroblastomatosis in a premature neonate with bilateral flank masses who died of respiratory failure 13 hours after birth; the lesions were bilateral and symmetrical.[88] Subsequently, another case of bilateral, diffuse, pancortical nephroblastomatosis was described by Murata et al.[138] The affected newborn was also premature and died of respiratory failure 1 hour after birth. In addition to the extensive bilateral renal lesions, the infant had other findings suggestive of the Perlman syndrome. A third example of panlobar nephroblastomatosis was reported by Regalado et al.[155] This patient, of 34 weeks' gestation, underwent prenatal sonography, which revealed oligohydramnios, ascites, bilateral renomegaly, and a small thorax. At necropsy, the kidneys had a cerebriform appearance lacking medullary pyramids; microscopic examination revealed a diffusely distorted architecture, inconspicuous proximal tubules, medullary and interstitial dysplasia, and nodules of perilobar nephrogenic rests. Other postmortem findings included Potter facies, hypoplastic lungs, and myxolipomas of the choroid plexus.

Massive nephroblastomatosis in infants has been treated by chemotherapy and radiation therapy, or by chemotherapy alone, with reversion to normal renal morphology.[50,83,115,184]

Nephroblastomatosis could be considered an example of both a malformation and a neoplasm, consistent with the idea of the "borderland of embryology and pathology" championed by Willis.[202]

Nephrogenic rests are observed in the fetus and newborn as an incidental finding in a surgical or postmortem kidney specimen from a patient with a non-neoplastic condition (e.g., hydronephrosis, dysplasia, double collecting systems, or congenital obstructive uropathy).[11,52] They are a rare cause of massive bilateral renomegaly, and may be found in an ipsilateral or contralateral kidney removed for a Wilms' tumor.[11,20,31,96,123,124] Dimmick et al. reviewed 60 cases of multicystic dysplastic kidneys and found rests in 6.7%, which is similar to the incidence of this lesion in the kidneys of other infants at their institution who have congenital obstructive uropathy.[52] Gaulier et al. described one case of panlobar nephroblastomatosis, occurring in a multicystic dysplastic kidney, which was detected antenatally by sonography as a right renal mass.[65] The mother had a history of hydramnios.

Rous et al. documented a case of nephrogenic rests that developed into nephroblastomatosis.[161] Hemihypertrophy and bilateral renomegaly with small, cortical, cyst-like lesions were noted on radiographic studies at birth. The diagnosis of nodular renal blastema (nephrogenic rests) was made following biopsy at 3 months of age. Follow-up examination at 12 months of age revealed progressive renal enlargement, deformed collecting systems, and multiple filling defects. Biopsies of both kidneys showed bilateral nephroblastomatosis with high mitotic activity that was histologically indistinguishable from Wilms' tumor. After a 13-month course of chemotherapy, the patient had a "third-look" operation. On gross examination the kidneys appeared normal, and biopsy studies showed small subcapsular nests of primitive tubules and infantile glomeruli, some with calcification.

Nephrogenic rests and nephroblastomatosis are found in association with a variety of syndromes, including thanatophoric dwarfism (a type of lethal, short-limbed chondrodysplasia), the Klippel-Trenaunay syndrome (cutaneous hemangiomas, varicose veins, and bony and soft tissue hypertrophy), trisomy 18 syndrome,[12,43,44,129] Perlman syndrome (familial nephroblastomatosis with visceromegaly, macrosomia, renal hamartomas, cryptorchidism, unusual facies, Wilms' tumor, and hydramnios),[79,147,148] and in newborn siblings.[121] Both nephroblastomatosis and del 11p13 occur with Wilms' tumor, suggesting an etiologic relationship.[85]

Perilobar nephrogenic rests, which were formerly designated as Wilms' tumor in situ or nodular renal blastema, are an incidental microscopic finding, occurring in every 100 to 200 necropsies performed on fetuses and on infants younger than 4 months of age (Fig. 11–15).[12,25,26,31,52,93] Multiple sections of kidney may be required to demonstrate these rests. Included in this category are entities such as tubular adenoma,[25] and sclerosing and nonsclerosing metanephric hamartoma.[31]

The results of the fourth National Wilms' Tumor Study showed that there was a high incidence of nephrogenic rests in kidneys with Wilms' tumors, both unilateral (29%) and bilateral (99%), as well as a high risk for developing a Wilms' tumor in the contralateral kidney when nephrogenic rests were found. Beckwith lists the risk figures as 26% for PLNR alone, 59% for ILNR alone, and 94% for combined ILNR and PLNR.[11]

According to Beckwith, most nephrogenic rests in infants regress and do not develop into a Wilms' tumor,[11] a situation that is, perhaps, analogous to neuroblastoma in situ.[11,25] The importance of the rests, in addition to being potentially malignant (perhaps representing the first mutational event in carcinogenesis), is that they are associated with the Beckwith-Wiedemann syndrome, hemihypertrophy, and Drash syndrome, a relatively high incidence of congenital heart disease, and certain chromosomal malformation syndromes (e.g., trisomies 13 and 18).[25,26,78] Moreover, the type of rest is associated with certain histologic forms of Wilms' tumor; for example, the perilobar rests are seen in conjunction with the blastemal or epithelial Wilms' tumors with little stroma, whereas the intralobar rests correlate with Wilms' tumors having prominent stroma; embryonic, nephron-like elements; and heterologous cell types. Actual progression of nephrogenic rests to nephroblastomatosis and subsequently to Wilms' tumor has been documented by serial biopsy studies.[114]

Occasionally, it is difficult or impossible to distinguish between Wilms' tumor and nephroblastomatosis. Neither the size of the lesion nor the microscopic appearance may be helpful in making this distinction.[11,12] Therefore, careful monitoring, with imaging studies performed at appropriate time intervals, is essential in the evaluation of young patients with the nephroblastomatosis complex. Prophylactic chemotherapy should be considered in certain selective cases.

CYSTIC TUMORS OF THE KIDNEY

Various cystic conditions of the kidney are found in the fetus and newborn. They include both true tumors and neoplastic-like entities of probable developmental origin.[151,152] Hydronephrosis and multicystic kidney are responsible for most abdominal masses in the perinatal period; therefore, it is important to keep these entities in mind when evaluating a cystic renal mass (see Fig. 11–1).[86,96] The cystic tumors to be discussed here include the cystic nephroma (multilocular cyst of the kidney); cystic, partially differentiated nephroblastoma; and cystic Wilms' tumor. Sometimes, the three conditions have been reported as the same entity under a variety of names, which merely adds to the diagnostic and nosologic confusion. It has been suggested that cystic nephroma, cystic partially differentiated nephroblastoma, and cystic Wilms' tumor are related, perhaps representing a continuum with cystic nephroma at the benign end, cystic partially differentiated nephroblastoma somewhere in the middle, and cystic Wilms' tumor at the malignant end.[3,11,100]

Cystic nephroma (multilocular cyst of the kidney) is rarely ever found in the fetus and neonate, but may be diagnosed later on in infancy and childhood (Fig. 11–16).[3,6,8,16,22,39,51,55,56,73,93,96,102] The author was unable to find a case report of a cystic nephroma occurring in an infant younger than 4 months of age. Compared to mesoblastic nephroma and Wilms' tumor, the lesion is relatively uncommon, accounting for less than 10% of all renal tumors occurring in the first year of life.[96] One of the youngest patients with this cystic lesion was a 4-month-old female infant who presented with seizures related to hypertension and an abdominal mass.[62] She died of sepsis 4 days after nephrectomy.

The controversy as to whether the multilocular cystic lesion represents a true neoplasm or a malformation of the kidney has not been completely resolved. Potter regarded multilocular cyst not as a neoplastic process, but as a segmental form of type II (IIA) cystic kidney in which the cysts involve only a segment of an otherwise normal kidney.[151,152] Tang et al. showed by electron microscopic studies that

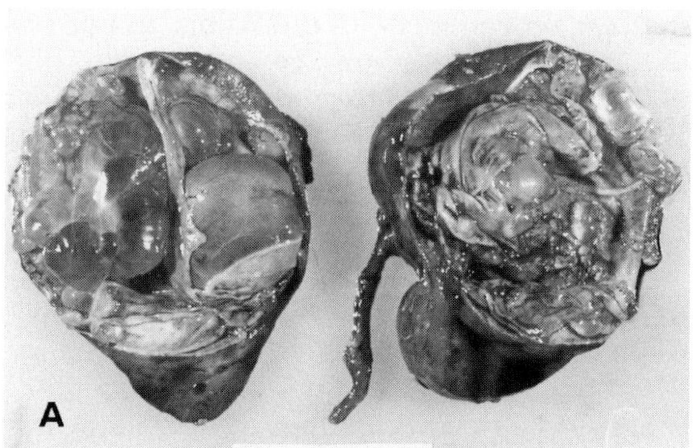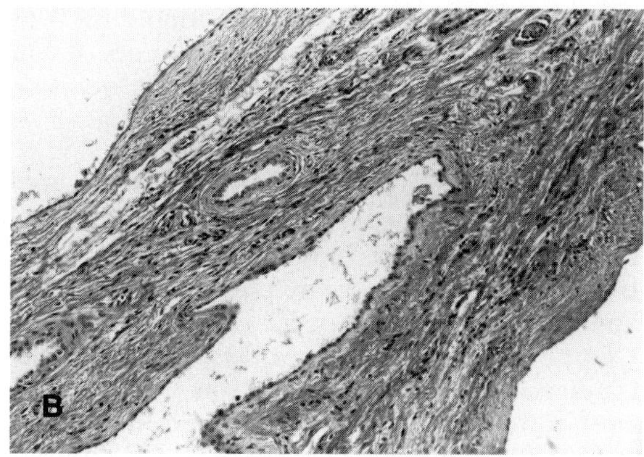

Figure 11–16. Multilocular cyst of the kidney. *A,* The surgical specimen (405 g, 13 × 10 cm) removed from a 2-year-old girl consists of a multiloculated cyst occupying most of the kidney. The lesion does not communicate with the renal pelvis. The cysts range in size from 0.2 cm up to 4 cm in diameter and contain clear, straw-colored fluid. They are well encapsulated and are surrounded by a capsule that is 2 to 3 mm thick. *B,* Cysts of various sizes are separated by fibrous connective tissue septa and are lined by cuboidal and flattened epithelium. No nephrogenic elements are present within the cyst walls (hematoxylin-eosin, ×120). (From Fobi M, Mahour GH, Isaacs H Jr. Multilocular cyst of the kidney. J Pediatr Surg 1979;14:282. Used by permission.)

the epithelial lining cells of the cysts resemble renal collecting tubule cells; they concluded from these observations that multilocular renal cyst represents a malformation resulting from a "segmental maldevelopment of the ureteric bud."[183] However, other investigators consider it to be a neoplasm rather than a malformation.[3,11,22,53,62,73,102,139] Nevertheless, in 1956, Boggs and Kimmelstiel established the criteria required for the diagnosis of cystic nephroma: (1) the lesion is multilocular; (2) most of the cysts are lined by epithelium; (3) the cysts do not communicate with the renal pelvis; (4) the adjacent renal tissue is normal except for pressure atrophy; and (5) nephrons are not present within the septa separating the cysts.[22]

Cystic nephroma (multilocular cyst) manifests clinically as an abdominal mass and occasionally is accompanied by hematuria.[6,22,56,62] Usually, the diagnosis is established preoperatively by imaging studies.[15,96] Most of these lesions are unilateral, but bilateral examples have been described.[39] Grossly, the cystic nephroma consists of a multicystic mass, situated in the upper or lower pole of the kidney, that is well demarcated from the renal pelvis by a discrete, light tan to white capsule (Fig. 11–16*A*). The cysts vary in size, contain clear fluid, and have thin fibrous septa which, by definition, lack nephrogenic elements on microscopic examination.[3,8,11,25,56,73,93,102,206] Moreover, skeletal muscle elements are not observed in the cyst walls.[56,73,102] Multilocular cysts are described in association with mesoblastic nephroma,

nephroblastomatosis complex, and Wilms' tumor.[3,96,102]

Cystic, partially differentiated nephroblastoma refers to another multicystic condition that is grossly identical to cystic nephroma but that differs microscopically from the latter because it contains immature or mature nephrogenic (metanephric) elements in the fibrous septa separating the cysts.[3,11,22,48,53,62,73,100,101,188,206] Skeletal muscle cells are present in the septa between the cysts, in addition to nephrogenic elements.[62,73,100]

An abdominal mass is the most common clinical presentation.[100] Cystic, partially differentiated nephroblastoma is described in the newborn and in the older child, and occurs most commonly in children younger than 2 years of age.[62,73,100,101] The neonate who presented with an abdominal mass and jaundice and was reported by Procainoy et al. is probably one of the earliest diagnosed cases.[153] The infant had hyperbilirubinemia and a consumptive coagulopathy, and bled into the tumor, which was successfully resected. Uson and colleagues reported a 3-week-old male infant who presented with an abdominal mass; the infant recovered following nephrectomy as the only treatment.[188] Dorai et al.[53] described another case report of unilateral, cystic, partially differentiated nephroblastoma with bilateral nephroblastomatosis in a 3-week-old girl. The patient had a favorable outcome following nephrectomy for the cystic lesion in the right kidney and chemotherapy for the perilobar nephroblastomatosis in the left. Joshi reviewed 17 patients, including 3 of his own, who were younger than 2 years of age and had cystic, partially differentiated nephroblastoma; none of the patients were found to have recurrences or metastases.[100] Fifteen infants and children for whom follow-up information was available survived; 8 of these patients underwent nephrectomy alone, and 7 were treated with nephrectomy plus radiation therapy and chemotherapy.[100] In the study by Ugarte and colleagues, 2 of the 24 infants with renal tumors (one of whom was 2 months of age) were diagnosed with partially differentiated cystic nephroma; both patients survived following surgical resection as did the two patients included in the study by Andrews.[3,187] One instance of local recurrence in a 4-month-old boy was reported by Joshi and Beckwith.[102]

Simple nephrectomy is recommended for the treatment of both cystic nephroma and cystic, partially differentiated nephroblastoma.[23,56,73,100,183] Partial nephrectomy should be considered in some patients with cystic nephroma.[39,96] Adjuvant chemotherapy and radiation therapy are contraindicated.

Cystic Wilms' tumor could be considered the third entity in the spectrum of cystic "neoplastic" conditions of the kidney. A well-differentiated Wilms' tumor with focal or multifocal cystic change sometimes creates difficulties in the differential diagnosis of a multicystic renal mass. Moreover, multilocular cyst can occur in the same kidney with a Wilms' tumor, but this is unusual.[96] Case 4 of Gonzalez-Crussi et al. (a 7-month-old boy) was extraordinary in that a solid polypoid nodule composed of a Wilms' tumor with triphasic histology was found amidst multiloculated cysts.[73] As with the other five cases of cystic nephroma in their study, neither metastases nor local recurrence occurred. Wilms' tumor originating from a multicystic, dysplastic kidney has also been described.[142] Kinoshita et al. have documented familial and nonfamilial cases of bilateral cystic Wilms' tumors associated with multiple congenital malformations and rhabdomyosarcoma as a second malignant lesion.[109] Currently, many surgeons perform needle biopsy rather than open biopsy as the primary diagnostic procedure in patients with Wilms' tumors. The cystic Wilms' tumor is a good example of why this procedure should not be considered. For instance, the diagnosis of the patient reported by Gonzalez-Crussi et al. (above) would likely have been missed with needle biopsy study because of sampling error.

The treatment of cystic conditions of the kidney is surgery, which results in cure in most instances.[26,100] Patients with the Wilms' tumor cystic variant should be treated according to one of the protocols recommended by the National Wilms' Tumor Study Group or an equivalent study, if indicated.

RHABDOID TUMOR OF THE KIDNEY

Formerly, rhabdoid tumor of the kidney was regarded as a form of Wilms' tumor, a "sarcomatoid Wilms' tumor," but the findings of the National Wilms' Tumor Study in 1978 showed that it is a distinctly different neoplasm, both clinically and pathologically.[13,17,194] The name "rhabdoid" was coined because microscopically, it resembles rhabdomyosarcoma although skeletal muscle elements are not demonstrated either by immunohistochemical or ultrastructural studies. To date, its histogenesis remains unclear.[63] This highly malignant neoplasm, characterized by early metastases, frequent recurrence, and a high mortality rate, occurs in the newborn and during the first year of life; indeed, more than 50% of rhabdoid tumors of the kidney are reported in infants (Table 11–6).[11,20,42,54,63,80,92,130,174,187,194] Rhabdoid tumor of the kidney is detected in utero by ultrasonography.[42]

Although rare, rhabdoid tumor is the third most common malignant renal tumor of the neonate, followed by clear cell sarcoma (see Tables 11–4, 11–6, and 11–7). The median age at diagnosis of 111 patients reviewed by the National Wilms' Tumor Study was 11 months, and rhabdoid tumor accounted for 2.5% of the total number of renal tumors.[194] In the older literature, some cases were reported as "neonatal metastasizing Wilms' tumor" before the entity was recognized.[106,197] This malignant tumor arises from the soft tissues, central nervous system, and other sites as well (see Chapters 4, 9, and 12).[174]

One interesting aspect of this tumor is its association with a second intracranial malignant lesion. However, no satisfactory explanation for this relationship has been presented. Medulloblastoma is listed most often as the second tumor and, less frequently, pineoblastoma, cerebral primitive neuroectodermal tumor (PNET), medulloepithelioma, ependymoma, and malignant astrocytoma.[29,42,63,174,182] Table 11–6 shows that almost one third of 16 new-

Table 11–6. 19 Newborn Rhabdoid Tumors of the Kidney*

Case No.	Age at Death	Initial Findings	Treatment	Comments	Reference(s)
1	Alive	Abdominal mass	S, CT, RT	Skin metastases 5 months after nephrectomy	Fung et al.[59]
2	6 mo	?Abdominal mass	S, CT	Widespread metastases	Haas et al.[82]
3	4 mo	?Abdominal mass	S, CT, RT	Pulmonary metastases at diagnosis	Haas et al.[82]
4	6 mo	Abdominal mass	S, CT	Metastases to lymph nodes, ovary, and fallopian tube	Sotelo-Avila et al.[174]
5	LTF	Abdominal mass, hematuria, hypertension	S, CT	Metastases to lungs and lymph nodes	Sotelo-Avila et al.[174]
6	18 mo	Abdominal mass, vomiting	S, CT, RT	Metastases to lymph nodes and gingiva; intracranial mass at 15 months of age	Sotelo-Avila et al.[174]
7	4 mo	Large head, abdominal mass	S, CT	Liver, lymph node RTK metastases; medulloblastoma	Kalousek et al.;[106] Bonnin et al.[29]
8	4 wks	Abdominal mass, hydrocephalus	S, CT	RTK metastases to liver, lymph nodes, adrenal, and bone marrow; medulloblastoma	Wexler et al.;[197] Bonnin et al.[29]
9	2 wks	?Abdominal mass	?	Medulloblastoma found at necropsy	Takagi et al.[182]
10	16 wks	Fever, abdominal mass	S, ?CT	Recurrence; metastases to lungs, liver, kidney, and retroperitoneum	Gururangan et al.[80]
11	7 wks	Abdominal mass	S	Recurrence; medulloblastoma noted at the age of 6 weeks; RTK metastases to liver, lymph nodes, and peritoneum	Gansler et al.[63]
12	14 wks	Intraocular metastasis and proptosis	S, BX, CT	Abdominal mass at the age of 11 weeks; metastases to liver and skin	Akhtar et al.[2]
13	80 days	Abdominal mass secondary to urinary bladder distention	S, CT	Bilateral RTKs; retrourethral rhabdoid tumor with metastases to bladder, prostate, ureter, rectum, and lung	Shimao et al.[170]
14	2 mo	Antenatal renal lesion detected by sonography; abdominal mass	S	Liver metastases; medulloblastoma	Chung et al.[42]
15	7 mo	Abdominal mass	S, CT	Metastases to lungs	Gonzalez-Crussi and Baum;[71a] Ugarte et al.[187]
16	Alive	Abdominal mass	S, CT, RT	Metastases to skin	Gonzalez-Crussi and Baum[71a]
17	2 mo	Posterior cervical mass	BX, RT	Metastases to lungs, liver, and cervical lymph nodes	Isaacs[94]
18	3 mo	Abdominal mass	S, CT, RT	No tumor at necropsy; patient died of sepsis	Isaacs[94]
19	LTF	Abdominal mass	S, CT		Isaacs[94]

*Selected from the literature.

RTK = rhabdoid tumor of the kidney; LTF = lost to follow-up; BX = biopsy; CT = chemotherapy; RT = radiation therapy; S = surgery.

Table 11–7. Five Neonatal Clear Cell Sarcomas of the Kidney*

Case No.	Status	Initial Findings	Treatment	Comments	Reference(s)
1	Alive	Hydramnios, abdominal mass	S, CT	Stage I	Suzuki et al.[181]
2	Alive	?Abdominal mass	S	?Stage I	Suzuki et al.[181]
3	Alive	?Abdominal mass	S	Stage I	Gonzalez-Crussi and Baum;[71a] Ugarte et al.[187]
4	Alive	Abdominal mass	S, CT, RT	Stage IV; metastases to the liver, other kidney, and scapula; protocolectomy performed for familial adenomatous polyposis coli	Uzoaru et al.[189]
5	Alive	Abdominal mass	S	Stage I	Kodet et al.[111]

*Selected from the literature.
LTF = lost to follow-up; BX = biopsy; CT = chemotherapy; RT = radiation therapy; S = surgery.

borns with rhabdoid tumor of the kidney had coexistent medulloblastoma.

In one study by Bonnin et al., two of seven patients with separate tumors arising from the kidney and the brain were younger than 3 months of age at presentation.[29] A progressive increase in head size and hydrocephalus were the initial manifestations in a 7-week-old boy who subsequently underwent surgical removal of a rhabdoid tumor of the kidney at the age of 3 months. Necropsy 1 month later revealed, in addition to rhabdoid tumor, metastases to the liver and to the abdominal and thoracic lymph nodes, and a cerebellar medulloblastoma with leptomeningeal metastases. This case had been identified 7 years earlier as "neonatal metastasizing Wilms' tumor" by Kalousek et al., before the entity had been defined.[106] Both the rhabdoid tumor of the kidney and cerebellar medulloblastoma were discovered shortly after birth in the second patient of Bonnin et al., at 24 hours and 36 hours postdelivery, respectively.[29] The infant died 2 weeks later. Postmortem examination revealed rhabdoid tumor metastases to the adrenal gland, liver, and bone marrow, and a large cerebellar medulloblastoma invading the brain stem.[29] Wexler and associates had reported this case 9 years previously, again as "neonatal metastasizing Wilms' tumor."[197] Gansler et al. described a similar case.[63] Their patient was a male neonate who presented with an abdominal mass and underwent a nephrectomy shortly after birth. Six weeks later, he was admitted to the hospital with bowel obstruction secondary to a massive intra-abdominal recurrent tumor. Concurrently, signs of increased intracranial pressure were noted, leading to the diagnosis of cerebel-

lar medulloblastoma. Widespread metastases from the rhabdoid tumor and a cerebellar medulloblastoma were found at necropsy. The rhabdoid tumor described by Chung et al. was detected by sonography on the day prior to birth and was removed on the second day of life.[42] Amazingly, no tumor was found on the initial sonogram performed 10 days prior to delivery, suggesting that the tumor grew very rapidly in utero. During a follow-up and metastatic evaluation at the age of 7 weeks, a posterior fossa tumor was discovered. Necropsy at 2 months of age revealed extensive local recurrence and hepatic metastases, in addition to a cerebellar medulloblastoma. One of the three newborns in the Children's Hospital, Los Angeles series who had rhabdoid tumor of the kidney presented with a posterior cervical mass; a biopsy was performed.[92] Further evaluation revealed a large, inoperable renal tumor. Postmortem examination showed multiple metastases to the lungs, liver, and lymph nodes.

Proptosis and intraocular metastasis mimicking retinoblastoma were the initial findings in one neonate.[2] Following enucleation, irradiation, and chemotherapy, an abdominal mass was discovered when the infant was 11 weeks old, at which time the diagnosis was changed to rhabdoid tumor of the kidney with metastases to the liver and eye. Shortly before death, at the age of 14 weeks, the patient developed cutaneous and gingival metastases. In another study, synchronous bilateral renal and retrourethral rhabdoid tumors, presumably three separate primaries, were described in a 52-day-old male infant by Shimao et al.[170] The patient presented with urinary bladder distention simulating a suprapubic abdominal mass. Subse-

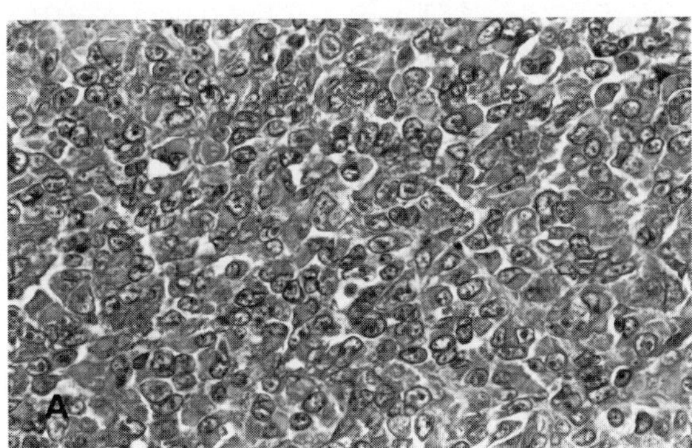 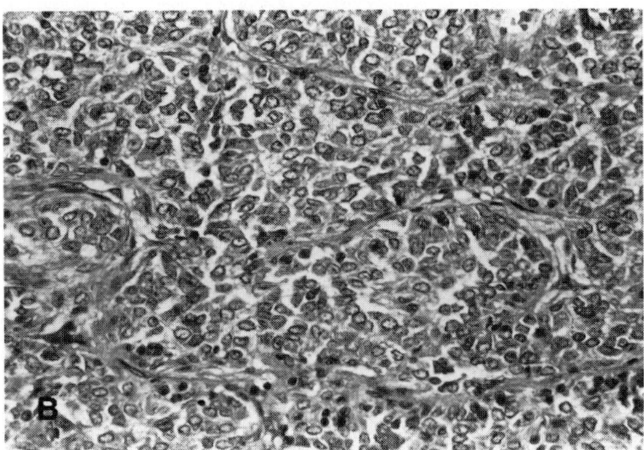

Figure 11–17. Rhabdoid tumor of the kidney. *A,* "Classic" pattern. The teardrop-shaped cells are seen to have vesicular nuclei, which characteristically contain a large nucleolus. In the cytoplasm, there are ill-defined, round to oval, hyaline bodies composed of intermediate filaments that are best demonstrated by electron microscopy (hematoxylin-eosin, ×250). The specimen was taken from a 2-year-old girl presenting with gross hematuria and an abdominal mass. *B,* Delicate, fibrovascular septa separate lobules of round to oval-shaped cells with vesicular nuclei and small nucleoli. The histologic appearance is consistent with the organoid pattern of rhabdoid tumor described by Weeks and colleagues.[194] This specimen was obtained from a 1-year-old boy with a renal mass and liver metastases (hematoxylin-eosin, ×200). (From Isaacs H Jr. Tumors of the Newborn and Infant. St. Louis: Mosby–Year Book, 1991.)

quently, an 83-g, 5 × 4 cm tumor was found in the right kidney, and two tumors were found in the left kidney. In addition, at necropsy, the retrourethal rhabdoid tumor was found to have invaded the bladder, prostate, ureter, and rectum. One of the few neonates with this malignant lesion who survived was reported by Fung and co-workers.[59] The 5-week-old male infant presented with symptoms of an upper respiratory infection, and a firm, nontender, 3 × 4 cm abdominal mass was discovered on physical examination. Following radical nephrectomy (stage I), the patient received radiation therapy and chemotherapy and recovered.

Hypercalcemia occurs in association with rhabdoid tumor of the kidney and mesoblastic nephroma, and is attributable to ectopic secretion of parathyroid hormone by the tumor.[80,98,163] Apparently, the hypercalcemia has no prognostic significance, but it can be used as a marker in some patients. Elevated lactic dehydrogenase levels correlate with tumor activity.[80] In contrast to Wilms' tumor, rhabdoid tumor expresses c-myc rather than the N-myc oncogene.[63]

Rhabdoid tumor has a tendency to be more hemorrhagic, necrotic, and cystic than a typical Wilms' tumor, but it may have a similar gross appearance.[11,13,17,59,94] The largest rhabdoid tumor in the Children's Hospital, Los Angeles neonatal study measured 11 cm in diameter, weighed 517 g, and occupied most of the kidney.[94] The main sites of metastases for renal rhabdoid tumors, in decreasing order of frequency, are the lungs, liver, lymph nodes, and brain.[174]

Rhabdoid tumor of the kidney displays a monomorphous growth pattern, with round to oval-shaped cells having a prominent eosinophilic cytoplasm, a large, slightly vesicular nucleus, and a characteristically big, single, round nucleolus (Fig. 11–17).[11,13,17,59,82,182] The cells contain a conspicuous, round, glassy to hyaline-appearing cytoplasmic inclusion which consists ultrastructually of a meshwork of intermediate filaments. Immunoperoxidase studies reveal that the filaments react positively with vimentin and cytokeratin but are unreactive with the skeletal muscle markers myoglobin and desmin.[59,82,165,182,191] Moreover, rhabdoid tumor cells are immunoreactive with laminin, a basement membrane glycoprotein, and peanut lectin.[182] Occasionally, neural markers are positive. Weeks and colleagues have described several other morphologic patterns observed in rhabdoid tumors, such as the organoid (Fig. 11–17B), epithelioid, sclerosing, lymphomatoid, and histiocytoid patterns.[194]

The survival rate for rhabdoid tumor of the kidney is dismal, regardless of clinicopathologic stage or form of therapy, and is less than 12% when diagnosed before the age of 2 years.[17,194] In one report of eight patients with this neoplasm who were 13 months of age or younger at diagnosis, all but one died within 1.5 years after diagnosis.[174] However, isolated

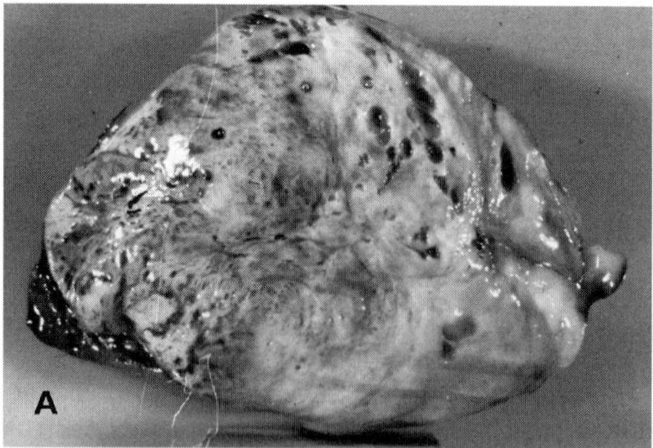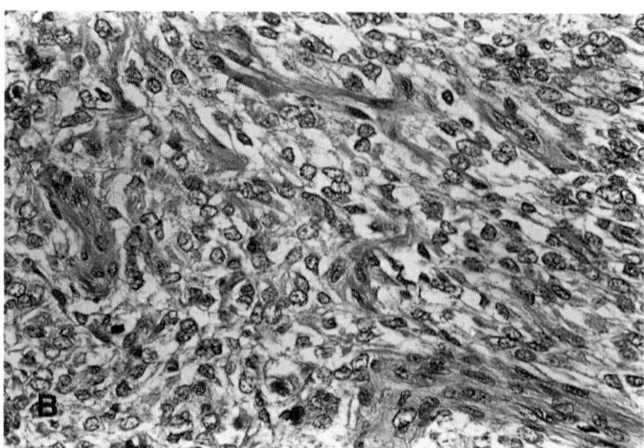

Figure 11–18. Clear cell sarcoma of the kidney. *A,* A tumor (735 g, 16.5 × 11.5 cm) was removed from the right kidney of a 15-month-old boy with an abdominal mass. The tumor is seen to have a soft, gray-white to gray-pink, cut surface. It had invaded the renal hilum and adjacent liver. *B,* These polygonal cells consist of water-clear cytoplasms and round to oval nuclei with finely dispersed chromatin and inconspicuous nucleoli (hematoxylin-eosin, ×200). (From Isaacs H Jr. Tumors of the Newborn and Infant. St. Louis: Mosby–Year Book, 1991.)

cases of newborns surviving following a combined treatment approach consisting of nephrectomy, chemotherapy, and radiation therapy have been reported.[59,80] Table 11–6, which lists 20 cases of rhabdoid tumor selected from the literature, shows an 11% survival rate: 2 patients living, 16 dead, and 2 lost to follow-up.

CLEAR CELL SARCOMA OF THE KIDNEY

Clear cell renal sarcoma is a unique malignant neoplasm that occurs much less frequently in the newborn than either Wilms' tumor or rhabdoid tumor (see Tables 11–4 through 11–7). Clear cell sarcoma accounts for 2.5% of the tumors enrolled in the National Wilms' Tumor Study. In the past, this malignant lesion was considered to be another Wilms' tumor variant, but several investigators have demonstrated that it is a distinct neoplasm, characterized histologically by the presence of clear cells, and clinically by a poor prognosis and a tendency to metastasize to the bones.[13,81,111,131,132,174] Clear cell sarcoma is found mostly in male patients, but it is not associated with any specific congenital anomaly, clinical condition, or malformation syndrome.[174] However, an association between congenital clear cell sarcoma and familial adenomatous polyposis coli has been noted.[189]

Several examples of clear cell sarcoma have been described in the newborn (see Table 11–7).[43,71a,111,181,187] Ugarte and colleagues reported one case of clear cell sarcoma occurring in a 9-

day-old male infant[187] but Lawler and Marsden reported no such neoplasm in their study of 30 infant renal tumors.[118]

The gross appearance of clear cell sarcoma is similar to that of Wilms' tumor, but bilateral renal lesions have not been described (Fig. 11–18A).[131] The tumor has a pink to yellowish to gray-white, soft, lobulated appearance with bands of necrosis but only rarely hemorrhage.[174] There is sharp demarcation from the adjacent normal kidney. The principal sites of metastases, in decreasing order of frequency, are bone (in more than 50% of the cases), lungs, liver, and lymph nodes.[174] On microscopic examination, the tumor shows a characteristic monomorphous appearance consisting of rows of round to oval, clear-staining cells separated by delicate septa (Fig. 11–18B). The nuclei are small and irregular and have a fine chromatin pattern and a vesicular appearance. Mitoses are seldom noted. There is a prominent vascular component. Some tumors show parallel rows of cells or pallisading that is reminiscent of a schwannoma. Other histologic findings include areas of fibrosis and stromal hyalinization mimicking osteoid, an epithelial trabecular arrangement resembling tubules, a storiform pattern, and cyst formations.[174,176] The tumor seems to surround or push aside preexisting glomeruli and tubules, which have an embryonic, metaplastic appearance.

Although the neoplasm is thought to be a sarcoma, neither the ultrastructural findings nor immunoperoxidase analyses appear to support this view.[174] Of the various immunohistochemical reagents, vimentin appears to be the only one that is consistently reactive; tumor cells per se are unreactive with muscle and cytokeratin antibodies.[111] Ultrastructurally, the cells have a primitive appearance, containing a few polyribosomes, mitochondria, and rough endoplasmic reticulum with dilated cisternae filled with electron-lucent material.[111] Electron microscopic and immunohistochemical studies are not particularly helpful in establishing the diagnosis, but are useful in excluding other renal neoplasms.[139] According to Haas and colleagues and Pettinato et al., areas resembling clear cell sarcoma are found in some mesoblastic nephromas.[81,149] At present, the histogenesis of the former malignant lesion remains an enigma.

The overall prognosis for children with clear cell sarcoma of the kidney is generally poor.[13,174] According to the findings of the second Wilms' Tumor Study, the tumor metastasizes early, and most patients die from metastatic disease.[11] Nevertheless, the prognosis for this malignant lesion in patients younger than 3 months of age is surprisingly good. Table 11–7 shows that four of the five newborns with clear cell sarcoma who were culled from the literature were classified as having group (stage) I disease at the time of diagnosis; all survived, including a fifth patient (stage IV) with metastatic disease.

OSSIFYING RENAL TUMOR OF INFANCY

Approximately 10 cases of ossifying renal tumor of infancy have been reported.[40,99,173,198] Typically, infants (usually male) present with hematuria and a calcified renal lesion that is demonstrated by imaging studies.[173,198] Chatten and colleagues proposed the term ossifying tumor, and suggested that it is a benign neoplastic condition rather than a reactive process.[40]

In 1980, the Children's Hospital of Philadelphia group reported two male infants, ages 3 and 4 months, who presented with gross hematuria and a calcified mass in the upper pole collecting system of the left kidney.[40] One patient underwent an upper pole partial nephrectomy, whereas the other was treated with total nephrectomy plus actinomycin D; both patients survived. The specimens consisted of rock-hard masses measuring 2 to 3 cm in diameter.

A 6-day-old male infant reported by Jerkins and Callihan had three episodes of gross hematuria.[99] Computed tomography (CT) scanning revealed a mass within the mid- and upper-pole region of the left kidney that displaced the calyces. An irregular, firm, grey-tan mass measuring 2 × 1.5 cm was found in the upper pole of the nephrectomy specimen.

Wheeler and associates described an 18-month-old boy who presented with a history of intermittent, sterile hematuria since 3 months of age.[198] A calcified renal mass, which measured 2 × 1.5 cm, was discovered in the upper and lower parts of the right renal pelvis on imaging studies. The lesion was attached to a renal papilla by a broad pedicle and was excised at the base of the pedicle. The kidney was not resected, and the child had an uneventful recovery.

Perhaps the most extensive review on this subject was published by Sotelo-Avila, Beckwith, and Johnson, who studied nine cases, including 4 of their own.[173] They confirmed the findings of previous investigators—namely, that ossifying renal tumors contain three main components: osteoid, osteoblasts, and spindle cells.

On histologic examination, the ossyfying renal tumor consists of a central nidus of mineralized osteoid admixed with polygonal cells having a plump nucleus, large nucleolus, and eosinophilic to amphophilic cytoplasm, features which are consistent with osteoblasts. The islands of osteoid are surrounded by mesenchyme composed of spindle-shaped cells that blend imperceptibly with the surrounding medulla. The polygonal cells seem to arise from the spindle cells. Variable perivascular fibrosis is present. Mitotic figures and cytologic atypia are absent.[40,99,173,198] The immunohistochemical studies performed by Wheeler et al. revealed strong reactivity of the tumor cells with vimentin, but no staining of the tumor cells per se with either epithelial or vascular markers, which instead stained adjacent renal tubules and blood vessels, respectively.[198]

The histogenesis of this neoplasm has not been determined. Because the mesenchymal component of the ossifying tumor is similar to CMN, one premise is that this tumor may be an unusual variant of CMN.[99,198] However, Sotelo-Avila and co-workers suggest that the spindle cell component represents hyperplastic, intralobar, nephrogenic rests related to the developing urothelium of the papilla and collecting ducts.[173]

The preferred treatment of ossifying renal tumor is conservative, with preservation of as much renal parenchyma as possible.[173] Radiation therapy and chemotherapy are definitely contraindicated.

MISCELLANEOUS RENAL TUMORS

Gonzales-Crussi et al. described a 180-g, cystic renal mass that was removed from a 3-month-old male infant. The mass was composed of many blood-filled cavernous spaces. Microscopic examination revealed plump cells with round, vesicular nuclei and a reticulin fiber pattern, which was interpreted as a hemangioendothelioma.[75]

In addition to angiomyolipoma, a distinctive cystic lesion composed of plump, hyperplastic, eosinophilic cells arises in the kidneys of newborns with tuberous sclerosis.[19,178] An unusual clear cell tumor of the kidney that is distinctly different from either clear cell sarcoma or renal cell carcinoma has been reported in a 7-month-old boy.[70] The tumor consisted of lobules of clear cells with regular, small, oval nuclei with a fine chromatin pattern and inconspicuous nucleoli, with little or no mitotic activity. Murphy et al. regard this lesion as a "hydropic cell variant of nephroblastoma."[139]

Although renal cell carcinoma is the major malignant tumor of the kidney in adults, it is the subject of only sporadic case reports during the first year of life.[36,110,150,154,167] Possibly the youngest patient recorded with this malignant lesion was a 3-month-old male infant with bilateral nodular tumors, imperforate anus, and rectourethral fistula.[110] Clinically, patients with renal cell carcinoma experience a rapidly progressive downhill course, similar to that of their adult counterpart. The primary mode of therapy is complete surgical excision, which resulted in cure in a 1-year-old boy.[122,154]

REFERENCES

1. Afshan AA, Finlay JL, Gerald WL, et al. Congenital mesoblastic nephroma with metastasis to the brain: A case report. Am J Pediatr Hematol Oncol 1994;16:361.
2. Akhtar M, Sackey K, Bakry M, et al. Malignant rhabdoid tumor of the kidney presenting as intraocular metastases. Pediatr Hematol Oncol 1991;8:33.
3. Andrews MJ Jr, Askin FB, Fried FA, et al. Cystic partially differentiated nephroblastoma and polycystic Wilms' tumor: A spectrum of related clinical and pathologic entities. J Urol 1983;129:577.
3a. Andrews PE, Kelalis PP, Haase GM. Extrarenal Wilms' tumor: Results of the National Wilms' Tumor Study. J Pediatr Surg 1992;27:1181.
4. Angulo JC, Lopez JI, Ereno C, et al. Hydrops fetalis and congenital mesoblastic nephroma. Child Nephrol Urol 1991;11:115.
5. Appuzio JJ, Unwin W, Adhate A, et al. Prenatal diagnosis of fetal renal mesoblastic nephroma. Am J Obstet Gynecol 1986;154:636.
6. Aterman K, Boustani P, Gillis DA. Solitary multilocular cyst of the kidney. J Pediatr Surg 1973;8:505.
7. Bader JL, Miller RW. U.S. cancer incidence and mortality in the first year of life. Am J Dis Child 1979;133:157.
8. Baldauf MC, Schulz DM. Multilocular cyst of the kidney: Report of three cases and review of the literature. Am J Clin Pathol 1976;65:93.
9. Barrantes JC, Toyn C, Muir KR, et al. Congenital mesoblastic nephroma: Possible prognostic and management value of assessing DNA content. J Clin Pathol 1991;44:317.
10. Beckwith JB. Mesenchymal renal neoplasm of infancy revisited. J Pediatr Surg 1974;9:803.
11. Beckwith JB. Pathological aspects of renal tumors in childhood. In Broecker BH, Klein FA (eds): Pediatric Tumors of the Genitourinary Tract, p 25. New York: Alan R. Liss, 1988.
12. Beckwith JB. Precursor lesions of Wilms' tumor: Clinical and biological implications. Med Pediatr Oncol 1993;21:158.
13. Beckwith JB. Wilms' tumor and other renal tumors of childhood: A selective review from the National Wilms' Tumor Study Pathology Center. Hum Pathol 1983;14:481.
14. Beckwith JB. Wilms' tumor and other tumors of childhood. In Finegold M (ed): Pathology of Neoplasia in Children and Adolescents, Major Problems in Pathology, Vol 18, p 232. Philadelphia: WB Saunders, 1986.
15. Beckwith JB, Kiviat NB. Multilocular renal cysts and cystic renal tumors. Am J Roentgenol 1980;136:435.
16. Beckwith JB, Kiviat NB, Bonadio JF. Nephrogenic rests, nephroblastomatosis, and the pathogenesis of Wilms' tumor. Pediatr Pathol 1990;10:1.
17. Beckwith JB, Palmer NF. Histopathology and prognosis of Wilms' tumor. Results of the first National Wilms' Tumor Study. Cancer 1978;41:1937.
18. Beckwith JB, Weeks DA. Congenital mesoblastic nephroma. When should we worry? Arch Pathol Lab Med 1986;110:98.
19. Bernstein J, Kissane JM. Hereditary disorders of the kidney. Perspect Pediatr Pathol 1973;1:132.
20. Berry PJ. Congenital tumours. In Keeling JW (ed): Fetal and Neonatal Pathology, 2nd ed, p 273. Berlin: Springer-Verlag, 1993.
21. Blank E, Neerhout RC, Burry KA. Congenital mesoblastic nephroma and polyhydramnios. J Am Med Assoc 1978;240:1504.
22. Boggs LK, Kimmelstiel P. Benign multilocular cystic nephroma: Report of two cases of so-called multilocular cyst of kidney. J Urol 1956;76:530.
23. Bolande RP. Commentary: Multicystic nephroma, what it is and its relationship to Wilms' tumor. Pediatr Radiol 1982;12:46.
24. Bolande RP. Congenital and infantile neoplasia of the kidney. Lancet 1974;2:1497.
25. Bolande RP. Developmental pathology. Am J Pathol 1979;94:627.
26. Bolande RP. Neoplasia of early life and its relationships to teratogenesis. In Rosenberg HS, Bolande RP (eds): Perspectives in Pediatric Pathology, Vol 3, p 145. Chicago: Year Book Medical Publishers, 1976.
27. Bolande RP, Brough JA, Izant RJ. Congenital mesoblastic nephroma of infancy: A report of 8 cases and the relationship to Wilms' tumor. Pediatrics 1967;40:272.

28. Bond JV. Wilms' tumour, hypospadias, and crpytorchidism in twins. Arch Dis Child 1977;52:243.

29. Bonnin JM, Rubenstein LJ, Palmer NF, et al. The association of embryonal tumors originating in the kidney and in the brain: A report of seven cases. Cancer 1984; 54:2137.

30. Bove KE, Koffler H, McAdams AJ. Nodular renal blastema: Definition and possible significance. Cancer 1969;24:323.

31. Bove KE, McAdams JA. The nephroblastomatosis complex and its relationship to Wilms' tumor: A clinicopathologic treatise. *In* Rosenberg HS, Bolande RP (eds): Perspectives in Pediatric Pathology, Vol 3, p 185. Chicago: Year Book Medical Publishers, 1976.

32. Broadbent VA. Malignant disease in the neonate. *In* Roberton NRC (ed): Textbook of Neonatology, 2nd ed, p 879. Edinburgh: Churchill Livingstone, 1992.

33. Cairney AEL, Greenberg M, Weksberg R. Wilms' tumor in three patients with Bloom syndrome. J Pediatr 1987;11:414.

34. Campbell AN, Chan HSL, O'Brien A, et al. Malignant tumours in the neonate. Arch Dis Child 1987;62:19.

35. Carpenter PM, Mascarello JT, Krous HF, et al. Congenital mesoblastic nephroma: Cytogenetic comparison to leiomyoma. Pediatr Pathol 1993;13:435.

36. Castellanos RD, Aron BS, Evans AT. Renal adenocarcinoma in children. Incidence, therapy and prognosis. J Urol 1974;111:534.

37. Chan HSL, Cheng M-Y, Mancer K et al. Congenital mesoblastic nephroma: A clinicoradiologic study of 17 cases representing the pathologic spectrum of the disease. J Pediatr 1987;111:64.

38. Chatten J. Epithelial differentiation in Wilms' tumor: A clinicopathologic appraisal. Perspect Pediatr Pathol 1976;3:225.

39. Chatten J, Bishop HC. Bilateral multilocular cysts of the kidney. J Pediatr Surg 1977;12:749.

40. Chatten J, Cromie WJ, Duckett JW. Ossifying tumor of infantile kidney: Report of two cases. Cancer 1980; 45:609.

41. Christmann D, Becmeur F, Marcellin L, et al. Mesoblastic nephroma presenting as a haemorragic cyst. Pediatr Radiol 1990;20:553.

42. Chung CJ, Cammoun D, Munden M. Rhabdoid tumor of the kidney presenting as an abdominal mass in a newborn. Pediatr Radiol 1990;20:562.

43. Coffin CM, Dehner LP. Congenital tumors. *In* Stocker JT, Dehner LP (eds): Pediatric Pathology, Vol 1, p 325. Philadelphia: JB Lippincott, 1992.

44. Coffin CM, Dehner LP. Nodular renal blastema and thanatophoric dwarfism. A newly reported association. Am J Pediatr Hematol Oncol 1982;4:428.

45. Coppes MJ, Sohl H, Teshima IE, et al. Wilms' tumor in a patient with Prader-Willi syndrome. J Pediatr 1993;122:730.

46. Craver R, Dimmick J, Johnson H, et al. Congenital obstructive uropathy and nodular renal blastema. J Urol 1986;136:305.

46a. Crom DB, Wilimas JA, Green AA, et al. Malignancy in the neonate. Med Pediatr Oncol 1989;17:101.

47. D'Angio GJ, Breslow N, Beckwith B, et al. Treatment of Wilms' tumor: Results of the third National Wilms' Tumor Study. Cancer 1989;64:349.

48. Datnow B, Daniel WW Jr. Polycystic nephroblastoma. JAMA 1976;236:2528.

49. Davis CF, Carachi R, Young DG. Neonatal tumors: Glasgow 1966–86. Arch Dis Child 63:1075, 1988.

50. deChadarevian J, Fletcher BD, Chatten J, et al. Massive infantile nephroblastomatosis: A clinical, radiological, and pathological analysis of four cases. Cancer 1977;39:2294.

51. Dehner LP: Neoplasms of the fetus and neonate. *In* Naeye RL, Kissane JM, Kaufman N (eds): Perinatal Diseases, International Academy of Pathology, Monograph No. 22, p 286. Baltimore: Williams and Wilkins, 1981.

52. Dimmick JE, Johnson HW, Coleman GU, et al. Wilms' tumorlet, nodular renal blastema and multicystic renal dysplasia. J Urol 1989;142:484.

53. Dorai CRT, Boucaut HAP, Le Quesne GW, et al. Unilateral cystic, partially differentiated nephroblastoma with nephroblastomatosis. Pediatr Surg Int 1994;9: 137.

54. Eftekhari F, Erly WK, Jaffe N. Malignant rhabdoid tumor of the kidney: Imaging features in two cases. Pediatr Radiol 1990;21:39.

55. Favara BE, Johnson W, Ito J. Renal tumors in the neonatal period. Cancer 1968;22:845.

56. Fobi M, Mahour GH, Isaacs H Jr. Multilocular cyst of the kidney. J Pediatr Surg 1979;14:282.

57. Fraumeni JF, Glass AG. Wilms' tumor and congenital aniridia. JAMA 1968;206:825.

58. Fu Y-S, Kay S. Congenital mesoblastic nephroma and its recurrence. Arch Pathol 1973;196:66.

59. Fung CHK, Gonzalez-Crussi F, Yonan TN, Martinez N. Rhabdoid Wilms' tumor: An ultrastructural study. Arch Pathol Lab Med 1981;105:521.

60. Gaddy CD, Gibbons MD, Gonzales ET Jr, et al. Obstructive uropathy, renal dysplasia and nodular renal blastema: Is there a relationship to Wilms' tumor? J Urol 1985;134:330.

60a. Gale GB, D'Angio GJ, Uri A, et al. Cancer in neonates: The experience at the Children's Hospital of Philadelphia. Pediatrics 1982;70:409.

61. Gallo GE, Chemes HE. The association of Wilms' tumor, pseudohermaphroditism and diffuse glomerular disease (Drash syndrome): Report of eight cases with clinical and morphologic findings and review of the literature. Pediatr Pathol 1987;7:175.

62. Gallo GE, Penchansky L. Cystic nephroma. Cancer 1977;39:1322.

63. Gansler T, Gerald W, Anderson G, et al. Characterization of a cell line derived from rhabdoid tumor of the kidney. Hum Pathol 1991;22:259.

64. Garmel SH, Crombleholme TM, Semple JP, et al. Prenatal diagnosis and management of fetal tumors. Semin Perinatol 1994;18:350.

65. Gaulier A, Boccon-Gibod L, Sabatier P, et al. Panlobar nephroblastomatosis with cystic dysplasia: An unusual case with diffuse renal involvement studied by immunohistochemistry. Pediatr Pathol 1993;13:741.

66. Gerber A, Gold JH, Bustamante S, et al. Congenital mesoblastic nephroma. J Pediatr Surg 1981;16:758.

67. Giangiacomo J, Kissane JM. Congenital Wilms' tumor. *In* Pochedly C, Baum ES, eds: Wilms' Tumor: Clinical and Biological Manifestations, p 103. New York: Elsevier, 1984.

68. Giangiacomo J, Penchansky L, Monteleone PL, et al. Bilateral neonatal Wilms' tumor with B–C chromosomal translocation. J Pediatr 1975;86:98.

69. Giulian BB. Prenatal ultrasonographic diagnosis of fetal renal tumors. Radiology 1984;152:69.

70. Glick AD, Tham KT, Leung NK, et al. Unusual clear cell tumor of the kidney in infancy. Am J Surg Pathol 1981;5:581.

71. Goldman SM, Garfinkel DJ, Oh KS, et al. The Drash

syndrome: Male pseudohermaphroditism, nephritis and Wilms' tumor. Radiology 1981;141:87.

71a. Gonzalez-Crussi F, Baum ES. Renal sarcomas of childhood. A clinicopathologic and ultrastructural study. Cancer 1983;51:898.

72. Gonzalez-Crussi F, Hsueh W, Ugarte N. Rhabdomyogenesis in renal neoplasia of childhood. Am J Surg Pathol 1981;5:525.

73. Gonzalez-Crussi F, Kidd JM, Hernandez RJ. Cystic nephroma: Morphologic spectrum and implications. Urology 1982;20:88.

74. Gonzalez-Crussi F, Sotelo-Avila C, Kidd JM. Malignant mesenchymal nephroma of infancy. Am J Surg Pathol 1980;4:185.

75. Gonzalez-Crussi F, Sotelo-Avila C, Kidd JM. Mesenchymal renal tumors in infancy: A reappraisal. Hum Pathol 1981;12:78.

76. Gormley TS, Skoog SJ, Jones RV, et al. Cellular congenital mesoblastic nephroma: What are the options? J Urol 1989;142:479.

77. Gray ES. Mesoblastic nephroma and non-immunological hydrops fetalis (Letter). Pediatr Pathol 1989;9:607.

78. Green DM, D'Angio GJ, Beckwith JB, et al. Wilms' tumor (nephroblastoma, renal embryoma). *In* Pizzo PA, Poplack DG (eds): Principles and Practice of Pediatric Oncology, 2nd ed, p 713. Philadelphia: JB Lippincott, 1993.

79. Greenberg F, Copeland K, Gresik MV. Expanding the spectrum of the Perlman syndrome. Am J Med Genet 1988;29:773.

80. Gururangan S, Bowman LC, Parham DM, et al. Primary extracranial rhabdoid tumors: Clinicopathologic features and response to ifosfamide. Cancer 1993;71:2653.

81. Haas JE, Bonadio JF, Beckwith JB. Clear cell sarcoma of the kidney with emphasis on ultrastructural studies. Cancer 1984;54:2978.

82. Haas JE, Palmer NF, Weinberg AG, et al. Ultrastructure of malignant rhabdoid tumor of the kidney: A distinctive renal tumor of children. Hum Pathol 1981;12:646.

83. Haddy TB, Bailie MD, Bernstein J, et al. Bilateral, diffuse nephroblastomatosis: Report of a case managed with chemotherapy. J Pediatr 1977;90:784.

84. Heidelberger KP, Ritchey ML, Dauser RC, et al. Congenital mesoblastic nephroma metastatic to brain. Cancer 1993;72:2499.

85. Heideman RL, McGavran L, Waldstein G. Nephroblastomatosis and deletion of 11p: The potential etiologic relationship to subsequent Wilms' tumor. Am J Pediatr Hematol Oncol 1986;8:231.

86. Henderson SC, Van Kolken RJ, Rahatzad M. Multicystic kidney with hydramnios. J Clin Ultrasound 1980;8:249.

87. Hilton C, Keeling JW. Neonatal renal tumors. Br J Urol 1973;46:157.

88. Hou LT, Holman RL. Bilateral nephroblastomatosis in a premature infant. J Pathol Bacteriol 1961;82:249.

89. Howell CG, Otherson HB, Kiviat NE, et al. Therapy and outcome in 51 children with mesoblastic nephroma: A report of the National Wilms' Tumor Study. J Pediatr Surg 1982;17:826.

90. Hrabovsky EE, Othersen HB, deLorimer A Jr, et al. Wilms' tumor in the neonate: A report from the National Wilms' Tumor Study. J Pediatr Surg 1986;21:385.

91. Isaacs H Jr. Congenital malignant tumors. *In* Reed GB, Claireaux AE, Bain AD (eds): Diseases of the Fetus and Newborn: Pathology, Radiology and Genetics, p 131. London: Chapman Hall, 1989.

92. Isaacs H Jr. Congenital and neonatal malignant tumors: A 28-year experience at Children's Hospital of Los Angeles. Am J Pediatr Hematol/Oncol 1987;9(2):121.

93. Isaacs H Jr. Neoplasms in infants: A report of 265 cases. Pathol Annu 1983;18(2):165.

94. Isaacs H Jr. Perinatal (congenital and neonatal) neoplasms: A report of 110 cases. Pediatr Pathol 1985;3:165.

95. Isaacs H Jr. Tumors. *In* Gilbert-Barness E (ed): Potter's Pathology of the Fetus and Infant. Vol 2, p 1242. St. Louis: Mosby–Year Book, 1996.

96. Isaacs H Jr: Tumors of the Newborn and Infant. St. Louis: Mosby–Year Book, 1991.

97. Jadresic L, Leake J, Gordon I, et al. Clinicopathologic review of twelve children with nephropathy, Wilms' tumor, and genital abnormalities (Drash syndrome). J Pediatr 1990;117:717.

98. Jayabose S, Iqbal K, Newman L, et al. Hypercalcemia in childhood renal tumors. Cancer 1988;61:788.

99. Jerkins GR, Callihan TR. Ossifying renal tumor of infancy. J Urol 1986;135:120.

100. Joshi VV. Cystic partially differentiated nephroblastoma: An entity in the spectrum of infantile renal neoplasia. Perspect Pediatr Pathol 1979;5:217.

101. Joshi VV, Banerjee AK, Yadav K, et al. Cystic partially differentiated nephroblastoma: An entity in the spectrum of infantile renal neoplasia. Cancer 1977;40:789.

102. Joshi VV, Beckwith JB. Multilocular cyst of the kidney (cystic nephroma) and cystic partially differentiated nephroblastoma: Terminology and criteria for diagnosis. Cancer 1989;64:466.

103. Joshi VV, Kay S, Milsten R. Congenital mesoblastic nephroma of infancy: Report of a case with unusual clinical behavior. Am J Clin Pathol 1973;60:811.

104. Joshi VV, Kaznicka J, Walters TR. Atypical mesoblastic nephroma: Pathologic characterization of a potentially aggressive variant of conventional congenital mesoblastic nephroma. Arch Pathol Lab Med 1986;110:100.

105. Kajtar P, Weisenbach J, Mehes K. Association of Wilms' tumour with spina bifida occulta. Eur J Pediatr 1990;149:594.

106. Kalousek DK, de Chadarevian JP, Mackie GG, et al. Metastatic infantile Wilms' tumor and hydrocephalus: A case report with a review of the literature. Cancer 1977;39:1312.

107. Kelly DR. Cystic cellular mesoblastic nephroma. Pediatr Pathol 1985;4:157.

108. King DR, Buck D, Kleinman PB, et al. Congenital mesoblastic nephroma. Am J Dis Child 1978;132:1139.

109. Kinoshita T, Nakamura Y, Kinoshita M, et al. Bilateral cystic nephroblastomas and botryoid sarcoma in a child with Dandy-Walker syndrome. Arch Pathol Lab Med 1986;110:150.

110. Kobayashi A, Hoshino H, Ohbe Y, et al. Bilateral renal cell carcinoma. Arch Dis Child 1970;45:141.

111. Kodet R, Stejskal J, Malis J, et al. Bone metastasizing renal tumor of childhood: A clinicopathological study of eleven cases from the Prague Pediatric Tumor Registry. Pathol Res Pract 1994;190:750.

112. Koop CE. Abdominal mass in the newborn infant. N Engl J Med 1973;289:569.

113. Koufos A, Grundy P, Morgan K, et al. Familial Wiede-

mann-Beckwith syndrome and a second Wilms' tumor locus both map to 11p15.5. Am J Hum Genet 1989; 44:711.

114. Kulkarni R, Bailie MD, Bernstein J. Progression of nephroblastomatosis to Wilms' tumor. J Pediatr 1980; 96:178.

115. Kumar APM, Pratt CB, Coburn TP, et al. Treatment strategy for nodular renal blastema and nephroblastomatosis associated with Wilms' tumor. J Pediatr Surg 1978;13:281.

116. Kurtz SM. A unique ultrastructural variant of Wilms' tumor: Its possible histogenetic implications. Am J Surg Pathol 1979;3:257.

117. Larson DM. Congenital mesoblastic nephroma. Am J Dis Child 1978;132:318.

118. Lawler W, Marsden HB. Bone metastases in children presenting with renal tumors. J Clin Pathol 1979;32:608.

119. Lemerle J, Tournade MF, Gerard-Marchant R, et al. Wilms' tumor: Natural history and prognostic factors. A retrospective study of 248 cases. Cancer 1976;37:2557.

120. Li FP, Williams WR, Gimbrere K, et al. Heritable fraction of unilateral Wilms' tumor. Pediatrics 1988;81:147.

121. Liban E, Kozenitzky IL. Metanephric hamartomas and nephroblastomatosis in siblings. Cancer 1970;25:885.

122. MacArthur CA, Isaacs H Jr, Miller JH, et al. Pediatric renal cell carcinoma: A complete response to recombinant interleukin-2 in a child with metastatic disease at diagnosis. Med Pediatr Oncol 1994;23:365.

123. Machin GA. Nephroblastomatosis and multiple bilateral nephroblastomata. Arch Pathol Lab Med 1978; 102:639.

124. Machin GA. Persistent renal blastema (nephroblastomatosis) as a frequent precursor of Wilms' tumor: A pathological and clinical review. Am J Pediatr Hematol/Oncol 1980;2:253, 353.

125. Magee JF, McFadden DE, Pantzar JT. Congenital tumors. In Dimmick JE, Kalousek DK (eds): Developmental Pathology of the Embryo and Fetus, p 235. Philadelphia: JB Lippincott, 1992.

126. Mahoney JP, Saffos RO. Fetal rhabdomyomatous nephroblastoma with a renal pelvic mass simulating sarcoma botryoides. Am J Surg Pathol 1981;5:297.

127. Malone PS, Duffy PG, Ransley PG, et al. Congenital mesoblastic nephroma, renin production, and hypertension. J Pediatr Surg 1989;24:599.

128. Manivel JC, Sibley RK, Dehner LP. Complete and incomplete Drash syndrome: A clinicopathologic study of five cases of a dysontogenetic-neoplastic complex. Hum Pathol 1987;18:80.

129. Mankad VN, Gray GF Jr, Miller DR. Bilateral nephroblastomatosis and Klippel-Trenaunay syndrome. Cancer 1974;33:1462.

130. Marsden HB, Lawler W. Primary renal tumors in the first year of life: A population based review. Virchows Arch [A] 1983;399:1.

131. Marsden HB, Lawler W, Kumar PM. Bone metastasizing renal tumor of childhood. Morphological and clinical characteristics from Wilms' tumor. Cancer 1978;42:1922.

132. Marsden HB, Lennox EL, Lawler W, et al. Bone metastases in childhood tumours. Br J Cancer 1980;41:875.

133. Mascarello JT, Cajulis TR, Krous HF, et al. Presence or absence of trisomy 11 is correlated with histologic subtype in congenital mesoblastic nephroma. Cancer Genet Cytogenet 1994;77:50.

134. Matsumura M, Nishi T, Sasaki Y, et al. Prenatal diagnosis and treatment strategy for congenital mesoblastic nephroma. J Pediatr Surg 1993;28:1607.

135. Meadows AT, Lichtenfeld JL, Koop CE. Wilms' tumor in three children of a woman with congenital hemihypertrophy. N Engl J Med 1974;291:23.

136. Miller RW, Fraumeni JF Jr, Manning MD. Association of Wilms' tumor with aniridia, hemihypertrophy and other congenital malformations. N Engl J Med 1964; 270:922.

137. Moore KL. The Developing Human: Clinically Oriented Embryology, 5th ed. Philadelphia: WB Saunders, 1993.

138. Murata T, Yoshida T, Takanari H, et al. Bilateral diffuse nephroblastomatosis, pancortical type: A case report with immunohistochemical investigations. Arch Pathol Lab Med 1989;113:729.

139. Murphy WM, Beckwith JB, Farrow GM. Tumors of the Kidney, Bladder, and Related Structures, Atlas of Tumor Pathology, Fascicle No. 11, Washington, DC. Armed Forces Institute of Pathology, 1994.

140. Nicholson DA, Gupta SC. Case report: Congenital mesoblastic nephroma occurring in a solitary kidney. Clin Radiol 1990;41:211.

141. Nisen PD, Rich MA, Gloster E, et al. N-myc oncogene expression in histopathologically unrelated bilateral pediatric renal tumors. Cancer 1987;61:1821.

142. Oddone M, Marino C, Sergi C, et al. Wilms' tumor arising in a multicystic kidney. Pediatr Radiol 1994; 24:236.

143. Ohmichi M, Tasaka K, Sugita N, et al. Hydramnios associated with congenital mesoblastic nephroma: A case report. Obstet Gynecol 1989;74:469.

144. Palmer N, Evans AE. The association of aniridia and Wilms' tumor: Methods of surveillance and diagnosis. Med Pediatr Oncol 1983;11:73.

145. Parkes SE, Muir KR, Southern L, et al. Neonatal tumours: A thirty-year population based study. Med Pediatr Oncol 1994;22:309.

146. Pastore G, Carli M, Lemerle J, et al. Epidemiological features of Wilms' tumor. Results of studies by the International Society of Paediatric Oncology (SIOP). Med Pediatr Oncol 1988;16:7.

147. Perlman M, Goldberg GM, Bar-Ziv J, et al. Renal hamartomas and nephroblastomatosis with fetal gigantism: A familial syndrome. J Pediatr 1973;83:414.

148. Perlman M, Levin M, Wittels B. Syndrome of fetal gigantism, renal hamartomas, and nephroblastomatosis with Wilms' tumor. Cancer 1975;35:1212.

149. Pettinato G, Manivel JC, Wick MR, et al. Classical and cellular (atypical) congenital mesoblastic nephroma: A clinicopathologic, ultrastructural, immunohistochemical and flow cytometric study. Hum Pathol 1989;20:682.

150. Pochedly C, Suwansirikul S, Penzer P. Renal-cell carcinoma with extrarenal manifestations in a ten-month-old child. Am J Dis Child 1971;121:528.

151. Potter EL. Normal and Abnormal Development of the Kidney, p 154. Chicago: Year Book Medical Publishers, 1972.

152. Potter EL, Craig JM. Pathology of the Fetus and Infant, 3rd ed, p 177. Chicago: Year Book Medical Publishers, 1975.

153. Procainoy RS, Giacomini CB, Mattos TC, et al. Congenital Wilms' tumor associated with consumption co-

agulopathy and hyperbilirubinemia. J Pediatr Surg 1986;21:993.

154. Raney RB Jr, Palmer N, Sutow WW, et al. Renal cell carcinoma in children. Med Pediat Oncol 1983;11:91.

155. Regalado JJ, Rodriquez MM, Bruce JH, et al. Bilateral hyperplastic nephromegaly, nephroblastomatosis, and renal dysplasia in a newborn: A variety of universal nephroblastomatosis. Pediatr Pathol 1994;14:421.

156. Reinberg Y, Anderson GF, Franciosi R, et al. Wilms' tumor and the VATER association. J Urol 1988;140:787.

157. Riccardi VM, Hittner H, Francke U. Aniridia caused by a heritable chromosome 11 deletion. Ophthalmol 1979;86:1173.

158. Riccardi VM, Sujansky E, Smith AC, et al. Chromosomal imbalance in the Aniridia-Wilms' tumor association: 11p interstitial deletion. Pediatrics 1978;61:604.

159. Richmond H, Dougall AJ. Neonatal renal tumors. J Pediatr Surg 1970;5:413.

160. Ritchey ML, Azizkhan RG, Beckwith JB, et al. Neonatal Wilms' tumor. J Pediatr Surg 1995;30:856.

161. Rous SN, Bailie MD, Kaufman DB, et al. Nodular renal blastema, nephroblastomatosis, and Wilms' tumor. Different points on the same disease spectrum? Urology 1976;8:599.

162. Rousseau-Merck MF, Nogues C, Nezelof C, et al. Infantile renal tumors with hypercalcemia. Characterization of intermediate filament clusters. Arch Pathol Lab Med 1983;107:311.

163. Rousseau-Merck MF, Nogues C, Roth A, et al. Hypercalcemic infantile renal tumors: Morphological, clinical and biological heterogeneity. Pediatr Pathol 1985;3:155.

164. Rubie H, Baunin C, Guitard J, et al. Tumeurs neonatales malignes. Rev Prat (Paris) 1993;43(17):2208.

165. Rutledge J, Beckwith JB, Benjamin D, et al. Absence of immunoperoxidase staining for myoglobin in the malignant rhabdoid tumor of the kidney. Pediatr Pathol 1983;1:93.

166. Sandstedt B, Delemarre JFM, Krul EJ, et al. Mesoblastic nephromas: A study of 29 tumours from the SIOP nephroblastoma file. Histopathology 1985;9:741.

167. Senga Y, Taguchi H, Aso T, et al. Undifferentiated renal cell carcinoma in infancy: Report of a case and review of the literature. Pediatr Pathol 1986;5:157.

168. Shannon RS, Mann JR, Harper E, et al. Wilms' tumor and aniridia: Clinical and cytogenetic features. Arch Dis Child 1982;57:685.

169. Shen SC, Yunis EJ. A study of the cellularity and ultrastructure of congenital mesoblastic nephroma. Cancer 1980;45:306.

170. Shimao S, Suzuki Y, Okada T. A case of bilateral Wilms' tumour of the kidneys and the retrourethral region. Eur J Pediatr 1984;143:158.

171. Slasky BS, Penkrot RJ, Bron KM. Cystic mesoblastic nephroma. Urology 1982;19:220.

172. Snyder HM, Lack EE, Chetty-Baktavizian A, et al. Congenital mesoblastic nephroma: Relationship to other renal tumors of infancy. J Urol 1981;126:513.

173. Sotelo-Avila C, Beckwith JB, Johnson JE. Ossifying renal tumor of infancy: A clinopathologic study of nine cases. Pediatr Pathol 1995;15:745.

174. Sotelo-Avila C, Gonzalez-Crussi F, deMello D, et al. Renal and extrarenal tumors in children: A clinicopathologic study of 14 patients. Semin Diagn Pathol 1986;3:151.

175. Sotelo-Avila C, Gonzalez-Crussi F, Fowler JW. Complete and incomplete forms of Beckwith-Wiedemann syndrome. Their oncogenic potential. J Pediatr 1980;96:47.

176. Sotelo-Avila C, Gonzalez-Crussi F, Sadowinski S, et al. Clear cell sarcoma of the kidney: A clinicopathologic study of 21 patients with long-term follow-up evaluation. Hum Pathol 1986;16:1219.

177. Sotelo-Avila C, Gooch WM. Neoplasms associated with the Beckwith-Wiedemann syndrome. *In* Rosenberg HS, Bolande RP (eds): Perspectives in Pediatric Pathology, Vol 3, p 255. Chicago: Year Book Medical Publishers, 1976.

178. Stapleton FB, Johnson D, Kaplan GW, et al. The cystic renal lesion of tuberous sclerosis. J Pediatr 1980;97:574.

179. Steinfeld AD, Crowley CA, O'Shea PA, et al. Recurrent and metastatic mesoblastic nephroma in infancy. J Clin Oncol 1984;2:956.

180. Stone MM, Beaver BL, Sun C-CJ, et al. The nephroblastomatosis complex and its relationship to Wilms' tumor. J Pediatr Surg 1990;25:933.

181. Suzuki H, Honzumi M, Itoh Y, et al. Clear-cell sarcoma of the kidney seen in a 3-day-old newborn. Z Kinderchir 1983;38:422.

182. Takagi M, Takakuwa T, Ushigome S, et al. Sarcomatous variants of Wilms' tumor: Immunohistochemical and ultrastructural comparison with classical Wilms' tumor. Cancer 1987;59:963.

183. Tang TT, Harb JM, Oechler HW, et al. Multilocular renal cyst: Electron microscopic evidence of pathogenesis. Am J Pediatr Hematol Oncol 1984;6:27.

184. Telander RL, Gilchrist GS, Burgert EO, et al. Bilateral massive nephroblastomatosis in infancy. J Pediatr Surg 1978;13:163.

185. Tomlinson GE, Argyle JC, Velasco S, et al. Molecular characterization of congenital mesoblastic nephroma and its distinction from Wilms' tumor. Cancer 1992;70:2358.

186. Tsuchida Y, Shimizu K, Hata J, et al. Renin production in congenital mesoblastic nephroma in comparison with that in Wilms' tumor. Pediatr Pathol 1993;13:155.

187. Ugarte N, Gonzalez-Crussi F, Hsueh W. Wilms' tumor: Its morphology under 1 year of age. Cancer 1981;48:346.

188. Uson AC, Rosario CD, Malicon MM. Wilms' tumor in association with cystic renal disease: Report of two cases. J Urol 1960;83:262.

189. Uzoaru I, Podbielski FJ, Chou P, et al. Familial adenomatous polyposis coli and clear cell sarcoma of the kidney. Pediatr Pathol 1993;13:133.

190. Vido L, Carli M, Rizzoni G, Calo L, et al. Congenital mesoblastic nephroma with hypercalcemia: Pathogenic role of prostaglandins. Am J Pediatr Hematol/Oncol 1986;8:149.

191. Vogel AM, Gown AM, Caughlan J, et al. Rhabdoid tumors of the kidney contain mesenchymal specific and epithelial specific intermediate filament proteins. Lab Invest 1984;50:232.

192. Waisman J, Cooper PH. Renal neoplasms of the newborn. J Pediatr Surg 1970;5:407.

193. Walker D, Richard GA. Fetal hamartoma of the kidney: Recurrence and death of a patient. J Urol 1973;110:352.

194. Weeks DA, Beckwith JB, Mierau GW, et al. Rhabdoid tumor of the kidney: A report of 11 cases from the National Wilms' Tumor Study Pathology Center. Am J Surg Pathol 1989;13:439.

195. Weinberg AG, Currarino G, Hurt GE Jr. Botryoid

Wilms' tumor of the renal pelvis. Arch Pathol Lab Med 1984;108:147.

196. Werb P, Scurry J, Ostor A, et al. Survey of congenital tumors in perinatal necropsies. Pathology 24:247, 1992.

197. Wexler HA, Poole CA, Fojaco RM. Metastatic neonatal Wilms' tumor: A case report with review of the literature. Pediatr Radiol 1975;3:179.

198. Wheeler RA, Moore IE, Atwell JD. An infantile ossifying renal tumour. Pediatr Surg Int 1994;9:135.

199. Wienk MATP, van Geijn HP, Copray FJA, et al. Prenatal diagnosis of fetal tumors by ultrasonography. Obstet Gynecol Surv 1990;45:639.

200. Wigger HJ. Fetal hamartoma of kidney: A benign symptomatic, congenital tumor, not a form of Wilms' tumor. Am J Clin Pathol 1969;51:323.

201. Wigger HJ. Fetal rhabdomyomatous nephroblastoma—A variant of Wilms' tumor. Hum Pathol 1976; 7:613.

202. Willis RA: The Borderland of Embryology and Pathology, 2nd ed. London: Butterworths, 1962.

203. Wockel W, Scheibner K, Lageman A. A variant of the Wiedemann-Beckwith syndrome. Eur J Pediatr 1981; 135:319.

204. Yazaki T, Akimoto M, Tsuboi N, et al. Congenital mesoblastic nephroma. Urology 1982;20:446.

205. Yokomori K, Hori T, Takemura T, et al. Demonstration of both primary and secondary renism in renal tumors in children. J Pediatr Surg 1988;23:403.

206. Young G, L'Heureux P, Dehner LP. Cystic nephroma (so-called polycystic Wilms' tumor) of childhood. A CT study. Am J Pediatr Hematol/Oncol 1979;1:179.

207. Zach TL, Cifuentes RF, Strom RL. Congenital mesoblastic nephroma, hemorrhagic shock and disseminated intravascular coagulation in a newborn infant. Am J Perinatol 1991;8:203.

LIVER TUMORS

12

Tumors and tumor-like conditions of the liver occur infrequently in the perinatal period, accounting for approximately 5% of the total number of neoplasms of various types occurring in the fetus and newborn (see Table 1–1).[9–11,23,67,107,144] Hemangioma is the most common of the primary hepatic tumors and tumor-like conditions, followed by mesenchymal hamartoma and hepatoblastoma (Table 12–1).[23,25,66,82,107] All three entities present clinically as an abdominal mass and can be detected antenatally by sonography.[42,118]

Including the total number of surgical and autopsy specimens, most hepatic lesions are metastatic rather than primary.[16,25] Neuroblastoma is the tumor that metastasizes most often to the liver in the fetus and newborn, followed by leukemia.[25,65,67] Yolk sac tumor arising from a sacrococcygeal teratoma and rhabdoid tumor of the kidney are additional examples of malignant lesions that can metastasize to the liver in this age group.[25,66]

During the first year of life, hepatoblastoma, rather than hepatocellular carcinoma, is the principal primary malignant hepatic tumor.[15,66,68,143] Hepatocellular carcinoma rarely occurs in patients younger than 6 years of age.[68,73,92,138] One of the few cases reported was a hepatocellular carcinoma occurring in a neonate with macronodular cirrhosis.[92]

The classification of liver tumors and tumor-like conditions used in this chapter is presented in Table 12–2.

EMBRYOLOGY

More than 30 years ago, Willis proposed that the liver blastema was capable of forming both epithelial and mesenchymal elements, resulting in variable predominance of one or more of these components.[147] He thought that this event might explain the wide variety of tumors and tumor-like conditions arising from the liver. It would be appropriate, then, at this juncture, to review briefly the embryology of the liver.

In the 4-week embryo, the liver, gallbladder, and bile ducts originate from the caudal portion of the foregut as a ventral bud of endoderm called the hepatic diverticulum.[98] The diverticulum expands into the mesenchyme (mesoderm) of the septum transversum as a mass of rapidly growing cells. The hepatic diverticulum develops into the liver cell cords, and the epithelial lining of the bile ducts and the mesenchyme of the septum transversum form the fibrous tissue, hematopoietic elements, and Kupffer cells (Fig. 12–1).[98]

HEMANGIOMA OF THE LIVER

Most hepatic hemangiomas are diagnosed before 6 months of age, and almost 50% appear within the first week of life (Figs. 12–2 and 12–3).[23,25,27,29,36,38,47,81,87,95,130,131,144] More hemangiomas occur in the liver than are actually recorded because many are asymptomatic or "silent" conditions that regress or are discovered as incidental clinical, imaging, or postmortem findings.[25] Some hemangiomas cause hepatomegaly or a mass lesion, whereas others may be life-threatening in the perinatal period owing to rupture and hemoperitoneum during delivery or high-output cardiac failure (see Fig. 12–3).[5,22,26,27,83,95,118,131,143] Other associated findings may include consumptive coagulopathy re-

Table 12–1. Newborn Hepatic Tumors and Tumor-Like Conditions, Children's Hospital, Los Angeles, 1960–1992*

Diagnosis	Number (%)	Alive	Dead	LTF
Hemangioma	10 (55.5)	5	3	2
Mesenchymal hamartoma	6 (33.3)	4	2	
Hepatoblastoma	1 (5.6)	1		
Solitary cyst	1 (5.6)	1		
	18 (100)	11 (61)	5	2

*Patients who underwent biopsy or partial resection, or who were diagnosed at necropsy.
LTF = lost to follow-up.

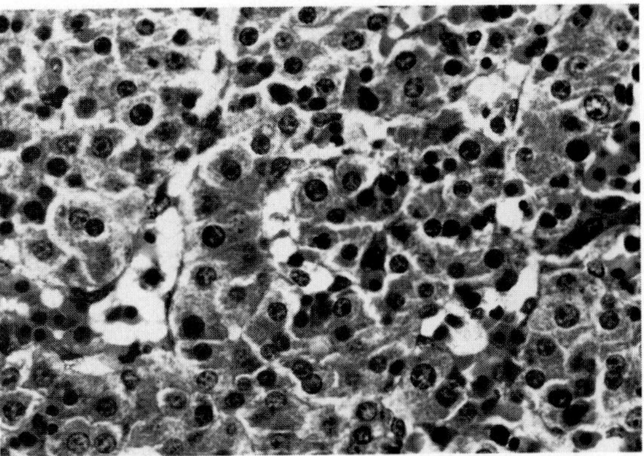

Figure 12–1. Developing liver (from a 14-mm human embryo). Hepatoblasts are composed of cells of variable size with regular, round nuclei and one or two prominent nucleoli. Irregularly arranged, early liver cell cord formations are bordered by sinusoids containing nucleated erythrocytes (hematoxylin-eosin, ×600). (From Isaacs H Jr. Tumors of the Newborn and Infant. St. Louis: Mosby–Year Book, 1991.)

sulting from disseminated intravascular coagulation (DIC), sequestration of platelets causing a bleeding diathesis (Kasabach-Merritt syndrome), and anemia (see Fig. 12–2).[5,27,67,83,127] High-output cardiac failure leading to in utero death at 33 weeks' gestation as a result of a hepatic hemangioma has been described by Nakamoto et al.[103] In one study, a palpable abdominal mass (n = 18) and cardiac failure (n = 11)

Table 12–2. Classification of Perinatal Liver Tumors and Tumor-Like Conditions

Hemangioma
  Capillary hemangioma
    ("hemangioendothelioma")
  Cavernous hemangioma
Mesenchymal hamartoma
Solitary unilocular cyst
Adenoma*
Focal nodular hyperplasia*
Hepatoblastoma
  Epithelial
  Mixed epithelial and mesenchymal
  Anaplastic
Hepatocellular carcinoma*
Germ cell tumors
  Teratoma
  Yolk sac tumor
Rhabdoid tumor
Sarcoma*
  Rhabdomyosarcoma
  Undifferentiated (embryonal) sarcoma
Metastatic neoplasms
  Neuroblastoma
  Leukemia
  Renal tumors (Wilms' tumor, rhabdoid tumor, and clear cell sarcoma)
  Yolk sac tumor

*Generally occurs in older children.
From Isaacs H Jr. Tumors of the Newborn and Infant. St. Louis: Mosby–Year Book, 1991.

were the most frequent presenting findings in 20 infants with hepatic hemangiomas.[131]

In about 50% of newborns, hepatic hemangiomas are associated with hemangiomas in the skin and other organs.[5,22,25,27,38,47,66,83,85,124,131] A large hepatic hemangioma should be a serious consideration in a neonate with cutaneous lesions, an abdominal mass, and congestive heart failure (see Fig. 12–3).[38,66] The fatal combination of cutaneous and hepatic hemangiomas, hydrops fetalis, hydramnios, and premature delivery has been reported by Shturman-Ellstein et al.[124] Placental edema and chorioangioma were also noted. The terminal clinical course was complicated by thrombocytopenia and DIC (Kasabach-Merritt syndrome) and pulmonary hyaline membrane disease.[124]

Hepatic hemangiomas can be detected antenatally by sonography.[42,48,60,109,110,121,124] They may be single or multiple, and may appear hypoechogenic, hyperechogenic, or mixed, depending on the amount of fibrosis and the stage of involution.[42] Hepatomegaly, hydramnios, and fetal hydrops are additional sonographic findings.[48,109,124]

Congenital malformations may also be observed in association with hepatic hemangioma. Werb et al. described two such cases in stillborn infants.[144] One infant had a 4-cm hemangioma and an omphalocele, and the other had two liver lesions in addition to anencephaly, rachischisis, partial gut malrotation, and a single umbilical artery. In another report,

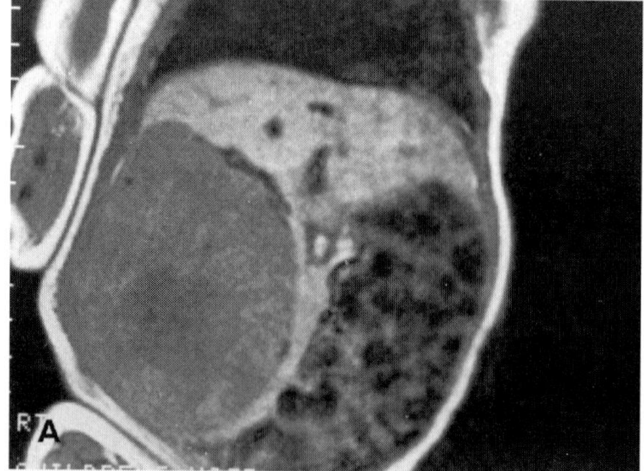

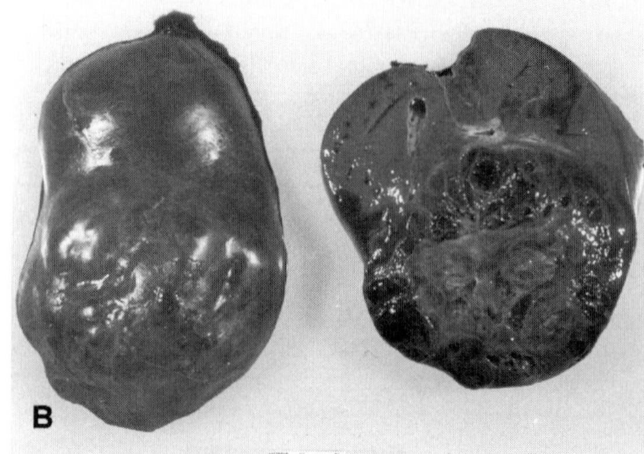

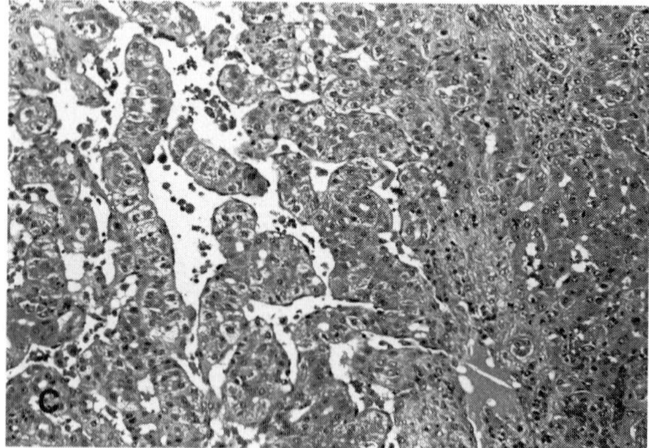

Figure 12–2. Hemangioma of the liver. _A,_ A magnetic resonance imaging (MRI) scan of a 6-day-old male infant with an abdominal mass and the Kasabach-Merritt syndrome demonstrates a large mass of variable density situated in the right lobe of the liver with features consistent with hemangioma. _B,_ The right lobe of the liver (225 g, 10 × 7 cm) contains a 6.5 × 6 cm hemorrhagic, spongy lesion. _C,_ The hemangioma is composed of both capillary and cavernous components (hematoxylin-eosin, ×240). (From Isaacs H Jr. Tumors of the Newborn and Infant. St. Louis: Mosby–Year Book, 1991.)

congenital heart disease and prune belly syndrome, respectively, occurred with hepatic hemangiomas in two neonates.[38] A necropsy, performed on a 6-hour-old term female infant who died during surgery for repair of a left diaphragmatic hernia, revealed a hemangioma arising in a heterotopic lobe of the liver in the left thorax.[122] Hepatic hemangioma has also been described in association with the Beckwith-Wiedemann syndrome, placental chorangioma, and dysmorphic kidneys.[36]

The histogenesis of hepatic hemangiomas and their soft tissue counterparts is controversial. One view is that they are actually neoplasms, and confusing terms, such as hemangioendothelioma, have been applied to some.[25,143] Another, perhaps more viable, explanation is that hemangiomas represent hamartomas (overgrowth of vessels normally present in their tissue of origin), or a local congenital malformation, or dysplasia of blood vessels.[67]

The typical gross appearance of a hepatic hemangioma is a single mass in the right or left lobe or, less often, multicentric lesions distributed throughout both lobes. The cut surface of the liver reveals a dark, reddish brown mass composed of blood vessels filled with blood (see Figs. 12–2 and 12–3).[25,82,87] Areas of fibrosis, calcification, and hemorrhage are variably present.

Hemangiomas are divided histologically into two main types—capillary and cavernous—depending only on the size of the vascular spaces, with the cavernous type having larger spaces than the capillary variety.[82] The vascular channels are lined by a single layer of plump, regular, endothelial cells. The pale-staining connective tissue stroma between the spaces varies in amount and contains small bile ducts and foci of extramedullary erythropoiesis. Apparently, with time, capillary hemangiomas become cavernous as the shunting increases and thrombosis, necrosis, and fibrosis leave large residual vessels.[82] Approximately two thirds of hemangiomas undergo spontaneous regression, characterized histologically by thrombosis, fibrosis, and calcification.[82] Both types of hemangiomas may coexist in the same lesion and may be accompanied by an arteriovenous malformation. Sometimes, it is difficult to distinguish some hemangiomas from mesenchymal hamartoma, as the two share certain characteristics, such as

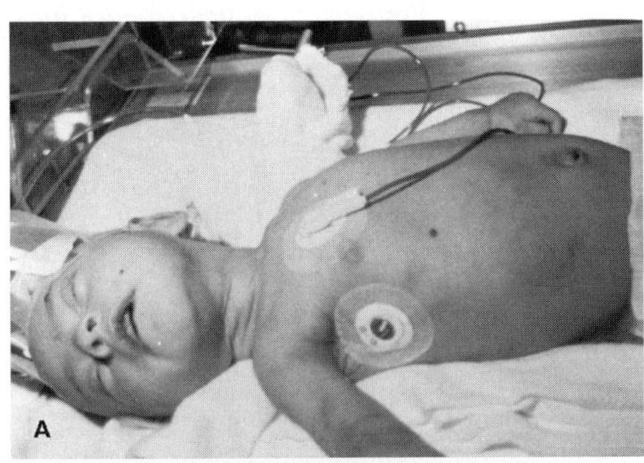

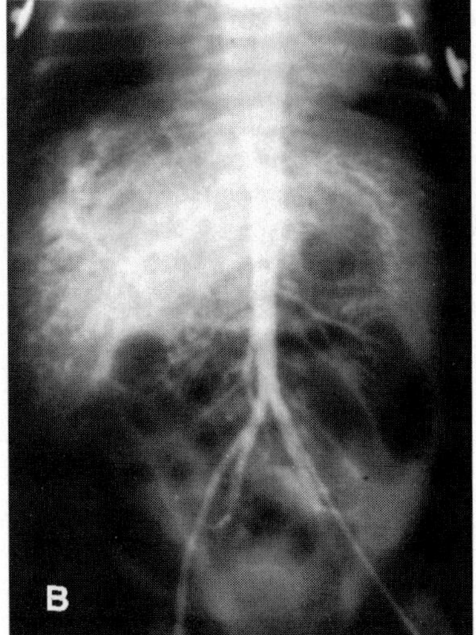

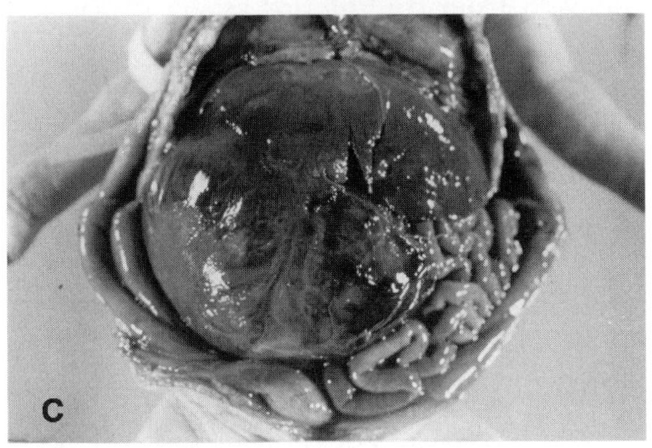

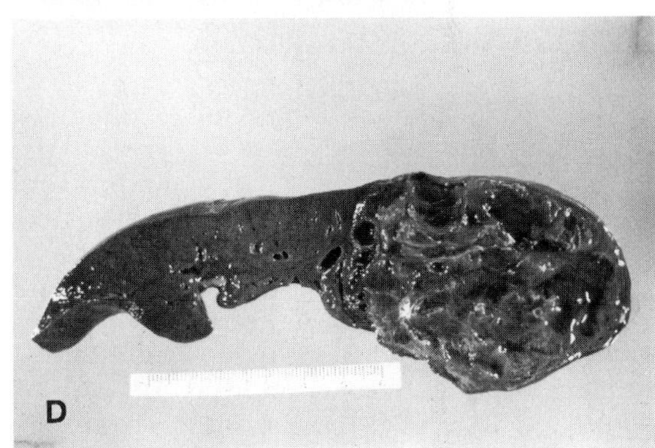

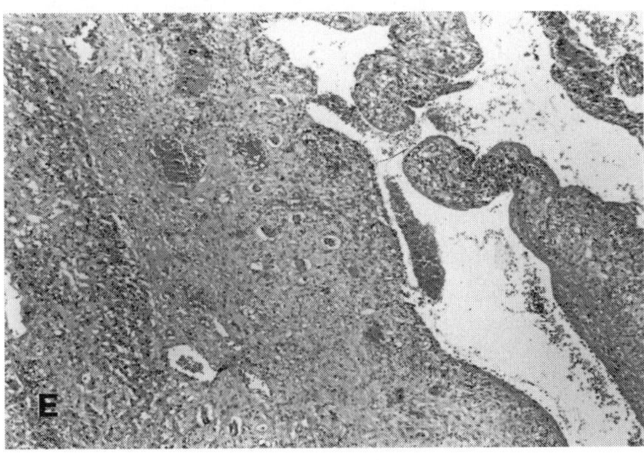

Figure 12–3. Hemangioma of the liver. *A,* A newborn with congestive heart failure and multiple cutaneous hemangiomas. *B,* An arteriogram demonstrates a highly vascular lesion occupying most of the right lobe of the liver. *C,* A postmortem photograph shows the hepatic hemangioma in situ arising from the right lobe. *D,* A cross-sectional view of the liver shows the sponge-like hemangioma. *E,* The cavernous hemangioma consists of large vascular channels. The adjacent parenchyma exhibits fibrosis and atrophy (hematoxylin-eosin, ×32). (From Pediatr Pathol 1985;3: 202–204, Isaacs H Jr., Taylor & Francis, Inc., Washington, DC. Reproduced with permission. All rights reserved.)

blood vessels, necrosis, and fibrous connective tissue stroma. A lymphangioendothelioma that practically replaced the entire liver in a newborn has been reported.[108]

A Children's Hospital, Los Angeles study (1950–1981) reviewed 12 infants who were 3 months of age or younger and had hepatic hemangiomas. Nine of the infants survived, two died, and one was lost to follow-up.[38] Four of the newborns underwent biopsy, one had a surgical resection, and seven were diagnosed on the basis of imaging studies. The results of a subsequent review (1960–1992) are shown in Table 12–1, which lists only those patients with hemangiomas who had a surgical procedure or were diagnosed at necropsy. A parallel study from the Department of Radiology revealed an 85% survival rate in 20 infants with hepatic hemangiomas who were treated in various ways (e.g., resection, embolization, ligation of the hepatic artery, or careful observation).[131]

Because noninvasive procedures are available, surgical exploration and biopsy, which may prove fatal, usually are not required for diagnosis.[87,95,131] However, when a relatively nondescript mass lesion is found in the liver and the imaging studies are equivocal, a biopsy study is indicated, particularly if a hepatoblastoma or other malignant lesion is suspected.[67] Davenport et al. recommend treating bilobar multifocal lesions by ligation of the hepatic artery and, if localized, by surgical resection to control the symptoms.[22] Generally, the prognosis is favorable, provided there are no major clinical complications.[5,25,94,95,130,131]

MESENCHYMAL HAMARTOMA

Mesenchymal hamartoma is the second most frequent benign hepatic lesion occurring in the perinatal period,[23,25,26,31,38,65,67,135,143] and recent studies suggest that it probably is not a true neoplasm (see Table 12–1).[84] More than 50% of the pediatric cases are observed in infants, and about 25% are found in newborns.[26,38,67,113,135,143] Five of seven patients with this condition in Keeling's study were 2 months of age or younger.[73] In a review of 30 infants and children with mesenchymal hamartoma, 7 (23%) were 3 months of age or younger.[135] The lesion was an incidental postmortem finding in three newborns, including one stillborn infant.

The pathogenesis of mesenchymal hamartoma is not completely understood. The name hamartoma implies that it is of developmental origin, rather than neoplastic.[25,143] Some propose that the lesion originates from the connective tissue of the portal tracts.[25,143] However, recent studies indicate that the lesion is reactive or developmental, rather than neoplastic, and that it may result from an anomalous blood supply to a liver lobule, leading to ischemia and subsequent cystic change and fibrosis.[84] Consistent with this premise is the fact that some hamartomas have necrotic centers and are attached to the liver by a pedicle.[84] Neither recurrence (once the lesion has been completely removed) nor malignant change has been reported.[25,65,66,132,135]

Most patients (50% to 80%) with mesenchymal hamartoma are younger than 1 year of age at the time of diagnosis, and they typically present with an abdominal mass or hepatomegaly

(Fig. 12–4).[25,38,40,67,78,143] Frequently, the diagnosis is suggested preoperatively by imaging studies (see Fig. 12–4A).[38,67,94,95,132] Moreover, the lesion can be detected prenatally by ultrasonography.[40,42,59,91,146] Fourcar et al. described a mesenchymal hamartoma that was discovered antenatally at 33 weeks' gestation, appearing as several large, hypoechoic masses occupying much of the liver.[40] Oligohydramnios and a thickened placenta were additional findings. Postmortem examination of the stillborn fetus showed an enlarged liver containing three large and several smaller cystic lesions. A patient of Hirata et al. had a more favorable outcome.[59] A multicystic mass and hydramnios were discovered on prenatal sonography at 38 weeks' gestation. At 6 days of age, a pedunculated mesenchymal hamartoma was successfully removed from the inferior aspect of the left lobe of the liver.

Jaundice in the neonate with a mesenchymal hamartoma is an unusual presentation. One female newborn was hospitalized with hepatomegaly, icterus (total bilirubin value of 11 mg/100 mL), and congestive heart failure.[38] She died at 15 days of age, and necropsy revealed a mesenchymal hamartoma partially obstructing the extrahepatic bile ducts, which probably accounted for the hyperbilirubinemia and jaundice. Other examples of this lesion causing heart failure in the neonate have been described.[128] Ruptured cystic mesenchymal hamartoma, manifested by neonatal ascites producing progressive respiratory distress, has been reported also.[44] At necropsy, a 6 × 5 cm cystic lesion containing a hematoma was found in the right lobe of the liver.

Generally, mesenchymal hamartoma does not occur in association with specific congenital malformations or other conditions,[143] but exceptions have been reported.[73,135] For example, a newborn in Keeling's study presenting with excessive oral mucous secretions and an abdominal mass; the infant was found to have a tracheoesophageal fistula and an annular pancreas, in addition to the hamartoma.[73] Stocker and Ishak reported that 5 of their 30 patients had various anomalies and diseases.[135]

Most mesenchymal hamartomas occur in the right lobe of the liver, but up to 10% arise from both lobes.[25,27,143] They are cured by surgical resection, provided that they are resectable, completely removed, and that there are no associated serious clinical problems, such as life-threatening congenital malformations, congestive heart failure, dehydration, electrolyte

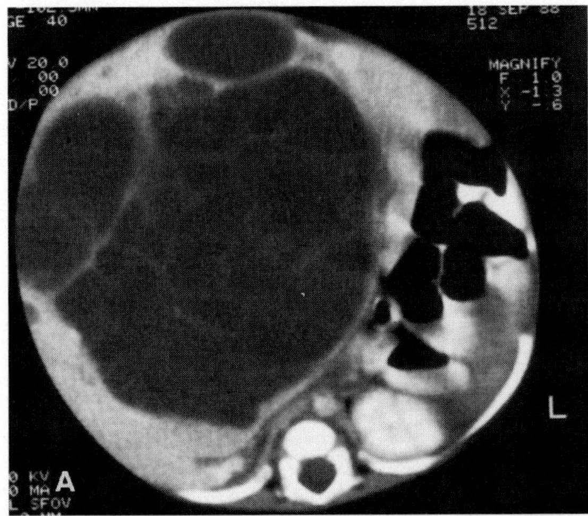

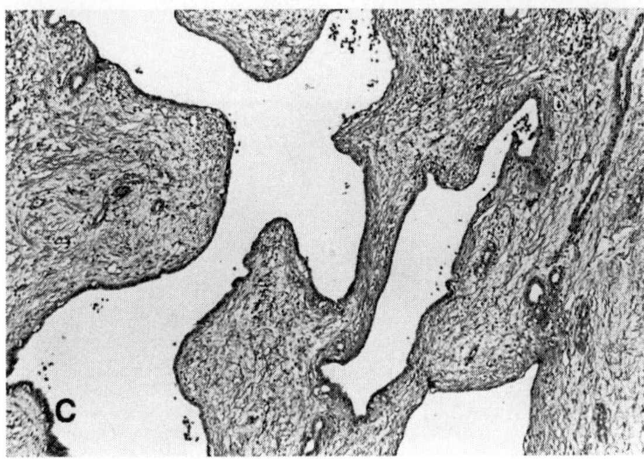

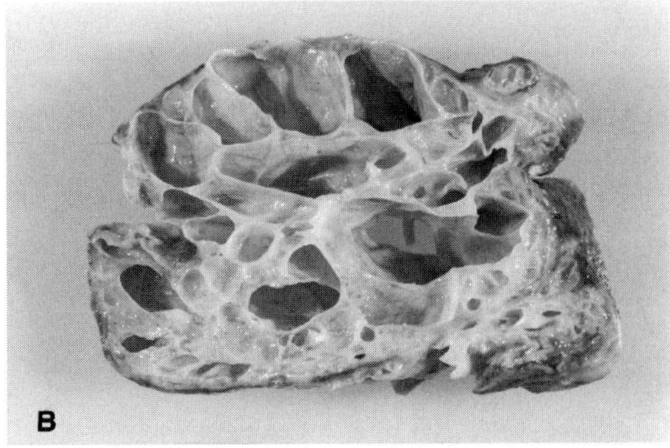

Figure 12–4. Mesenchymal hamartoma. *A,* A CT scan reveals a large, benign, cystic lesion within the liver of a 6-month-old boy with a rapidly growing abdominal mass that was first noticed at 4 months of age. *B,* Only a small portion of the lesion, which weighed more than 1 kg and occupied the right and left lobes of the liver, is shown. The lesion consists of multiple large cysts (filled with clear fluid) separated by white fibrous connective tissue septa. *C,* The cysts are lined by cuboidal and endothelial cells separated by fibrovascular septa. The interstitial connective tissue contains a few small bile ducts. These cysts fill with fluid, presumably lymph and bile, and may expand at an alarming rate, mimicking a malignant tumor (hematoxylin-eosin, ×120). (From Isaacs H Jr. Tumors of the Newborn and Infant. St. Louis: Mosby–Year Book, 1991.)

imbalances,[46] pulmonary compromise, or fatal operative complications.[46,67,82]

Often, a mesenchymal hamartoma can be diagnosed from its characteristic gross appearance, which consists of a well-circumscribed, demarcated, multiloculated, cystic mass with a light gray or pale white, bosselated external surface (see Figs. 12–4*B* and 12–5*A*).[25,26,37,67] Usually, the adjacent liver is normal in appearance. Occasionally, it occurs as pedunculated mass arising from the surface of the liver and, therefore, has a tendency to undergo torsion and hemorrhagic necrosis.[59] The specimens range in size from 100 g to more than 1 kg.[67,135] The cut surface of the hamartoma shows multiple cysts varying in diameter from a few millimeters to 6 cm or more, with grey-white, smooth, and glistening linings and clear, pale yellow fluid within (see Fig. 12–4). Some specimens consist of multiple large cysts, whereas others are composed mostly of fibrous connective tissue solid components and only a few small cysts. Some have large necrotic centers (see Fig. 12–5).

Histologically, the multilocular cysts are lined by endothelium, sometimes by cuboidal bile duct epithelium, or by no epithelium (see Figs. 12–4 and 12–5). The cysts are surrounded by dense or pale, myxoid, fibrous, connective tissue septa containing blood vessels and small bile ducts.[25,28,31,67] The periphery of the lesion is either encircled by a thick, fibrous capsule or it may blend imperceptibly with the immediately adjacent liver parenchyma, which sometimes shows compression, fibrosis, and atrophy. Electron microscopy reveals that mesenchymal hamartoma is composed mainly of connective tissue, fibroblasts, and bile ducts, and that the hepatocytes are normal.[25,28] As mentioned earlier, in some instances, it may be difficult to distinguish between a mesenchymal hamartoma and a hemangioma of the liver because the vascular component of the former may resemble the latter.

Complete surgical excision is curative, but there is a definite risk for operative mortality.[31,38,78,87,135] Instances of recurrence or malig-

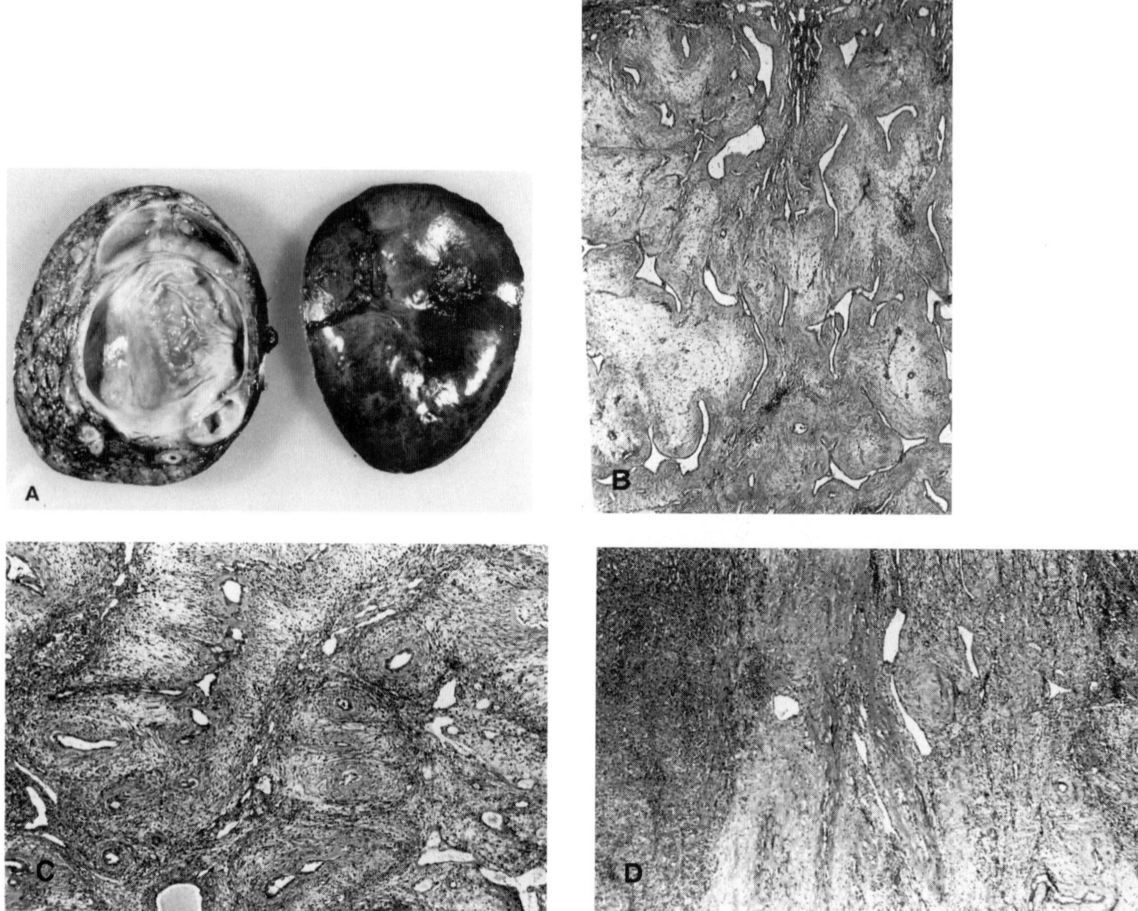

Figure 12–5. Mesenchymal hamartoma. *A,* A cystic lesion weighing 643 g and measuring 14.5 × 13 cm was removed from the liver of a 2-year-old girl with an abdominal mass. These cysts vary in size, have a smooth lining, and are separated by fibrous connective tissue septa. *B,* The capsule of the liver is at the top of the photomicrograph. The cysts vary in size and in shape, forming slit-like structures, and are surrounded by fibrous connective tissue, which is dense in some areas and myxoid-appearing in others (hematoxylin-eosin, ×30). *C,* The cysts are lined by regular cuboidal cells, by endothelium, or by no epithelium. Small bile ducts are seen (hematoxylin-eosin, ×60). *D,* Foci of necrosis are present in the upper left corner (hematoxylin-eosin, ×48).

nant change have not been documented in the young.[67,132,135]

HEPATOBLASTOMA

Hepatoblastoma is the leading primary hepatic malignant lesion during the first year of life.[7,11,16,25,26,39,52,67,68,71,107,118] For the entire pediatric population, more than 50% of hepatoblastomas are diagnosed in infants, and less than 10% are found in newborns.[11,39,52,67,73,142,143] Although the number of cases reported in the infant and older child exceed all benign hepatic lesions combined, in the newborn, hemangioma and mesenchymal hamartoma are by far the most prevalent (see Table 12–1).[16,25,65–67,79,107,143]

Of 129 infants and children with hepatoblastoma reviewed by Exelby and colleagues, 11 (8.5%) were younger than 6 weeks of age, and 3 (2.3%) were neonates.[39] The Children's Hospital, Los Angeles experience was similar in that, of 46 hepatoblastomas removed from children of all ages during a 27-year period (1960–1986), a little more than 50% occurred in infants and one (2.6%) was congenital.[64] Similar frequency figures for the neonate were obtained by Campbell et al. and by Rubie et al.[11,119] Misugi et al. reviewed 24 primary hepatic malignant tumors in infants and children, including 5 hepatocellular carcinomas in children 6 years of age and older and 19 hepatoblastomas in younger children, 4 of whom were newborns.[96]

Typically, hepatoblastoma presents as an up-

Adenomatoid transformation of the renal
  epithelium
Aicardi syndrome
Alpha$_1$-antitrypsin deficiency
Beckwith-Wiedemann syndrome
Cystathioninuria
Fetal alcohol syndrome
Hemihypertrophy
Hydrops fetalis
Isosexual precocity
Maternal contraceptive use
Osteoporosis
Intestinal adenomatous polyposis
Polyhydramnios
Stillbirth
Trisomy 18
Umbilical hernia
Wilms' tumor

Adapted from Stocker JT, Ishak KG. Hepatoblastoma. *In* Okuda K, Ishak KG (eds): Neoplasms of the Liver. New York: Springer-Verlag, 1987. Used by permission.

per abdominal mass arising as a single focus, more often from the right lobe of the liver than the left (see Fig. 12–8).[25,39,68,79,126] The tumor can be detected on antenatal ultrasonography.[42,105,140] In addition to abdominal distention, which is the second most common sign, other manifestations may include respiratory distress and/or gastrointestinal symptoms secondary to a massively enlarged liver,[10] sexual precocity in older male infants,[79,101,102] nonimmune fetal hydrops,[72] polyhydramnios,[20,72,140] spontaneous rupture with hemoperitoneum,[20,53,79,126,140] and occasionally, anemia and jaundice.[72,126] The various clinical conditions associated with hepatoblastoma are listed in Table 12–3.

In one case, hepatoblastoma was responsible for compression of the inferior vena cava, leading to fetal hydrops and intrauterine death at 36 weeks' gestation.[4] At necropsy, the tumor occupied the fossa of the absent gallbladder. Kazzi et al. described a similar case of a newborn with a hepatoblastoma that was diagnosed antenatally; this infant survived 2 days.[72] Hydrops fetalis, consumptive coagulopathy associated with massive hemorrhage into the tumor, and anemia were present at birth. In another case, the combination of hepatoblastoma (detected antenatally), adrenal cytomegaly, nephromegaly, and pancreatic nesidioblastosis raised the possibility of the Beckwith-Wiedemann syndrome, although the affected neonate did not have either macroglossia or omphalocele.[105] Another unique manifestation of this neoplasm occurred in a 1-month-old male infant who presented with signs of brain metas-

tases—namely, twitching, left hemiparesis, and projectile vomiting—noted shortly after birth.[73] In addition to neuroblastoma and leukemia, hepatoblastoma is one of the perinatal malignant lesions responsible for placental metastases and fetal death.[8,33,116]

Various congenital anomalies and malformation syndromes occur in association with hepatoblastoma (see Tables 12–3 and 12–4).[52,53,58,68,82] Hemihypertrophy (in 2% to 3% of affected patients), the Beckwith-Wiedemann syndrome, and intestinal adenomatous polyposis syndrome are cited most often.[7,26,41,43,45,53,58,72,82,86,105,119,143] The combination of hepatoblastoma and familial adenomatous polyposis, an autosomal dominant disorder, has also been reported.[45,53,76,86] Ophthalmoscopic examination of the affected individual reveals hypertrophy of the retinal pigment epithelium, which appears to be a sensitive and specific marker for the polyposis gene.[45] Although the hepatoblastoma in these individuals is usually diagnosed before the age of 5 years, the intestinal polyposis may not become apparent until the second decade of life.[45] It should be mentioned that some of the same congenital malformations and syndromes are noted also in patients with Wilms' tumor.[129]

Hepatoblastoma has been described in siblings in a variety of clinical settings, including the fetal alcohol syndrome, in association with maternal use of contraceptives, in trisomy 18, and in patients with Wilms' tumor and in newborns with adenomatoid malformation of the renal epithelium.[5,53,75,77,79,82,88,115] Aicardi syndrome (spasms in flexion, agenesis of the corpus callosum, and multiple ocular malformations) was described in a 2-month-old female infant with hepatoblastoma.[137] Other examples of clinical conditions coexisting with hepatoblastoma are shown in Table 12–3.

Almost all patients with hepatoblastoma have significantly elevated serum alpha-fetoprotein (AFP) levels, which makes this a useful diagnostic marker.[1,26,39,53,102,105,119,120,126,143] However, AFP values are normally elevated during the first month of life, and it is important to remember that levels are also increased in patients with yolk sac tumor, the main perinatal malignant germ cell tumor (see Table 2–4). Blair et al. compiled a useful table listing the AFP reference values for infants ranging in age from birth to 5 months and for those of gestational ages ranging from 26 to 43 weeks, taking into account the effect of prematurity of these values.[6] According to these authors, the alpha-globulin reaches a peak level of 3,000,000 U/mL at

Table 12–4. 21 Fetal and Newborn Hepatoblastomas*

Case No.	Age at Death	Initial Findings	Treatment	Comment(s)	Reference(s)
1	Stillborn	—	—	Hydrops fetalis; absent gallbladder	Benjamin et al.[4]
2	1 day	Abdominal mass, hydramnios, anemia	S	Rupture of tumor with hemoperitoneum	Cremin and Nuss[20]
3	15 min	Hydramnios, abdominal distention and shock†	—	Rupture of tumor with hemoperitoneum	Van de Bor et al.[140]
4	5 wks	Abdominal distention, hepatomegaly	S	Adenomatoid transformation of the renal epithelium‡	Knowlson and Cameron[77]
5	3 mos	Seizures, abdominal mass	S	Agenesis of the corpus callosum (Aicardi syndrome)	Tanaka et al.[137]
6	Stillborn	—	—	Metastases to the lungs, placenta, and cord—other	Robinson and Bolande[116]
7	3 mos	Abdominal mass	S	Operative death	Gonzalez-Crussi et al.[52]
8	37 hrs	Abdominal mass	S	Operative death, lung metastases, horseshoe kidney	Gonzalez-Crussi et al.[52]
9	2 mos	Abdominal mass	S	Operative death	Gonzalez-Crussi et al.[52]
10	2 days	Hydramnios, fetal hydrops, abdominal mass†	—	Anemia, consumptive coagulopathy, hemorrhage into tumor, pulmonary hyaline membrane disease	Kazzi et al.[72]
11	Alive	Jaundice, abdominal distention, hemoperitoneum	S	Ruptured tumor	Sirota et al.[126]
12	2 wks	Abdominal distention, hepatic mass†	CT	Tumor considered inoperable; ?BWS: adrenal cytomegaly, nephromegaly, nesidioblastosis	Orozco-Florian[105]
13	5 days	Abdominal mass	S	—	Weinberg[142]
14	2 mos	Abdominal mass	S	Undifferentiated component	Weinberg[142]
15	Alive	Abdominal mass	S, CT, RT	Undifferentiated component	Weinberg[142]
16	1 year	?Abdominal mass	S, CT, RT	Brain metastases	Campbell[11]
17	12 wks	Abdominal distention	BXs, CT	Intra-abdominal metastases	Keeling[73]
18	5 wks	Vomiting, abdominal distention	S	Died few hours after laparotomy	Keeling[73]
19	3 mos	Twitching, hemiparesis, projectile vomiting	S	Pulmonary and cerebral metastases	Keeling[73]
20	?3 mos	Abdominal mass, hemihypertrophy	S, CT	Pulmonary metastases	Rubie[119]
21	Alive	Abdominal mass	S	—	Isaacs[66]

*Including patients 3 months of age or younger who were selected from the literature.
†Tumor is detected antenatally by ultrasonography.
‡Cuboidal or columnar epithelium lines Bowman's capsule and extends a short distance down the related proximal tubule.
BWS = Beckwith-Wiedemann syndrome; S = surgery; CT = chemotherapy; RT = radiation therapy; BXs = biopsies.

about 14 weeks' gestation, declining thereafter to 50,000 U/mL at birth, and finally reaching adult levels of 10 U/mL at 6 to 8 months of age. High serum cholesterol values in infants and children with hepatoblastoma are correlated with a poor prognosis.[100]

The gross appearance of hepatoblastoma is a single, round mass that replaces a part or almost the entire lobe of the liver, measuring 10 to 20 cm or more in diameter (Fig. 12–6). Usually, the tumor is well circumscribed and well demarcated from the adjacent normal liver by a whitish-gray, fibrous pseudocapsule. The appearance of the cut surface varies, but it is gen-

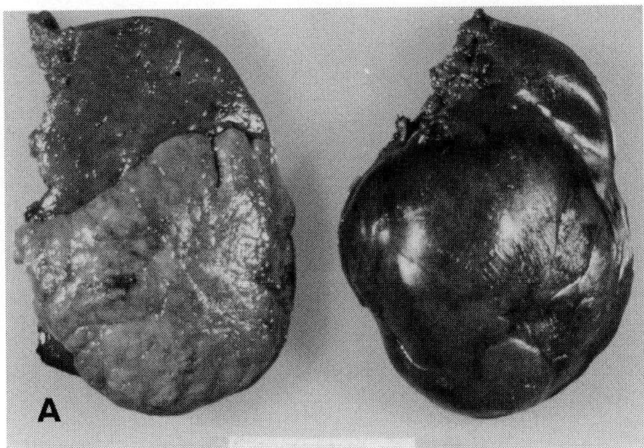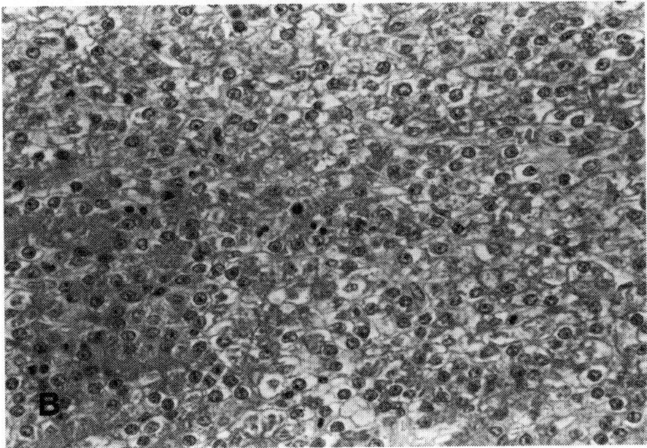

Figure 12–6. Fetal epithelial hepatoblastoma. *A,* The right lobe of the liver (347 g, 13 × 7 cm) from a 1-year-old boy with an abdominal mass and an elevated serum AFP level (6× the normal value). The lobe contains a 9 × 7 cm, soft, tannish-yellow bulging mass. *B,* The tumor is composed of uniform, small cells. Both light and dark cells and transition forms between the two types of fetal hepatoblasts are noted (hematoxylin-eosin, ×600). (From Isaacs H Jr. Neoplasms in infants: A report of 265 cases. Pathol Annu 1983;18(2):165. Used by permission.)

erally light tan or cream-colored and soft in consistency, with or without grey myxoid areas and yellow necrotic zones. Tiny white foci of osteoid are noted in some of the mixed hepatoblastomas.[25,26,67,68,79,143]

Hepatoblastoma is classified histologically into two main types—epithelial or mixed—depending on whether mesenchymal elements are present (Table 12–5).[18,25,52,68,79,142,143] The epithelial components occurring in both the epithelial and mixed hepatoblastomas are subdivided further into four main cell types designated as fetal, embryonal, macrotrabecular, and small cell undifferentiated ("anaplastic"). As the name implies, the fetal cell type resembles fetal liver cells and consists of small, regular cells with minimal nuclear atypia and a low mitotic rate; these cells form narrow cords with bordering sinusoids and prominent foci of hematopoiesis (see Fig. 12–6). In addition, the fetal type has both light and dark cells, with the former containing more glycogen and lipid

Table 12–5. Histologic Classification of Hepatoblastoma

Epithelial
  Fetal pattern
  Embryonal pattern
  Macrotrabecular pattern
  Small cell undifferentiated ("anaplastic")
    pattern
  Mixed epithelial and mesenchymal
  Mixed with teratoid components*

*Tissues from all three germ layers.
From Pediatr Pathol 1992;12:169, Conran RM, Hitchcock CL, Waclawiw MA, et al., Taylor & Francis, Inc., Washington, DC. Reproduced with permission. All rights reserved.

than the latter, as demonstrated by both histochemical and ultrastructural studies.[143]

Embryonal epithelial hepatoblastoma is composed of more atypical, more variable, and larger cells than are noted in the fetal type; moreover, the tumors have a tendency to grow in a more solid pattern (Figs. 12–7 through 12–9).[51,52] Frequent mitoses are noted. Sometimes, tubule formations are found that resemble bile ductules or embryonic tubules, similar to those seen in Wilms' tumor. Both fetal and embryonal cell types may coexist in the same tumor with transition zones between the two. Electron microscopic studies reveal that the

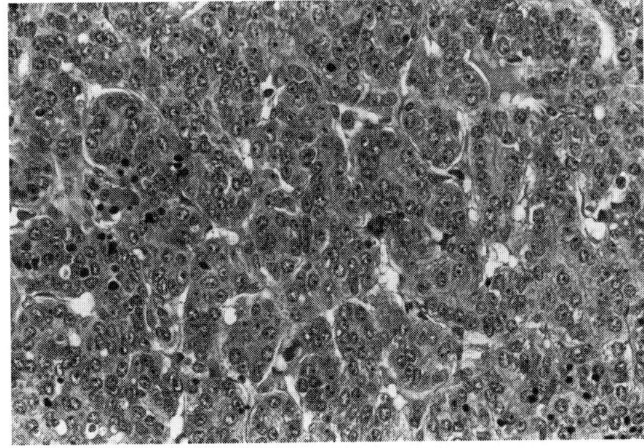

Figure 12–7. Embryonal epithelial hepatoblastoma. The tumor consists of cord-like and pseudoacinar structures. The cells show slight to moderate variation in nuclear size and shape, and several mitoses are noted. The cells with small, round, darkly staining nuclei are nucleated erythrocytes. The tumor appeared in a male newborn with signs of increasing respiratory distress and abdominal distention noted at birth. The tumor measured 11 × 9.5 cm (hematoxylin-eosin, ×600). (From Isaacs H Jr. Tumors of the Newborn and Infant. St. Louis: Mosby–Year Book, 1991.)

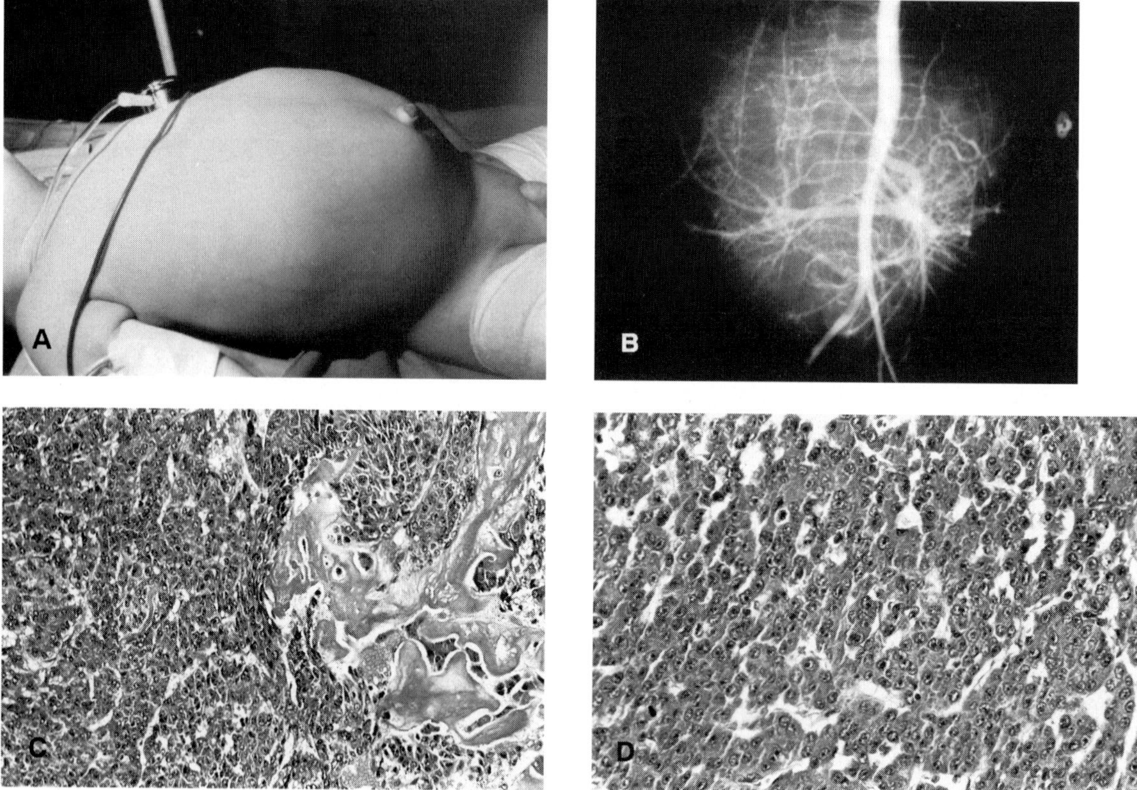

Figure 12–8. Embryonal mixed hepatoblastoma. *A,* A 5-month-old male infant with a 3-month history of progressive abdominal distention. The huge abdominal mass arising from the liver is depicted. *B,* An arteriogram reveals involvement of almost the entire liver. *C,* A biopsy study showed a mixed hepatoblastoma with both osteoid and epithelial components, the latter consisting of fetal and embryonal cell types (hematoxylin-eosin, ×300). *D,* Higher magnification of the embryonal hepatoblasts reveals greater irregularity in nuclear configuration and cell size as compared to the fetal hepatoblastoma pictured in Figure 12–6*B* (hematoxylin-eosin, ×600). (From Isaacs H Jr. Tumors of the Newborn and Infant. St. Louis: Mosby–Year Book, 1991.)

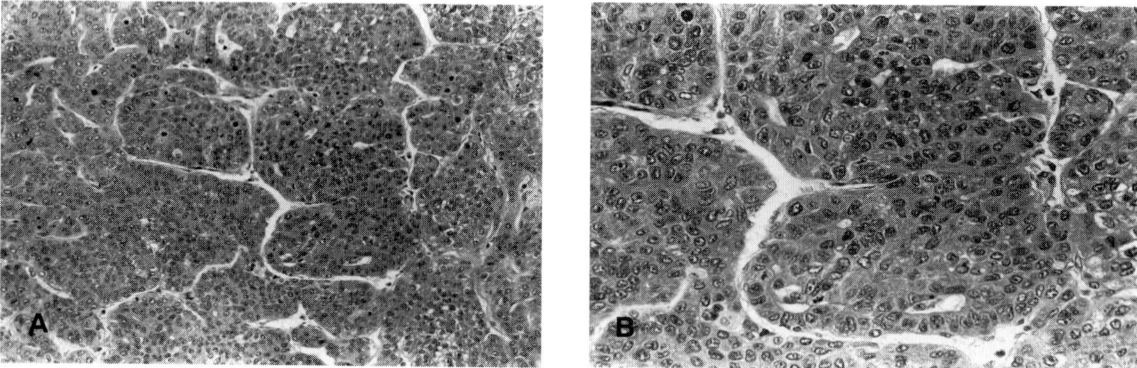

Figure 12–9. Embryonal hepatoblastoma. *A,* The macrotrabecular pattern is characterized by trabeculae (cords) greater than 10 cells thick and composed of embryonal hepatoblasts (hematoxylin-eosin, ×150). *B,* At higher magnification, the trabecular and pseudoacinar formations are shown in greater detail. This morphologic pattern of hepatoblastoma is difficult to distinguish from hepatocellular carcinoma (hematoxylin-eosin, ×300).

embryonal hepatoblast is a more primitive cell, containing fewer organelles than the fetal hepatoblast.[61,143] The pattern of cytokeratin expression of hepatoblastoma was studied in detail by Van Eyken et al.[141] Embryonic and fetal type tumor cells stain positively for cytokeratins numbers 8 and 18, as well as for the bile duct cytokeratin 19. Tumor cells associated with osteoid express vimentin and the cytokeratins 7, 18, and 19. The type of epithelial component present in hepatoblastomas is more important in terms of the prognosis than whether there are mesenchymal elements.[66]

Sometimes it is difficult, on the basis of microscopic findings, to distinguish between an embryonal epithelial hepatoblastoma with the "macrotrabecular" pattern and hepatocellular carcinoma, which tends to be multifocal and associated with an underlying condition, such as cirrhosis. However, distinguishing the two is important, for hepatocellular carcinoma has a poorer prognosis and is treated differently.[52,53,143] The macrotrabecular pattern is characterized by trabeculae (cords) that are greater than 10 cells thick and are composed of embryonal hepatoblasts (see Fig. 12–9).[52]

The rare small cell undifferentiated ("anaplastic") pattern, representing the least differentiated form of hepatoblastoma according to Gonzalez-Crussi, is observed usually during the first 6 months of life.[49] Microscopically, it consists of small, round, darkly staining cells with vesicular nuclei showing little evidence of liver cell differentiation by hematoxylin-eosin staining; characteristically, pools of mucoid material that is rich in acid mucopolysaccharide are present between the cells.[18,49,69,79] Ultrastructural studies confirm the liver cell origin of the tumor.[49,69] The cells contain abundant glycogen, a prominent endoplasmic reticulum, tonofilaments, desmosomes, and canalicular microvilli. The tumor cells are cytokeratin-positive but stain negatively for vimentin, desmin, S-100 protein, and neuron-specific enolase (NSE).[49] When fetal or embryonal epithelial components are found in the tumor, the diagnosis of the small cell undifferentiated pattern can be made with confidence. A chromosomal translocation—t(10;22)—has been described for this variant.[56] The 5-month-old male infant with a small cell undifferentiated hepatoblastoma depicted by Joshi et al. had a markedly elevated serum AFP level prior to surgery.[69]

Electron microscopic examination of the tumor in question may be helpful in distinguishing between hepatoblastoma and hepatocellular carcinoma.[25,56,61] Ultrastructurally, the cells of the former are less mature compared to the latter, as they contain fewer cytoplasmic organelles and less well-developed microvilli. Hepatoma is extremely rare in the newborn.[92,138]

In addition to the epithelial components described earlier, mixed hepatoblastomas contain mesenchymal elements consisting mostly of spindle-shaped fibroblastic cells with a pale-staining myxoid stroma and small foci of osteoid, bone, and, less often, cartilage or skeletal muscle located within nests of fetal or embryonic epithelium. Osteoid is the most common differentiated tissue, being found in 20% to 35% of hepatoblastomas (Fig. 12–8C).[27] Evidently, osteoid is formed by the mesenchymal cells of the tumor.[25,125,143] The number of cases of "pure" epithelial versus mixed hepatoblastoma varies, but in most series, the epithelial type predominates.[25,52,66,79] The presence of a mesenchymal component apparently has no effect on prognosis.[68,143] The term "teratoid" is used for mixed hepatoblastomas with tissues from all three germ layers, such as cartilage, skeletal muscle, and intestinal and keratinizing stratified squamous epithelium.[18,89] Deposits of melanin pigment are often present in these tumors. Hepatoblastoma with a yolk sac tumor component was documented in a 6-month-old male infant.[21]

All four newborn hepatoblastomas reported by Misugi et al. consisted of embryonal type epithelium (3 of the 4 had, in addition, fetal-type epithelium), and two contained osteoid (mixed type).[96] Pulmonary metastases occurred in two, and there were no survivors. The distribution of tumor histologic types—that is, fetal versus embryonal, and epithelial versus mixed mesenchymal—in the 21 newborns listed in Table 12–4 is similar to that reported by Misugi et al.[96]

The sites of metastases of hepatoblastoma, in decreasing order of frequency, are the lungs, abdomen, brain, lymph nodes, and vena cava.[39] Metastases may be present at the time of diagnosis, or they may occur late in the course of the disease.[73] Campbell et al. described a patient with a hepatoblastoma noted at birth who was treated by resection, irradiation, and chemotherapy but who died of brain metastases 1 year later.[11] In contrast, Gonzalez-Crussi and coworkers described a newborn with macrotrabecular-pattern hepatoblastoma who had bone marrow metastases at the time of diagnosis.[52]

The survival of infants and children with hepatoblastoma depends on three main factors: complete resection of the tumor, absence of

Table 12–6. Staging Classification
for Hepatoblastoma

Stage	Description
I	Complete resection
II	Microscopic residual tumor, no nodal involvement; no spilled tumor
III	Gross residual tumor, nodal involvement, or spilled tumor
IV	Metastatic disease

metastases, and absence of embryonal or undifferentiated cell types ("unfavorable histology").[55,79,142,143] If the tumor is small and is completely resected before it has metastasized (i.e., stage I), then the patient has the best chance for survival (Table 12–6). Only the patients in whom the primary treatment is complete resection of the neoplasm survive. One exception is the patient with the small cell undifferentiated variant, which has a particularly poor prognosis, as it metastasizes early in the course of the disease, regardless of the therapeutic regimen.[5,16,25,49,69]

Generally, the outcome of hepatoblastoma in the fetus and newborn is dismal. Table 12–4 is a compilation of 21 cases of fetal and newborn hepatoblastomas selected from the literature for which clinical information was given. Table 12–4 shows that, of 21 patients, only 3 (14%) survived. Hepatic resection in these young patients is associated with a high mortality because the tumors tend to be large and unresectable and the neonate is, by nature, clinically unstable. Intrapartum rupture and hemorrhage are frequent complications. Metastases may be present at the time of diagnosis (see Table 12–4).

PRIMARY SARCOMAS OF THE LIVER

Embryonal rhabdomyosarcoma and undifferentiated (embryonal) sarcoma are the two main primary malignant mesenchymal tumors of the liver in childhood.[3,27,50,136,143] Hepatic sarcomas are noted rarely in the newborn and infant.[82,136] Although embryonal sarcoma may occur during the first year of life, it affects primarily older children (6 to 10 years of age), whereas rhabdomyosarcoma occurs predominantly in younger children between the ages of 2 and 4 years.[24,25,27,50,74] Angiosarcoma of the

liver is the subject of an anecdotal case report.[2,104]

Although rare, undifferentiated sarcoma should be considered in the differential diagnosis of a primary liver tumor in the young. An abdominal mass and pain are the main clinical findings.[136] According to the Armed Forces Institute of Pathology report of 31 cases of undifferentiated sarcoma of the liver in adults and children, 3 patients were 2 months of age at the time of presentation, and 1 was diagnosed at birth.[136] Imaging studies reveal a space-occupying lesion, usually situated in the right lobe of the liver, with solid and cystic areas.

The tumors are large, measuring 30 cm or more in diameter, and have a fibrous pseudocapsule.[25,143] The cut surface has a tan to light gray, gelatinous appearance with extensive necrosis and cyst formation. Microscopically, there is an abundant, pale-staining, myxoid stroma with clusters of small, dark, round, oval, or spindle-shaped cells. Large tumor cells with bizarre nuclei and characteristic eosinophilic-staining cytoplasmic spherules are seen. Mitoses are common. Entrapped liver cells and bile ducts are noted about the periphery. Vascular invasion by tumor cells is an important diagnostic finding. Reactivity to vimentin and the histiocytic markers lysozyme and alpha$_1$-antitrypsin is generally positive, but AFP testing yields negative results. The tumor may be focally positive to desmin.[3] Ultrastructurally, embryonal sarcomas are composed principally of fibroblastic cells with spindle-shaped cytoplasms containing well-developed, rough endoplasmic reticulum; primitive-appearing mesenchymal cells with scanty cytoplasm and few organelles; histiocytoid cells with lysosomal granules and microvillous-like cytoplasmic projections; and myofibroblastic cells with serrated nuclei, abundant rough endoplasmic reticulum, filamentous condensations beneath the cytoplasmic membrane, and focal basal lamina formation.[3]

The prognosis of patients with undifferentiated sarcoma is guarded. Few patients live longer than 18 months after diagnosis.[3,25,53,62,136,143]

The liver is rarely the primary site of embryonal rhabdomyosarcoma, which originates from the intrahepatic bile ducts or from the extrahepatic biliary system.[25,62,143] The child presents with an abdominal mass, which is accompanied by jaundice if the biliary tract is obstructed. When the sarcoma is found in one of the major bile ducts, it forms tiny, pale, gray-tan, grape-like, polypoid masses that fill the ductal lumen, similar to those arising from hollow viscera elsewhere. The histologic appearance is that of a botryoid embryonal rhabdomyosarcoma, consisting of polypoid projections composed of a pale, myxoid stroma with a cellular rind of small, dark, round, or spindle-shaped cells situated beneath the bile duct epithelium. Cytoplasmic cross-striations may be evident upon hematoxylin-eosin staining, but desmin and other skeletal markers show positivity and the ultrastructural characteristics are diagnostic. (For further discussion, see Chapter 4, "Soft Tissue Tumors.") When the tumor arises from the liver parenchyma, it forms a light grey-tan, gelatinous-appearing, intrahepatic mass with foci of necrosis and hemorrhage.

Historically, the prognosis of intrahepatic rhabdomyosarcoma has been poor because it metastasizes early to the lungs, brain, and lymph nodes, and it is often difficult to resect because of its location.[25] Recently, the prognosis has improved somewhat.[62]

RHABDOID TUMOR OF THE LIVER

Rhabdoid tumor is a highly aggressive, malignant neoplasm that most often arises from the kidney in children. It is characterized by a high rate of recurrence and early metastases, and is refractory to therapy.[54,63] The histogenesis of the tumor has not yet been determined. Histologically, rhabdoid tumor consists of a round or oval vesicular nucleus containing a large nucleolus, as well as characteristic cytoplasmic eosinophilic inclusions consisting of intermediate filaments that can be demonstrated by ultrastructural studies (see Chapter 11, "Renal Tumors").[106] Some of these highly malignant tumors also occur in association with brain tumors, particularly primitive neuroectodermal tumor (PNETs) (see Chapter 9, "Brain Tumors").

Rhabdoid primary tumors in the liver have been documented in the neonate.[13,106,107] Bilateral pulmonary metastases were present at the time of diagnosis in a 3-month-old male infant who presented with an abdominal mass. The patient did not respond to therapy (excisional biopsy plus chemotherapy) and died at 5 months of age. Rhabdoid tumor of the liver was an incidental necropsy finding in a 14-day-old male infant with a large, cerebral PNET.[13] Chang and colleagues proposed that, because rhabdoid tumor cells were found in the cerebral PNET, the liver lesion represented a metastasis rather than a second malignant lesion.[13]

GERM CELL TUMORS

Germ cell tumors metastatic to the liver—namely, yolk sac tumor from the sacrococcygeal area or testis—are observed more frequently than primary tumors during the first year of life.[25,66,143] Although few in number, cases of teratoma of the liver are reported more often than primary yolk sac tumor.[19,25,34,57,97,117,139,143] Teratoma of the liver occurs more often in the newborn and infant than in older children and adults.[117] Indeed, 25% of hepatic teratomas are found at birth.[19] Robinson and Nelson described a hepatic teratoma in a stillborn anencephalic fetus.[117] The tumor occupied 25% of the liver in the right lobe and contained squamous epithelium, peripheral nerve, and skeletal elements.[117] Serum AFP levels may be markedly elevated in infants with this tumor.[139] Hepatic teratomas typically are cystic; are composed of mature and, to a lesser extent, immature neuroglial elements; and usually lack malignant germ cell tumor components. Yolk sac tumor is observed rarely in combination with hepatoblastoma.[21] Surgical excision results in cure, provided no residual tumor is left behind.

LIVER CELL ADENOMA AND FOCAL NODULAR HYPERPLASIA

Adenoma and focal nodular hyperplasia are considered to be benign proliferations of liver cells that occur more often in adults than in infants and children.[12,25,27,30,38,114,133,143,145] Marks et al. detected a 4 × 4 cm hepatic adenoma on prenatal sonography that was subsequently confirmed at postmortem examination.[90] The newborn had no other associated anomalies. Resnick et al. described a similar case of a newborn who survived, and a second patient, a 2-day-old male infant, who presented with neonatal jaundice and who died following an attempt at surgical excision.[114] In their study of eight infants and children with hepatic adenoma, two were congenital. One newborn adenoma had a well-formed fibrous capsule that separated the tumor from the adjacent compressed liver parenchyma, and the other had a thin, incomplete, fibrous capsule. Histologically, the tumor cells were arranged in sheets and formed tra-

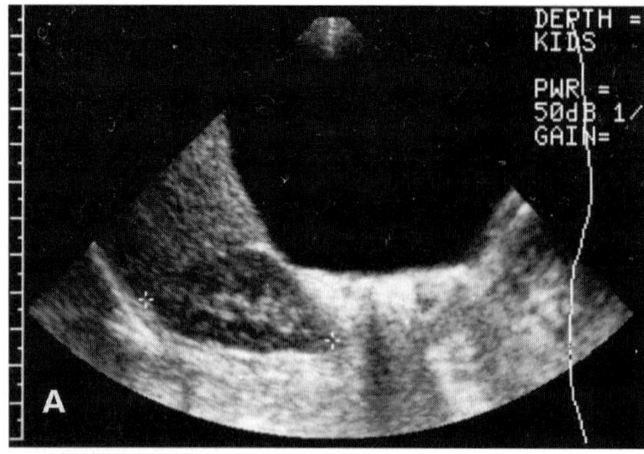

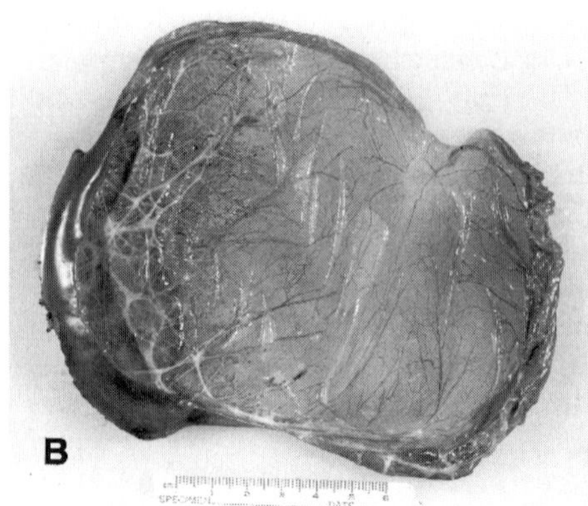

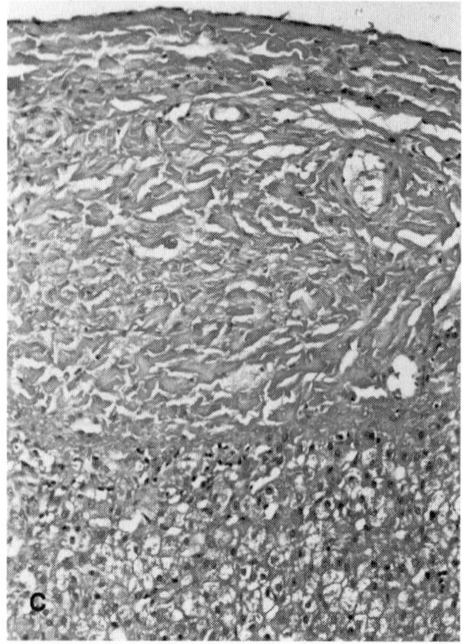

Figure 12–10. Unilocular cyst of the liver. *A,* A sonogram of an 11-month-old girl with a history of abdominal distention reveals a cystic mass occupying the abdominal cavity without a definite site of origin. *B,* The cyst (1.1 kg, 18 cm in diameter) has a smooth lining. *C,* The hepatic cyst is lined by both cuboidal and flattened epithelium resting on a thick layer of fibrous connective tissue. The underlying liver parenchyma is unremarkable (hematoxylin-eosin, ×300).

beculae 2 to 3 cells in thickness separated by sinusoidal spaces lined by endothelial cells.[114]

Focal nodular hyperplasia is a benign condition of the liver characterized by hepatocytes separated by a stellate scar situated in the center of the lesion.[25,30,37,38,133,143] The etiology is unknown. Most cases in children occur between the ages of 7 and 14 years.[30,133,143] One newborn had, in addition to this lesion, multiple congenital malformations, including gastroschisis, absence of the anterior portion of the diaphragm, rib anomalies, hypoplasia of the left lung, and agenesis of the gall bladder.[133] The youngest patient in Edmondson's classic review, who was 7 months of age, presented with a right upper quadrant mass that moved on respiration.[37] Focal nodular hyperplasia is cured by surgical excision.

Nodular regenerative hyperplasia is an uncommon liver lesion in infants and children, presenting as hepatomegaly and/or splenomegaly, with or without portal hypertension.[99] It may be an incidental finding at postmortem examination, and has been reported in association with other conditions, such as Wilms' tumor, mental retardation, VATER syndrome (vertebral defects, imperforate anus, tracheoesophageal fistula, and radial and renal dysplasia), renal angiomyolipoma, and anticonvulsant therapy.[99] The entire liver may be replaced by multiple, tan to yellow, nonencapsulated nodules varying in size from a few millimeters to a few centimeters. Histologically, the nodules are composed of hepatocytes slightly larger than normal, which cause compression atrophy of the adjacent parenchyma.

MISCELLANEOUS TUMORS AND TUMOR-LIKE CONDITIONS

Several unusual hepatic tumors occur in infants. A fatal cystic malignant neoplasm,

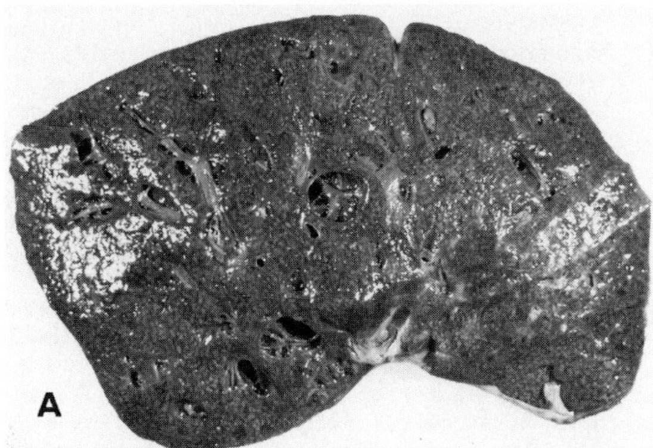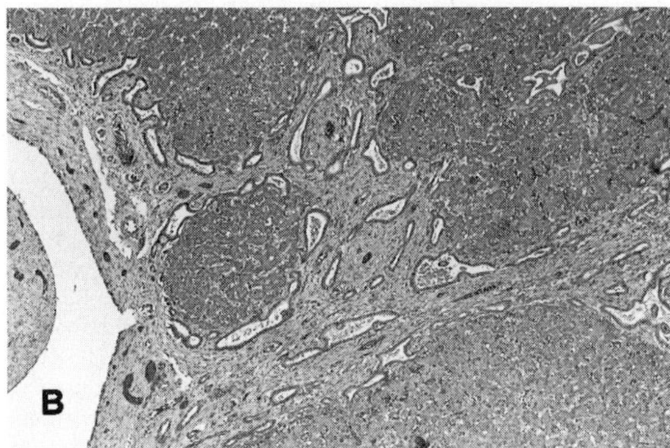

Figure 12–11. Infantile polycystic disease of the kidneys and liver (autosomal recessive). *A,* The gross appearance of the liver with multiple cysts. The patient and his cystic kidneys are pictured in Figure 11–3*C. B,* Microscopic examination reveals angulated, branching, cystically dilated bile ducts and portal fibrosis (hematoxylin-eosin, ×48).

thought to be derived from mesothelium, was found in a 6-month-old girl.[32] Two cases have been reported, one in a 5-week-old female infant, of a small cell malignant tumor resembling neuroblastoma by light and electron microscopy, but differing from small cell undifferentiated ("anaplastic") hepatoblastoma.[111] Angiomyolipomas of the liver have been demonstrated by ultrasonography in infants with tuberous sclerosis.[70] Usually, the lesions are clinically silent and may be found in the kidneys, as well.

Occasionally, hepatic ("nonparasitic") cysts reach an enormous size and are responsible for an abdominal mass in the fetus and newborn (Fig. 12–10).[14,35,67,93,112] Chung described a solitary, unilocular, hepatic cyst that was detected prenatally at 27 weeks' gestation.[14] By the end of gestation, the cyst had grown to 11 cm in diameter, displacing the left lobe of the liver, and was successfully resected. Quillin and McAlister[112] and Merine and co-workers[93] reported similar cases, manifesting as large, cystic, abdominal masses present at birth. Donovan and colleagues reviewed the Boston Children's Hospital experience over a 63-year period.[35] They collected 30 cases of hepatic cysts, 50% of which involved patients younger than 3 months of age and 8 of which were diagnosed during the first week of life. From their study, no definite conclusion could be drawn regarding etiology of the cysts. Infantile polycystic disease of the kidneys and liver may be apparent at birth and is manifested by renohepatomegaly (Fig. 12–11).

Inflammatory pseudotumor (inflammatory myofibroblastic tumor) of the liver has also been reported in the newborn.[17,123] The male patient described by Coffin et al. had an 8-cm mass that involved the liver and peritoneum. The mass was excised, but it recurred and persisted for more than 2 years at the time of writing.[17] The patient was well otherwise. Three main histologic patterns are described for this "nebuloma": one that resembles nodular fasciitis, another that resembles fibrous histiocytoma, and a third that is similar to that of a desmoid or scar.[17] The immunohistochemical findings suggest that the spindle cells comprising the lesion are myofibroblasts, in that they are reactive with vimentin, muscle-specific actin, and smooth muscle actin. Although the lesions recur if not completely excised, they do not metastasize. The lesions are probably inflammatory and "reactive" in nature.

REFERENCES

1. Alpert ME, Seeler RA. Alpha-fetoprotein in embryonal hepatoblastoma. J Pediatr 1970;77:1058.
2. Alt B, Hafez GR, Trigg M, et al. Angiosarcoma of a liver and spleen in an infant. Pediatr Pathol 1985;4:331.
3. Aoyama C, Hachitanda Y, Sato JK, et al. Undifferentiated (embryonal) sarcoma of the liver: A tumor of uncertain histogenesis showing divergent differentiation. Am J Surg Pathol 1991;15:615.
4. Benjamin E, Lendon M, Marsden HB. Hepatoblastoma as a cause of intrauterine fetal death. Case report. Br J Obstet Gynaecol 1981;88:329.
5. Berry PJ. Congenital tumours. *In* Keeling JW (ed): Fetal and Neonatal Pathology, 2nd ed, p 273. Berlin: Springer-Verlag, 1993.
6. Blair JI, Carachi R, Gupta R, et al. Plasma α-fetoprotein reference ranges in infancy: Effect of prematurity. Arch Dis Child 62:362, 1987.
7. Bolande RP. Developmental pathology. Am J Pathol 1979;94:627.

8. Bond JV. Neuroblastoma metastatic to the liver in infants. Arch Dis Child 1976;51:879.

9. Borch K, Jacobsen T, Olsen JH, et al. Neonatal cancer in Denmark 1943–1985. Pediatr Hematol Oncol 1992;9:209.

10. Broadbent VA. Malignant disease in the neonate. *In* Roberton NRC (ed): Textbook of Neonatology, 2nd ed, p 879. Edinburgh: Churchill Livingstone, 1992.

11. Campbell AN, Chan HSL, O'Brien A, et al. Malignant tumours in the neonate. Arch Dis Child 1987;62:19.

12. Chandra RS, Kapur SP, Kelleher J Jr, et al. Benign hepatocellular tumors in the young: A clinicopathologic spectrum. Arch Pathol Lab Med 1984;108:168.

13. Chang C-H, Ramirez N, Sakr WA. Primitive neuroectodermal tumor of the brain associated with malignant rhabdoid tumor of the liver: A histologic, immunohistochemical and electron microscopic study. Pediatr Pathol 1989;9:307.

14. Chung W. Antenatal detection of hepatic cyst. J Clin Ultrasound 1986;14:217.

15. Clatworthy HW Jr, Schiller M, Grosfeld JL. Primary liver tumors in infancy and childhood. 41 cases previously treated. Arch Surg 1974;109:143.

16. Coffin CM, Dehner LP. Congenital tumors. *In* Stocker JT, Dehner LP (eds): Pediatric Pathology, Vol 1, p 325. Philadelphia: JB Lippincott, 1992.

17. Coffin CM, Watterson J, Priest JR, et al. Extrapulmonary inflammatory myofibroblastic tumor (inflammatory pseudotumor): A clinicopathologic and immunohistochemical study of 84 cases. Am J Surg Pathol 1995;19:859.

18. Conran RM, Hitchcock CL, Waclawiw MA, et al. Hepatoblastoma: The prognostic significance of histologic type. Pediatr Pathol 1992;12:167.

19. Craig JR, Peters RL, Edmondson HA. Tumors of the liver and intrahepatic bile ducts, Atlas of Tumor Pathology, Fascicle 26, 2nd Series. Washington, DC: Armed Forces Institute of Pathology, 1989.

20. Cremin BJ, Nuss D. Calcified hepatoblastoma in a newborn. J Pediatr Surg 1974;9:913.

21. Cross SS, Variend S. Combined hepatoblastoma and yolk sac tumor of the liver. Cancer 1992;69:1323.

22. Davenport M, Hansen L, Heaton ND, et al. Hemangioendothelioma of the liver in infants. J Pediatr Surg 1995;30:44.

23. Davis CF, Carachi R, Young DG. Neonatal tumors: Glasgow 1966–86. Arch Dis Child 1988;63:1075.

24. Davis GL, Kissane JM, Ishak KG. Embryonal rhabdomyosarcoma (sarcoma botryoides) of the biliary tree. Cancer 1969;24:333.

25. Dehner LP. Hepatic tumors in the pediatric age group: A distinctive clinico-pathologic spectrum. Perspect Pediatr Pathol 1978;4:217.

26. Dehner LP. Neoplasms of the fetus and neonate. *In* Naeye RL, Kissane JM, Kaufman N (eds): Perinatal Diseases, International Academy of Pathology, Monograph No. 22, p 286. Baltimore: Williams and Wilkins, 1981.

27. Dehner LP. Pediatric Surgical Pathology, 2nd ed. Baltimore: Williams and Wilkins, 1987.

28. Dehner LP, Ewing SL, Sumner HW. Infantile mesenchymal hamartoma of the liver: Histologic and ultrastructural observations. Arch Pathol 1975;99:379.

29. Dehner LP, Ishak KG. Vascular tumors of the liver in infants and children. Arch Pathol 1971;92:101.

30. Dehner LP, Parker ME, Franciosi RA, et al. Focal nodular hyperplasia and adenoma of the liver. A pediatric experience. Am J Pediatr Hematol Oncol 1979;1:85.

31. De Maioribus CA, Lally KP, Sim K, et al. Mesenchymal hamartoma: A 35-year review. Arch Surg 1990;125:598.

32. DeStephano DB, Wesley JR, Heidelberger KP, et al. Primitive cystic hepatic neoplasm of infancy with mesothelial differentiation: Report of a case. Pediatr Pathol 1985;4:291.

33. Dimmick JE. Liver disease in the perinatal infant. *In* Wigglesworth JS, Singer DB (eds): Textbook of Fetal and Perinatal Pathology, Vol 2, p 981. London: Blackwell, 1991.

34. Dische MR, Gardner HA. Mixed teratoid tumors of the liver and neck in trisomy 13. Am J Clin Pathol 1978;69:631.

35. Donovan MJ, Kozakewich H, Perez-Atayde A. Solitary nonparasitic cysts of the liver: The Boston Children's Hospital experience. Pediatr Pathol Lab Med 1995;15:419.

36. Drut R, Drut RM, Toulouse JC. Hepatic hemangioendotheliomas, placental chorangiomas, and dysmorphic kidneys in Beckwith-Wiedemann syndrome. Pediatr Pathol 1992;12:197.

37. Edmondson HA. Differential diagnosis of tumors and tumor-like lesions of liver in infancy and childhood. Am J Dis Child 1956;91:168.

38. Ehren H, Mahour GH, Isaacs H Jr. Benign liver tumors in infancy and childhood: Report of 48 cases. Am J Surg 1983;145:325.

39. Exelby PR, Filler RM, Grosfeld JL. Liver tumors in children in particular reference to hepatoblastoma and hepatocellular carcinoma: American Academy of Pediatrics Surgical Section Survey—1974. J Pediatr Surg 1975;10:329.

40. Foucar E, Williamson RA, Yiu-Chiu V, et al. Mesenchymal hamartoma of the liver identified by fetal sonography. AJR 1983;140:970.

41. Fraumeni JF Jr, Miller RW, Hill JA. Primary carcinoma of the liver in childhood: An epidemiologic study. J Natl Cancer Inst 1978;40:1087.

42. Garmel SH, Crombleholme TM, Semple JP, et al. Prenatal diagnosis and management of fetal tumors. Semin Perinatol 1994;18:350.

43. Geiser CF, Baez A, Schindler AM. Epithelial hepatoblastoma associated with congenital hemihypertrophy and cystathioninuria. Pediatr 1970;46:66.

44. George JC, Cohen MD, Tarver RD, et al. Ruptured cystic mesenchymal hamartoma: An unusual cause of neonatal ascites. Pediatr Radiol 1994;24:304.

45. Giardiello FM, Offerhaus GJA, Krush AJ, et al. Risk of hepatoblastoma in familial adenomatous polyposis. J Pediatr 1991;119:766.

46. Gold JH, Guzman IJ, Rosai J. Benign tumors of the liver: Pathologic examination of 45 cases. Am J Clin Pathol 1978;70:6.

47. Golitz LE, Rudikoff J, O'Meara OP. Diffuse neonatal hemangiomatosis. Pediatr Dermatol 1986;3:145.

48. Gonen R, Fong K, Chiasson DA. Prenatal sonographic diagnosis of hepatic hemangioendothelioma with secondary nonimmune hydrops fetalis. Obstet Gynecol 1989;73:485.

49. Gonzalez-Crussi F. Case 1. Undifferentiated small cell ("anaplastic") hepatoblastoma. Pediatr Pathol 1991;11:155.

50. Gonzalez-Crussi F. Undifferentiated (embryonal) liver sarcoma of childhood: Evidence of leiomyoblastic differentiation. Pediatr Pathol 1983;1:281.

51. Gonzalez-Crussi F, Manz HJ. Structure of a hepatoblastoma of pure epithelial type. Cancer 1972;29:1272.

52. Gonzalez-Crussi F, Upton MP, Mauer HS. Hepatoblastoma: Attempt at characterization of histologic subtypes. Am J Surg Pathol 1982;6:599.

53. Greenberg M, Filler RM. Hepatic tumors. *In* Pizzo PA, Poplack DG (eds): Principles and Practice of Pediatric Oncology, 2nd ed, p 697. Philadelphia: JB Lippincott, 1993.

54. Gururangan S, Bowman LC, Parham DM, et al. Primary extracranial rhabdoid tumors: Clinicopathologic features and response to ifosfamide. Cancer 71: 2653, 1993.

55. Haas JE, Muczynski KA, Krailo M, et al. Histopathology and prognosis in childhood hepatoblastoma and hepatocarcinoma. Cancer 1989;64:1082.

56. Hansen K, Bagtas J, Mark HF, et al. Undifferentiated small cell hepatoblastoma with a unique chromosomal translocation: A case report. Pediatr Pathol 1992;12:457.

57. Hart WR. Primary endodermal sinus (yolk sac) tumor of the liver: First reported case. Cancer 1975;35:1453.

58. Hartley AL, Birch JM, Kelsey AM, et al. Epidemiological and familial aspects of hepatoblastoma. Med Pediatr Oncol 1990;18:103.

59. Hirata GI, Matsunaga MI, Medearis AL, et al. Ultrasonographic diagnosis of a fetal abdominal mass: A case of a mesenchymal liver hamartoma and a review of the literature. Prenat Diagn 1990;10:507.

60. Horgan JG, King DL, Taylor JKW. Sonographic detection of prenatal liver mass. J Clin Gastroenterol 1984; 6:277.

61. Horie A, Kotoo Y, Hayashi I. Ultrastructural comparison of hepatoblastoma and hepatocellular carcinoma. Cancer 1979;44:2184.

62. Horowitz ME, Etcubanas E, Webber BL, et al. Hepatic undifferentiated (embryonal) sarcoma and rhabdomyosarcoma in children: Results of therapy. Cancer 1987;59:396.

63. Hunt SJ, Anderson WD. Malignant rhabdoid tumor of the liver. A distinct clinicopathologic entity. Am J Clin Pathol 1990;94:645.

64. Isaacs, H Jr. Congenital and neonatal malignant tumors: A 28-year experience at Children's Hospital of Los Angeles. Am J Pediatr Hematol/Oncol 1987; 9(2):121.

65. Isaacs H Jr. Neoplasms in infants: A report of 265 cases. Pathol Annu 1983;18(2):165.

66. Isaacs H Jr. Perinatal (congenital and neonatal) neoplasms: A report of 110 cases. Pediatr Pathol 1985;3: 165.

67. Isaacs H Jr. Tumors of the Newborn and Infant: St. Louis: Mosby–Year Book, 1991.

68. Ishak KG, Glunz PR. Hepatoblastoma and hepatocarcinoma in infancy and childhood: Report of 47 cases. Cancer 1967;20:396.

69. Joshi VV, Kaur P, Ryan B, et al. Mucoid anaplastic hepatoblastoma. A case report. Cancer 1984;54:2035.

70. Jozwiak S, Pedich M, Rajszys P, et al. Incidence of hepatic hamartomas in tuberous sclerosis. Arch Dis Child 1992;67:1363.

71. Kasai M, Watanabe I. Histologic classification of liver cell carcinoma in infancy and childhood and its clinical evaluation: A study of 70 cases collected in Japan. Cancer 1970;25:551.

72. Kazzi NJ, Chang C-H, Roberts EC, et al. Fetal hepatoblastoma presenting as non-immune hydrops. Am J Perinatol 1989;6:278.

73. Keeling JW. Liver tumours in infancy and childhood. J Pathol 1971;103:69.

74. Keating S, Taylor GP. Undifferentiated (embryonal) sarcoma of the liver: Ultrastructural and immunohistochemical similarities with malignant fibrohistiocytoma. Hum Pathol 1985;16:693.

75. Khan A, Bader JL, Hoy GR, et al. Hepatoblastoma in a child with fetal alcohol syndrome. Lancet 1979;1: 1403.

76. Kingston JE, Herbert A, Draper GJ, et al. Association between hepatoblastoma and polyposis coli. Arch Dis Child 1983;58:959.

77. Knowlson GTG, Cameron AH. Hepatoblastoma with adenomatoid renal epithelium. Histopathology 1979; 3:201.

78. Lack EE. Mesenchymal hamartoma of the liver. A clinical and pathologic study of nine cases. Am J Pediatr Hematol Oncol 1986;8:91.

79. Lack EE, Neave C, Vawter GF. Hepatoblastoma: A clinical and pathological study of 54 cases. Am J Surg Pathol 1982;6:693.

80. Lack EE, Neave C, Vawter GF. Hepatocellular carcinoma. A review of 32 cases in childhood and adolescence. Cancer 1983;52:1510.

81. Laird WP, Friedman S, Koop CE, et al. Hepatic hemangiomatosis. Am J Dis Child 1976;130:657.

82. Landing BH. Tumors of the liver in childhood. *In* Okuda K, Peters RL (eds): Hepatocellular Carcinoma. New York: John Wiley and Sons, 1976.

83. Larcher VF, Howard ER, Mowat AP. Hepatic haemangiomata: Diagnosis and management. Arch Dis Child 1981;56:7.

84. Lennington WJ, Gray GF Jr, Page DL. Mesenchymal hamartoma of liver: A regional ischemic lesion of a sequestered lobe. Am J Dis Child 1993;147:193.

85. Leonidas JC, Strauss L, Beck AR. Vascular tumors of the liver in newborns. Am J Dis Child 1973;125:507.

86. Li FP, Thurber WA, Seddon J, et al. Hepatoblastoma in families with polyposis coli. JAMA 1987;257:2475.

87. Luks FI, Yazbeck S, Brandt ML, et al. Benign liver tumors in children: A 25 year experience. J Pediatr Surg 1991;26:1326.

88. Mamlok V, Nichols M, Lockart L, et al. Trisomy 18 and hepatoblastoma. Am J Med Genet 1989;33:125.

89. Manivel C, Wick MR, Abenoza P, et al. Teratoid hepatoblastoma: The nosologic dilemma of solid embryonic neoplasms of childhood. Cancer 1986;57:2168.

90. Marks F, Thomas P, Lustig I, et al. In utero sonographic description of a fetal liver adenoma. J Ultrasound Med 1990;9:119.

91. Mason BA, Hodges W, Goodman JR. Antenatal sonographic detection of a rare solid hepatic mesenchymal hamartoma. J Maternal-Fetal Med 1992;1:134.

92. McGoldrick JP, Boston VE, Glasgow JFT. Hepatocellular carcinoma associated with macronodular cirrhosis in a neonate. J Pediatr Surg 1986;21:277.

93. Merine D, Nussbaum AR, Sanders RC. Solitary nonparasitic hepatic cyst causing abdominal distension and respiratory distress in a newborn. J Pediatr Surg 1990;25:349.

94. Miller JH, Greenspan BS. Integrated imaging of hepatic tumors in childhood. Part I: Malignant lesions (primary and metastatic). Radiology 1985;154:83.

95. Miller JH, Greenspan BS. Integrated imaging of hepatic tumors in childhood. Part II: Benign lesions (congenital, reparative, and inflammatory). Radiology 1985;154:91.

96. Misugi K, Okajima H, Misugi N, et al. Classification of primary malignant tumors of the liver in infancy and childhood. Cancer 1967;20:1760.

97. Misugi K, Reiner CB. A malignant true teratoma of the liver. Arch Pathol 1965;80:409.

98. Moore KL. The Developing Human—Clinically Oriented Embryology, 5th ed. Philadelphia: WB Saunders, 1993.

99. Moran CA, Mullick FG, Ishak KG. Nodular regenerative hyperplasia of the liver in children. Am J Surg Pathol 1991;15:449.

100. Muraji T, Woolley MM, Sinatra F, et al. The clinical implication of hypercholesterolemia in infants and children with hepatoblastoma. J Pediatr Surg 1985;20:228.

101. Murthy ASK, Vawter GF, Lee ABH, et al. Hormonal bioassay of gonadotropin-producing hepatoblastoma. Arch Pathol Lab Med 1980;104:513.

102. Nakagawara A, Ikeda K, Tsuneyoshi M, et al. Hepatoblastoma producing both alpha-fetoprotein and human chorionic gonadotropin. Clinicopathologic analysis of four cases and a review of the literature. Cancer 1985;56:1636.

103. Nakamoto SK, Dreilinger A, Dattel B, et al. The sonographic appearance of hepatic hemangioma in utero. J Ultrasound Med 1983;2:239.

104. Noronha R, Gonzalez-Crussi F. Hepatic angiosarcoma in a child. Am J Surg Pathol 1984;8:863.

105. Orozco-Florian R, McBride JA, Favara BE, et al. Congenital hepatoblastoma and Beckwith-Wiedemann syndrome: A case study including DNA ploidy profiles of tumor and adrenal cytomegaly. Pediatr Pathol 1991;11:131.

106. Parham DM, Peiper SC, Robicheaux G, et al. Malignant rhabdoid tumor of the liver. Arch Pathol Lab Med 1988;112:61.

107. Parkes SE, Muir KR, Southern L, et al. Neonatal tumours: A thirty-year population based study. Med Pediatr Oncol 1994;22:309.

108. Peters ME, Gilbert-Barness EF, Rao B, et al. Lymphangioendothelioma of the liver in a neonate. J Pediatr Gastroenterol Nutr 1989;9:115.

109. Petrovic O, Haller H, Rukavina B, et al. Prenatal diagnosis of a large liver cavernous hemangioma associated with polyhydramnios (Letter). Prenatal Diagn 1992;12:70.

110. Platt LD, Devore GR, Bennet P, et al. Antenatal diagnosis of a fetal liver mass. J Ultrasound Med 1983;2:521.

111. Platt MS, Agamanolis DP, Krill CE Jr, et al. Occult hepatic sinusoid tumor of infancy simulating neuroblastoma. Cancer 1983;52:1183.

112. Quillin SP, McAlister WH. Congenital solitary nonparasitic cyst of the liver in a newborn. Pediatr Radiol 1992;22:543.

113. Raffensberger F, Gonzalez-Crussi F, Sheehan T. Mesenchymal hamartoma of the liver. J Pediatr Surg 1983;18:585.

114. Resnick MB, Kozakewich HPW, Perez-Atayde AR. Hepatic adenoma in the pediatric age group: Clinicopathological observations and assessment of cell proliferative activity. Am J Surg Pathol 1995;19(10):1181.

115. Riikonen P, Tuominen L, Seppa A, et al. Simultaneous hepatoblastoma in identical male twins. Cancer 1990;66:2429.

116. Robinson HB Jr, Bolande RP. Case 3. Fetal hepatoblastoma with placental metastases. Pediatr Pathol 1985;4:163.

117. Robinson RA, Nelson L. Hepatic teratoma in an anencephalic fetus. Arch Pathol Lab Med 1986;110:655.

118. Romero R, Oilu G, Jeanty P, Ghidini A, Hobbins JC. Prenatal Diagnosis of Congenital Anomalies, p 34. Norwalk: Appleton & Lange, 1988.

119. Rubie H, Baunin C, Guitard J, et al. Tumeurs neonatales malignes. Rev Prat (Paris) 1993;43(17):2208.

120. Seppala M, Ruoslahti E. Alpha-fetoprotein: Physiology and pathology during pregnancy and application to antenatal diagnosis. J Perinatal Med 1973;1:104.

121. Sepulveda WH, Donetch G, Giuliano A. Prenatal sonographic diagnosis of fetal hepatic hemangioma. Eur J Obstet Gynecol Reprod Biol 1993;48:73.

122. Shah KD, Beck AR, Jhaveri MK, et al. Infantile hemangioendothelioma of heterotopic intrathoracic liver associated with diaphragmatic hernia. Hum Pathol 1987;18:754.

123. Shek TWH, Ng IOL, Chan KW. Inflammatory pseudotumor of the liver: Report of four cases and review of the literature. Am J Surg Pathol 1993;17:231.

124. Shturman-Ellstein R, Greco MA, Myrie C, Goldman EK. Hydrops fetalis, hydramnios and hepatic vascular malformation associated with cutaneous hemangioma and chorangioma. Acta Paediatr Scand 1978;67:239.

125. Silverman JF, Fu Y, McWilliams NB, et al. An ultrastructural study of mixed hepatoblastoma with osteoid elements. Cancer 1975;36:1436.

126. Sirota L, Freud N, Dulitzki F, et al. Hemoperitoneum as the presenting sign of hepatoblastoma in a newborn. Pediatr Surg Int 1992;7:131.

127. Slopec LL, Lakatau DJ. Non-immune fetal hydrops with hepatic hemangioepithelioma and Kasabach-Merritt syndrome: A case report. Pediatr Pathol 1989;9:987.

128. Smith WL, Ballantine TVN, Gonzalez-Crussi F. Hepatic mesenchymal hamartoma causing heart failure in the neonate. J Pediatr Surg 1978;13:183.

129. Sotelo-Avila C, Gooch WM. Neoplasms associated with the Beckwith-Wiedemann syndrome. In Rosenberg HS, Bolande RP (eds): Perspectives in Pediatric Pathology, Vol 3, p 255. Chicago: Year Book Medical Publishers, 1976.

130. Stanley P, Gates GF, Eto RT, et al. Hepatic cavernous hemangiomas and hemangioendotheliomas in infancy. Am J Radiol 1977;129:317.

131. Stanley P, Geer GD, Miller JH, et al. Infantile hepatic hemangiomas: Clinical features, radiologic investigations, and treatment of 20 patients. Cancer 1989;64:936.

132. Stanley P, Hall TR, Woolley MM, et al. Mesenchymal hamartomas of the liver in childhood: Sonographic and CT findings. AJR 1986;147:1035.

133. Stocker JT, Ishak KG. Focal nodular hyperplasia of the liver: A study of 21 pediatric cases. Cancer 1981;48:336.

134. Stocker JT, Ishak KG. Hepatoblastoma. In Okuda K, Ishak KG (eds): Neoplasms of the Liver. New York: Springer-Verlag, 1987.

135. Stocker JT, Ishak KG. Mesenchymal hamartoma of the liver: Report of 30 cases and review of the literature. Pediatr Pathol 1983;1:245.

136. Stocker JT, Ishak KG. Undifferentiated (embryonal) sarcoma of the liver. Cancer 1978;42:336.

137. Tanaka T, Takakura H, Takashima S, et al. A rare case of Aicardi syndrome with severe brain malformation and hepatoblastoma. Brain Dev 1985;7:507.

138. Todani T, Tabuchi K, Watanabe Y, et al. Carcinoma arising in the wall of congenital bile duct cysts. Cancer 1979;44:1134.

139. Todani T, Tabuchi K, Watanabe Y, et al. True hepatic

teratoma with high alpha-fetoprotein in serum. J Pediatr Surg 1977;12:591.

140. Van de Bor M, Verway RA, van Pel R. Acute polyhydramnios associated with fetal hepatoblastoma. Eur J Obstet Gynecol Reprod Biol 1985;20:65.

141. Van Eyken P, Sciot R, Callea F, et al. A cytokeratin-immunohistochemical study of hepatoblastoma. Hum Pathol 1990;21:302.

142. Weinberg AG, Finegold MJ. Primary hepatic tumors of childhood. Hum Pathol 1983;14:512.

143. Weinberg AG, Finegold MJ. Primary hepatic tumors in childhood. *In* Finegold M (ed): Pathology of Neoplasia in Children and Adolescents, Major Problems in Pathology, Vol 18, p 333. Philadelphia: WB Saunders, 1986.

144. Werb P, Scurry J, Ostor A, et al. Survey of congenital tumors in perinatal necropsies. Pathology 1992;24:247.

145. Wheeler DA, Edmondson HA, Reynolds TB. Spontaneous liver cell adenoma in children. Am J Clin Pathol 1986;85:6.

146. Wienk MATP, van Geijn HP, Copray FJA, et al. Prenatal diagnosis of fetal tumors by ultrasonography. Obstet Gynecol Surv 1990;45:639.

147. Willis RA. The Borderland of Embryology and Pathology, 2nd ed, p 442. London: Butterworths, 1962.

ADRENOCORTICAL TUMORS

13

The embryology of the adrenal gland, tumor-like conditions, adrenocortical adenoma, and carcinoma are the subjects discussed in this chapter.

The adrenal cortex is the source of several tumors and tumor-like conditions with unusual clinical manifestations in the newborn.[3,19,30,31,36,69,77,86,92,96] Adrenocortical neoplasms are uncommon in this age group and throughout childhood as well.[24,30] Relatively few examples of adrenal cysts, cortical adenomas, and carcinomas have been described, some in association with the Beckwith-Wiedemann syndrome, hemihypertrophy, cancer family syndrome (Li-Fraumeni), or other tumors (Table 13–1).[17,72,75,80,101–103,107] Overall, the adrenal medulla is a far more common site for tumors in the fetus and newborn than the cortex; in fact, the incidence ratio of neuroblastoma to adrenocortical tumors is about 10:1 in children.[31,32] Adrenocortical hyperplasia associated with the adrenogenital and Cushing's syndromes occurs more often than true adrenocortical neoplasms in the first year of life.[25,54,86]

EMBRYOLOGY OF THE ADRENAL CORTEX

The adrenal gland consists of two components, the cortex and medulla, which are embryologically and biochemically distinct. The cortex arises from the embryonic mesoderm and secretes steroid hormones, whereas the medulla develops from the neural crest and produces catecholamines.[42,83,86,92]

The adrenal cortex is first observed at the 9-mm stage (sixth week of gestation) as a prolifer-ation of the coelomic mesothelium between the root of the mesentery and the upper end of the mesonephros of the developing gonad. This cluster of cells descends into the underlying mesenchyme, forming the fetal (provisional) cortex. Approximately at the same time, cells from the neural crest migrate into the center of the fetal cortex to form the medulla (see Fig. 6–1). Several days later, a second mesothelial proliferation is added to the surface of the fetal cortex that will form the peripheral rim of the permanent cortex (definitive or adult zone) of the adrenal.[42,83] By the 12th week of gestation, the two cortices are easily recognizable; the outer cortex is made up of a thin rim of regular, small, cuboidal cells, whereas the central fetal zone comprising the bulk of the gland consists of prominent anastomosing cords of large, polyhedral, acidophilic cells separated by sinusoids.[42,92] Owing to the presence of the fetal cortex, which constitutes more than 75% of the gland, the adrenal is relatively large in the fetus and newborn as compared to the size of the kidney. The permanent cortex is essentially nonfunctional throughout the first 3 months of gestation, but begins to show hormonal activity at about the 25th week.[42] By contrast, the dominant fetal cortex begins steroid synthesis from the seventh week on, increasing through the next trimesters until birth.[42] Histologic differentiation of the permanent cortex into the zona glomerulosa and fasciculata is evident at birth, but the zona reticularis is not well defined until about the third year of life.[81,83] Both steroid metabolism and the development of the adrenal cortex in the fetus are dependent on the fetal-placental maternal unit.[73] Throughout most of gestation, fetal adrenocor-

Table 13–1. Tumors Associated with the Beckwith-Wiedemann Syndrome

---

Adrenocortical adenoma and carcinoma
Nephroblastomatosis
Wilms' tumor
Hepatoblastoma
Astrocytoma (glioblastoma, optic glioma)
Rhabdomyosarcoma
Cardiac fibroma
Neuroblastoma-ganglioneuroma
Pancreatoblastoma
Umbilical myxoma

From Beckwith;[11] Sotelo-Avila, Gonzalez-Crussi, and Fowler;[101] Sotelo-Avila and Gooch;[102] and Orozco-Florian, McBride, Favara et al.[89]

tical steroid synthesis is under the influence of both maternal and placental hormones.

METABOLISM

Adrenocortical hormones are subdivided into three main categories: glucocorticoids, mineralocorticoids, and sex steroids (androgens and estrogens) (Fig. 13–1). The zona glomerulosa secretes the mineralocorticoids aldosterone and deoxycorticosterone, the cells of the zona fasciculata secrete the glucocorticoids cortisone and cortisol, and the cells of the zona reticularis synthesize the sex steroids (androgens and estrogens).[86,109] Moreover, the zona reticularis and fasciculata act together as a functional unit, synthesizing both glucocorticoids and sex steroids. The cortical cells of all three zones are controlled by adrenocorticotropic hormone (ACTH).

Biosynthesis of steroid hormones from cholesterol proceeds through the formation of an intermediate, pregnenolone, which has the cholesterol ring and a two-carbon side chain (see Fig. 13–1). Pregnenolone is the precursor of progesterone, the progestational hormone of the corpus luteum and placenta, and this compound, in turn, is the precursor of the androgens (male hormones) androsterone and testosterone, of the estrogens (female sex hormones) estradiol and estrone, and of the adrenocortical hormones corticosterone and aldosterone.[54,81,86,117] If there is an enzymatic defect or block in one or more of the biosynthetic steps in the metabolic pathway (e.g., as in congenital adrenal hyperplasia) precursor steroids synthesized before the block accumulate in excess and produce characteristic clinical findings (e.g., virulism and salt loss). Cortical nodular hyperplasias, adenomas, and carcinomas may secrete an excess of one or more steroid hormones, resulting in certain endocrinopathies (e.g., virulism, Cushing's syndrome, and hypertension).

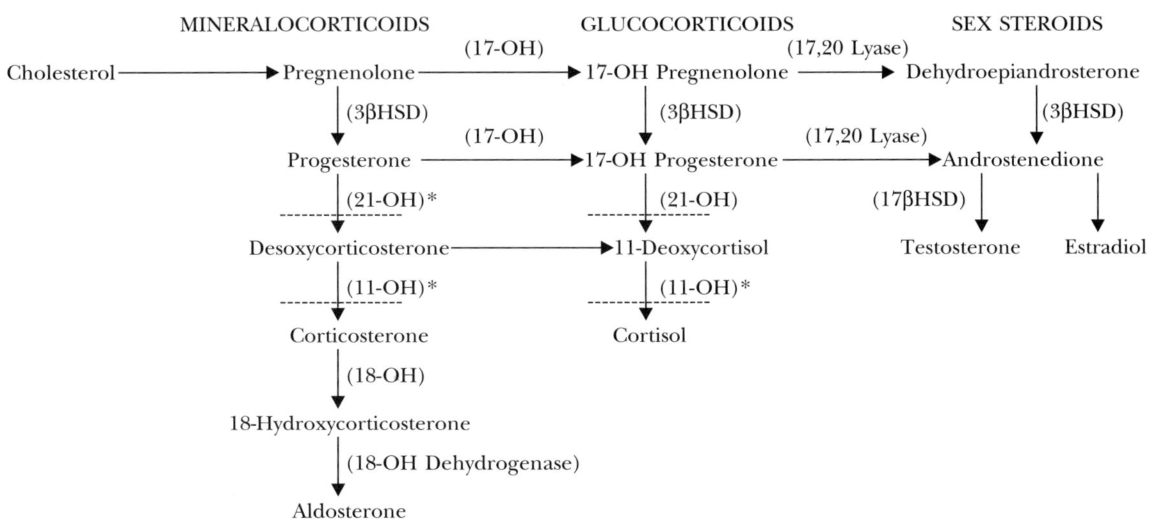

Enzyme abbreviations: 3βHSD = 3β-hydroxysteroid dehydrogenase; 17βHSD = 17β-hydroxysteroid dehydrogenase; 17-OH = 17-hydroxylase; 11-OH = 11-hydroxylase; 18-OH = 18-hydroxylase; 21-OH = 21-hydroxylase; --------------- = enzyme block. *Most common enzyme defects associated with the adrenogenital syndrome.

Figure 13–1. Adrenocortical steroid biosynthetic pathways. (From New MI, del Balzo P, Crawford C, et al. The adrenal cortex. *In* Kaplan SA (ed): Clinical Pediatric Endocrinology, p 181. Philadelphia: WB Saunders, 1990. Used by permission; and Hughes IA. Congenital and acquired disorders of the adrenal cortex. Clin Endocrinol Metab 1982;11[1]:89. Used by permission.)

ULTRASTRUCTURE OF THE ADRENAL CORTEX

Adrenocortical cells from all three zones—the zona glomerulosa, fasciculata, and reticularis—have certain ultrastructural features in common.[21,38,81] The cytoplasm of these cells contains an abundance of smooth- and rough-surfaced endoplasmic reticulum, ribosomes, and large lipid droplets with spherical or irregular outlines. The Golgi apparatus is prominent. Mitochondria are numerous and contain lamellar, tubular, or vesicular cristae; they have a round, oval, or elongated configuration with a fine structure characteristic of most steroid-secreting cells. The distribution and morphology of organelles, particularly the mitochondria and endoplastic reticulum, vary from one cortical zone to the next. Ultrastructurally, demarcation between the three zones is not always well defined. The reader is referred to the reviews by Ghadially,[38] Carney,[21] and Mininberg and colleagues[81] for a more detailed discussion of the ultrastructural features of the adrenal cortex.

ADRENOCORTICAL HYPERPLASIA

Hyperplasia and neoplasms of the adrenal cortex occur in the newborn. The excess hormone secretion associated with these conditions results in recognizable clinical syndromes, with the manifestations depending on the type(s) of steroid produced.[54,86,109] The hormone excess produces one or more characteristic findings (or a combination): Cushing's syndrome from hypersecretion of glucocorticoids; hypertension and hypokalemia from excess mineralocorticoids; or virilization or feminization from increased levels of androgens and estrogens, respectively.[86,109] Inherited enzyme defects in steroid hormone biosynthesis are responsible for most adrenocortical disorders in infants and children.[54,86] Congenital adrenal hyperplasia (adrenogenital syndrome) and Cushing's syndrome are the two principal endocrine diseases associated with adrenocortical hyperplasia, with the former being far more common than the latter.[31,54,86]

Congenital Adrenal Hyperplasia (Adrenogenital Syndrome)

Congenital adrenal hyperplasia is an autosomal recessive disease caused by one of the five

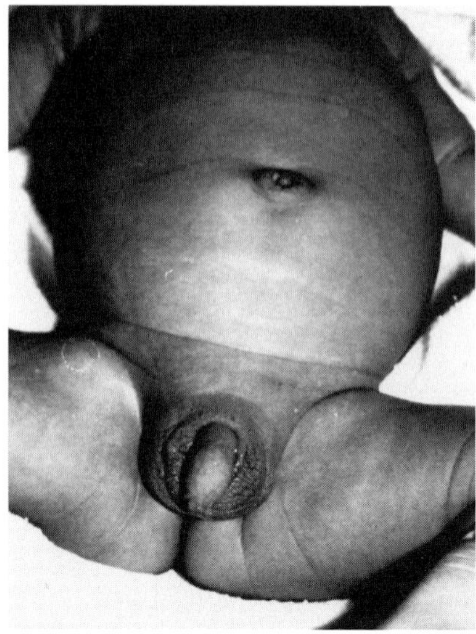

Figure 13–2. Congenital adrenal hyperplasia (adrenogenital syndrome). This female newborn with this syndrome has striking clitoral enlargement, labial fusion ("scrotalization"), and hyperpigmentation. Congenital adrenal hyperplasia is one of the most common causes of ambiguous genitalia. (Courtesy of Francine Kaufman, MD, Division of Endocrinology and Metabolism, Children's Hospital, Los Angeles, CA.)

or more known enzymatic defects (blocks) in cortisol biosynthesis from cholesterol (see Fig. 13–1).[54,57,81,86,117] It is the most frequent cause of ambiguous genitalia in the newborn (Fig. 13–2).[81] Neonatal screening studies indicate a frequency ranging from 1 in 5000 to 1 in 15,000, which is relatively common for an inborn error of metabolism.[117] Cortisol is synthesized principally in the zona fasciculata of the adrenal cortex. The secretion of cortisol is regulated by a negative feedback mechanism that involves this steroid and ACTH. Low cortisol levels lead to increased ACTH production by the pituitary gland which, in turn, produces continued stimulation of the adrenal cortex. The end result of this adrenal-pituitary imbalance is bilateral adrenocortical hyperplasia and increased cortical steroid synthesis, along with excessive secretion of sex hormones and other steroids, depending on the enzymatic block. If not treated promptly, some forms of congenital adrenal hyperplasia can be fatal in the newborn.

Deficiency of the 21-hydroxylase enzyme accounts for more than 90% of cases of congenital adrenal hyperplasia (Figs. 13–2 and 13–3).[25,31,42,54,57,86,117] Next in frequency is 11-hydroxylase deficiency. The genetic defect of congenital adrenal hyperplasia is localized to the 6p

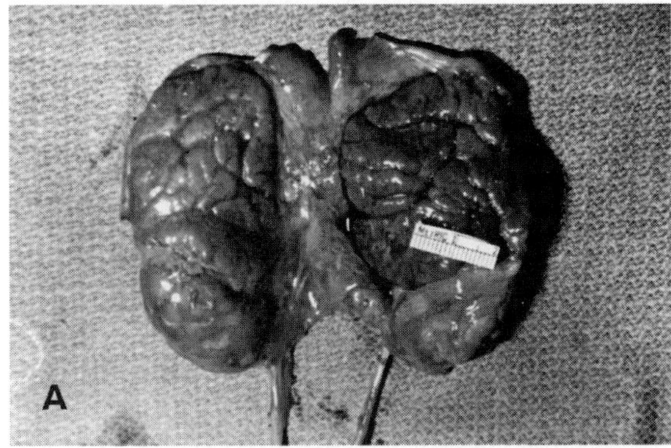

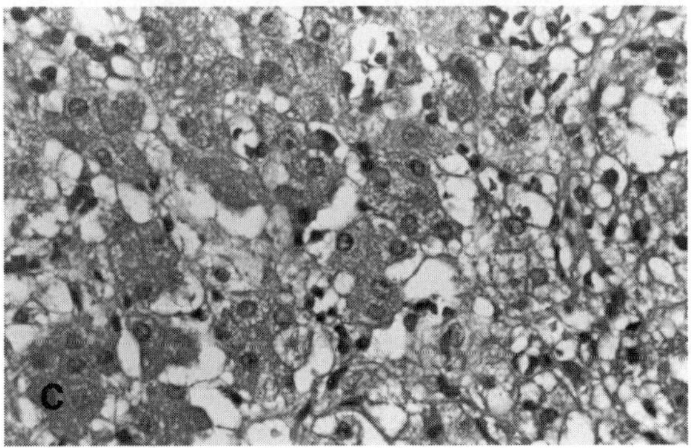

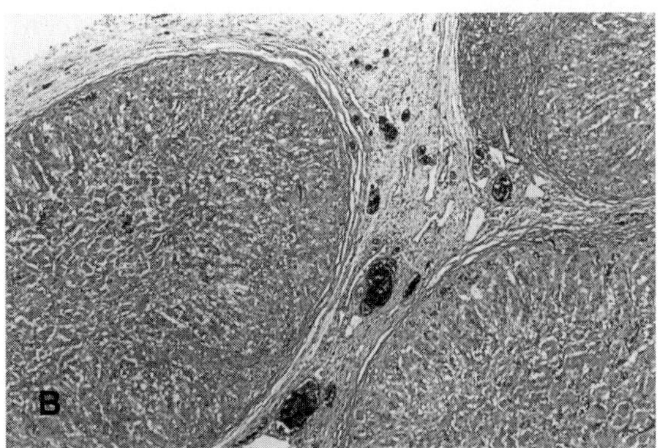

Figure 13–3. Congenital adrenal hyperplasia. *A,* Kidneys and adrenals from a 3-year-old boy with the salt-losing form of congenital adrenal hyperplasia secondary to 21-hydroxylase deficiency. The kidneys are dwarfed by huge, convoluted adrenals *(top),* which together weigh 25 g and have a wrinkled, cerebriform appearance. *B,* The cortex is thrown into numerous folds. The hyperplasia involves primarily the zona fasciculata and zona reticularis. The zona glomerulosa is abnormally small in size (hematoxylin-eosin, ×30). *C,* The adrenocortical cells are large, vacuolated, and filled with lipid. The darker staining cells in the left half of the field have eosinophilic-staining cytoplasms (hematoxylin-eosin, ×300).

chromosome for the 21-hydroxylase deficiency and the 8q chromosome for the 11-hydroxylase deficiency.[86] The 21-hydroxylase defect is closely linked to the human leukocyte antigen (HLA) major histocompatibility complex situated on the short arm of chromosome 6.[117]

Cortisol is not synthesized effectively in patients with the 21-hydroxylase defect, as 17-hydroxyprogesterone is not converted to 11-deoxycortisol, the immediate precursor of cortisol (see Fig. 13–1).[117] The lack of negative feedback then leads to high levels of ACTH and, in turn, to the hypersecretion of steroid precursors proximal to the 21-hydroxylation step. These precursors are converted to androgens and, in two thirds of patients with the 21-hydroxylase defect, the mineralocorticoid aldosterone. Androgens regulate the growth and development of both the male and female external genitalia of the fetus, but not the internal female organs (the uterus, fallopian tubes, and ovaries).[117]

Virilization is the end result of high levels of circulating androgens and is the most important physical finding in newborns with both the 11- and 21-hydroxylase enzyme defects. It is manifested in the female by clitoral hypertrophy (a phallus-like clitoris), labial fusion, and sometimes, scrotalization of the labia majora (see Fig. 13–2).[54,86,92,117] The internal female organs are essentially normal. The presence of ambiguous genitalia should alert the clinician to the possibility of the diagnosis of the adrenogenital syndrome, the discovery of which may be life-saving.[117] Virilization in the male newborn is not as obvious as it is in the female, and may not become noticeable in the former until the baby is several months old. It should be kept in mind that virilization that is present at birth secondary to an adrenal neoplasm can be mistaken for the adrenogenital syndrome.[91]

In roughly one half to two thirds of patients with the classic 21-hydroxylase defect, aldosterone synthesis is impaired.[117] This form of the disease is called the salt-wasting type of congenital adrenal hyperplasia.[81,117] "Simple virilizing disease" is the term used for infants and children without impaired aldosterone synthesis. Excessive salt loss from the renal tubules, secondary to low levels of aldosterone, leads to feeding difficulties, vomiting, hypovolemia, and shock. If left untreated, the salt-losing type results in death within the first weeks of life.[25,117]

Prenatal detection of 21-hydroxylase deficiency can be accomplished by measuring elevated levels of 17-hydroxyprogesterone in amniotic fluid collected between 14 and 20 weeks' gestation in pregnant women at risk.[54] Virilization and hypertension without salt-wasting are characteristically found in the female newborn with 11-hydroxylase deficiency.[86]

Adrenocortical tumors associated with congenital adrenal hyperplasia generally appear later in childhood and adulthood, and in this age group, are the subject of a few case reports.[8]

In the Children's Hospital, Los Angeles series of 74 patients with congenital adrenal hyperplasia secondary to 21-hydroxylase deficiency reported over a 25-year period, 36 patients presented at birth with the simple virilizing form, and 38 presented with the salt-losing form.[25] During the same period, seven children with virilizing adrenocortical tumors were observed at the hospital, a ratio of hyperplasia to neoplasm of 12:1. Among the 36 patients with the simple virilizing form, there were twice as many females affected as males. This finding is attributed to the fact that the enzymatic defect is easier to detect in the female because virilization is more obvious at birth. None of the infants or children in the series reported by Collipp and colleagues had the 11-hydroxylase, 3-B dehydrogenase, or the other rarer enzyme defects that have been described.[54,86] Moreover, the study pointed out that there is a high incidence (22%) of associated congenital anomalies in patients with congenital adrenal hyperplasia—namely, cardiovascular, genitourinary, and gastrointestinal defects.

The diagnosis of 21-hydroxylase deficiency in the newborn is established by determining the serum 17-hydroxyprogesterone level.[81,117] This steroid, which is the substrate for the 21-hydroxylases enzyme, is sufficiently elevated at birth so the test can be done on umbilical cord blood. The prenatal diagnosis of congenital adrenal hyperplasia is established by amniotic fluid analysis.[81] Urinary levels of 17-hydroxyprogesterone and 17-ketosteroids (chiefly derived from androgens) are elevated in patients with the 21-hydroxylase deficiency, but serum sterol determinations are more accurate.

Recently, sonography has been used for the diagnosis of congenital adrenal hyperplasia, particularly in newborns with ambiguous genitalia. The cerebriform pattern of the adrenals observed on sonography appears to be specific for the disease.[5]

The adrenal glands of patients with congenital adrenal hyperplasia have a striking and distinctive gross appearance.[31,42,67,92] First of all, the adrenals are usually enlarged, weighing as much as 15 g or more than the normal expected weight, which is 3 to 10 g.[92] Typically, the cortex is thrown into numerous folds or convolutions, giving the gland a wrinkled or cerebriform external surface that is even more evident on cross section (Fig. 13–3A).

Microscopic examination reveals cortical hyperplasia, which is sometimes nodular in configuration, with increased numbers of eosinophilic cells extending out toward the cortical surface (Figs. 13–3B and C). The cortical cells show a decreased amount of lipid as compared to normal cells.[30,92] Adrenal cytomegaly has been described in a newborn with congenital adrenal hyperplasia and transposition of the great vessels.[4] Ultrastructurally, the cells of the hyperplastic nodules closely resemble those of the zona reticularis.[38] They show abundant smooth endoplastic reticulum, and spherical and elongated mitochondria with tubulovesicular cristae.[38] Despite these findings, electron microscopy cannot be utilized to distinguish adrenocortical hyperplasia from either adenoma or carcinoma.[38]

Adrenocortical Hyperplasia Associated with Cushing's Syndrome

Adrenocortical hyperplasia occurs also in infants who do not have a known enzymatic block in steroid metabolism. Cushing's syndrome develops when there is excessive cortisol production by a neoplasm or as a result of hyperplasia of the adrenal cortex.[54,57,78,86] The syndrome should be distinguished from Cushing's disease, which results from excessive ACTH secretion by a basophilic adenoma of the anterior pituitary gland which, in turn, leads to excessive production of cortisol by the adrenal cortex. Nevertheless, the clinical signs and symptoms of both the syndrome and disease are essentially the same. For all practical purposes, Cushing's disease does not occur in the newborn.[1,40,41,65,74,78,94] Rarely, Cushing's syndrome is familial.[2] Arce et al. described a family in whom 4 of 7 siblings had the syndrome appearing at puberty. Adrenocortical carcinoma was found in one sibling, and adenomatous hyperplasia was diagnosed in three.[2]

Infants and newborns with Cushing's syndrome have either primary adrenocortical hyperplasia or a functioning neoplasm of the adrenal.[31,65,67,74,86,90] Most such disorders in this age group are associated with adrenocortical carcinoma, although several examples of cortical adenoma and hyperplasia have been described. Klevit et al. reviewed 20 patients with Cushing's syndrome in infancy, including one of their own.[65] More than 50% (11 of 20) had adrenocortical carcinoma, 5 had an adenoma, and 4 had nodular hyperplasia.[65] A comparable review of 27 cases was reported by Gilbert and Cleveland (1924–1969) with similar findings.[40] The final diagnoses included carcinoma in 11 infants, adenoma in 10 patients, and hyperplasia in 6. Their youngest patient was a 1-month-old with bilateral adrenal hyperplasia.

Clinical Findings

The presenting signs and symptoms of an infant with Cushing's syndrome secondary to either adrenal hyperplasia or neoplasm are variable. They may appear abruptly or gradually, and they may be subtle or obvious.[65,87] In most series, obesity is the most frequent presenting sign in the young.[57,65,74,90] Other clinical findings include "moon facies" with plump cheeks, buffalo hump, and hypertension as observed in older individuals.[65,74] Excessive weight gain, even though there is failure of normal growth, is characteristic of this condition in the infant.[86] Additional features of Cushing's syndrome in this age group are worth mentioning.[41] Virulism is a more common sign in infancy than in older children. Insulin-resistant diabetes is found in all age groups, and although the pathogenesis is not well understood, the diabetes is usually cured by removal of the adrenal tumor. Hypertension accompanies the syndrome, and its pathogenesis is also unknown. The effects of high blood pressure can be severe and, if not corrected, heart failure may result.

The onset of symptoms of Cushing's syndrome associated with adrenocortical nodular hyperplasia beginning in the neonatal period is uncommon, but it has been reported.[1,40,65,87,90] For example, one of Loridan and Senior's patients with nodular hyperplasia had clinical symptoms at birth.[74] Aarskog and Tveteraas described a female infant who developed symptoms of the syndrome at 1 month of age and subsequently had a total bilateral adrenalectomy at the age of 4 months. Less than 4 years after surgery, the clinical manifestations of McCune-Albright's syndrome appeared— namely, skin pigmentation, polyostotic fibrous dysplasia, and sexual precocity.[1] The patient depicted by Klevit et al. had "failed to thrive" since birth.[65] Diabetes mellitus and severe osteoporosis were documented at 4 and 7 weeks of age, respectively. By 12 weeks of age, the infant had an obvious plethoric moon-shaped facies, a thoracodorsal fat pad, and evidence of virilization. Exploratory laparotomy at the age of 13 weeks revealed enlarged, irregularly nodular, adrenal glands. A striking retardation of skeletal maturation, with a bone age less than term, suggested to O'Bryan et al. a prenatal onset of Cushing's syndrome in their 8-week-old patient.[87]

Laboratory findings in young patients with Cushing's syndrome include leukocytosis with lymphopenia and eosinopenia, and often, a diabetic glucose tolerance curve.[57,74] Imaging studies show decreased muscle mass and increased subcutaneous fat, osteoporosis, retarded bone age, and lack of a thymic shadow.[65,74]

Pathologic Findings

The adrenal glands observed in infants with Cushing's syndrome associated with adrenocortical nodular hyperplasia are usually, but not always, enlarged, and are characterized by the presence of numerous, irregular, ill-defined nodularities that can be seen on both the external and cut surfaces.[1,65,74,78,87,92] Histologically, the hyperplastic nodules vary in size and involve mostly the zona fasciculata. They consist of active-appearing cortical cells of various sizes with varying degrees of lipid vacuolization. The intervening cortical tissue between the nodules tends to be atrophic. In the newborn, fetal cortical cells may comprise the nodules.[31,65] On microscopic examination, the adrenal glands of a 3-month-old male reported by Klevit et al.[65] showed a well-developed adult (permanent) cortex composed of zona glomerulosa and zona fasciculata and a prominent, wide, fetal cortex. Distributed throughout the glands were hyperplastic nodules composed of fetal cortical cells surrounded by atrophic permanent cortex.

The ultrastructural findings in adrenocortical hyperplasia, adenoma, and carcinoma associated with Cushing's syndrome are practically the same.[38,47,67,97] The cells show an abundant, smooth endoplasmic reticulum forming tubular networks and smooth-walled vesicles. The mitochondria have a distinctive pleomorphic appearance. They are round, oval, or elongated, and contain both tubular and lamellar

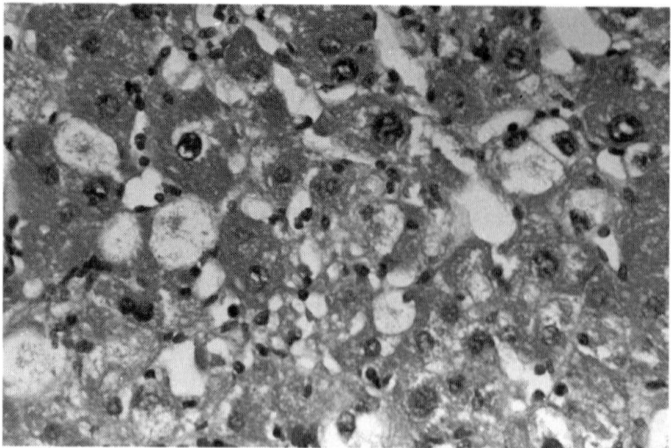

Figure 13–4. Adrenocortical cytomegaly. Large, peculiar-appearing cells with huge nuclei are present within the developing fetal adrenal cortex. Focal infiltrates of lymphocytes are noted. This was an incidental necropsy finding in a 4-day-old male infant with the Pena-Shokar syndrome (dysmorphic facies, multiple joint contractures, and pulmonary hypoplasia) (hematoxylin-eosin, ×300).

cristae; giant mitochondria may also be present.[38]

Bilateral, pigmented, nodular cortical hyperplasia ("primary pigmented nodular adrenocortical disease") is a rare cause of Cushing's syndrome in children and adults, but to the author's knowledge, it has not been reported in infants.[17,60] The youngest patient with this type of nodular hyperplasia in the Mayo Clinic review of 28 patients (including 4 patients of their own) was 4 years old.[98]

A discussion of the treatment of adrenocortical hyperplasia is beyond the scope of this book.

ADRENOCORTICAL CYTOMEGALY

Large, peculiar-looking, adrenocortical cells were first described by Kampmeier in 1927[59] and were reported later in a detailed study by Craig and Landing,[27] who also noted similar cells in the developing fetal cortex of stillborns and infants up to 2 months of age. Adrenal cytomegaly, a term coined by Potter and Craig,[92] is defined as the presence of large, bizarre-looking, eosinophilic cells with huge nuclei distributed focally or diffusely within the fetal cortical zone.[27,88,92] The cytomegalic cells are found only in the fetal cortex and are thought to arise from the large, single cells noted early in the developing fetal cortex.[27] They may occur singly, or in large numbers as wedge-shaped clusters extending to the surface of the adrenal, or as collections of cells distributed diffusely throughout the fetal cortex (Figs. 13–4, 13–5E, and 13–6E).

Craig and Landing reported 37 cases of adrenocortical cytomegaly from the Children's Hospital of Boston series,[27] and Potter and Craig described more than 20 cases from the Chicago Lying-in Hospital series.[92] The frequency of adrenal cytomegaly was 3% for the 1-day to 1-month age group, and 6.5% for stillborns. In the study of Aterman and co-workers, 16 of 300 (5.3%) newborns had the lesion.[4] However, the incidence of cytomegaly was considerably lower in several other reviews, including that of Beatty and Hawes[9] (11 of 1243 [0.9%]); Bech[10] (25 of 927 [2.7%]); Nakamura and colleagues[84] (17 of 1000 [1.7%]); and Favara et al.[35] (23 of 2711 [0.8%]). In Bech's series, the oldest patient with the lesion was 7 days of age.

An increased incidence of adrenal cytomegaly is noted in fetuses and newborns in association with erythroblastosis fetalis, maternal toxemia, multiple pregnancies, congenital heart malformations, hemihypertrophy, and in particular, Beckwith-Wiedemann syndrome (see Figs. 13–5 and 13–6).[4,7,9,10,16,27,67,84,88,92,103] In the study of Aterman and associates, 11 of 16 (69%) neonates with cytomegaly had erythroblastosis fetalis.[4] The most characteristic and consistent histologic feature of the adrenal gland in patients with the Beckwith-Wiedemann syndrome is diffuse, bilateral cytomegaly of the fetal cortex.[11,16,56,95,99,103] Cytomegaly is described in essentially every patient with this syndrome whose adrenals are examined microscopically. Familial examples of adrenal cytomegaly associated with the Beckwith-Wiedemann syndrome have been reported as well. Borit and Kosek describe a female newborn with the Beckwith-Wiedemann syndrome and adrenal cytomegaly.[16] Previously, the infant's 23-year-old mother had delivered a premature male infant who died shortly after birth with the same lesion.

There is a significant association between adrenal cytomegaly and congenital malformations.[4,9,10,13,88] Of 25 patients in Bech's review, 9 (36%) had cardiac anomalies, such as truncus arteriosus, atrial and ventricular septal defects, and various types of atresias.[10] Cardiac defects were found in 5 of 23 patients in the Johns Hopkins series.[88]

Adrenal cytomegaly is reported in fetuses and newborns in association with a wide variety of other conditions, such as pancreatic islet and Leydig cell hyperplasia,[88] idiopathic adrenal hypoplasia,[10,42] congenital rubella syndrome,[100] maternal diabetes,[27] and congenital adrenal hyperplasia.[4,27] It is noteworthy that 3 of 17 patients with cytomegaly in the study of

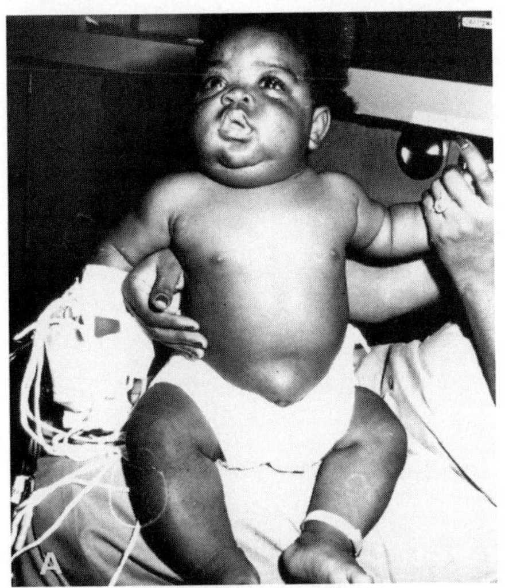

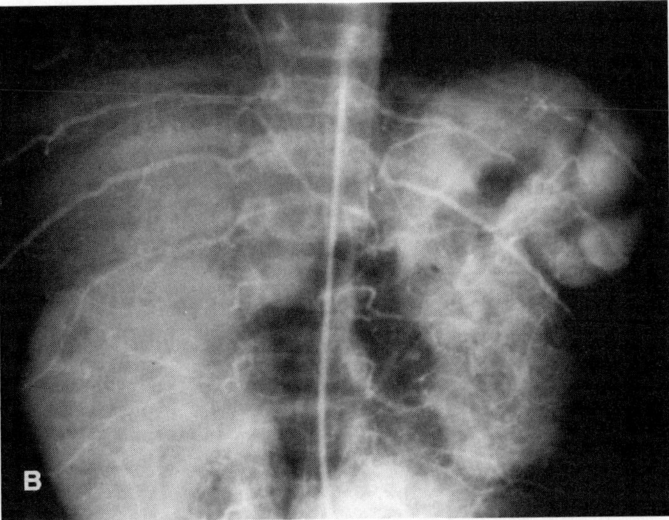

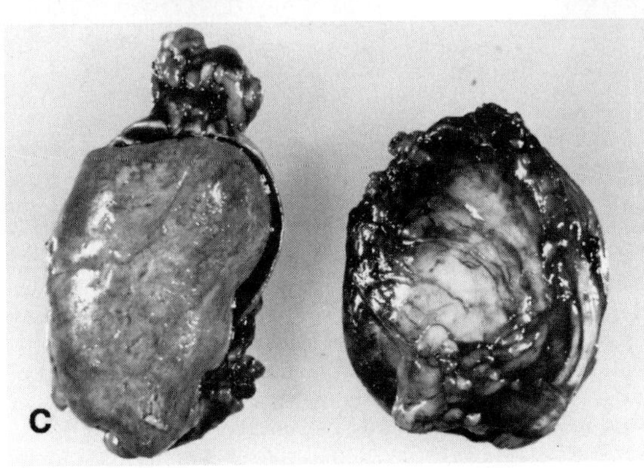

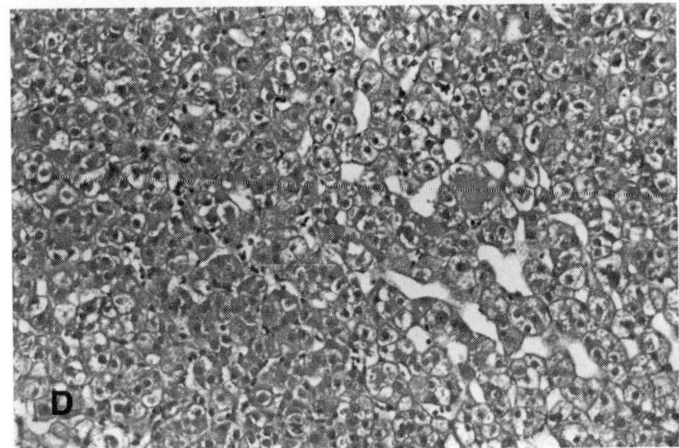

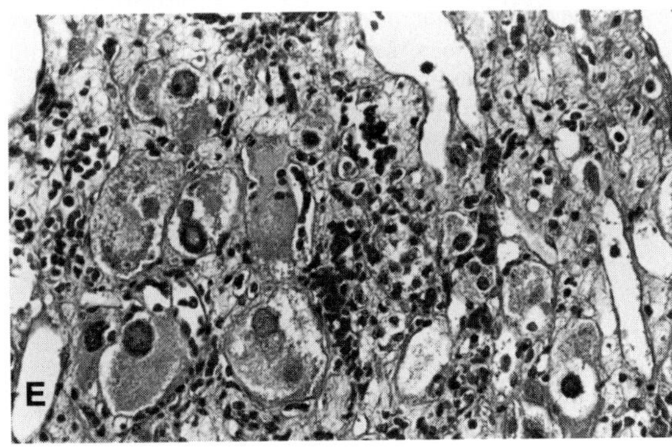

Figure 13–5. Adrenocortical adenoma. *A,* An 8-month-old girl presented with obesity, hypertension, acne (Cushing's syndrome) and a right adrenal mass. Hemihypertrophy is present on the right. *B,* An arteriogram shows a right suprarenal mass and an enlarged right kidney as compared to the left. *C,* The adrenal has been replaced by a 21-g, 5.5 × 3.5 cm tumor with a bright orange-tan, smooth, bulging, cut surface. *D,* Microscopic examination reveals nests and cords of clear, vacuolated cells with regular nuclei and cells with eosinophilic cytoplasms and more variable nuclei. Neither mitoses nor nuclear atypia are seen (hematoxylin-eosin, ×150). *E,* A focus of adrenal cytomegaly is present in the residual fetal cortex, which normally involutes at the age of 3 months (hematoxylin-eosin, ×300). Hemihypertrophy is associated with an increased incidence of adrenal tumors.

Nakamura and colleagues[84] and 6 of 23 in Oppenheimer's series[88] had pancreatic islet cell hyperplasia manifested clinically by neonatal hypoglycemia, which was presumbly the cause of death. It is conceivable that some of these patients had the "incomplete" form of Beckwith-Wiedemann syndrome.

The association of adrenal cytomegaly and neoplasms is well documented, particularly those associated with the Beckwith-Wiedemann syndrome and hemihypertrophy (see Table 13–1 and Figs. 13–5 and 13–6).[9,89,101] The neonate with disseminated metastatic adrenocortical carcinoma, described by Sherman and coworkers, had marked adrenal cytomegaly involving both glands.[99] The authors commented on the striking resemblance of the cytomegalic cells to those of adrenocortical carcinoma and proposed an etiologic relationship. A newborn with hepatoblastoma detected prenatally had,

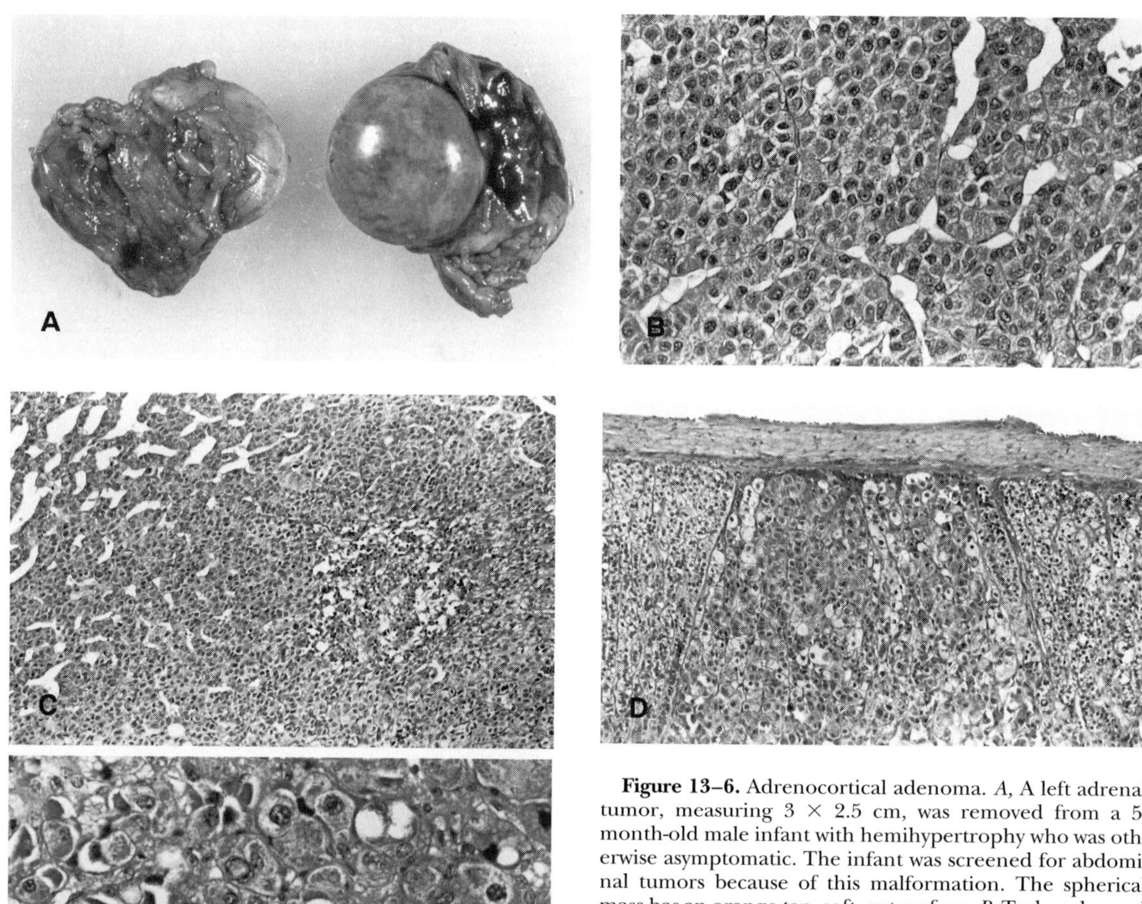

Figure 13–6. Adrenocortical adenoma. *A,* A left adrenal tumor, measuring 3 × 2.5 cm, was removed from a 5-month-old male infant with hemihypertrophy who was otherwise asymptomatic. The infant was screened for abdominal tumors because of this malformation. The spherical mass has an orange-tan, soft, cut surface. *B,* Trabeculae and cords of tumor cells are separated by vascular channels. Slight nuclear pleomorphism is noted (hematoxylin-eosin, ×300). *C,* An area of necrosis is present (hematoxylin-eosin, ×120). *D,* A section of adrenal cortex not involved by tumor reveals the adrenal capsule and zonae glomerulosa and fasciculata situated on either side of a wedge-shaped area of adenomatous hyperplasia (hematoxylin-eosin, ×120). *E,* The residual fetal cortex with a focus of adrenocortical cytomegaly is depicted (hematoxylin-eosin, ×300).

in addition to adrenal cytomegaly, nephromegaly (nephroblastomatosis) and pancreatic nesidioblastosis at necropsy.[89] However, this patient did not have either macroglossia or an omphalocele.

In most instances, the external appearance of the adrenals is normal, and the presence of cytomegaly is an unexpected microscopic finding on postmortem examinations performed on fetuses, stillborns, and newborns.[4,9,16,27,35,84,88,92] In only 1 of the 57 cases in Craig, Landing, and Potter's review was there any abnormality suspected from the gross appearance, and this was because of the difference in size between the two adrenals.[27,92] About 50% of the time, when both glands are examined, only one is found to have the cytomegalic cells.[84]

The huge nuclei of the cytomegalic cells have a dumbbell shape and a polylobar configuration. They are irregular, darkly basophilic-staining, and are composed of spherical, acidophilic, inclusion-like bodies and vacuoles. The cytoplasm stains uniformly eosinophilic, similar to the rest of the fetal cortical cells, and contains circumscribed masses of finely granular material. There is a peripheral rim of small vacuoles, giving the cell a characteristic foamy appearance. Like the smaller cells of the fetal cortex, the cytomegalic cells have a polygonal outline (Figs. 13–4 through 13–6).[27,84,92] Electron microscopic studies show that the nuclear inclusions actually represent invaginations of portions of the cytoplasm into the nucleus surrounded by double membranes.[16,84] The cytoplasm is packed with numerous mitochondria, vesicles, microsomes, and lysosomes, and the cytoplasmic granular material appears to be a lipochrome pigment.[31,84]

The cytomegalic cells show degenerative and involutionary changes similar to those observed in the ordinary fetal cortical cells.[27] The nuclear alterations seen include loss and fraying of the nuclear membrane, with fragmentation, pyknosis, and karyorrhexis. The cytoplasmic membrane becomes ill defined. Fatty infiltration, fading of the eosinophilic cytoplasm, and eccentric location of the nuclear remnants are other changes that may occur. Inflammatory infiltrates composed of neutrophils and large mononuclear cells are found in the rapidly involuting areas of the fetal cortex.[27]

The cause of adrenal cytomegaly is unknown. One proposal is that it is a manifestation of adrenal cortical hyperactivity in utero or in the newborn period.[31,84,88] For example, it could represent an exaggerated response to ACTH stimulation. Others believe that it is the result of a reactive or degenerative process.[4,67] Craig and Landing suggested that these atypical-looking cells may, in some instances, represent the precursor of masculinizing adrenal cortical carcinoma because the nuclei of the carcinoma cells in the adrenal closely resemble those of the cytomegalic cells seen in the newborn.[27] Sherman and co-workers[99] described an example of congenital metastasizing adrenocortical carcinoma associated with diffuse cytomegaly of the fetal cortex. In retrospect, the infant probably had the Beckwith-Wiedemann syndrome. The authors mentioned that the morphologic features of the cytomegalic cells were similar to those seen in the carcinoma cells. Another interesting hypothesis is that cytomegaly represents an in situ carcinoma of the fetal adrenal cortex that is destined, in most instances, to disappear at about the same time as involution of the fetal cortex.[103] This situation would be comparable to neuroblastoma and Wilms' tumor (nephrogenic rests) in situ. Some reports seem to support the neoplasia concept,[103] whereas others do not.[9,35] Bech suggested a viral etiology on the basis of the necrotic and inflammatory changes that are generally present.[10]

Using DNA quantitation by image analysis, Favara et al. noted significantly large amounts of DNA in the adrenocortical cytomegalic cells, more than 25 times the normal amount in some instances; the term they used to describe this phenomenon was polyploidization.[35] Cytomegaly with a high nuclear DNA content is found also in the pancreatic islets, acinar, and pituitary cells of these patients. The authors suggest that the increased amount of DNA in the cells of various organs is a response to physiologic demand, and not a specific marker for neoplasia.[35] Flow cytometric studies were performed by Camuto et al. on fetal adrenals with cortical cytomegaly the increased DNA content was interpreted to be the result of sustained hyperactivity followed by exhaustion secondary to some unknown stress.[20a] In earlier studies, Craig and Landing[27] and Aterman and colleagues[4] inferred that adrenal cytomegaly might represent polyploidy resulting from prolonged stimulation. Nevertheless, the etiology and significance of adrenal cytomegaly remain enigmatic.

ADRENOCORTICAL TUMORS

Incidence

Adrenocortical tumors are exceptionally uncommon in the pediatric age group, occurring in less than 15 children per year in the United States[80] and in less than 3 per year in England.[46] They may produce signs and symptoms in the newborn, particularly in the case of adrenal cortical carcinoma (Table 13–2). Female patients are affected much more often than male patients, with a ratio of almost 3:1.[20,36,41,46,52,52a,67] More than 50% of cortical tumors are found in children younger than 3 years of age. When they occur in the newborn, they are histologically similar to those noted in older children.[3,20,30,42,49,67,104,115] Carcinomas occur more frequently in the newborn than do adenomas. Eleven of the 14 (85%) adrenocortical tumors listed in Table 13–2 were diagnosed as carcinoma.

Clinical Findings

Virilization, Cushing's syndrome, and an abdominal mass are the main presenting findings in the newborn with adrenal tumors (see Table 13–2).[3,18,19,30,37,41,44,52,52a,54,55,63,77,86,91,93,96,99] Almost 50% of newborns present with an abdominal mass (see Table 13–2). The other clinical manifestations depend largely upon the type of hor-

Table 13–2. 14 Newborn Adrenocortical Tumors*

Case No.	Sex	Histologic Diagnosis	Presenting Findings	Associated Conditions	Therapy	Status	Reference
1	F	ACA, bilateral†	C, M		—	D	Powell et al.[93]
2	F	ACC	C, M		S	D	Guin and Gilbert[44]
3	F	ACC†‡; lung, brain, and pancreas metastases	Cyanosis, apnea	B-W	—	D	Sherman et al.[99]
4	F	ACC	V, HPN		S	D	Burrington and Stephens[18]
5	F	ACA	C, M, HPN	Monilial endocarditis and sepsis	S	D	Giombetti et al.[41]
6	M	ACT†	C, M, HPN	Adrenal ganglioneuroma	—	D	Gershanik et al.[37]
7	F	ACC	V, M		S, RT	L§	Artigas et al.[3]
8	F	ACC	V, M		S	D	Artigas et al.[3]
9	F	ACC; lung metastases	V, ambiguous genitalia		S, CT	D	Pigeon et al.[91]
10	M	ACC	V, HPN	CVA, acne	S	L	Hutchinson and Heyn[55]
11	M	ACC‡	Skin and brain metastases	HH, ?B-W, Wilms' tumor‖	S	L	Saracco et al.[96]
12	F	ACC, bilateral	C; liver metastasis		S	L	Holcombe et al.[52a]
13	M	ACC‡	Skin metastases		S, CT	?LTF	Butler et al.[19]
14	F	ACC‡; lung, skin, skeletal, and lymph node metastases	Skin metastases		BX	D	Mann et al.[77]

*Occurring in infants 3 months of age or younger who were selected from the literature.
†Diagnosed at necropsy.
‡Nonfunctioning adrenocortical carcinoma.
§Alive after recurrence.
‖Second malignant lesion.
C = Cushing's syndrome; V = virilization; HPN = hypertension; M = abdominal mass; ACA = adrenocortical adenoma; ACC = adrenocortical carcinoma; ACT = adrenocortical tumor; L = living; D = dead; LTF = lost to follow-up; HH = hemihypertrophy; B-W = Beckwith-Wiedemann syndrome; BX = biopsy; CVA = cerebrovascular accident; CT = chemotherapy; S = surgery; RT = radiation therapy.

mone(s) secreted by the tumor.[86] Virilization is present in one third and Cushing's syndrome in another third. However, the three main findings may be seen alone or in combination (see Table 13–2). Metastases to the skin or other sites may be the presenting findings in this age group, and may not be associated with endocrine manifestations. Hyperaldosteronism and feminizing signs, described infrequently in older children, for all practical purposes are not observed in younger children.

Neoplasms of the adrenal cortex have in common with Wilms' tumor and hepatoblastoma an increased association with hemihypertrophy and the Beckwith-Wiedemann syndrome, suggesting a common etiology, possibly of genetic origin (see Tables 13–1 and 13–2).[15,17,30,36,74,80] Tumors associated with the Beckwith-Wiedemann syndrome are listed in Table 13–1.

Cytogenetic studies show that a locus exists on chromosome 11p15 (a deletion or loss of heterozygosity) which is found in both adrenocortical carcinoma and with the Beckwith-Wiedemann syndrome.[50,51,118] Loss of tumor suppressor genes at loci on the short arm of chromosome 11 (p) also may be involved with the formation of other childhood malignant lesions, such as hepatoblastoma, Wilms' tumor, and possibly, rhabdomyosarcoma.[50,66] Moreover, certain families with children who have adrenocortical tumors exhibit an increased susceptibility to malignant disease as part of the SBLA cancer family syndrome (sarcoma, breast and brain tumor, leukemia, laryngeal and lung cancer, and adrenocortical carcinoma), which is probably transmitted in an autosomal dominant fashion.[46,72,75]

Congenital anomalies of the genitourinary tract, hamartomas, and brain tumors—namely, astrocytoma and medulloblastoma—have been reported in affected patients, particularly with virilizing cortical tumors.[17,36,71,86] It is recommended that those infants and children with hemihypertrophy and/or the Beckwith-Wiedemann syndrome should be followed closely by physical examinations and imaging studies at least every 6 months to facilitate early diagnosis of tumor formation.[119]

The investigation of a patient suspected of having an adrenocortical tumor should include imaging studies of the abdomen and measurement of urinary steroid levels. A suprarenal mass, with or without calcification, that displaces the kidney downward and laterally is the characteristic finding on computed tomography (CT) scanning. Abdominal sonography and CT scanning are recommended for determining the location of a tumor.[19,29,58,68] If a tumor is discovered in the adrenal, a CT scan of the lungs is mandatory.[29] Analyses of 24-hour urine specimens for increases in 17-ketosteroids, particularly dehydroepiandrosterone, and 17-hydroxysteroids are helpful, especially when the steroid production is independent of pituitary control after dexamethasone suppression.[40,52,52a,54,55,86] Usually, steroid secretion is suppressed in patients with congenital adrenal hyperplasia, but not in those with a neoplasm. Urinary 17-ketosteroid levels are usually significantly elevated in patients with cortical carcinoma.[52] Ultimately, the final diagnosis rests on microscopic examination of the tumor.

Most adrenal tumors are encapsulated even when malignant. Both adenomas and carcinomas may have large cells with bizarre hyperchromatic nuclei. The histologic distinction between a benign and malignant adrenocortical tumor is not always clear, which makes it difficult to predict prognosis on the basis of histologic findings alone. Pathologists disagree with regard to distinguishing between hyperplasia, adenomatous hyperplasia, and adenoma, a problem shared with several endocrine neoplasms in other organs (see Chapter 14, "Pancreatic Tumors").[31,97]

The study of adrenocortical tumors is further complicated by the fact that, in some published reports, it is not stated whether a neoplasm is an adenoma or carcinoma, but rather the vague term "adrenocortical tumor" is used. For this reason, estimates of the actual numbers of benign and malignant tumors, based on the literature, are not always accurate.

Adrenocortical Adenoma

An adrenocortical adenoma may be responsible for Cushing's syndrome, with or without virilization in newborns, but nodular hyperplasia and cortical carcinoma are more common causes (see Table 13–2).[18,31,40,41,44,49,63] There is a significant female predominance of about 4 to 1 in young patients with adenoma.

Cortical adenoma is a single, encapsulated mass that is usually surrounded by a thin, fibrous capsule. The cut surface is smooth and bulging, varying in color from tannish-gray to tannish-yellow, to orange brown (see Figs. 13–5 and 13–6). As a rule, cyst formations, hemorrhage, and necrosis are not seen except in some of the larger specimens. Adjacent to the adenoma, the atrophic adrenal cortex may be compressed into an almost paper-thin, orange-tan shell. The largest of the two specimens removed from infants in the Children's Hospital, Los Angeles series weighed 21 g and measured 4 cm in greatest dimension. However, tumors weighing as much as 100 to 200 g have been recorded in older children.[31,115]

Microscopic examination reveals cords and clusters of round, oval to polygonal cells having the appearance of adrenocortical cells surrounded by a prominent sinusoidal network (see Figs. 13–5 and 13–6). Two types of cells are found in adenomas removed from young patients with clinical signs and symptoms of Cushing's syndrome and virilization. One type is morphologically similar to the eosinophilic compact cells of the zona reticularis and is observed in patients with virilization. The other type, often associated with Cushing's syndrome, is a larger cell with a vacuolated, spongy appearance attributable to increased lipid content and comparable to cells of the zona fasciculata.[115] Frequently, blending of the two types of cells occurs, which is the author's experience. Moderate variation in cell size is noted, and focally giant cells with atypical nuclei may be present. However, areas of necrosis, anaplasia, and significant mitotic activity usually are not observed.[33] Capsular and vascular invasion, two important criteria of malignancy, generally are absent, but the latter is sometimes difficult to evaluate, particularly in adrenocortical and in other endocrine neoplasms, because of the inherent intimate relationship between tumor cells and the adjacent vascular channels.

The ultrastructural features of adrenocortical adenoma, carcioma, and hyperplasia associated with virilization are practically the same and have been described by Ghadially,[38] Hashida and colleagues,[47] Lack et al.,[67] and Sasano and colleagues.[97] The cells in these three conditions resemble the cells of the fetal cortex and zona reticularis.[38,97] The organelles showing the characteristic morphologic changes are the mitochondria and the smooth- and rough-surfaced endoplasmic reticulum, which are the principal sites for steroid hormone biosynthesis from cholesterol in the adrenal cortical cell. The smooth- and rough-surfaced endoplasmic reticula are abundant. The mitochondria are spherical or elongated, containing prominent tubular and vesicular cristae.[38,97] According to Ghadially, the mitochondria and the smooth endoplasmic reticulum are more common and better developed in adenomas and hyperplastic nodules as compared to carcinomas; however, only a few carcinoma cells may contain these characteristic structures.[38] Despite these findings, electron microscopy is not particularly useful in distinguishing adrenocortical hyperplasia from either adenoma or carcinoma.[38]

Adrenocortical Carcinoma

Adrenocortical carcinoma is a rare neoplasm in children and is even less prevalent in the newborn.[19,26,31,33,44,52,52a,62,63,67,69,113] Among all childhood malignant diseases, its incidence is estimated at 0.2% to 0.4%.[31,46,52,52a,67] Adrenocortical carcinoma is recorded more frequently than adenoma in the newborn, in a ratio of 5.5 to 1 (see Table 13–2). Two age peaks have been noted for cortical carcinoma, one in infancy and the other in adolescence.[31] Female predominance is at least 2 to 1 or more in patients with functioning tumors. Signs and symptoms of virilization and/or Cushing's syndrome and an abdominal mass are the presenting findings; most tumors are endocrinologically active, and virilization is found in one third of newborns (see Table 13–2).[18,67,113,115] Metastastases, particularly to the skin and liver, are the initial signs of disease in about 25% of newborns (see Table 13–2).[19,52,77,96]

"Nonfunctioning" adrenocortical carcinomas occur in the newborn, and some of these present with metastasis as the initial finding (see Table 13–2).[19,67,96,113] Table 13–2 shows that three newborns with clinically nonfunctioning malignant lesions had cutaneous nodular metastases as the initial presentation. One of these is a patient, reported by Saracco et al., who was born with multiple, red, cutaneous nodules distributed over his back, neck, and scalp as the main clinical finding.[96] Subsequent evaluation with imaging studies revealed a right adrenal tumor and cerebral metastases. One of the skin nodules and the adrenal tumor were excised and diagnosed as adrenocortical carcinoma. Surprisingly both the skin and brain metastases spontaneously resolved by 4 months of age. Other coexistent conditions in this patient included hemihypertrophy, possible Beckwith-Wiedemann syndrome, and a Wilms' tumor, which was removed when the patient was 1 year of age.[96]

Adrenocortical carcinoma may affect more than one child in a sibship,[36,71,76,80] and may occur in families with certain malignant diseases.[72,75,80] The various tumors that have been described in family cancer syndromes also are found excessively in patients as second malignant diseases, an observation that would certainly indicate a genetic influence.[80] Hemihypertrophy, the Beckwith-Wiedemann syndrome, the cancer family ("SBLA") syndrome, genitourinary malformations, and brain and liver tumors are reported more often in patients with adrenocortical carcinoma than in the general population; this association is described also in children with Wilms' tumor and hepatoblastoma.[31,36,46,51,72,75,80,101,102] As with Wilms' tumor, various urinary tract malformations occur in patients with adrenocortical carcinoma. They include polycystic, hypoplastic, and medullary sponge kidneys and collecting system duplications.[67]

Adrenal carcinomas tend to be larger than adenomas, ranging in diameter from 5 to 20 cm, with some weighing more than 100 g.[31,67,115] Most of these are encapsulated, but extension through the capsule into the adjacent tissues is sometimes seen, particularly in the larger malignant lesions. The cut surfaces are soft, lobular, and vary in color and consistency. Some tumors have a mushy, light tan-gray appearance, whereas others are firm and yellow-orange to tan. Prominent fibrous bands are observed in the latter and are considered one of the features of malignancy. Large areas of necrosis, hemorrhage, and cystic degeneration, with or without calcification, typically are seen in adrenocortical carcinomas.[31,67]

Analogous to the adrenocortical adenoma, the carcinoma cells resemble cells of the adrenal cortex. Typically, the tumor cells are arranged in nests and cords, situated adjacent to prominent vascular structures. Some carcinomas consist of cells with compact eosinophilic cytoplasms, whereas others have larger cells composed of clear or vaculated cytoplasms owing to abundant lipid droplets, similar to those described for the adenoma. Mixtures of the two cell types are also seen. Sometimes, the tumor cells resemble the peculiar-looking giant cells of adrenal cortical cytomegaly found incidentally in stillborns and neonates with a variety of conditions. These bizarre-appearing giant tumor cells are observed both in adenomas and in carcinomas (see the earlier section on adrenal cytomegaly). Poorly differentiated adrenocortical carcinomas are unusual in the first year of life. The electron microscopic findings are similar to those of adrenocortical adenoma, but the organelles in the carcinoma are not as numerous and are not as well developed as in the former (see the previous section on adrenocortical adenoma).

The histologic criteria proposed for diagnosing adrenocortical carcinoma include capsular and vascular invasion, trabecular and solid growth patterns, broad fibrous bands, increased mitotic rate, single cell necrosis, and extreme pleomorphism.[18,20,24,31,33,53,55,61,62,64,67,69,79,97,105,115] Nonhistologic factors, such as a tumor weight of more than 200 g and weight loss in the patient, have been used as indicators of malignancy.[31,48,49,53,105]

Immunohistochemical studies and DNA content (ploidy) do not appear to be particularly helpful in distinguishing between benign and malignant adrenal cortical neoplasms.[67,79] Moreover, DNA content (ploidy) does not seem to be a reliable index of malignancy and outcome.[79] Contrary to what would be expected, the DNA content of some carcinomas has been shown to be diploid, whereas the DNA content of some adenomas has been shown to be aneuploid, and vice versa.[23,67,96] However, Taylor and co-workers determined, on the basis of their DNA flow cytometric studies, that DNA ploidy may be of some prognostic value.[108] Nevertheless, more data are needed to evaluate the usefulness of immunohistochemical and DNA content analysis in the study of these uncommon, unpredictable tumors.

It should be mentioned that there is considerable difference of opinion regarding the assessment of the malignancy of adrenocortical tumors in the pediatric age group. Hawkins and Cagle[48] and others[20] believe that tumors in the young, like many other childhood neoplasms, are different biologically from those found in adults. Morphologic features considered to be predictors of malignant behavior— namely, necrosis, vascular and capsular invasion, nuclear pleomorphism, high mitotic rate, and broad fibrous bands—may be seen in both adrenocortical adenomas and carcinomas, and

are probably not useful in distinguishing between the two. Some adrenocortical tumors of the newborn behave in a benign fashion, regardless of histologic characteristics. Apparently, the only reliable criteria for malignancy are a tumor size greater than 200 g and development of metastases.[20,48,69] Several histologic parameters (listed earlier) may assist in assessing malignancy, even in children. A high mitotic rate is thought to be one of the most reliable indicators of malignancy.[53,67,79,112,115,116] The size of the tumor, however, is not always helpful in predicting malignancy, as small tumors have been known to metastasize, whereas some of the larger ones have not.

Newborns with adrenocortical carcinoma have a somewhat better prognosis than adolescents and adults with this disease, as evidenced by survival rates of 31% and 17%, respectively (Table 13–2).[14,20,79] Moreover, some adenomas have been overdiagnosed as carcinomas, which merely confuses the issue when evaluating both age groups.[24,67]

Local spread within the abdomen connotes a poor outcome. The most frequent sites of metastases of adrenocortical carcinoma, in decreasing order of frequency, are the lung, liver, peritoneum, regional lymph nodes, kidney, and brain.[29,31,52,52a,67,85,86] Recurrence of tumor or death secondary to metastases generally occur within 2 years of diagnosis.[85] However, some deaths have been reported as late as 5 years after the original diagnosis.[69]

Although the curative value of surgical resection in the absence of metastatic disease is proven, the efficacy of chemotherapy following surgery remains controversial.[113] At present, there is no convincing evidence that adjuvant chemotherapy improves survival once the tumor has metastasized.

ADRENAL CYST

Adrenal cysts have been described in newborns, but are more common in adults.[31,70,120] Approximately 5% occur in children, and less than 30 cases have been reported in neonates.[6,31,39,70,82,106,110,111,114,120] These cysts may present as abdominal masses or they may be discovered as an incidental finding on imaging studies performed for some other reason (Fig. 13–7).[6,39,106,110,120] Many are asymptomatic and spontaneously resolve. Adrenal cysts should be considered in the differential diagnosis of a cys-

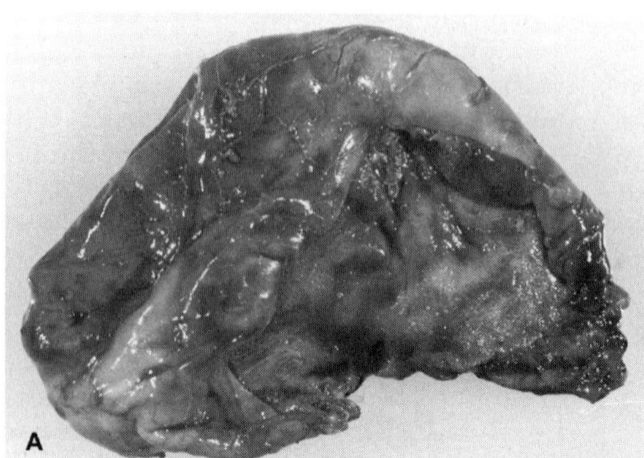

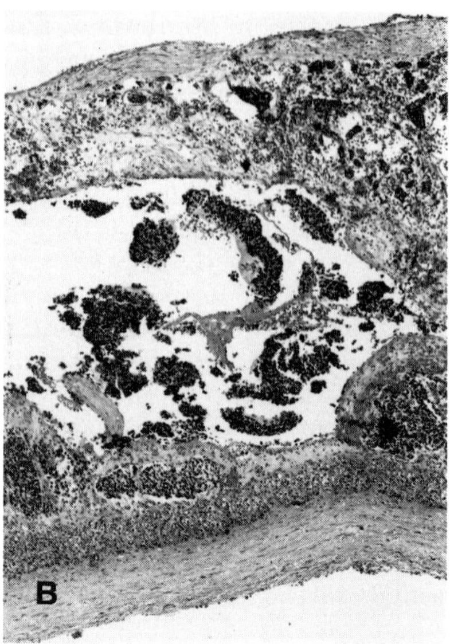

Figure 13–7. Adrenal cyst. *A,* An adrenal cyst, measuring 6 × 5 cm after removal of 20 mL of serosanguinous fluid, was removed from a 12-day-old female neonate with an abdominal mass. The left adrenal is expanded by a central cystic cavity. *B,* The cyst is rimmed by atrophic adrenal tissue containing small nests of neuroblastoma (hematoxylin-eosin, ×120). Besides a solid mass, neuroblastoma can manifest within the adrenal as hemorrhage or as a cyst. (From Isaacs H Jr. Tumors of the Newborn and Infant. St. Louis: Mosby–Year Book, 1991.)

tic abdominal mass in the fetus and newborn (Table 1–2).[111]

Unusual manifestations of this lesion have been reported. Levin et al. described a neonate with an adrenal cyst that appeared as a chest wall mass and extended into the thorax, destroying an adjacent rib by pressure, thus mimicking the findings of a metastatic tumor.[70]

Most adrenal cysts are considered to be sequelae of perinatal adrenal hemorrhage, which is found in up to 1% of newborns in whom postmortem examinations are performed.[39,43,70,111,114] Trauma associated with delivery is regarded as the most important cause, but other less common etiologies, such as infection, neoplasms (namely, leukemia and neuroblastoma), hemorrhagic disease of the newborn, incompatible blood transfusion, and adrenal vein thrombosis have been implicated.[70]

The adrenal is about one third the size of the kidney at birth, making it more susceptible to injury during delivery. Hemorrhage into the adrenal in the neonate is more often right-sided than left-sided because of its proximity to the liver and vertebrae, but it may be bilateral. When hemorrhage occurs, parenchymal necrosis and distention of the gland within its thin capsule result. Complications of adrenal hemorrhage include rupture into the peritoneal cavity, leading to an acute abdomen and shock, and a mass lesion in the retroperitoneal space.

If it remains localized, jaundice, a sudden decline in hemoglobin values, compression of the adjacent abdominal viscera, and, rarely, adrenal insufficiency may result.[43,70,111]

Adrenal cysts seldom arise from a hematoma within a tumor such as neuroblastoma (see Fig. 6–2). In situ neuroblastoma coexistent with an adrenal cyst was found in 3 of the 13 cases reported by Beckwith and Perrin,[12] in 2 of the 6 patients reported by Guin and colleagues,[45] in the 10-day-old female neonate presenting with an abdominal mass who was reported by Tubergen and Heyn,[110] and the neonate with an adrenal cystic mass described by Croitoru et al.[28]

Bilateral adrenal cysts associated with fatal congenital adrenocortical insufficiency have been reported, as in the case described by Moore and Cermak.[82] At postmortem examination, both of the adrenals of this 5-month-old male infant were replaced by cysts measuring 2 cm in diameter, having thin walls, and containing brown fluid. This finding suggests that destructive adrenal hemorrhage was responsible for the cyst formation. The newborn with bilateral hemorrhagic adrenal cysts reported by Wagner[114] survived, but subsequently developed bilateral abdominal masses and adrenal insufficiency, which required maintenance adrenocortical replacement therapy.

The characteristic features of an adrenal cyst,

observed on plain roentgenograms and sonograms of the abdomen or on CT scans, include a suprarenal cystic defect, with or without peripheral curvilinear calcification in the wall of the cyst, and downward displacement of the adjacent kidney and other viscera, such as the intestines.[39,70,106,111,114,120]

Pathologic Findings

Organization of adrenal hemorrhage may lead to a large cyst, occasionally one as big as an orange.[111] On examination of a cross section, the cysts may be unilocular or multilocular, varying in diameter from 2 to 11 cm.

Microscopically, the cyst wall consists of fibrous connective tissue with clusters of adrenocortical cells. The wall lacks an epithelial lining, and focal calcification is sometimes present. The cyst contents are variable and may be composed of fibrin, necrotic debris, and erythrocytes. If the lesion is secondarily infected, inflammatory granulation tissue or pus may be present as well.[34,39,70] A 28-day-old female infant with an abdominal mass, reported by Favara et al.,[34] was found to have hemosiderin and calcification in the wall of the adrenal abscess. This finding suggested that adrenal hemorrhage resulting from trauma or hypoxia may have provided a nidus for bacterial seeding during a septicemic episode, leading to the adrenal abscess.[34] As mentioned earlier, adrenal cysts have been found in association with neuroblastoma (see Fig. 13–7)[106,110] and adrenocortical cytomegaly[6,31] in the newborn.

Excision of an adrenal cyst is usually followed by survival. According to Van De Water and Fonkalsrud, all of the infants in whom resection was not performed have had an unfavorable outcome.[111]

REFERENCES

1. Aarskog D, Tveteraas E. McCune-Albright's syndrome following adrenalectomy for Cushing's syndrome. J Pediatr 1968;73:89.
2. Arce B, Licea M, Hung S, et al. Familial Cushing's syndrome. Acta Endocrinol 1978;87:139.
3. Artigas JLR, Niclewicz ED, Silva APG, et al. Congenital adrenal cortical carcinoma. J Pediatr Surg 1976;11:247.
4. Aterman K, Kerenyi N, Lee M. Adrenal cytomegaly. Virchows Arch [A] 1972;355:105.
5. Avni EF, Rypens F, Smet MH, et al. Sonographic demonstration of congenital adrenal hyperplasia in the neonate: The cerebriform pattern. Pediatr Radiol 1993;23:88.
6. Barron SH, Emanuel B. Adrenal cyst: A case report and a review of the pediatric literature. J Pediatr 1961;59:592.
7. Bartman J, Driscoll SG. Fetal adrenal cortex in erythroblastosis fetalis. Arch Pathol 1969;87:343.
8. Bauman A, Bauman CG. Virilizing adrenocortical carcinoma: Development in a patient with salt-losing congenital adrenal hyperplasia. JAMA 1982;248:3140.
9. Beatty EC, Hawes CR. Cytomegaly of the adrenal gland. Am J Dis Child 1955;89:463.
10. Bech K. Cytomegaly of the foetal adrenal cortex. Acta Pathol Microbiol Scand 1971;79:279.
11. Beckwith JB. Macroglossia, omphalocele, adrenal cytomegaly, gigantism and hyperplastic visceromegaly. Birth Defects: Original Article Series 1969;5:188.
12. Beckwith JB, Perrin EV. In situ neuroblastomas: A contribution to the natural history of neural crest tumors. Am J Pathol 1963;43:1089.
13. Birdwell TR, Dimmette RM. Cytomegaly of the adrenal gland. An interesting finding: Report of three cases. Am J Clin Pathol 1967;47:585.
14. Bolande RP. Developmental pathology. Am J Pathol 1979;94:627.
15. Bolande RP. Neoplasia of early life and its relationships to teratogenesis. In Rosenberg HS, Bolande RP (eds): Perspectives in Pediatric Pathology, Vol 3, p 145. Chicago: Year Book Medical Publishers, 1976.
16. Borit A, Kosek J. Cytomegaly of the adrenal cortex: Electron microscopy in Beckwith's syndrome. Arch Pathol 1969;88:58.
17. Burke BA. The pituitary, pineal, adrenal, thyroid and parathyroid glands. In Stocker JT, Dehner LP (eds): Pediatric Pathology, Vol 2, p 941. Philadelphia: JB Lippincott, 1992.
18. Burrington JD, Stephens CA. Virilizing tumors of the adrenal gland in childhood: Report of eight cases. J Pediatr Surg 1969;4:291.
19. Butler H, Bick R, Morrison S. Unsuspected adrenal masses in the neonate. Adrenal cortical carcinoma and neuroblastoma: Report of two cases. Pediatr Radiol 1988;18:237.
20. Cagle PT, Hough AJ, Pysher TS, et al. Comparison of adrenal cortical tumors in children and adults. Cancer 1986;57:2235.
20a. Camuto PM, Wolman SR, Perle MA, et al. Flow cytometry of fetal adrenal glands with adrenocortical cytomegaly. Pediatr Pathol 1989;9:551.
21. Carney JA. Adrenal gland. In Sternberg SS (ed): Histology for Pathologists, p 321. New York: Raven Press, 1992.
22. Chan HSL. Carcinoma of the adrenal gland in children—A study of 12 patients. In Humphrey FB, Grindley LP, Dehner LP, et al. (eds): Adrenal and Endocrine Tumors in Children. Boston: Martinus Nijhoff Publishers, 1984.
23. Cibas ES, Medeiros LJ, Weinberg DS, et al. Cellular DNA profiles of benign and malignant adrenocortical tumors. Am J Surg Pathol 14:948, 1990.
24. Coffin CM, Dehner LP. Congenital tumors. In Stocker JT, Dehner LP (eds): Pediatric Pathology, Vol I, p 325. Philadelphia: JB Lippincott, 1992.
25. Collipp PJ, Irani NG, Plachte F. Congenital anomalies and congenital adrenal hyperplasia. Calif Med 1966;104:278.
26. Cooper JD, Maldonado L, Earll JM. Adrenocortical carcinoma with virilism in an infant under 1 year of age. Am J Dis Child 1967;113:730.
27. Craig JM, Landing BH. Anaplastic cells of fetal adrenal cortex. Am J Clin Pathol 1951;21:940.

28. Croitoru DP, Sinsky AB, Laberge J-M. Cystic neuroblastoma. J Pediatr Surg 1992;27:1320.

29. Daneman A, Chan HSL, Martin DJ. Adrenal carcinoma and adenoma in children: A review of 17 patients. Pediatr Radiol 1983;13:11.

30. Dehner LP. Neoplasms of the fetus and neonate. *In* Naeye RL, Kissane JM, Kaufman N (eds): Perinatal Diseases, International Academy of Pathology, Monograph No. 22, p 286. Baltimore: Williams and Wilkins, 1981.

31. Dehner LP. Pediatric Surgical Pathology, 2nd ed, p 550. Baltimore: Williams and Wilkins, 1987.

32. Dehner LP, Franciosi RA. Adrenocortical neoplasia in the pediatric age group. A clinicopathologic study of seven cases. *In* Humphrey FB, Grindley LP, Dehner LP, et al. (eds): Adrenal and Endocrine Tumors in Children, p 291. Boston: Martinus Nijhoff Publishers, 1984.

33. Evans HL, Vassilopoulou-Sellin R. Adrenal cortical neoplasms: A study of 56 cases. Am J Clin Pathol 1996; 105:76.

34. Favara BE, Akers DR, Franciosi RA. Adrenal abscess in a neonate. J Pediatr 1970;77:682.

35. Favara BE, Steele A, Grant JH, et al. Adrenal cytomegaly: Quantitative assessment by image analysis. Pediatr Pathol 1991;11:521.

36. Fraumeni JF Jr, Miller RW. Adrenocortical neoplasms with hemihypertrophy, brain tumors, and other disorders. J Pediatr 1967;70:129.

37. Gershanik JJ, Elmore M, Levkoff AH. Congenital occurrence of adrenal cortical tumor, ganglioneuroma and toxoplasmosis. Pediatrics 1973;51:705.

38. Ghadially FN. Diagnostic Electron Microscopy of Tumours, 2nd ed, p 291. London: Butterworths, 1985.

39. Ghandur-Mnaymneh L, Slim M, Muakassa K. Adrenal cysts: Pathogenesis and histological identification with a report of 6 cases. J Urol 1979;122:87.

40. Gilbert MG, Cleveland WW. Cushing's syndrome in infancy. Pediatrics 1970;46:217.

41. Giombetti R, Hagstrom JWC, Landey S, et al. Cushing's syndrome in infancy: A case complicated by monilial endocarditis. Am J Dis Child 1971;122:264.

42. Gray ES. The endocrine system. *In* Keeling JW (ed): Fetal and Neonatal Pathology, 2nd ed, p 502. Berlin: Springer-Verlag, 1993.

43. Gross M, Kottmeier PK, Waterhouse K. Diagnosis and treatment of neonatal adrenal hemorrhage. J Pediatr Surg 1967;2:308.

44. Guin GH, Gilbert EF. Cushing's syndrome in children associated with adrenal cortical carcinoma. A case report with review of the literature. Am J Dis Child 1956; 92:297.

45. Guin GH, Gilbert EF, Jones B. Incidental neuroblastoma in infants. Am J Clin Pathol 1969;51:126.

46. Hartley AL, Birch JM, Marsden HB, et al. Adrenal cortical tumors: Epidemiological and familial aspects. Arch Dis Child 1987;62:683.

47. Hashida Y, Kenny FM, Yunis EJ. Ultrastructure of the adrenal cortex in Cushing's disease in children. Hum Pathol 1970;1:595.

48. Hawkins HP, Cagle PT. Adrenal cortical neoplasms in children (Correspondence and Corrections). Am J Clin Pathol 1992;98:382.

49. Hayles AB, Hahn HB Jr, Sprague RG, et al. Hormone-secreting tumors of the adrenal cortex in children. Pediatrics 1966;37:19.

50. Henry I, Grandjouan S, Coullin P, et al. Tumor specific loss of 11p15.5 alleles in del 11p13 Wilms' tumor and in familial adrenocortical carcinoma. Proc Natl Acad Sci 1989;86:3247.

51. Henry I, Jeanpierre M, Couillin P, et al. Molecular definition of the 11p15.5 region involved in Beckwith-Wiedemann syndrome and probably in predisposition to adrenocortical carcinoma. Hum Genet 1989; 81:273.

52. Hogan TF, Gilchrist KW, Westring DW, et al. A clinical and pathological study of adrenocortical carcinoma: Therapeutic implications. Cancer 1980;45: 2880.

52a. Holcombe JH, Pysher TJ, Kirkland RT. Functioning adrenocortical tumors in childhood. *In* Humphrey GB, Grindley LP, Dehner LP, et al. (eds): Adrenal and Endocrine Tumors in Children, p 277. Boston: Martinus Nijhoff Publishers, 1984.

53. Hough AJ, Hollifield JW, Page DL, et al. Prognostic factors in adrenal cortical tumors. A mathematical analysis of clinical and morphologic data. Am J Clin Pathol 1979;72:390.

54. Hughes IA. Congenital and acquired disorders of the adrenal cortex. Clin Endocrinol Metab 1982;11(1): 89.

55. Hutchinson RJ, Heyn RM. Adrenocortical carcinoma in children. *In* Humphrey FB, Grindley LP, Dehner LP, et al. (eds): Adrenal and Endocrine Tumors in Children, p 306. Boston: Martinus Nijhoff Publishers, 1984.

56. Irving IM. Exomphalos with macroglossia: A study of 11 cases. J Pediatr Surg 1967;2:499.

57. Job J-C, Chaussain J-L. The adrenals. *In* Job J-C, Pierson M (eds): Pediatric Endocrinology, p 275. New York: John Wiley, 1981.

58. Jones GS, Shah KJ, Mann JR. Adreno-cortical carcinoma in infancy and childhood: A radiological report of ten cases. Clin Radiol 1985;36:257.

59. Kampmeier OF. Giant epithelial cells of the human fetal adrenal. Anat Rec 1927;37:95.

60. Kaplowitz PB, Carpenter R, Newsome HH Jr, et al. Cushing's syndrome resulting from primary pigmented nodular adrenocortical disease. Am J Dis Child 1986;140:1072.

61. Kay R, Schumacher OP, Tank ES. Adrenocortical carcinoma in children. J Urol 1983;130:1130.

62. Kay S. Hyperplasia and neoplasia of the adrenal gland. Pathol Annu 1976;11:103.

63. Kenny FM, Hashida Y, Askari A, et al. Virilizing tumors of the adrenal cortex. Am J Dis Child 1968;115: 445.

64. King DR, Lack EE. Adrenal cortical carcinoma: A clinical and pathological study of 49 cases. Cancer 1979; 44:239.

65. Klevit HD, Campbell RA, Blair HR, et al. Cushing's syndrome with nodular adrenal hyperplasia in infancy. J Pediatr 1966;68:912.

66. Koufos A, Hansen MF, Copeland NG, et al. Loss of heterozygosity in three embryonal tumors suggests a common pathogenetic mechanism. Nature 1985;316: 330.

67. Lack EE, Mulvihill JJ, Travis WD, et al. Adrenal cortical neoplasms in the pediatric and adolescent age group: Clinicopathologic study of 30 cases with emphasis on epidemiological and prognostic factors. Pathol Annu 1992;27(1):1.

68. Lee PDK, Winter RJ, Green OC. Virilizing adrenocortical tumors in childhood: Eight cases and review of the literature. Pediatrics 1985;76:437.

69. Lefevre M, Gerard-Marchant R, Gubler JP, et al. Adre-

nal cortical carcinoma in children: 42 patients treated from 1958 to 1980 at Villejuif. *In* Humphrey FB, Grindley LP, Dehner LP, et al. (eds): Adrenal and Endocrine Tumors in Children, p 265. Boston: Martinus Nijhoff Publishers, 1984.

70. Levin SE, Collins DL, Kaplan GW, et al. Neonatal adrenal pseudocyst mimicking metastatic disease. Ann Surg 1974;179:186.

71. Levine GW. Adrenocortical carcinoma in two children with subsequent primary tumors. Am J Dis Child 132:238, 1978.

72. Li FP, Fraumeni JF. Rhabdomyosarcoma in children: Epidemiologic study and identification of a family cancer syndrome. J Natl Cancer Inst 1969;43:1365.

73. Lockitch G, Halstead AC, Dimmick JE. Endocrine system. *In* Dimmick JE, Kalousek DK (eds): Developmental Pathology of the Embryo and Fetus, p 707. Philadelphia: JB Lippincott, 1992.

74. Loridan L, Senior B. Cushing's syndrome in infancy. J Pediatr 1969;75:349.

75. Lynch HT, Katz DA, Bogard PJ, et al. The sarcoma, breast, cancer and adrenocortical carcinoma syndrome revisited. Am J Dis Child 1985;139:134.

76. Mahloudji D, Ronaghy H, Dutz W. Virilizing adrenal carcinoma in two sibs. J Med Genet 1971;8:160.

77. Mann JR, Cameron AH, Gornall P, et al. Transplacental carcinogenesis (adrenocortical carcinoma) associated with hydroxyprogesterone hexanoate. Lancet 1983;2:580.

78. McArthur RG, Bahn RC, Hayles AB. Primary adrenocortical nodular dysplasia as a cause of Cushing's syndrome in infants and children. Mayo Clin Proc 1982; 57:58.

79. Medeiros LJ, Weiss LM. New developments in the pathologic diagnosis of adrenal cortical neoplasms: A review. Am J Clin Pathol 1992;97:73.

80. Miller RM. Peculiarities in the occurrence of adrenal cortical carcinoma. Am J Dis Child 1978;132:235.

81. Mininberg DT, Levine LS, New MI. Current concepts in congenital adrenal hyperplasia. Pathol Annu 1982; 17(2):179.

82. Moore FP, Cermak EG. Adrenal cysts and adrenal insufficiency in an infant with fatal termination. J Pediatr 1950;36:9.

83. Moore KL. The Developing Human—Clinically Oriented Embryology, 5th ed. Philadelphia: WB Saunders, 1993.

84. Nakamura Y, Yano H, Nakashima T. False intranuclear inclusions in adrenal cytomegaly. Arch Pathol Lab Med 1981;105:358.

85. Neblett WW, Frexes-Steed M, Scott HW Jr. Experience with adrenocortical neoplasms in childhood. Am Surg 1987;53:117.

86. New MI, del Balzo P, Crawford C, et al. The adrenal cortex. *In* Kaplan SA (ed): Clinical Pediatric Endocrinology, p 181. Philadelphia: WB Saunders, 1990.

87. O'Bryan RM, Smith RW Jr, Fine G, et al. Congenital adrenocortical hyperplasia with Cushing's syndrome. JAMA 1964;187:257.

88. Oppenheimer EH. Adrenal cytomegaly: Studies by light and electron microscopy. Arch Pathol 1970;90: 57.

89. Orozco-Florian R, McBride JA, Favara BE, et al. Congenital hepatoblastoma and Beckwith-Wiedemann syndrome: A case study including DNA ploidy profiles of tumor and adrenal cytomegaly. Pediatr Pathol 1991;11:131.

90. Perlmutter M, Apfel AZ, Avin J, et al. Cushing's syndrome in infancy: Report of a case. Metabolism 1962; 11:946.

91. Pigeon B, Ryckewaert P, Massin B. Corticosurrenalome virilisant de l'enfant a propos d'une observation neo-natale. Pediatrie 1985;40:309.

92. Potter EL, Craig JM. Pathology of the Fetus and Infant, 3rd ed, p 330. Chicago: Year Book, 1975.

93. Powell LW Jr, Newman S, Hooker JW. Cushing's syndrome: Report of a case in an infant 12 weeks old. Am J Dis Child 1955;90:417.

94. Raiti S, Grant DB, Williams DI, et al. Cushing's syndrome in childhood: Postoperative management. Arch Dis Child 1972;47:597.

95. Roe TF, Kershnar AK, Weitzman JJ, et al. Beckwith's syndrome with extreme organ hyperplasia. Pediatrics 1973;52:372.

96. Saracco S, Abramowsky C, Taylor S, et al. Spontaneously regressing adrenal cortical carcinoma in a newborn: A case report with DNA ploidy analysis. Cancer 1988;62:507.

97. Sasano N, Ojima M, Masuda T. Endocrinologic pathology of functioning adrenocortical tumors. Pathol Annu 1980;15(2):105.

98. Shenoy BV, Carpenter PC, Carney JA. Bilateral primary pigmented nodular adrenocortical disease: Rare cause of the Cushing syndrome. Am J Surg Pathol 1984;8:335.

99. Sherman FE, Bass LW, Fetterman GH. Congenital metastasizing adrenal cortical carcinoma associated with cytomegaly of the fetal adrenal cortex. Am J Clin Pathol 1958;30:439.

100. Singer DB, Rudolph AJ, Rosenberg HS, et al. Pathology of the congenital rubella syndrome. J Pediatr 1967;71:665.

101. Sotelo-Avila C, Gonzalez-Crussi F, Fowler JW. Complete and incomplete forms of Beckwith-Wiedemann syndrome. Their oncogenic potential. J Pediatr 1980; 96:47.

102. Sotelo-Avila C, Gooch WM. Neoplasms associated with the Beckwith-Wiedemann syndrome. *In* Rosenberg HS, Bolande RP (eds): Perspectives in Pediatric Pathology, Vol 3, p 255. Chicago: Year Book Medical Publishers, 1976.

103. Sotelo-Avila C, Singer DB. Syndrome of hyperplastic fetal visceromegaly and neonatal hypoglycemia (Beckwith's syndrome): A report of seven cases. Pediatrics 1970;46:240.

104. Stewart DR, Jones PHM, Jolleys A. Carcinoma of the adrenal gland in children. J Pediatr Surg 1974;9:59.

105. Tang CK, Gray GF. Adrenocortical neoplasms: Prognosis and morphology. Urology 1975;5:691.

106. Tank ES, Bartlett JD, Herwig KR, et al. Surgery of the adrenal glands in infancy and childhood. J Urol 1971; 106:280–286.

107. Tank ES, Kay R. Neoplasms associated with hemihypertrophy. Beckwith-Wiedemann syndrome and aniridia. J Urol 1980;124:266.

108. Taylor SR, Roederer BS, Murphy RF. Flow cytometric DNA analysis of adrenocortical tumors in children. Cancer 1987;59:2059.

109. Telander RL, Wolf SA, Simmons PS, et al. Endocrine disorders of the pancreas and adrenal cortex. Mayo Clin Proc 1986;61:459.

110. Tubergen DG, Heyn RM. In situ neuroblastoma associated with an adrenal cyst. J Pediatr 1970;76:451.

111. Van De Water JM, Fonkalsrud EW. Adrenal cysts in infancy. Surgery 1966;60:1267.

112. Van Slooten H, Schaberg A, Smeenk D, et al. Morpho-

logic characteristics of benign and malignant adrenocortical tumors. Cancer 1985;55:766.

113. Visconti EB, Peters RW, Cangir A, et al. Unusual case of adrenal cortical carcinoma in a female infant. Arch Dis Child 1978;53:342.

114. Wagner AC. Bilateral hemorrhagic pseudocysts of the adrenal glands in a newborn. Am J Roentgenol Radium Ther Nucl Med 1961;86:540.

115. Weatherby RP, Carney JA. Pathologic features of childhood adrenocortical tumors. _In_ Humphrey FB, Grindley LP, Dehner LP, et al. (eds): Adrenal and Endocrine Tumors in Children, p 217. Boston: Martinus Nijhoff Publishers, 1984.

116. Weiss LM, Medeiros LJ, Vickery AL Jr. Pathologic features of prognostic significance in adrenocortical carcinoma. Am J Surg Pathol 1989;13:202.

117. White PC, New MI, Dupont B. Congenital adrenal hyperplasia. N Engl J Med 1987;316:1519.

118. Yano T, Linehan M, Anglard P, et al. Genetic changes in human adrenocortical carcinomas. J Natl Cancer Inst 1989;81:518.

119. Zaitoon MM, Mackie GG. Adrenal cortical tumors in children. Urology 1978;12:645.

120. Zivkovic SM, Jancic-Zguricas M, Jokanovic R, et al. Adrenal cysts in the newborn. J Urol 1983;129:1031.

14

PANCREATIC TUMORS

True neoplasms of the pancreas are seldom found in the newborn.[14,19,21,24,35,44,51,53,54,59,65,68,88] Lesions arising from islet cells—namely nesidioblastosis and islet cell adenoma—are seen more often than exocrine tumors in this age group (Table 14–1).[5,10,23,24,33,36,46,50,54,64,68,69,71–73,82,93] The pluripotential, "embryonic" tumor of the pancreas, the so-called pancreatoblastoma, a neoplasm that is unique to infants and children, is the subject of several case reports and some debate (see Table 14–1).[9,25,42,52–54,60,63,66] Table 14–2 is a proposed classification for the various pancreatic tumors and tumor-like conditions occurring in the fetus and newborn.

EMBRYOLOGY

The pancreas develops as two endodermal outgrowths or primordial buds, one from the dorsal wall of the duodenum and the other from the ventral wall adjacent to the hepatic duct.[34,46,57,62] The dorsal bud grows into the dorsal mesentery, which is to the left of the developing portal vein and which forms the body and tail of the pancreas. The ventral bud, which becomes the future head of the pancreas, is swept around into the dorsal mesentery when the duodenal loop is rotated clockwise. After this event occurs, the ventral bud is situated on the right side of the dorsal pancreas. The two primordia fuse at 6 to 7 weeks of gestation, occupying the second portion of the duodenum. At the same time, the ventral (main) and the dorsal (accessory) ducts communicate with one another. Eventually, the hepatic duct becomes the common bile duct.

Both the endocrine and exocrine pancreas arise from endodermal buds, whereas the connective tissue stroma and septae originate from adjacent splanchnic mesenchyme (mesoderm).[57] Primitive pancreatic ducts and acini develop by repeated sproutings from the endodermal buds (Fig. 14–1). Acini, which eventually secrete digestive enzymes, arise as cell clusters around the ends and the sides of these primitive ducts during the third month of fetal life.[62] Proliferation of acini continues after birth.[46,62] Concomitantly, groups of islet cells develop and arise as sprouts from the walls of the pancreatic ducts. Subsequently, they separate from the ductal epithelium and lie in between the acini. In the fourth month, a second generation of islet cells begins to appear as individual or small clusters of cells. The cell clusters gradually increase in size, becoming more centrally located in the lobule, and are surrounded by acini as the fetus matures; they eventually become mature islets of Langerhans. Histochemical studies show that there are at least four types of endocrine cells in the pancreas which appear as early as 9 weeks of gestation: alpha cells secreting glucagon, beta cells secreting insulin, delta cells secreting somatostatin, and gamma cells secreting gastrin.[34,62]

Histologic examination of the normal pancreas at birth shows increased numbers of islet cells distributed diffusely throughout the lobule as single cells and as clusters of cells, in addition to the islets of Langerhans; this is a different histologic picture from that observed in the older infant and child.[34,47] The islets become larger and more consolidated by the age of 6 weeks. Knowledge of this diffuse pattern of development in the fetal and newborn endocrine pancreas is important in evaluating a pancreas for the presence of nesidioblastosis or other conditions caused by an excess of islet

Table 14–1. 26 Newborn Pancreatic Tumors*

Case No.	Diagnosis	Age at Death	Initial Findings	Comment(s)	Reference
1	Pancreatoblastoma	Alive	Hypoglycemia, mass, nephromegaly	BWS, Wilms' tumor	Koh et al.[53]
2	Pancreatoblastoma	?Alive	Cystic abdominal mass on antenatal sonography	BWS, adrenal tumor	O'Hara[60]
3	Pancreatoblastoma	Alive	Cystic abdominal mass on antenatal sonography	BWS, HH	Potts et al.[63]
4	Pancreatoblastoma	12 days	Cleft lip, abdominal mass, hypoglycemia	BWS	Drut and Jones[25]
5	Pancreatoblastoma	Alive	Jaundice, abdominal mass	Hepatic adenoma, cirrhosis	Rich et al.[66]
6	Pancreatoblastoma	Stillborn	—	Incidental necropsy finding	Potter and Craig[62]
7	Pancreatoblastoma	At birth	—	Incidental necropsy finding	Potter and Craig[62]
8	Pancreatoblastoma	Stillborn	—	Incidental necropsy finding; dysmorphic facies and clubfoot	Klimstra et al.[52]
9	Pancreatoblastoma	Alive	Incidental mass	Recurrence at 7 months of age; received chemotherapy	Klimstra et al.[52]
10	Islet cell adenoma ("insulinoma")	Alive	Hypoglycemia, seizures, hypotonia	—	Carney[13]
11	Islet cell adenoma	Alive	Hypoglycemia, seizures	Microcephaly, cortical blindness, delayed developmental milestones	Kirkland et al.[50]
12	Islet cell adenoma	Alive	Cyanosis, hypoglycemia	—	Rickham[67]
13	Islet cell tumor	Alive	Hypoglycemia, seizures	Retarded with seizures	Rich et al.[65]
14	Islet cell tumor	Alive	Hypoglycemia, seizures	—	Rich et al.[65]
15	Islet cell tumor	Alive	Hypoglycemia, seizures	Retarded with seizures	Rich et al.[65]
16	Islet cell tumor	Alive	Hypoglycemia, seizures	Retarded with seizures	Rich et al.[65]
17	Islet cell tumor	Alive	Hypoglycemia, seizures	—	Rich et al.[65]
18	Islet cell tumor	Alive	Hypoglycemia, seizures	Retarded with seizures	Rich et al.[65]
19	Islet cell tumor	Alive	Hypoglycemia, seizures	—	Rich et al.[65]
20	Islet cell tumor	3 days	Hypoglycemia, seizures	—	Rich et al.[65]
21	Islet cell tumor	Alive	Hypoglycemia, seizures	—	Grant and Barbor[33]
22	Cystadenoma	Alive	Abdominal mass, vomiting	—	Jenkins and Othersen[49]
23	Cystadenoma	Alive	Abdominal mass	—	Romansky (see Fig. 14–4)
24	Hamartoma	3 months	Abdominal mass, hypoglycemia	—	Burt et al.[10]
25	Hemangioma	Alive	Jaundice, bleeding disorder, abdominal mass	—	Tunell[84]
26	Fibromatosis	1 month	Jaundice, abdominal mass	—	Amann and Klingenberg[1]

*Includes patients younger than 3 months of age who have been selected from the literature.
BWS = Beckwith-Wiedemann syndrome; HH = hemihypertrophy.

Table 14–2. Classification of Perinatal Pancreatic Tumors and Tumor-Like Conditions

Endocrine

    Nesidioblastosis
    Hyperplasia
    Adenomatous hyperplasia
    Islet cell adenoma (insulinoma)

Exocrine

    Cystadenoma
    Ductal adenocarcinoma*
    Acinar adenocarcinoma*
    Hamartoma

Pluripotential

    Pancreatoblastoma

Mesenchymal

    Hemangioma
    Lymphangioma
    Fibromatosis

Metastatic neoplasms

    Neuroblastoma
    Leukemia
    Wilms' tumor
    Rhabdoid tumor
    Yolk sac tumor

Miscellaneous

    Extramedullary hematopoiesis
    Lymphocytic infiltration

*Usually not observed in the newborn.

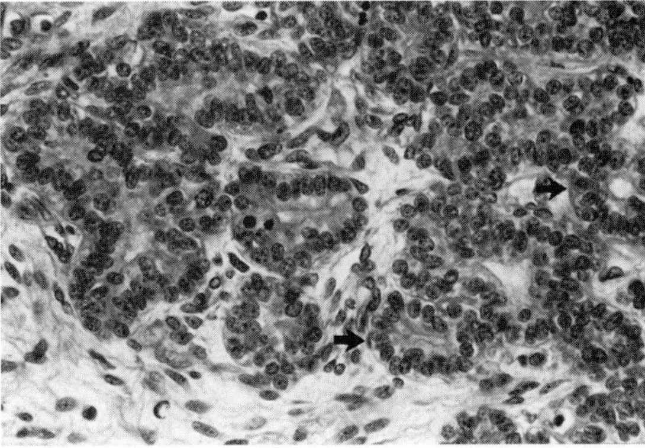

Figure 14–1. Developing pancreas (from an embryo of an estimated 10 to 12 weeks' gestation). Acini (*arrows*) are budding off from proliferating ducts (hematoxylin-eosin, ×250).

cells in this age group.[23,34] Moreover, it is necessary to perform immunohistochemical studies for insulin and other islet cell hormonal peptides before an abnormality of islet cells can be diagnosed.[34] Taguchi and co-workers recommend neuron-specific enolase (NSE) immunostaining to demonstrate the distribution of pancreatic islet cells.[80]

NESIDIOBLASTOSIS

In 1938, Laidlaw coined the controversial term "nesidioblastosis" to describe the neoformation of islets of Langerhans from pancreatic duct epithelium.[55] The term is derived from the Greek words *nesidion*, for islet, and *blastos*, for germ. He also proposed the term "nesidioblastoma" for an adenoma composed of islet cells. In 1971, Yakovac and colleagues were among the first to describe nesidioblastosis in a group of 12 infants with intractable hypoglycemia.[93] They demonstrated, by histochemical analysis,

the presence of single islet cells, or clusters of 2 to 6 islet cells, that were separate from the islets of Langerhans located in acini and in small pancreatic ducts (Fig. 14–2). This observation has since been confirmed by others.[3,4,23,24,30–32,34,39,41,56,58,73,79,80,90–92] The association of nesidioblastosis and congenital neuroblastoma has been reported by Grotting and colleagues, who suggest that this combination represents a "complex neurocristopathy."[37]

THE PANCREAS IN THE BECKWITH-WIEDEMANN SYNDROME

The syndrome of omphalocele-macroglossia-gigantism was first recognized by Beckwith in the United States in 1963[6] and at approximately the same time in Europe by Wiedemann.[89] Since then, more than 100 cases have been described, and extensive reviews on this subject have been published.[25,26,70,74–78,89] The Beckwith-Wiedemann syndrome is recognizable at birth and is characterized by a group of findings that include omphalocele, macroglossia, visceromegaly, microcephaly, gigantism, and hyperinsulinemic hypoglycemia (Fig. 14–3).[70,74,75,78] The syndrome is associated with a defect in the short arm of chromosome 11 (11p).[85,87] Individuals with this autosomal-recessive condition have a significantly increased risk for the development of certain benign and malignant tumors (see Chapter 13, "Adrenal Tumors," and Table 13–1.[26,60,74,75] When hemihypertrophy is associated with the syndrome, this risk increases.[25,77] Adenomatous hyperplasia of islet cells with nesidioblastosis is one of the hall-

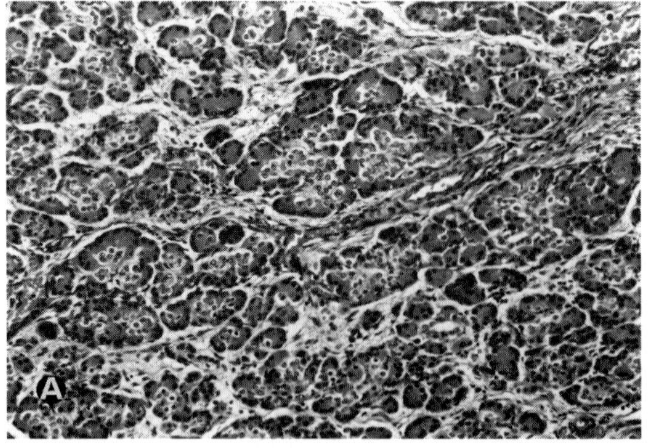
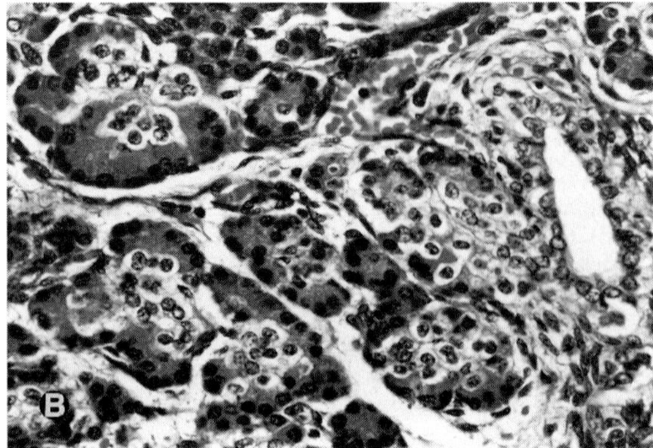
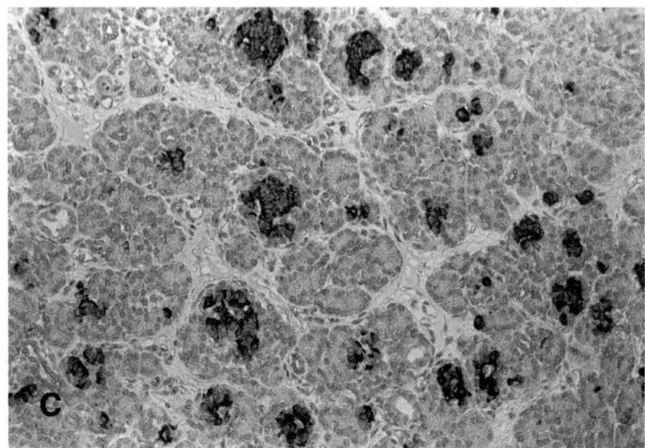

Figure 14–2. Nesidioblastosis (pancreas from a 650-g fetus). *A,* Clusters of single or several islet cells that are separate from the islets of Langerhans are situated within acini and small pancreatic ducts (hematoxylin-eosin, ×100). *B,* Higher magnification reveals islet cells within acini and in the wall of a small pancreatic duct (hematoxylin-eosin, ×250). *C,* Insulin immunoperoxidase staining demonstrates the distribution of islet cells (×100).

marks of the Beckwith-Wiedemann syndrome in the pancreas (see Fig. 14–3),[23,45] and pancreatoblastoma is the exocrine tumor associated with this syndrome.[25,53,60,74]

Severe hypoglycemia occurs in almost 50% of neonates with the Beckwith-Wiedemann syndrome, and may prove fatal.[3,8,12,23,78] This association was observed in the Children's Hospital, Los Angeles study, in which 4 of 16 infants with hyperinsulinemic hypoglycemia had the syndrome. The pancreases of the four patients had striking islet hyperplasia and hypertrophy and nesidioblastosis on microscopic examination.[23] In areas where the islet tissue was confluent and occupied a larger area than the acinar pancreas, the lesion was called adenomatous hyperplasia (Fig. 14–3,*C* and *D*). One female newborn in the series was seen at 14 days of age with severe hypoglycemia and a right upper quadrant abdominal mass, which, on exploratory laparotomy, proved to be an enlarged, nodular pancreas with the histologic features just described (see Fig. 14–3).[23,70] Other findings in this patient were adrenal cortical hyperplasia and cytomegaly, as well as nephrogenic rests (nodular renal blastema).[70] Similar clini-

cal and pathologic findings have been reported in these patients by others.[78]

ISLET CELL ADENOMA

Islet cell adenoma ("islet cell tumor," "insulinoma," "nesidioblastoma") is uncommon in the newborn and infant.[13,29,33,45,50,64,65,67,69,71,74] Rich et al.[65] collected from the literature 31 cases of infants younger than 9 months of age, including 8 of their own, from 1945 to 1978. They found that the tumor occurs more often in male patients than in female patients, with a ratio of about 2.7:1.[65] The tumors are responsible for persistent hypoglycemia and, if not treated promptly, may lead to seizures and permanent brain damage.[65]

Table 14–1 presents an assorted collection of 26 newborn pancreatic tumors culled from the literature, with islet cell adenomas comprising almost half (48%) of the reported cases. Although 11 of the 12 (92%) newborns with this tumor survived, 5 (42%) had serious sequelae—namely, seizures, mental retardation, and blindness.

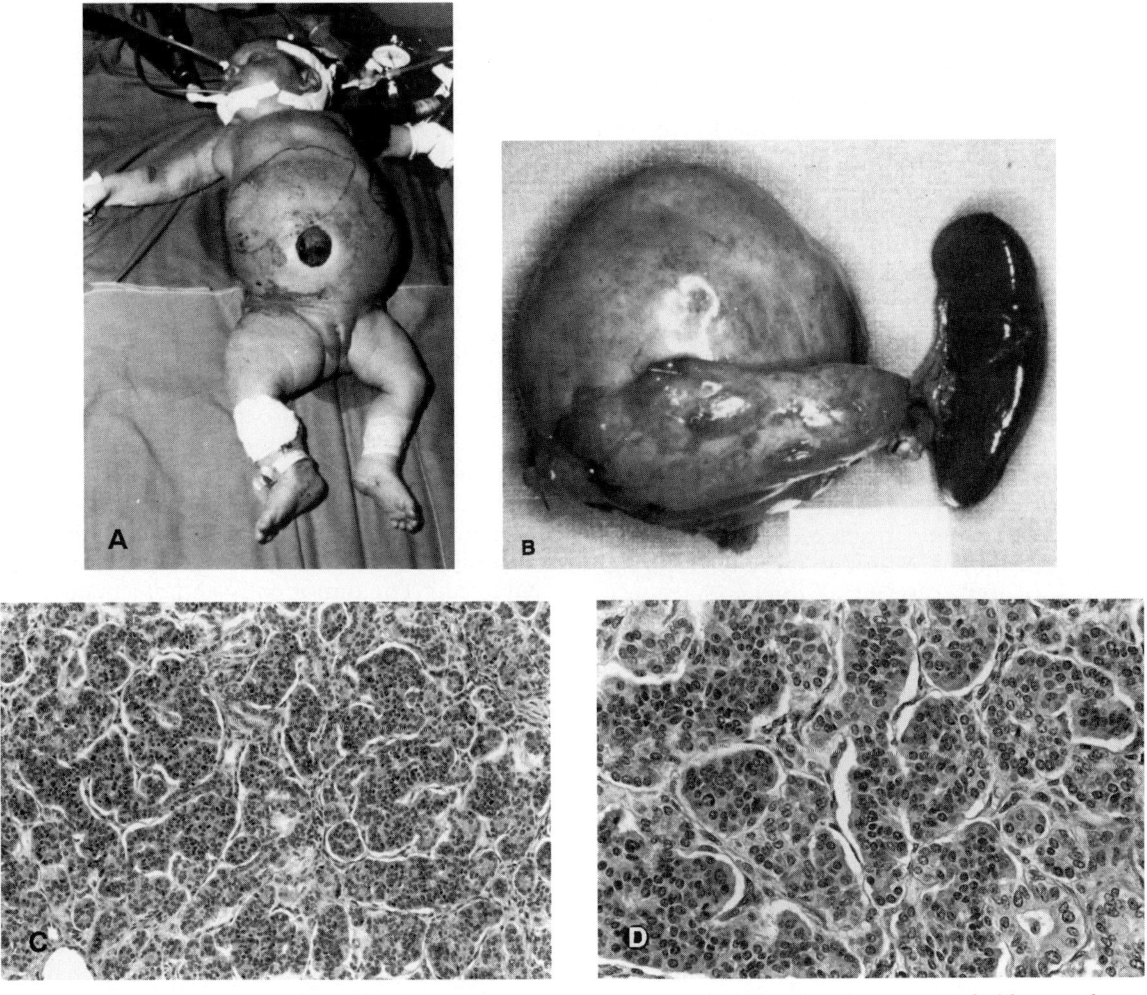

Figure 14–3. Pancreas in the Beckwith-Wiedemann syndrome. *A,* A 3-week-old female infant presented with severe hypoglycemia, right hemihypertrophy, omphalocele, and abdominal visceromegaly. The enlarged liver and pancreas are outlined on the patient's abdomen. *B,* The excised portion of the pancreas with its enlarged midportion (weighing 71 g) and the spleen are shown. *C,* The pancreas shows a jumbled (dysplastic) mixture of islet cells (mostly), acini, and small ducts (hematoxylin-eosin, ×100). *D,* At higher magnification, the disorganized proliferation of ductal and islet tissue can be seen. The distinction between the cell types is unclear. Adenomatous hyperplasia is a term used to describe this lesion, in which islet tissue is confluent and occupies a larger area than the acinar pancreas (hematoxylin-eosin, ×200). Biopsy examination of the enlarged right adrenal revealed fetal cortical cytomegaly. Subcapsular nephrogenic rests were found at renal biopsy. At 8 months of age, she developed an umbilical myxoma. (*A* and *B:* Courtesy of Jordon Weitzman, MD, Department of Surgery, Children's Hospital, Los Angeles, CA.) (*C* and *D:* From Roe TF, Kershnar AK, Weitzman JJ, et al. Beckwith's syndrome with extreme organ hyperplasia. Reproduced by permission of Pediatrics, Vol 52, page 372, copyright 1973.)

Most islet cell adenomas are found in the head of the pancreas, but some are situated in the body and tail.[65] Typically, islet cell adenomas are small in size, measuring between 0.1 and 1 cm in diameter.[13,24,34,43,50,65] Sometimes, the nodules are neither seen nor are palpable on the external surface of the pancreas, and multiple cross-cut sections are then required to demonstrate the tumor, which has a variable-appearing cut surface, described as reddish-tan to white, and gritty. Serial sectioning of the par-affin block(s) of the excised specimen may be necessary to find tiny lesions.

Microscopically, the adenoma is composed of nests of islet cells, and it is separated from acinar tissue by a thin, fibrous capsule with small ducts at the periphery of the nests.[13,24] Delicate fibrous connective tissue septae divide the tumor into small lobules. The term nesidioblastoma has been given because of the intimate relationship of the islet cells to the small pancreatic ducts.[13] Recall that, in the development of the pancreas, islet cells arise as sprouts from the walls of the ducts (see the earlier section on embryology). Immunoperoxidase staining and ultrastructural findings indicate that the tumors are composed primarily of beta cells and ductal cells.[13,50,65] Congenital islet cell adenomas may be associated with nesidioblastosis.[3,32] The studies of Amendt and co-workers show that function tests, such as the oral glucose tolerance, diazoxide, somatostatin, and C-peptide suppression tests, do not distinguish the hyperinsulinism caused by nesidioblastosis from that due to an adenoma.[2]

Successful treatment of an islet cell adenoma is based on prompt recognition and early excision of the tumor.[65,67] Resection can be accomplished readily if the lesion is easily palpable, but if the tumor is small and deeply embedded in pancreatic tissue, this may result in technical surgical problems. Although there is a high rate of survival (90%), serious sequelae develop in more than one third of the patients (see Table 14–1).

EXOCRINE TUMORS OF THE PANCREAS

Neoplasms arising from the exocrine pancreas in patients younger than 3 months of age are rare.[14,20–22,24,38,51,59] Cystadenoma, hamartoma, pancreatoblastoma, and pancreatic ductal adenocarcinoma are examples of the types of tumors that have been described.[10,25,36,49,53,54,60,66,68,74] Pancreatoblastoma, which probably should be considered a pluripotential neoplasm composed of acinar, islet, and ductular elements, is the most frequent malignant lesion re-

ported, accounting for one third of the total number of newborn pancreatic neoplasms (see Table 14–1).

Cystadenoma

Cystadenoma of the pancreas is a benign, well-circumscribed, multilocular cystic neoplasm presenting as an abdominal mass (Fig. 14–4).[14,24,36,49] The lesion is relatively uncommon, for only about 200 cases have been reported in all ages, most of them occurring in older women.[14] To date, five histologically documented cystadenomas occurring in the first year of life have been described. One of the youngest of those affected was a 2-day-old female infant, reported by Jenkins and Othersen, who presented with vomiting and an abdominal mass.[49] The tumor consisted of a cystic mass occupying the head and body of the pancreas, measuring 12 cm in diameter, and containing amber fluid. Another tumor, removed from a 6-month-old female infant at the Children's Hospital of Michigan, weighed 350 g, measured 9.5 × 9 cm, and consisted of multiloculated cysts of varying sizes that were filled with serous fluid.[14] Histologically, the cysts were lined by a single layer of regular cuboidal or columnar epithelium separated by fibrous septae. The 4-month-old male infant with cystadenoma in the series by Grosfeld et al. was cured by an 80% distal pancreatectomy.[36] A 3-week-old female infant with an abdominal mass was noted by Romansky. The mass, a cystic tumor weighing 440 g and measuring 8 × 14 cm, was removed from the body of the pancreas (see Fig. 14–4).

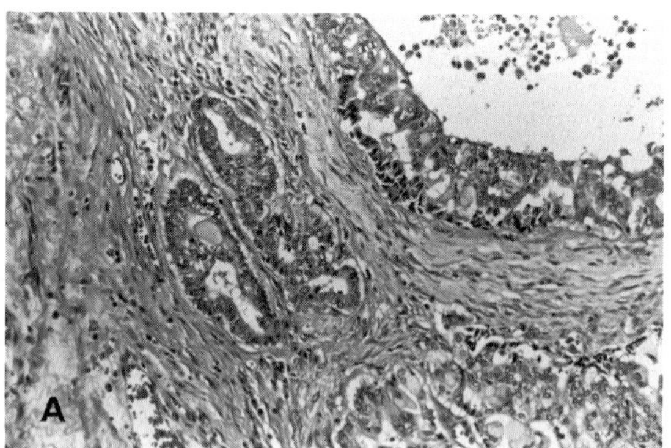
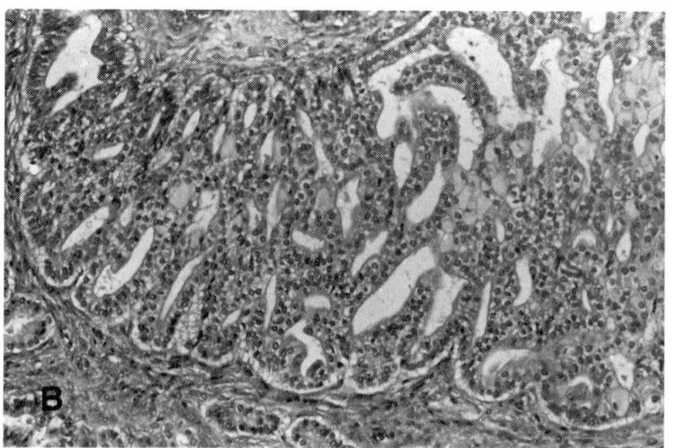

Figure 14–4. Cystadenoma of the pancreas. *A*, A 3-week-old female infant had a 440-g cystic tumor, measuring 13 × 14 cm, arising from the body of the pancreas. The wall of the cyst is lined by several rows of vacuolated epithelial cells. Acinar structures are present within the wall (hematoxylin-eosin, ×150). *B*, The tumor consists of cuboidal to columnar cells with regular, round nuclei and vacuolated cytoplasms forming glandular and duct-like structures (hematoxylin-eosin, ×48). (Courtesy of Stephen G. Romansky, MD, Department of Pathology, Long Beach Memorial Medical Center, Long Beach, CA.)

Hamartoma

Burt and colleagues described an unusual example of a pancreatic adenoma, occurring in a premature newborn, which presented as an abdominal mass with refractory hypoglycemia.[10] At surgery, a markedly enlarged, macronodular pancreas measuring 11 × 4.8 cm was found. Microscopically, the lesion consisted primarily of groups of ductal elements surrounded by broad connective tissue septa. Small foci of both acinar and islet cells were interspersed between groups of proliferating ducts.[10] Although hypoglycemia was noted, the presence of acinar cells in the tumor excluded the diagnosis of a "pure" islet cell adenoma.

Adenocarcinoma of the Pancreas

Pancreatic adenocarcinoma is a common neoplasm in adults, but rarely occurs in neonates and infants.[16,20,22,24,36,54,81] Moynan and associates described three cases that occurred in the first year of life, one in a 3-month-old infant.[59] Of 28 pediatric cases of pancreatic malignant lesions described by Welch, 5 (18%) occurred in infants.[88] The clinical presentation of affected young patients is similar to that of adults: an abdominal mass (the most common sign), with or without jaundice or abdominal pain.[54,88] The diagnosis is rarely, if ever, made preoperatively.[66] Metastases may already be present at the time of exploratory laparotomy, and are usually found in the liver and regional lymph nodes.[62,68,81] Welch reviewed the world literature prior to 1986 and found 28 cases of pancreatic malignant disease in infants and children.[88] He mentioned that the review of this subject was made difficult because of the varied terminology used for these tumors. Of 28 infants and children in the review, 4 were younger than 1 year of age, and the youngest with an adenocarcinoma was 3 months old. Controversy persists regarding the term pancreatoblastoma because the tumor has some histologic features in common with pancreatic ductal adenocarcinoma; moreover, in the early literature, the two diagnoses were used interchangeably.[54] It is conceivable that some of the earlier cases that were diagnosed as adenocarcinoma were actually examples of pancreatoblastoma, which is more common in infancy.

Ductal adenocarcinoma is the leading tumor of the pancreas in most age groups, accounting for approximately 80% of the malignant lesions affecting this organ.[20,22] It is primarily a tumor of adults. The youngest patient with adenocarcinoma in Taxy's[81] review of 15 pediatric cases was a 7-month-old female infant (described initially by Corner[19] in 1943), who presented with a large tumor in the head of the pancreas. The tumor metastasized to the liver, regional lymph nodes, and pleura. The carcinoma had a distinctive gross appearance, consisting of a firm, grey to white, ill-defined mass with infiltrating borders, and was situated in the head, the usual site for this tumor. Some ductal adenocarcinomas are multifocal and are located throughout the body of the pancreas. Larger tumors show foci of necrosis and cyst formation. Microscopically, they display atypical duct-like structures surrounded by a dense fibrous stroma.[22,24,54]

The papillary-cystic tumor, a pancreatic neoplasm of uncertain histogenesis, occurs primarily in adolescent females, and to the author's knowledge, has not been observed in the first year of life.[24,46,54,61] One of the youngest patients reported to have this tumor was 2 years of age.[61]

Acinar adenocarcinoma is considerably less common than ductal adenocarcinoma.[20,21,24,54] In the series of Cubilla and Fitzgerald, only 1% of pancreatic malignant lesions were classified as the acinar cell type.[21] According to the author's review, pure acinar adenocarcinoma has not been described in the first year of life. The youngest patient with this diagnosis in the Children's Medical Center, Boston study of eight patients was a 15-month-old boy who presented with melena and hematemesis resulting from invasion of the duodenum by the tumor.[54] A solid, circumscribed, lobular tumor with a yellow-white cut surface are the characteristic gross findings.[54] The histologic features of acinar cell adenocarcinoma include relatively uniform cells with abundant acidophilic cytoplasm and distinct cytoplasmic borders occurring in acini, cords, clusters of cells, and sometimes, rosette-like structures.[20,24,54] The histochemical and ultrastructural findings have been presented by Ulich and co-workers,[86] Lack et al.,[54] and Taxy.[81] The diagnosis is established by finding cytoplasmic granules that show periodic acid-Schiff (PAS) positivity or by demonstrating electron-dense zymogen granules, measuring up to 1000 nm in diameter.[54,81]

Pancreatoblastoma

The term pancreatoblastoma ("infantile carcinoma of the pancreas") was coined in 1977 by Horie et al. to describe a unique childhood tumor with distinct histologic features and a much better prognosis than adult pancreatic carcinomas.[42] However, the use of this term has been questioned by some.[9,84] The tumor was described originally in older children and adolescents.[9,28,42,59,83]

Pancreatoblastoma is detected antenatally by sonography (see Table 14–1).[60,63] In addition, several newborn cases have been reported.[17,25,52,53,60,63,65,68,77] Microscopically, the tumors are distinguished by a lobular growth pattern, acinar and ductular formations, and central nodules of squamous cells.[17,25,52]

The neonate with pancreatoblastoma depicted by Rich et al. presented with a right upper quadrant abdominal mass and jaundice at 3 weeks of age.[66] Imaging studies revealed a cystic lesion arising from the retroperitoneal area. At surgery, a tumor measuring 6 cm in diameter was removed from the head of the pancreas. The child was alive, well, and free of disease 4 years following surgery. Similarly, Robey and colleagues described a 3-week-old premature male infant with a firm, right upper quadrant pancreatoblastoma, which was seen on CT scan and ultrasonogram as an irregularly enhancing, central mass extending from the retroperitoneal area almost to the anterior abdominal wall. The child was free of disease 9 months after removal of the tumor.[68]

At the Chicago Lying-in Hospital, two pancreatoblastomas, composed primarily of acinar cells and a few ductular elements, were found incidentally at postmortem examination in a stillborn and a newborn infant; the tumors measured 1 and 1.5 cm, respectively. Both tumors were well demarcated and were situated in the head of the pancreas.[62] No other history was given.

Klimstra et al. reviewed 55 cases, including 14 of their own.[52] Two of the authors' patients were 3 months of age or younger. One was a stillborn female infant with dysmorphic features, a club foot, and a 1.5-cm tumor that was discovered at necropsy. The other was a 3-month-old female infant with a 10.5-cm pancreatic mass that was discovered incidentally and was subsequently resected. The pancreatoblastoma of the latter recurred 7 months after surgery; she survived following chemotherapy (see Table 14–1).

In the first year of life, pancreatoblastoma occurs predominantly in male patients, and more than 50% of the patients have the Beckwith-Wiedemann syndrome (see Table 14–1). Several cases have been reported with this association. O'Hara and colleagues[60,63] described a

10-day-old neonate with this syndrome who had an intra-abdominal cystic tumor detected by sonography at 32 weeks' gestation. In the 19-day-old male neonate reported by Koh et al.,[53] a 110-g multicystic abdominal mass measuring 7.5 cm in diameter was discovered on a routine follow-up postnatal examination. The lesion was successfully resected, but the patient subsequently developed a Wilms' tumor at 17 months of age. The child was living and well 2 years after nephrectomy.[17,53] Drut and Jones reported a case of a 12-day-old male infant with the Beckwith-Wiedemann syndrome who was noted to have a mid to upper abdominal mass at birth. Postmortem examination revealed a cystic pancreatoblastoma measuring 10 cm in diameter.[25] Other histologic findings included diffuse nesidioblastosis and islet cell adenomatous hyperplasia in the pancreas. Both adrenals displayed fetal cortical cytomegaly, the hallmark of this syndrome.

Pancreatoblastomas are described as encapsulated, occasionally cystic masses that are situated most often in the head of the pancreas, but sometimes in the body of the pancreas.[42,52,53] The surgical specimen from the neonate reported by Robey and associates consisted of a 77-g tumor measuring 6 cm in diameter. The lesion occupied the head of the pancreas and had a central, yellow zone with several cysts, necrosis, and hemorrhage surrounded by a white, firm, peripheral rim.[68] On histologic examination, pancreatoblastomas display a characteristic organoid growth pattern. Bands of cellular fibrous connective tissue divide the epithelial components, which consist of solid nests and peripheral acinar duct–like formations, into lobules.[52] Central nodules of squamous cells are surrounded by small, round, darkly staining cells.[17,42,52]

Alpha$_1$-antitrypsin positivity, demonstrated by the immunoperoxidase technique, suggests an acinar cell component.[7,25] In addition, Klimstra et al. have reported strong reactivity with keratin and epithelial membrane antigen (EMA).[52] According to Cooper and Lake, esterase and esteroprotease are strongly reactive in the squamous cell areas, which they believe to be a helpful indicator for establishing the diagnosis.[17] The pancreatoblastomas studied immunohistochemically by Klimstra et al. showed acinar, ductal, and endocrine differentiation.[52]

Ultrastructurally, the tumor cells contain zymogen-like granules, luminal microvilli, junctional complexes, and a lamellar arrangement of the granular endoplasmic reticulum, similar to that observed in normal pancreatic acinar cells.[17,25,42,52,81] Endocrine differentiation, in the form of neurosecretory granules, has also been described.[9,52]

An analogy has been drawn between pancreatoblastoma and other embryonic tumors ("embryomas"), such as Wilms' tumor and neuroblastoma. It has been suggested that the tumor arises from a totipotential cell of pancreatic duct origin called the "pancreatoblast."[25,28,36,44,45,52,60,70] Carrying this idea further, it is conceivable that islet cells (e.g., those in nesidioblastosis or islet cell adenoma) could originate from the pancreatoblast as well.

Adenocarcinoma of the pancreas has a poor outcome in all age groups, with an overall survival rate of only 1% to 4%.[9,18,22,36] However, certain types of pediatric pancreatic malignant lesions, such as the papillary-cystic (solid) tumor of the adolescent female and the pancreatoblastoma, have a much better prognosis than does adult ductal adenocarcinoma.[9,11,36,42,61] Most studies indicate that primary resection of pancreatic tumors in infants and children is the treatment of choice (as it is in adults), if this can be accomplished.[9,11,27,35,36,48,68,83,88] The prognosis for pancreatoblastoma is generally good, and complete surgical resection results in cure.[9,53,59,63,66,68,83] Of the nine cases of pancreatoblastoma reviewed and tabulated in Table 14–1, one third were incidental necropsy findings. Of the six newborns treated by surgery, five survived (83%) and 1 died of sepsis. The overall survival of newborns with benign and malignant pancreatic tumors listed in Table 14–1 is 73%.

MISCELLANEOUS TUMORS AND TUMOR-LIKE CONDITIONS

Nonepithelial, mesenchymal, pancreatic tumors of the newborn have been the subject of a few case reports. Hemangioma and fibromatosis involving the pancreas have been reported.[1,15,84] Tunell has described a hemangioma ("hemangioendothelioma"), occurring in a 3-month-old infant, which caused jaundice and obstruction of the duodenum and the common bile duct.[84] Extensive leukemic infiltration can occur with congenital leukemia[45] (personal observation), and the retroperitoneal, small, round cell tumors, such as rhabdomyosarcoma, rhabdoid tumor, and neuroblastoma, can metastasize to the pancreas.[24]

In the fetus and newborn, foci of extramedul-

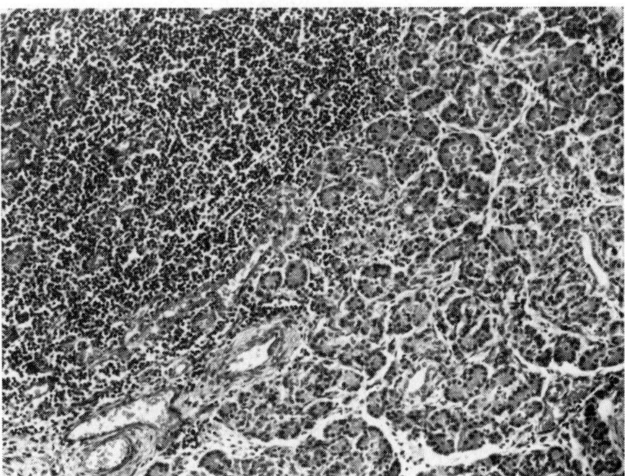

Figure 14–5. Lymphocytic infiltration of the pancreas. This section of the head of the pancreas (from a 650-g fetus) reveals extensive infiltration by lymphocytes, which are small, round, and regular, without atypical features (hematoxylin-eosin, ×120). This benign, probably reactive lesion may be mistaken for leukemia-lymphoma.

lary erythropoiesis and myelopoiesis are found in the pancreas and may be seen even at term. Sometimes, this finding is extensive, and then may be mistaken for congenital leukemia (see Chapter 7, "Leukemia"). Excessive myelopoiesis has been described in patients with a generalized leukemoid reaction associated with infection and trisomies 18 and 21.[34] Lymphocytic infiltrates normally located in the head of the pancreas have been noted in premature and term infants examined postmortem. Occasionally, the infiltrates may be so extensive that they have been misinterpreted as lymphoma, rather than reaction to some other condition, such as degenerating islet tissue (Fig. 14–5).[34,45,62]

REFERENCES

1. Amann FW, Klingenberg A. Localized congenital fibromatosis of the head of the pancreas as a cause of neonatal icterus. Z Kinderchir 1974;14:403.
2. Amendt P, Kohnert KD, Kunz J. The hyperinsulinaemic hypoglycaemias in infancy: A study of six cases. Eur J Pediatr 1988;148:107.
3. Aynsley-Green A. Hypoglycemia in infants and children. Clin Endocrinol Metab 1982;11(1):159.
4. Aynsley-Green A, Polak JM, Bloom SR, et al. Nesidioblastosis of the pancreas: Definition of the syndrome and the management of severe neonatal hyperinsulinaemic hypoglycaemia. Arch Dis Child 1981;56:496.
5. Becker K, Wendel U, Pryzrembel H, et al. Beta cell nesidioblastosis. Eur J Pediatr 1978;127:75.
6. Beckwith JB. Extreme cytomegaly of the adrenal fetal cortex, omphalocele, hyperplastic kidneys and pancreas, and Leydig cell hyperplasia: Another syndrome?

Presented at Annual Meeting of Western Society for Pediatric Research, Los Angeles, CA, November 11, 1963.

7. Benjamin E, Wright DH. Adenocarcinoma of the pancreas in childhood: A report of two cases. Histopathology 1980;4:87.

8. Bolande RP. Developmental pathology. Am J Pathol 1979;94:623.

9. Buchino JJ, Castello FM, Nagaraj HS. Pancreatoblastoma: A histochemical and ultrastructural analysis. Cancer 1984;53:963.

10. Burt TB, Condon VR, Matlak ME. Fetal pancreatic hamartoma. Pediatr Radiol 1983;13:287.

11. Camprodon R, Quintanilla E. Successful long-term results with resection of pancreatic carcinoma in children. Favorable prognosis for an uncommon neoplasm. Surgery 1984;95:420.

12. Carcassonne M, DeLarue A, LeTourneau JN. Surgical treatment of organic pancreatic hypoglycemia in the pediatric age. J Pediatr Surg 1983;18:75.

13. Carney CN. Congenital insulinoma (nesidioblastoma): Ultrastructural evidence for histogenesis from pancreatic ductal epithelium. Arch Pathol Lab Med 1976;100:352.

14. Chang CH, Perrin EV, Hertzler J, et al. Cystadenoma of the pancreas with cytomegalovirus infection in a female infant. Arch Pathol Lab Med 1980;104:7.

15. Chappell JS. Benign hemangioendothelioma of the head of the pancreas treated by pancreaticoduodenectomy. J Pediatr Surg 1973;8:431.

16. Coffin CM, Dehner LP. Congenital tumors. _In_ Stocker JT, Dehner LP (eds): Pediatric Pathology, Vol 1, p 325. Philadelphia: JB Lippincott, 1992.

17. Cooper JE, Lake BD. Use of enzyme histochemistry in the diagnosis of pancreatoblastoma. Histopathology 1989;15:407.

18. Cooperman AM. Cancer of the pancreas: A dilemma in treatment. Surg Clin North Am 1981;61:107.

19. Corner BD. Primary carcinoma of the pancreas in an infant aged seven months. Arch Dis Child 1943;18:106.

20. Cubilla A, Fitzgerald PJ. Classification of pancreatic cancer (non-endocrine). Mayo Clin Proc 1979;54:449.

21. Cubilla AL, Fitzgerald PJ. Morphological patterns of primary nonendocrine human pancreas carcinoma. Cancer Res 1975;35:2234.

22. Cubilla A, Fitzgerald PJ. Pancreas cancer. I. Duct adenocarcinoma: A clinical-pathologic study of 380 patients. Pathol Annu 1978;13(1):241.

23. Dahms BB, Landing BH, Blascovics M, et al. Nesidioblastosis and other islet cell abnormalities in hyperinsulinemic hypoglycemia of childhood. Hum Pathol 1980;11:641.

24. Dehner LP. Pediatric Surgical Pathology, 2nd ed, p 546. Baltimore: Williams and Wilkins, 1987.

25. Drut R, Jones MC. Congenital pancreatoblastoma in Beckwith-Wiedemann syndrome: An emerging association. Pediatr Pathol 1988;8:331.

26. Emery LG, Shields M, Shah NR, et al. Neuroblastoma associated with Beckwith-Wiedemann syndrome. Cancer 1983;52:176.

27. Fonkalsrud EW, Wilkerson JA, Longmire WP. Pancreatoduodenectomy for islet cell tumor of the pancreas in infancy and childhood. JAMA 1966;197:586.

28. Frable WJ, Still WJS, Kay S. Carcinoma of the pancreas, infantile type. A light and electron microscopic study. Cancer 1971;27:667.

29. Francois R, Pradon M, Sherrer M, et al. Hypoglycemia due to pancreatic cell adenoma: Report of two cases in young children. J Pediatr 1962;60:721.

30. Goossens A, Gepts W, Saudubray JM, et al. Diffuse and focal nesidioblastosis: A clinicopathological study of 24 patients with persistent neonatal hyperinsulinemic hypoglycemia. Am J Surg Pathol 1989;13:766.

31. Gould VE, Memoli VA. Nesidiodysplasia and nesidioblastosis of infancy: Structural and functional correlations with the syndrome of hyperinsulinemic hypoglycemia. Pediatr Pathol 1983;1:7.

32. Grampa G, Gargantini L, Grigolato PG, et al. Hypoglycemia in infancy caused by beta cell nesidioblastosis. Am J Dis Child 1974;128:226.

33. Grant DB, Barbor PRH. Islet-cell tumour causing hypoglycaemia in a newborn infant. Arch Dis Child 1970;45:434.

34. Gray ES. The endocrine system. _In_ Keeling JW (ed): Fetal and Neonatal Pathology, 2nd ed, p 499. Berlin: Springer-Verlag, 1993.

35. Grosfeld JL, Clatworthy HW, Hamoudi AB. Pancreatic malignancy in children. Arch Surg 1970;101:370.

36. Grosfeld JL, Vane DW, Rescoria FJ, et al. Pancreatic tumors in childhood: Analysis of 13 cases. J Pediatr Surg 1990;25:1057.

37. Grotting JC, Kassel S, Dehner LP. Nesidioblastosis and congenital neuroblastoma. Arch Pathol Lab Med 1979;103:642.

38. Gundersen AE, Janis JF. Pancreatic cystadenoma in childhood: Report of a case. J Pediatr Surg 1969;4:478.

39. Habbick BF, Cram RW, Miller KR. Neonatal hypoglycemia resulting from islet cell adenomatosis: Successful treatment with total pancreatectomy. Am J Dis Child 1977;131:210.

40. Hamoudi AB, Misugi K, Grosfield GL, et al. Papillary epithelial neoplasm of the pancreas in a child. Report of a case with electron microscopy. Cancer 1970;26:1126.

41. Heitz PU, Kloppel G, Hacki WH, et al. Nesidioblastosis: The pathologic basis of persistent hyperinsulinemic hypoglycemia in infants: Morphologic and quantitative analysis of seven cases based on specific immunostaining and electron microscopy. Diabetes 1977;26:632.

42. Horie A, Yano Y, Kotoo Y, et al. Morphogenesis of pancreatoblastoma, infantile carcinoma of the pancreas: Report of two cases. Cancer 1977;39:247.

43. Irving IM: Abdominal tumours. _In_ Lister J, Irving IM (eds): Neonatal Surgery, 3rd ed, p 122. London: Butterworths, 1990.

44. Iseki M, Suzuki T, Koizumi Y, et al. Alpha-fetoprotein producing pancreatoblastoma. A case report. Cancer 1986;57:1833.

45. Jaffe R. The pancreas. _In_ Stocker JT, Dehner LP (eds): Pediatric Pathology, Vol 2, p 791. Philadelphia: JB Lippincott, 1992.

46. Jaffe R. The pancreas. _In_ Wigglesworth JS, Singer DB (eds): Textbook of Fetal and Perinatal Pathology, Vol 2, p 1021. Oxford: Blackwell, 1991.

47. Jaffe R, Hashida Y, Yunis EJ. Pancreatic pathology in hyperinsulinemic hypoglycemia of infancy. Lab Invest 1980;42:356.

48. Jaksic T, Yaman M, Thorner P, et al. A 20-year review of pediatric pancreatic tumors. J Pediatr Surg 1992;27:1315.

49. Jenkins JM, Othersen HB Jr. Cystadenoma of the pancreas in a newborn. J Pediatr Surg 1992;27:1569.

50. Kirkland J, Ben-Menachem Y, Akhtar M, et al. Islet cell tumor in a neonate: Diagnosis by selective angiography and histological findings. Pediatrics 1978;61:790.

51. Kissane JM. Tumors of the exocrine pancreas in childhood. *In* Humphrey GB, Grindy GB, Dehner LP, et al. (eds): Pancreatic Tumors in Children, p 99. Boston: Martinus Nijhoff Publishers, 1982.

52. Klimstra DS, Wenig BM, Adair CF, et al. Pancreatoblastoma: A clinicopathologic study and review of the literature. Am J Surg Pathol 1995;19(2):1371.

53. Koh THHG, Cooper JE, Newman CL, et al. Pancreatoblastoma in a neonate with Wiedemann-Beckwith syndrome. Eur J Pediatr 1986;145:435.

54. Lack EE, Cassady JR, Levey R, et al. Tumors of the exocrine pancreas in children and adolescents. Am J Surg Pathol 1983;7:319.

55. Laidlaw GF. Nesidioblastoma, the islet cell tumor of the pancreas. Am J Pathol 1938;14:125.

56. Misugi K, Misugi N, Sotos J, et al. The pancreatic islet of infants with severe hypoglycemia. Arch Pathol 1970;89:208.

57. Moore KL. The Developing Human—Clinically Oriented Embryology, 5th ed. Philadelphia: WB Saunders, 1993.

58. Moreno LA, Turck D, Gottrand F, et al. Familial hyperinsulinism with nesidioblastosis of the pancreas: Further evidence for autosomal recessive inheritance. Am J Med Genet 1989;34:584.

59. Moynan RW, Neerhout RC, Johnson TS. Pancreatic carcinoma in childhood: Case report and review. J Pediatr 1964;65:711.

60. O'Hara D. Pancreatoblastoma—Does it exist? Pediatr Pathol 1985;3:118 (Abstract).

61. Pettinato G, Manivel JC, Ravetto C, et al. Papillary cystic tumor of the pancreas: A clinicopathologic study of 20 cases with cytologic, immunohistochemical, ultrastructural and flow cytometric observations and a review of the literature. Am J Clin Pathol 1992;98:478.

62. Potter EL, Craig JM. Pathology of the Fetus and Infant, 3rd ed, p 344. Chicago: Year Book Medical Publishers, 1975.

63. Potts SR, Brown S, O'Hara MD. Pancreatoblastoma in a neonate associated with Beckwith-Wiedemann syndrome. Z Kinderchir 1986;41:56.

64. Rawlinson DG, Christiansen RO. Light and electron microscopic observations on a congenital insulinoma. Cancer 1973;32:1470.

65. Rich RH, Dehner LP, Okinaga K, et al. Surgical management of islet-cell adenoma of infancy. Surgery 1978;84:519.

66. Rich HR, Weber JL, Shandling B. Adenocarcinoma of the pancreas in the neonate managed by pancreatoduodenectomy. J Pediatr Surg 1986;21:806.

67. Rickham PP. Islet cell tumors in childhood. J Pediatr Surg 1975;10:83.

68. Robey G, Daneman A, Martin DJ. Pancreatic carcinoma in a neonate. Pediatr Radiol 1983;13:284.

69. Robinson MJ, Clark AM, Gold H, et al. Islet cell adenoma in the newborn: Report of two patients. Pediatrics 1971;48:232.

70. Roe TF, Kershnar AK, Weitzman JJ, et al. Beckwith's syndrome with extreme organ hyperplasia. Pediatrics 1973;52:372.

71. Salinas ED, Mangurten HH, Roberts SS, et al. Functioning islet cell adenoma in the newborn: Report of a case with failure of diazoxide. Pediatrics 1968;41:646.

72. Schiller M, Krausz M, Meyer S, et al. Neonatal hyperinsulinism—Surgical and pathologic considerations. J Pediatr Surg 1980;15:16.

73. Schwartz SS, Rich BH, Lucky AW, et al. Familial nesidioblastosis: Severe neonatal hypoglycemia in two families. J Pediatr 1979;95:44.

74. Sotelo-Avila C, Gonzalez-Crussi F: Congenital tumours. *In* Wigglesworth JS, Singer DB (eds): Textbook of Fetal and Perinatal Pathology, Vol 1, p 455. Oxford: Blackwell, 1991.

75. Sotelo-Avila C, Gonzalez-Crussi F, Fowler JW. Complete and incomplete forms of Beckwith-Wiedemann syndrome: Their oncogenic potential. J Pediatr 1980;96:47.

76. Sotelo-Avila C, Gonzalez-Crussi F, Starling KA. Wilms' tumor in a patient with an incomplete form of Beckwith-Wiedemann syndrome. Pediatr 1980;66:121.

77. Sotelo-Avila C, Gooch WM. Neoplasms associated with the Beckwith-Wiedemann syndrome. Perspect Pediatr Pathol 1976;3:255.

78. Sotelo-Avila C, Singer DB. Syndrome of hyperplastic fetal visceromegaly and neonatal hypoglycemia (Beckwith's syndrome): A report of seven cases. Pediatrics 1970;46:240.

79. Stanley CA, Baker L. Hyperinsulinism in infants and children: Diagnosis and therapy. Adv Pediatr 1976;23:315.

80. Taguchi T, Suita S, Hirose R. Histological classification of nesidioblastosis: Efficacy of immunohistochemical study of neurone-specific enolase. J Pediatr Surg 1991;26:770.

81. Taxy JB. Adenocarcinoma of the pancreas in childhood: Report of a case and a review of the English language literature. Cancer 1976;37:1508.

82. Thomas CG Jr, Underwood LE, Carney CN, et al. Neonatal and infantile hypoglycemia due to insulin excess. New aspects of diagnosis and surgical management. Ann Surg 1976;185:505.

83. Tsukimoto I, Watanabe K, Lin JB, et al. Pancreatic carcinoma in children in Japan. Cancer 1973;31:1203.

84. Tunell WP. Hemangioendothelioma of the pancreas obstructing the common bile duct and duodenum. J Pediatr Surg 1976;11:827.

85. Turleau C, de Grouchy J, Chavin-Colin F, et al. Trisomy 11p15 and Beckwith-Wiedemann syndrome. A report of 2 cases. Hum Genet 1984;67:219.

86. Ulich T, Cheng L, Lewin KJ. Acinar-endocrine cell tumor of the pancreas. Report of a pancreatic tumor containing both zymogen and neuroendocrine granules. Cancer 1982;50:2099.

87. Waziri M, Patil SR, Hanson JW, et al. Abnormality of chromosome 11 in patients with features of Beckwith-Wiedemann syndrome. J Pediatr 1983;102:873.

88. Welch KJ. The pancreas. *In* Welch KJ, Randolph JG, Ravitch MM, et al. (eds): Pediatric Surgery, 4th ed, Vol 2, p 1096. Chicago: Year Book, 1986.

89. Wiedemann HR. Tumours and hemihypertrophy associated with Wiedemann-Beckwith syndrome. Eur J Pediatr 1983;141:129.

90. Witte DP, Greider MH, DeSchryver-Kecskemeti K, et al. The juvenile human pancreas: Normal versus idiopathic hyperinsulinemic hypoglycemia. Semin Diagn Pathol 1984;1:30.

91. Woo D, Scopes JW, Polak JM. Idiopathic hypoglycemia in sibs with morphological evidence of nesidioblastosis of the pancreas. Arch Dis Child 1976;51:528.

92. Woolf DA, Leonard JV, Trembath RC, et al. Nesidioblastosis: Evidence for autosomal recessive inheritance. Arch Dis Child 1991;66:529.

93. Yakovac WC, Baker L, Hummeler K. Beta cell nesidioblastosis in idiopathic hypoglycemia of infancy. J Pediatr 1971;79:226.

15

THYROID TUMORS

TERATOMA

Teratoma is the major thyroid neoplasm affecting the newborn and infant. Neonates with this tumor often have a maternal history of polyhydramnios and an obvious, sometimes gigantic, cervical mass that causes airway compression, respiratory symptoms, and sometimes, stillbirth (Fig. 15–1). Histologically, these tumors are composed of mature tissues of various types and immature neuroglial elements (see Chapter 2, "Germ Cell Tumors").

CARCINOMA

Thyroid carcinoma has been described in children,[3,6,10] but during the first year of life, it is unusual, being the subject of an isolated case report. Thyroid carcinoma has been reported as an incidental postmortem finding in stillborns. An occult, 3-mm, papillary carcinoma was noted in a stillborn male of 34 weeks' gestation with facial anomalies by Mills and Allen,[8] and a follicular variant of papillary carcinoma was reported in a 38-week stillborn infant by Coffin and Dehner.[2] Moreover, this malignant lesion has been described in infants who have had palpable thyroid nodules at birth.[8,10] Metastastatic thyroid carcinoma has not been documented in the perinatal period.

MEDULLARY THYROID CARCINOMA

The risk of early spread of medullary thyroid carcinoma is significant in the multiple endocrine neoplasia syndrome, type 2b (MEN 2b) (mucosal neuroma syndrome).[1,4,7] Affected individuals with MEN 2b have fleshy, everted lips ("blubbery lips"), nodules on the lips and tongue, and a predisposition for medullary carcinoma and pheochromocytoma.[4] Occasionally, the oral nodules (mucosal neuromas) are present at birth, which can lead to early detection, not only of thyroid cancer, but also of pheochromocytoma. One of the youngest patients with medullary thyroid carcinoma associated with MEN 2b was a 15-month-old female infant.[9] Calcitonin is an important chemical marker used to detect the presence of the tumor before clinical signs appear.[7]

CYSTS ASSOCIATED WITH VESTIGIAL REMNANTS

Cysts may develop anywhere along the course of the thyroglossal duct, from the base of the tongue to the neck inferior to the hyoid bone, usually in the midline. They may be present at birth, but are more commonly noted later. Eventually, the cyst enlarges, often rupturing and forming a draining sinus. Thyroglossal duct cyst has been responsible for death in the neonate owing to respiratory obstruction.[5] Microscopically, the epithelial lining of the cyst consists of columnar, respiratory, squamous epithelium or a mixture. When chronically infected, the cyst epithelium may be replaced by inflammatory granulation tissue. Small nests of thyroid follicles are found adjacent to the cyst in less than 50% of specimens.

Branchial cysts are remnants of the branchial clefts, which normally disappear during development. The cysts, which do not appear until later childhood and adolescence, cause a painless swelling (unless infected) on the lateral

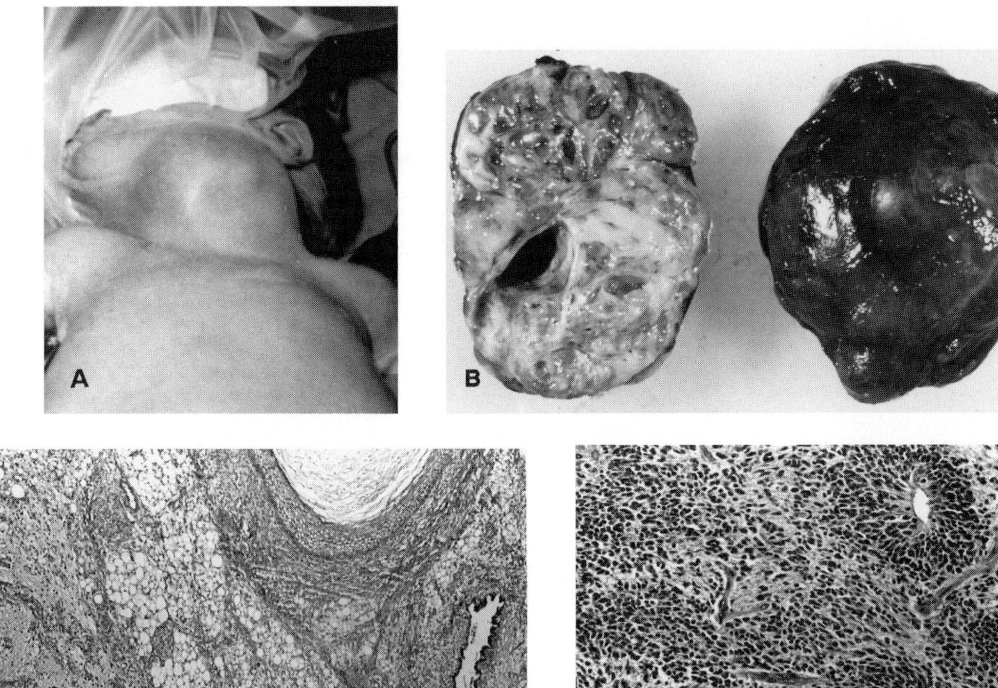

Figure 15–1. Thyrocervical teratoma. *A,* A midline neck mass in a 6-day-old male infant. *B,* The tumor, weighing 28 g and measuring 5.5 × 4.9 cm, is composed of solid and cystic areas. *C,* Keratinized, stratified, squamous and ependymal-type epithelium, fat, and brain tissue are present (hematoxylin-eosin, ×100). *D,* Immature neuroglial elements constitute a large part of the neoplasm (hematoxylin-eosin, ×100). Teratoma is the most common tumor involving the thyroid of the fetus and newborn. (*A:* From Isaacs H Jr. Neoplasms in infants: A report of 265 cases. Pathol Annu 1983;18(2):165. Used by permission.)

side of the face and neck. Small, preauricular cysts and sinuses are manifested as pits in the skin of the face anterior to the ear. Histologically, the cysts are lined by stratified squamous epithelium, respiratory epithelium, or a mixture of the two. Moreover, the cyst may be replaced by inflammatory tissue if it becomes infected. The preauricular sinuses often have small islands of elastic cartilage in their walls. The branchial cysts characteristically contain lymphoid nodules and mucous glands.

REFERENCES

1. Bigner SH, Mendelsohn G, Wells SA Jr, et al. Medullary carcinoma of the thyroid in the multiple endocrine neoplasia IIA syndrome. Am J Surg Pathol 1981;5:459.
2. Coffin CM, Dehner LP. Congenital tumors. *In* Stocker JT, Dehner LP (eds): Pediatric Pathology, Vol I, p 325. Philadelphia: JB Lippincott, 1992.
3. Franssila KO, Harach HR. Occult papillary carcinoma of the thyroid in children and young adults. A systemic autopsy study in Finland. Cancer 1986;58:715.
4. Gorlin RJ, Sedano HO, Vickers RA, et al. Multiple mucosal neuroma, pheochromocytoma and medullary carcinoma of the thyroid: A syndrome. Cancer 1968; 22:293.
5. Hanzlick RL. Thyroglossal duct cyst causing death in a four week old infant. J Forensic Sci 1984;29:345.
6. Hung W, August GP, Randolph JJ, et al. Solitary thyroid nodules in children and adolescents. J Pediatr Surg 1982;17:225.
7. Kaufman FR, Roe TF, Isaacs H Jr, et al. Metastatic medullary thyroid carcinoma in young children with mucosal neuroma syndrome. Pediatrics 1982;70:263.
8. Mills SE, Allen MS Jr. Congenital occult papillary carcinoma of the thyroid gland. Hum Pathol 1986;17:1179.
9. Moyes CD, Alexander FW. Mucosal neuroma syndrome presenting in a neonate. Dev Med Clin Neurol 1977;19:518.
10. Winship T, Rosvoll RV. Thyroid carcinoma in childhood: Final report on a 20 year study. Clin Proc Child Hosp 1970;26:327.

16

CARDIAC TUMORS

Cardiac tumors (Table 16–1) seldom occur in the perinatal period. Rhabdomyomas, by far the most common tumor of the heart in the fetus and newborn, are probably hamartomas rather than true neoplasms. Next in frequency are teratoma and fibroma, followed by myxoma (see Tables 16–2 to 16–8). Because of their location, however, tumors and hamartomas of the heart may severely compromise blood flow, interfere with myocardial function, and cause arrhythmias, leading to their clinical discovery, stillbirth, or sudden death.[7,44,79,111] Solid tumor metastasis to the heart is found more often than primary tumors in the older child and adult, as compared to the newborn, in which age group it rarely occurs.[20,79]

INCIDENCE

Primary cardiac tumors are diagnosed in approximately 1 in 10,000 (0.01%) routine necropsies of patients of all ages.[79] Nadas and Ellison, reporting from the Boston Children's Hospital Medical Center, culled 11,000 necropsies over a 53-year period and found six infants, two of whom were newborns, with primary cardiac tumors (0.05%).[79] Both newborns had rhabdomyomas. A study of The Hospital for Sick Children, London reported a similar figure of 0.04%.[105] The review included two neonates with rhabdomyoma and 1 fibroma and 1 myxoma in an older infant. Of the primary cardiac tumors listed in the Armed Forces Institute of Pathology series for patients younger than 1 year of age, 45 were benign and 2 were malignant, the former comprising 28 rhabdomyomas, 9 teratomas, 6 fibromas, 1 hemangioma, and 1 mesothelioma of the atrioventricular

node and the latter comprising 1 rhabdomyosarcoma and 1 fibrosarcoma.[76] Van der Hauwaert collected 22 cases occurring in infants and children from an Association of European Paediatic Cardiologists survey.[111] The newborn cases accounted for almost one fourth of the total of 22, and comprised 4 rhabdomyomas and 1 teratoma. The youngest patient with a cardiac fibroma in their series was 5 months of age. The New England Regional Infant Cardiac Program review showed that, of 2251 infants surveyed with the diagnosis of congenital heart disease, 9 had cardiac tumors (0.4%), including 3 intrapericardial teratomas, 4 rhabdomyomas, and 2 fibromas.[46] The Hospital for Sick Children, Toronto study consisted of 16 patients with primary tumors, 6 of which occurred in newborns, including 4 rhabdomyomas, 1 fibroma, and 1 myxoma.[20] Using antenatal sonography, Groves et al. detected 11 fetal cardiac tumors (10 rhabdomyomas and 1 intrapericardial teratoma) from a series of more than 10,000 scans.[54] They noted a high rate of intrauterine death, as only 3 of 7 infants survived when the pregnancy was allowed to continue.

Some tumors (e.g., myxoma) are found most often in adults, but occasionally are observed in the newborn and infant.[20,56,76,92] Most childhood atrial myxomas occur in adolescence.[30] Other neoplasms, such as fibromas and intracardiac teratomas, are seldom noted in adults, but are among the more common lesions in infants and children.[7] During the first year of life, rhabdomyoma and pericardial teratoma are responsible for more than 75% of the primary cardiac tumors.[6,12,20,46,76,81] In Table 16–2, a survey of 91 fetal and newborn cardiac lesions shows that rhabdomyoma accounts for more than half

Table 16–1. Cardiac Tumors and Tumor-Like Conditions of the Fetus and Newborn

Rhabdomyoma
Teratoma
Fibroma
Myxoma
Hemangioma
Rhabdomyosarcoma
Fibrolipoma
Hemangiopericytoma
Oncocytic cardiomyopathy
Metastatic lesions
    Neuroblastoma
    Leukemia

(51%), whereas teratoma represents 21%, followed by fibroma (11%) and myxoma (8%).

CLINICAL FINDINGS

Fetal cardiac tumors can be detected by antenatal ultrasonography (Fig. 16–1).[21,49,53,54,58,86,93,115] Three main manifestations of fetal cardiac tumors have been described: arrhythmias produced by a conduction defect or abnormal pacemaker function; fetal hydrops resulting from congestive heart failure; or stillbirth following obstruction of blood flow by an intracavitary tumor.[53–55,86] Cardiac arrhythmia is the most frequent sign, and it is a definite indication for antenatal sonography, which may demonstrate the tumor.[55] Cardiomegaly, congestive

Table 16–2. Distribution and Survival of 91 Fetal and Newborn Cardiac Tumors and Tumor-Like Conditions*

Tumor	Number (%)	Survival (%)	
		Living	*Dead*
Rhabdomyoma	46 (50.5)	21	25 (46)
Teratoma	19 (20.9)	16	3 (84)
Fibroma	11 (12.1)	1	10 (9)
Myxoma	7 (7.7)	1	6 (14)
Hemangioma	4 (4.4)	4	0 (100)
Rhabdomyosarcoma	3 (3.3)	0	3 (0)
Fibrolipoma	1 (1.1)	0	1 (0)
	91 (100)	43	48 (47)†

*Compiled from Tables 16–3 to 16–8, consisting of 91 newborn cases selected from the literature.
†Overall survival: 43/91 × 100 = 47%.

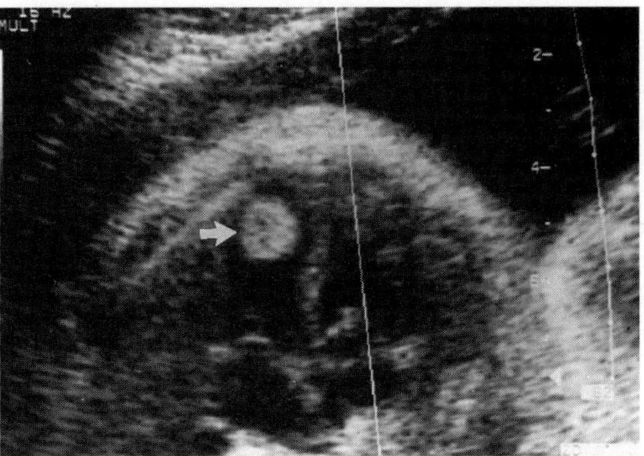

Figure 16–1. Cardiac rhabdomyoma. An ultrasonogram of a fetus at 32 weeks' gestation demonstrates a round, echogenic mass (*arrow*) bulging into the cavity of the left ventricle. Several additional tumors were visible in other views. The infant was diagnosed as having tuberous sclerosis, but survived. (Courtesy of Val Catanzarite, MD, Perinatology, Sharp Memorial Hospital, San Diego, CA.)

heart failure, pericardial effusion, a murmur, and arrhythmias are the most common findings in the newborn (see Tables 16–3 to 16–8).

Cardiac tumors may imitate other conditions in the neonate, such as sepsis and congenital heart disease (e.g., hypoplastic left heart syndrome, subaortic stenosis, mitral stenosis, and tricuspid insufficiency).[44,50,66,78,92,100] Primary tumors in a malformed heart have been documented, but the concurrence is unusual and, when present, adversely affects the surgical management and prognosis for that patient.[14,50,86,92] A tumor should be considered in the differential diagnosis in a fetus or newborn with unexplained murmurs, congestive heart failure, or arrhythmias.[6]

A cardiac neoplasm may be the initial manifestation of certain genetic disorders, such as tuberous sclerosis, neurofibromatosis, the Gorlin syndrome (nevoid-basal cell carcinoma syndrome), familial myxomas, and the Beckwith-Wiedemann syndrome.[22,52,75,85,113] A family history of tuberous sclerosis in the mother or other family members is a definite indication for antenatal sonography.[54] Gorlin reviewed 250 patients with cardiac fibroma and noted that 4% had the nevoid-basal cell carcinoma syndrome.[52] The term "syndrome myxoma" has been applied to describe a group of patients whose cardiac myxomas are associated with pigmented skin lesions and peripheral and endocrine tumors.[113] The cutaneous lesions of this syndrome include lentiginosis, myxomas, neurofibromas, and blue nevi.

Early diagnosis of cardiac tumors in the fetus and newborn is accomplished through the use of sonography, echocardiography, cineangiography, and cardiac catheterization. Surgical resection can be performed, even in the newborn. Certain tumors—notably, intrapericardial teratomas, hemangiomas, and myxomas—can be successfully removed, as can obstructive intracavitary rhabdomyomas, provided the lesions are not extensive or inoperable.[6,7,111]

RHABDOMYOMA

Cardiac rhabdomyomas occur predominantly in infants and children, with about 75% of those affected being 1 year of age or younger.[7,76] Rhabdomyoma is the leading cardiac tumor of the fetus and newborn, followed by teratoma and fibroma* (see Table 16–2). Cardiac rhabdomyoma may be found unexpectedly at postmortem examination of a stillborn or of a newborn with nonimmune fetal hydrops.[7,48,54,55,61,111] In the study by McAllister and Fenoglio, 3 of 28 (11%) infants with rhabdomyomas were stillborn.[76] Table 16–3 shows that 6 of 46 (13%) were stillborn, which is comparable to the findings of the Armed Forces Institute of Pathology study. Recurrent arrhythmias or sudden unexpected death may be the result of rhabdomyomas that interfere with the conduction system or obstruct left or right ventricular blood flow.[7,64,79,81] Cardiomegaly, congestive heart failure, and murmurs are other clinical findings (see Table 16–3).[7,76,79]

In the fetus, cardiac arrhythmia is the most frequent sign, and is an indication for ultrasonography, which may demonstrate the tumor.[3,15,48,53,54,114] However, 50% of prenatally diagnosed rhabdomyomas are asymptomatic and are discovered on routine ultrasonographic scans (see Table 16–3).[21,49] Rhabdomyomas may be detected in fetuses as young as 22 weeks' gestation.[114] The tumor is rarely noted in association with congenital heart malformations.[50,92]

Although they may occur independently, rhabdomyomas are only one manifestation of tuberous sclerosis, a phakomatosis (a hereditary condition involving the central nervous system, eye, and skin) that is transmitted as an autosomal dominant trait of variable expression

(see Figs. 16–1 and 16–2). The disease is classically manifested by the triad of mental retardation, epilepsy, and angiofibromas of the face, which may not become apparent until later in infancy. More than one third of infants and children with cardiac rhabdomyomas have been reported to have tuberous sclerosis, and the reverse is also probably true.[30,41,57,81] Webb and associates suggest that the incidence of rhabdomyomas in patients with tuberous sclerosis is much higher than this figure, approaching 60%, and that at least 80% of children with rhabdomyomas have tuberous sclerosis.[114] Of 46 fetuses and newborns with cardiac rhabdomyomas selected from the literature, 22 (48%) had evidence of tuberous sclerosis (see Table 16–3).

Not only is a history of tuberous sclerosis in the mother or in other family members an indication for antenatal sonographic studies, but also the discovery of fetal rhabdomyoma should suggest to the physician that both parents should be investigated for evidence of the disease.[49]

Other manifestations of tuberous sclerosis may be present in the patient with rhabdomyoma. Skin lesions, such as "mountain ash" maculae and adenoma sebaceum (angiofibromatous hamartoma), may be apparent at birth. When present, cortical and subependymal tubers (gliomas) may be detected by imaging studies or macroscopically at necropsy.[7,49,82,111] Although the kidneys are grossly normal, microscopic examination may show multiple cysts. Renal angiomyolipomas, consisting of vascular smooth muscle and adipose tissue elements, occur later in life.

Rhabdomyomas consist of one or more white to yellow-tan, circumscribed nodules in the myocardium, situated most often within the ventricles and in the ventricular septum. Additionally some occur in the subepicardial region and in the atria. In about 50% of the affected patients, rhabdomyomas are intracavitary, producing obstruction.[7,11,35,41,48,50,55,66,67,72,79,81,82,99,103,111]

Usually designated rhabdomyomas or hamartomas because of the presence of striated myofibrils, these lesions are considered to be focal or diffuse overgrowths of cardiac muscle, showing only mildly abnormal changes and not true neoplasia. They have a characteristic histologic appearance consisting of large, round or oval cells with small, central nuclei and a thin peripheral rim of cytoplasm. Connecting the nucleus with the cell wall are delicate radiating strands responsible for the designation of "spi-

---

*References: 6, 10–12, 15, 20, 21, 24, 31, 35, 41, 44–48, 50, 53–55, 59, 67, 72–74, 79, 80, 87, 89, 92, 94, 97–99, 101–103, 105, 107–109, 111, 112, 117, 118.

Table 16–3. 46 Fetal and Newborn Cardiac Rhabdomyomas*

Case No.	Age at Death	Tuberous Sclerosis	Location	Initial and Associated Findings	Reference
1	Alive	+	IVS	U/S screen	DiLollo et al.[34]
2	3 mos	+	IVS	Cardiomegaly, murmur, CHF, arrhythmia	Schmaltz and Apitz[95]
3	3 days	–	LV, IVS	Cardiomegaly, CHF	Kuehl et al.[66]
4	3 days	–	LV, IVS	Cardiomegaly, CHF	Kuehl et al.[66]
5	1 week	+	LV	Arrhythmia	Isaacs[62]
6	Alive	+	IVS	Arrhythmia	Smythe et al.[107]
7	Alive	+	RV, LV	Murmur	Smythe et al.[107]
8	Alive	+	LV	Murmur	Smythe et al.[107]
9	Alive	–	LV	Murmur	Smythe et al.[107]
10	Alive	+	Multiple	U/S screen	Smythe et al.[107]
11	Alive	+	Multiple	Arrhythmia, U/S screen	Smythe et al.[107]
12	Alive	–	Multiple	Murmur	Smythe et al.[107]
13	Alive	+	LV, IVS	FH, U/S screen	Smythe et al.[107]
14	Alive	+	IVS	Arrhythmia, murmur	Alkalay et al.[3]
15	Alive	–	IVS	Cyanosis, arrhythmia	Bjorkhem et al.[15]
16	Alive	+	Multiple	Arrhythmia, murmur, U/S screen	Bjorkhem et al.[15]
17	3 weeks	+	Multiple	CHF, murmur	Bjorkhem et al.[15]
18	Stillborn	–	Multiple	Arrhythmia, hydrops, U/S screen	Geva et al.[48]
19	Stillborn	–	LA, IVS	Hydrops, unexpected necropsy finding	Geva et al.[48]
20	Stillborn	–	IVS	Hydramnios, hydrops, U/S screen	Kleinman et al.[65]
21	Stillborn	–	LV	Hydrops, U/S screen	Iliff et al.[61]
22	4 days	+	Multiple	Died after repair of TEF; necropsy finding	Van der Hauwaert[111]
23	6 weeks	–	RV	Dyspnea, cyanosis, cardiomegaly, RVH	Van der Hauwaert[111]
24	2 days	+	IVS	CHF, cyanosis, cardiomegaly, RBBB	Van der Hauwaert[111]
25	15 days	–	IVS	Cardiomegaly, murmur, arrhythmia	Van der Hauwaert[111]
26	1 day	–	RV	Respiratory distress, congenital anomalies	Chan et al.[20]
27	1 day	–	Multiple	Cardiomegaly, cyanosis, cardiac defects	Chan et al.[20]
28	3 days	–	LV	Cardiomegaly, respiratory distress, cardiac defects	Chan et al.[20]
29	Alive	+	RV, LV	Cardiomegaly, murmur	Chan et al.[20]
30	Alive	–	IVS	Cardiomegaly, murmur	Arciniegas et al.[5,6]
31	Alive	–	IVS	Cardiomegaly, murmur	Arciniegas et al.[5,6]
32	9 days	–	IVS	Cardiomegaly, murmur	Arciniegas et al.[5,6]
33	Alive	–	IVS	Cardiomegaly, murmur	Arciniegas et al.[5,6]
34	2 days	+	Multiple	Cardiomegaly, murmur, respiratory distress	Bini et al.[12]
35	3 mos	–	Multiple	Cardiomegaly, bradycardia	Bini et al.[12]
36	2 days	+	IVS	Cardiomegaly, CHF	Bini et al.[12]
37	2 days	+	IVS, LA, LV	Hydrops, CHF, cardiomegaly, murmur, U/S screen	Guereta et al.[55]
38	Alive	+	Multiple	Murmur, bradycardia, CHF	Marx et al.[74]
39	Alive	–	RA, RV	Arrhythmia	Marx et al.[74]
40	Alive	+	Multiple	U/S screen	Marx et al.[74]
41	Alive	+	Multiple	Murmur, bradycardia, CHF	Marx et al.[74]
42	Alive	–	Multiple	Bradyarrhythmia, U/S screen	Gresser et al.[53]
43	Stillborn	–	IVS	"Dysplastic tricuspid valve"	Russell et al.[92]
44	2 mos	+	RV	Cardiomegaly, cyanosis, dyspnea, murmur	Simcha et al.[105]
45	3 mos	–	IVS	Cardiomegaly, cyanosis, murmur, LBBB	Simcha et al.[105]
46	Stillborn	–	IVS	Hydrops, U/S screen	DeVore et al.[32]

*Selected from the literature.

CHF = congestive heart failure; FH = family history of tuberous sclerosis; LV = left ventricle; LA = left atrium; RV = right ventricle; RVH = right ventricular hypertrophy; RA = right atrium; IVS = interventricular septum; TEF = tracheoesophageal fistula; RBBB = right bundle branch block; LBBB, left bundle branch block; U/S screen = tumor(s) detected on antenatal sonography.

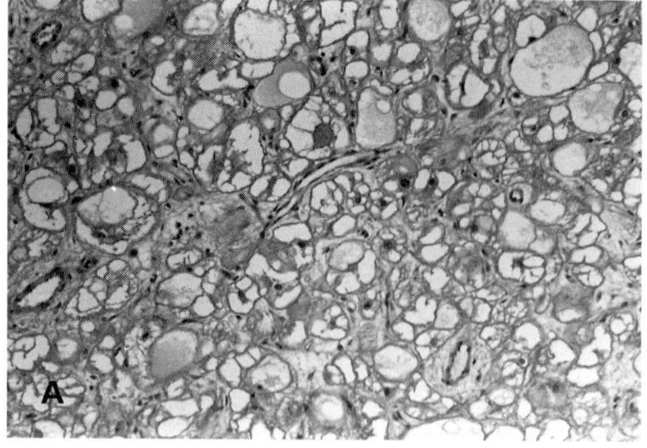

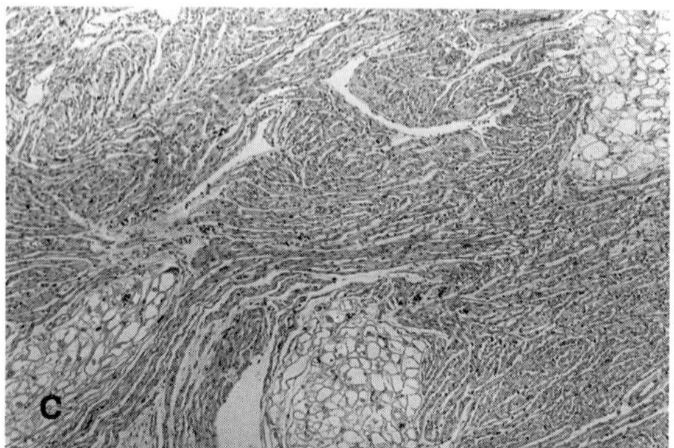

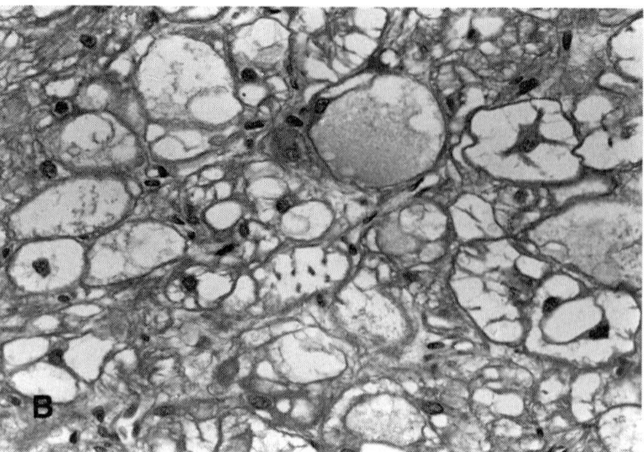

Figure 16–2. Cardiac rhabdomyoma. A 6-week-old male infant developed an arrhythmia at 1 week of age. Cardiac catheterization revealed a tumor in the posterior wall of the left ventricle. At the time of surgery, 4 g of yellow-white and lobulated tissue was excised. *A,* These large myocardial cells have cytoplasms distended by glycogen-filled vacuoles. Some contain central nuclei with delicate strands extending from the nucleus to the cell wall. These are the so-called "spider cells," which are considered pathognomonic for cardiac rhabdomyoma (hematoxylin-eosin, ×120). *B,* The spider cells are shown at higher magnification (hematoxylin-eosin, ×200). *C,* At postmortem examination, the patient had several additional cardiac rhabdomyomas (hematoxylin-eosin, ×60). Numerous glial nodules were found in the cerebrum and basal ganglia. (*A* and *B:* From Isaacs H Jr. Tumors of the Newborn and Infant. St. Louis: Mosby–Year Book, 1991.)

der cells'' (Fig. 16–2*A* and *B*). Cross-striations are detected in these strands and at the periphery of the cells. The intervening vacuoles are filled with glycogen, which is recognizable with appropriate staining. Such cells are scattered in small groups throughout the musculature, as well as in masses in grossly visible tumors (Fig. 16–2*C*). Electron microscopy confirms the presence of cross-striations and abundant beta glycogen within the cells.[40,104] Other ultrastructural features include leptofibrils, a poorly developed sarcoplasmic reticulum, and scattered desmosomes.[40]

Spontaneous regression of cardiac rhabdomyomas has been documented rather frequently (see Fig. 16–1).[3,44,54,74,107,114] Smythe et al. studied nine patients, three of whom were diagnosed prenatally and six of whom were diagnosed before 8 months of age, who had a total of 24 rhabdomyomas.[107] Measurements showed at least some evidence of regression in all 24 tumors, with 20 of 24 resolving completely. A comparable study by Farooki et al. confirmed these observations.[39] These researchers studied four newborns with 12 cardiac rhabdomyomas and found that all tumors, except those in the

right atrium, displayed spontaneous regression. Because of this tendency, surgical intervention is recommended only for those patients with severe hemodynamic compromise or for those with persistent arrhythmias.[44,107] Although spontaneous regression occurs, the prognosis for affected patients remains guarded.[107] The mortality rate for 46 fetuses and newborns with cardiac rhabdomyomas was reported to be greater than 50% (25 of 46) (see Tables 16–2 and 16–3).

TERATOMAS OF THE HEART AND PERICARDIUM

Teratoma is a rare primary tumor of the heart or pericardium at any age.[1,2,5,6,20,25,28,29,44,46,54,62,69,71,76,90,110,111,115,119] Nearly two thirds of teratomas are found in infants, and it is the second most common primary cardiac tumor (following rhabdomyoma) in the newborn (see Table 16–2).[76,90,111] Cardiac teratomas arise from either the pericardium or from within the heart. Most occur in the pericardium and are attached to the great vessels, as compared to

Table 16–4. 19 Fetal and Newborn Cardiac Teratomas

Case No.	Age at Death	Location	Initial Findings	Reference
1	Stillborn	Pericardium	Hydramnios, fetal hydrops, U/S screen	Rasmussen et al.[83]
2	Alive	Pericardium	Tachypnea, cyanosis, CHF	Rasmussen et al.[83]
3	Alive	Pericardium	Cardiomegaly, respiratory distress, CHF	Rasmussen et al.[83]
4	Alive	Pericardium	Cardiomegaly, respiratory distress	Rasmussen et al.[83]
5	15 hrs	IVS, IAS	Cyanosis, murmur, CHF	Rasmussen et al.[83]
6	Alive	RV	Murmur, arrhythmia	Costas et al.[25]
7	Alive	Pericardium	Cyanosis, respiratory distress, pericardial effusion	Agozzino et al.[1]
8	3 mos	Pericardium	Respiratory distress, pericardial effusion	Agozzino et al.[1]
9	Alive	Pericardium	Respiratory distress, cardiomegaly, pericardial effusion	Zerella and Halpe[119]
10	Alive	Pericardium	Respiratory distress, mediastinal mass, pericardial effusion	Lubin et al.[71]
11	Alive	Pericardium	Respiratory distress, pericardial effusion	Reynolds et al.[90]
12	Alive	Pericardium	Respiratory distress, pericardial effusion	Reynolds et al.[90]
13	Alive	Pericardium	Respiratory distress, pericardial effusion	Weber et al.[115]
14	Alive	Pericardium	Cyanosis, bradycardia, pericardial effusion	Aldousany et al.[2]
15	Alive	Pericardium	Pericardial effusion, U/S screen	De Geeter et al.[29]
16	Alive	Pericardium	Respiratory distress, pericardial effusion	Deenadayalu et al.[28]
17	Alive	Pericardium	Pericardial effusion	Lintermans et al.[69]
18	Alive	Pericardium	Pericardial effusion	Sumner et al.[110]
19	Alive	Pericardium	Respiratory distress	Isaacs[62]

CHF = congestive heart failure; RV = right ventricle; IAS = interatrial septum; IVS = interventricular septum; U/S screen = tumor(s) detected on antenatal sonography.

the atrium or ventricle, where less than a dozen cases have been reported (Table 16–4 and Fig. 16–3).[25,82,111,116] Of 19 cases of teratomas listed in Table 16–4, 17 were intrapericardial in location, and 2 were within the heart, one in the right ventricle and another in the intraatrial and intraventricular septum.

The main clinical findings in newborns and infants with intrapericardial teratomas are respiratory distress, cardiomegaly, and congestive heart failure, which may be accompanied by cyanosis and a cardiac murmur (see Table 16–4).[25,111] Pericardial effusion, which is present in virtually all patients, sometimes leads to life-

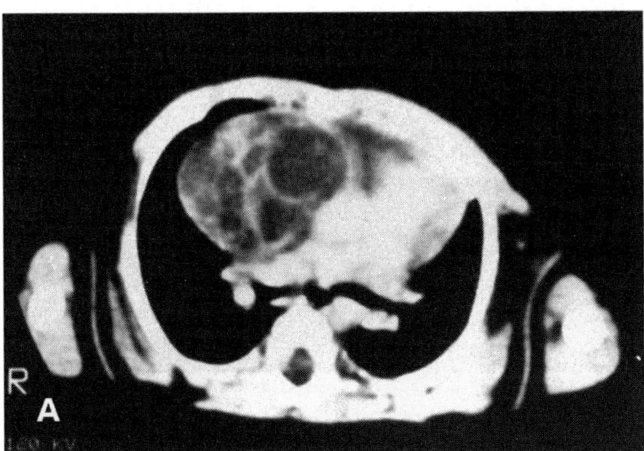
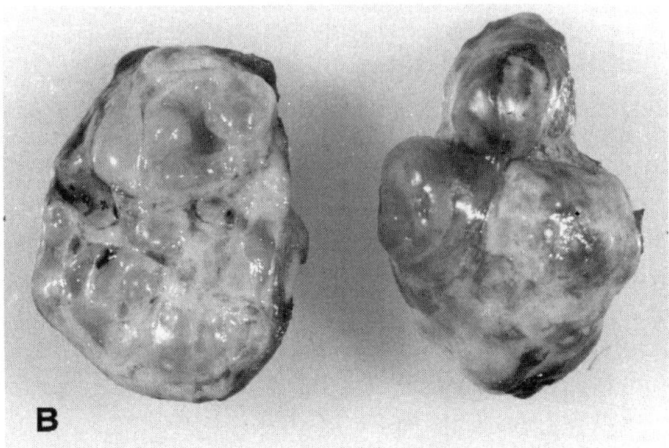

Figure 16–3. Intrapericardial teratoma. *A,* A CT scan of the chest of a 2-month-old male infant who presented with increasing respiratory distress showed a nodular, cystic density arising from the pericardium and bulging into the right pleural cavity. *B,* The tumor, weighing 27.5 g and measuring 5.5 × 3.6 cm, was situated within the pericardial cavity and was attached to the aorta. It has a lobulated appearance and contains multiple cysts. Both mature and immature elements were present on histologic examination (see Chapter 2, "Germ Cell Tumors"). (From Isaacs H Jr. Tumors of the Newborn and Infant. St. Louis: Mosby–Year Book, 1991.)

threatening tamponade. Pericardial teratoma is the leading cause of massive pericardial effusion in the neonate and, therefore, should be given prime consideration in the differential diagnosis.[90,119] However, it should be remembered that hemangioma is another perinatal cardiac tumor producing pericardial effusion and tamponade (see Table 16–7).[16,18,91] Occasionally, teratoma is responsible for sudden, unexpected death.[7,76]

Cardiac teratoma may be detected both antenatally and postnatally by sonography. Angiocardiography and/or computerized tomography (CT) scans usually are not required to demonstrate the lesion.[2,54] Frequently, nonimmune hydrops is present in the fetus and newborn with a teratoma.[26,54,81]

Intrapericardial teratomas are attached to the root of the pulmonary artery and aorta and encroach on the adjacent atria or ventricle, depending on their size. The tumor has a smooth, lobulated surface (see Fig. 16–3). On cross-section examination, it consists of numerous, multiloculated cysts with intervening solid areas. The intracardiac tumors arise from the atrial and/or ventricular wall as nodular masses projecting into the cardiac chamber(s).[25,76,82,111]

Histologically, pericardial and intracardiac teratomas are essentially the same as those found in other locations, with all three germ layers being represented in most instances. The cysts are lined by a variety of epithelia, including stratified squamous, cuboidal, mucin-secreting, or respiratory epithelium. The more solid areas contain mature or immature neuroglial tissue, thyroid, pancreas, smooth and skeletal muscle, and foci of cartilage and bone. Practically all the pericardial and intracardiac teratomas reported in the newborn and infant are composed of benign mature tissues, as just described, with or without immature neuroglial elements.[7,62,115] Agozzino et al. described a newborn with a teratoma who had a fatal recurrence 2 months following the initial surgery.[1] The authors believed that the recurrence was malignant, but their published photomicrographs show typical-appearing, immature, neuroglial elements, without evidence of either embryonal carcinoma or yolk sac tumor.

Early recognition of a cardiac teratoma is important because most can be cured by surgical resection. These lesions have been successfully removed from both neonates and infants.[2,7,25,71,76,119] Compared to other cardiac tumors of the fetus and newborn, with the exception of hemangioma, teratomas are associated with the highest survival rate (see Table 16–2). Table 16–4 shows that, of 19 patients with teratomas, 16 survived (84%) and 3 died, 1 a stillborn, 1 secondary to disease recurrence, and a third from congestive heart failure.

FIBROMA

Although uncommon, cardiac fibromas are found more often in infants and children than in adults. Of 29 published cases collected by Van der Hauwaert, 11 (38%) were described in infants;[111] 5 of 17 (30%) patients reported in the Armed Forces Institute of Pathology series[76] were younger than 1 year of age. In the newborn, cardiac fibromas rank third in frequency, following rhabdomyoma and teratoma (see Table 16–2).[6,8,12,20,31,36,46,47,51,73,88,92,96,100,105,111,117,118]

Cardiac fibroma is considered to be a tumor of connective tissue origin, arising from fibroblasts and myofibroblasts and having the same gross and microscopic appearance and biologic behavior as its soft tissue counterpart (see Chapter 4, "Soft Tissue Tumors"). Other names applied to this tumor include fibromatosis, myofibromatosis, fibrous hamartoma, and congenital mesoblastic tumor.[23,51,76]

The clinical findings depend on the location and extent of the tumor (Table 16–5).[44,79] Fibromas arising from the ventricular septum may involve the conduction system, resulting in arrhythmias, such as ventricular fibrillation. Cardiomegaly (the most frequent manifestation) and sudden, unexpected death occur with tumors situated both in the free wall of the ventricle and in the septum. Moreover, at either location, the lesion may obstruct the inflow or outflow tract of the ventricle, leading to progressive congestive heart failure.[7,44,118] When fibromas occur in the left ventricle, the signs and symptoms of obstruction often relate to the left side of the heart.[79] For example, in the cases described by Gonzalez-Crussi and colleagues[51] and by Freedom et al.,[44] the findings suggested the hypoplastic left heart syndrome. In the patient reported by McCue et al., subaortic stenosis was suspected.[78] In the series of McAllister and Fenoglio, the fibromas in all five infants arose from the ventricular septum.[76] The causes of death in these patients were listed as congestive heart failure (n = 2), sudden unexpected death (n = 2), and ventricular fibrillation (n = 1). Table 16–5 shows that the interventricular septum is the most common site of origin in the newborn (7 of 9 cases).

Table 16–5. 11 Fetal and Newborn Cardiac Fibromas

Case No.	Age at Death	Location	Initial Findings and Associated Conditions	Reference
1	7 wks	IVS	Cardiomegaly, ventricular fibrillation	McCallister and Fenoglio[76]
2	8 wks	IVS	Cardiomegaly, CHF	McCallister and Fenoglio[76]
3	3 mos	IVS	Sudden, unexpected death	McCallister and Fenoglio[76]
4	1 day	LV	Cardiomegaly, murmur, respiratory distress, CHF	McCallister and Fenoglio[76]
5	5 days	IVS	Cyanosis, murmur, cardiomegaly	Gonzalez-Crussi et al.[51]
6	2 days	IVS, apex*	Respiratory distress, murmur, cardiomegaly, hypoplastic mitral valve	Gonzalez-Crussi et al.[51]
7	Alive	RA	Cyanosis	Sharratt et al.[100]
8	4 days	IVS	Respiratory distress, murmur, CHF	Yabek et al.[118]
9	12 days	IVS	Respiratory distress, cardiomegaly, cystic renal dysplasia	Schwartz et al.[96]
10	1 day	LV	Murmur, CHF, respiratory distress	Chan et al.[20]
11	4 wks	LV	CHF, Gorlin syndrome	Coffin[22]

*Two tumors were found at necropsy.

CHF = congestive heart failure; LV = left ventricle; RA = right atrium; IVS = interventricular septum.

Associated extracardiac malformations or syndromes are seldom present, but the tumor has been observed in association with cleft lip and palate,[9] the Beckwith-Wiedemann syndrome,[85] and the basal cell nevus syndrome (Gorlin-Goltz syndrome).[22,23,52,113] The neonate with a cardiac fibroma reported by Schwartz et al. had bilateral cystic renal dysplasia.[96] In cases of congenital generalized (visceral) fibromatosis, fibromas also can occur in the heart and are associated with a poor prognosis[63,91a] (see Chapter 4, "Soft Tissue Tumors").

Cardiac fibromas are usually solitary, arising from the myocardium of the ventricular septum or free wall of the right or left ventricle (predominantly the left).[7,76] Exceptions do occur, however. Two separate fibromas, one arising from the apex and another from the interventricular septum, were found in a newborn described by Gonzalez-Crussi and co-workers.[51] Cardiac fibromas have a firm, white, myxoid or trabeculated gross appearance and measure 5 cm or more in diameter.[22] The tumor is unencapsulated, blending imperceptibly with the adjacent myocardium. Foci of calcification may be observed within the center of the lesion.[7,51,76,96] Histologically, the tumor is composed of variable numbers of spindle-shaped fibroblastic cells surrounded by abundant collagen fibers. Mitoses are rarely noted. Central areas show foci of calcification, elastic fibers, and cystic change. Characteristically entrapped myocardial fibers are present within the tumor.[7,51,76,81,96] Immunohistochemical staining reveals diffuse vimentin reactivity and focal smooth muscle actin reactivity.[22] Ultrastructural studies also suggest a fibroblastic rather than a myofibroblastic, origin for the tumor.[22,96]

Spontaneous regression has not been observed in cardiac fibromas, and operative intervention is required for cure.[44] The mortality rate for this tumor in the perinatal period is high, as only 1 of the 11 newborns included in Table 16–5 survived.

MYXOMA

Myxoma is the leading primary tumor of the heart in adults, but it is the subject of only a few case reports in the newborn (Table 16–6).[17,19,20,33,56,76,84,92,100,105] One of the youngest patients recorded was a stillborn infant.[84] Most myxomas in the pediatric age group occur during adolescence.[30]

In the Armed Forces Institute of Pathology study of 130 patients with cardiac myxoma, 9% of the patients were 15 years old or younger.[76] The youngest patient was 4 years old. There were nine infants with cardiac tumors in The Hospital for Sick Children, Toronto series; two had myxomas. One myxoma occurred in an 11-day-old male infant with various congenital anomalies who presented with congestive heart failure and cyanosis. Another case involved a 4-month-old male infant with congestive heart failure and cardiomegaly.[20] The myxoma was located in the left ventricle in the former and in the right atrium in the latter. The patient of Simcha et al. was a 4-month-old male infant

Table 16–6. 7 Fetal and Newborn Cardiac Myxomas

Case No.	Age at Death	Location	Initial and Associated Findings	Reference
1	11 days	LV	Cardiomegaly, cyanosis, CHF	McCallister and Fenoglio[76]
2	4 days	RA	Cardiomegaly, cyanosis, murmur, double-chambered right ventricle	Russell et al.[92]
3	Alive	RA	Sepsis	Sharratt et al.[100]
4	10 hrs	RA	Hydramnios, hydrops, CHF, paradoxical systemic embolization	Dianzumba and Char[33]
5	3 mos	RA	Sudden death	Hals and Sandnes[56]
6	11 days	LV	Cyanosis, CHF, cardiomegaly, multiple congenital anomalies	Chan et al.[20]
7	2 mos	PV	Cardiomegaly, murmur, CHF, arrhythmia, pulmonary stenosis	Catton et al.[19]

CHF = congestive heart failure; LV = left ventricle; RA = right atrium; PV = pulmonary valve.

who presented with cyanosis, dyspnea, a systolic murmur, and cardiomegaly. Angiocardiography revealed a large tumor emanating from the right ventricle; this was confirmed at surgery and at necropsy.[105] Sudden death in a 3-month-old girl was attributed to a 4 × 2.5 cm atrial myxoma occluding the tricuspid valve orifice and apparently producing a "ball valve" phenomenon.[56] The female newborn with a right atrial myxoma reported by Russell et al. had, in addition, a double-chambered right ventricle;[92] cyanosis, a systolic murmur, and cardiomegaly were noted shortly after birth. Catton and associates described a myxoma involving the pulmonary valve that produced severe stenosis, cardiomegaly, and congestive heart failure in a 2-month-old infant.[19] In another patient, a large, calcified, right atrial myxoma obstructing the tricuspid valve was reponsible for multiple paradoxical emboli (see Table 16–6).[33]

The clinical findings associated with cardiac myxoma depend on the cardiac chamber involved by the neoplasm. Adult studies show that most myxomas are located in the left atrium (75%) and in the right atrium (18%).[76] According to Table 16–6, which lists seven newborns with myxomas who were selected from the literature, the right atrium appears to be the most common site in this age group (4 of 7), followed, in order of frequency, by the left ventricle (2 of 7) and pulmonary valve (1 of 7). When the tumor arises from the left side of the heart, it is responsible for signs and symptoms of mitral valve disease, particularly, mitral stenosis; when it originates from the right side, it is

manifested by tricuspid or pulmonary valvular disease and conduction disturbances.[7] In one newborn, tumor emboli developed secondary to a right atrial myxoma.[33]

Myxomas are characteristically polypoid, soft, gelatinous, friable, grayish-white, and mucoid, having a broad base of attachment.[7,76] The tumors contain foci of hemorrhage or thrombus formation. They vary in size from 0.5 cm in diameter in a newborn to 15 cm or more in the adult.[19,76,92] The tumor may occupy the atrium and protrude through the atrioventricular valve into the ventricular cavity, producing stenosis or insufficiency of the mitral valve and aortic stenosis. When myxomas arise from the right atrium (usually near the limbus of the fossa ovalis), they may extend through the tricuspid valve and cause pulmonary stenosis.[7,76]

Histologically, myxomas are composed of stellate and polygonal cells, which are sometimes multinucleated, with a scanty pink cytoplasm embedded in a loose, myxoid matrix that is rich in acid mucopolysaccharide.[7,17,33,76] The surrounding matrix contains elastic fibers and collagen. Endothelial cells often cover the surface, forming small vascular spaces or invaginations into the interior of the tumor; the cells stain positively for the vascular markers QBEnd and factor VIII/von Willebrand factor.[17,77] Small foci of extramedullary hematopoiesis and calcification may be present. The tumor extends in the underlying subendocardium and surrounds individual atrial myocardial fibers.[7]

Myxomas are thought to originate from the subendocardial multipotential mesenchymal

Table 16–7. 4 Fetal and Newborn Cardiac Hemangiomas

Case No.	Status	Diagnosis	Location	Initial Findings	Reference
1	Alive	Hemangioma	RA	Pericardial effusion, respiratory distress	Cartegena et al.[18]
2	Alive	Hemangioma	RA	Pericardial effusion	Burke et al.[16]
3	Alive	Hemangioma	RA	Pericardial effusion,* fetal hydrops, multiple cutaneous hemangiomata	Riggs et al.[91]
4	Alive	Hemangioma	RA	Pericardial effusion, respiratory distress	Ilbawi et al.[60]

*Tumor detected on antenatal sonography.
RA = right atrium.

cell, and thus have the potential for diverse differentiation along several cell lines.[77] Ultrastructural studies reveal that more than one cell type is involved.[42,77] Tumor cells may show some features of myofibroblasts and fibroblasts (prominent, rough endoplasmic reticulum), smooth muscle cells (basal lamina, microfilaments, dense bodies, pinocytotic vesicles), or endothelial cells (Weibel-Palade bodies). Other cells have an undifferentiated appearance, composed of only a few rudimentary organelles and filamentous structures.[42,77]

Complete surgical excision, if this can be accomplished, is the treatment of choice.[76] As would be anticipated, the tumor does recur if it is not completely removed. Most myxomas occurring in the newborn and infant have proved fatal.[19,20,33,56,92,105] In the series listed in Table 16–6, only 1 of 7 (14%) newborns with this neoplasm survived.

CARDIAC HEMANGIOMA

Cardiac hemangiomas are exceedingly rare, and are the subject of only a few case reports (Table 16–7).[16,18,60,76,91] Historically, most have been diagnosed at necropsy.[60] In older children and adults, hemangiomas may occur at any location in the heart, such as the ventricles, atrium, epicardial surface, and pericardium.[76] However, the right atrium appears to be the primary site involved in the newborn (see Table 16–7).[76] Pericardial effusion is the most common clinical manifestation and is present in practically all cases (see Table 16–7). In one case, an atrial hemangioma and fetal hydrops were detected by antenatal sonography at 32 weeks' gestation.[91] Multiple cutaneous hemangiomas were present in a neonate with a right atrial lesion.[91] Generally, cardiac hemangiomas in the infant are associated with a good prognosis.[16,18,60,76,91] The four newborns listed in Table 16–7 and the one described by McAllister and Fenoglio[76] were all cured by surgical resection.

CARDIAC RHABDOMYOSARCOMA

Primary rhabdomyosarcoma of the heart is described infrequently in the newborn[95] and in the infant.[37,70,76,79] This ultimately fatal condition may present clinically with congestive heart failure and/or an arrhythmia. If the tumor ex-

Table 16–8. Miscellaneous Cardiac Tumors of the Fetus and Newborn

Case No.	Age at Death	Diagnosis	Location	Initial Findings	Reference
1	3 wks	Rhabdomyosarcoma	RV	Cyanosis, murmur, respiratory distress	Schmaltz and Apitz[95]
2	4 mos	Rhabdomyosarcoma	RV	CHF, cardiomegaly	Engle and Glenn[37]
3	4 mos	Rhabdomyosarcoma	RV	Respiratory distress, cyanosis, pericardial effusion (tamponade)	Longino and Meeker[70]
4	2 days	Fibrolipoma	RA	Murmur, multiple congenital anomalies, trisomy 18*	Marx et al.[74]

*Tumor detected on antenatal sonography.
RV = right ventricle; RA = right atrium; CHF = congestive heart failure.

tends into the cardiac chamber, it produces obstruction and cardiac murmurs that change in intensity.[76] The right ventricle is a favored site for cardiac rhabdomyosarcomas in the young (Table 16–8). The clinical picture may resemble that of pulmonary or tricuspid stenosis associated with a right-to-left shunt at the atrial level; this was the initial impression in a case involving a newborn with primary right ventricular rhabdomyosarcoma.[95] Engle and Glenn described a 4-month-old male infant who presented with a sudden onset of heart failure.[37] Exploratory thoracotomy revealed a rhabdomyosarcoma, involving primarily the right ventricle, which had invaded the left ventricle and surrounded the left coronary artery, obstructing it. Extensive metastases were noted in the lungs, thymus, and regional lymph nodes.

ONCOCYTIC CARDIOMYOPATHY

Myocardial hamartomas, which are morphologically distinct from rhabdomyomas, are found in infants and young children who present with refractory tachyarrhythmias or sudden death.[13,64] This lesion of unknown etiology has been given a variety of names, including histiocytoid cardiomyopathy, Purkinje cell tumor, oncocytic cardiomyopathy, focal lipid cardiomyopathy, and idiopathic infantile cardiomyopathy.[13,64] The condition is associated with extracardiac anomalies, particularly involving the eye, brain, and skin. Microphthalmia with linear skin defects (''MLS'') is a recently recognized syndrome consisting of congenital linear skin defects and ocular abnormalities in female patients who are monosomic for Xp22.[13] Not every child with the syndrome has the cardiac hamartoma. Bird et al. described 49 patients with MLS and oncocytic cardiomyopathy who were younger than 28 months of age; 15 of them were symptomatic before 3 months of age, and 5 showed symptoms on onset within the first week of life.[13]

On histologic examination, oncocytic cardiomyopathy is characterized by collections of large, round to polygonal cells within the myocardium that are composed of a coarsely granular or foamy, pale cytoplasm. If large enough, yellow-tan nodules may be observed on gross examination of the myocardium. Ultrastructurally, the granules correspond to numerous mitochondria, some containing inclusions (hence the name ''oncocytic''). The exact cell of origin—that is, whether it is a myocyte or a Pur-

kinje cell—has not been settled. Some patients with this lesion have been cured with electrophysiologic mapping and surgical excision.[64]

MISCELLANEOUS CONDITIONS

Pericardial hemangiopericytoma was reported in a newborn by Lazarus et al.[68] Fibrosarcoma and rhabdoid primary tumors in the heart have been recorded in infants.[76,106] Pericardial effusion was the initial sign in a 6-month-old female infant with a rhabdoid tumor of the left ventricle extending into the pericardial space.[106] Despite chemotherapy, the infant died 3 months after diagnosis.

Glandular inclusions, lined by ciliated columnar epithelium and situated within the fetal myocardium of the left ventricle, have been mentioned occasionally.[4] They appear to be endodermal heterotopias of congenital origin. The glandular structures are reactive with epithelial membrane and carcinoembryonic antigens and do not communicate with the pericardium.

REFERENCES

1. Agozzino L, Vosa C, Arciprete P, et al. Intrapericardial teratoma in the newborn. Int J Cardiol 1984;5:21.
2. Aldousany AW, Joyner JC, Price RA, et al. Diagnosis and treatment of intrapericardial teratoma. Pediatr Cardiol 1987;8:51.
3. Alkalay AL, Ferry DA, Lin B, et al. Spontaneous regression of cardiac rhabdomyoma in tuberous sclerosis. Clin Pediatr 1987;26:532.
4. Aqel NM, Shousha S. Glandular inclusions in the fetal myocardium. Histopathology 1994;24:85.
5. Arciniegas E, Hakimi M, Farooke QZ, et al. Intrapericardial teratoma in infancy. J Thorac Cardiovasc Surg 1980;79:306.
6. Arciniegas E, Hakimi M, Farooke QZ, et al. Primary cardiac tumors in children. J Thorac Cardiovasc Surg 1980;79:582.
7. Arey JB. Cardiovascular Pathology in Infants and Children, p 372. Philadelphia: WB Saunders, 1984.
8. Aryanpur I, Nazarian I, Razmara M, et al. Calcified right ventricular fibroma causing outflow obstruction. Am J Dis Child 1976;130:1265.
9. Back LM, Brown AS, Barot LR. Congenital cardiac tumors in association with orofacial clefts. Ann Plastic Surg 1988;20:558.
10. Balian AA, Hogan TF. Cardiac tumors. *In* Moller JH, Neal WA (eds): Fetal, Neonatal and Infant Cardiac Disease, p 869. Norwalk: Appleton & Lange, 1990.
11. Bass JL, Breningstall GN, Swaiman KF. Electrocardiograph incidence of cardiac rhabdomyoma in tuberous sclerosis. Am J Cardiol 1985;55:1379.
12. Bini RM, Westaby S, Bargeron LM Jr, et al. Investiga-

tion and management of primary cardiac tumors in infants and children. J Am Coll Cardiol 1983;2:351.

13. Bird LM, Krous HF, Eichenfield LF, et al. Female infant with oncocytic cardiomyopathy and microphthalmia with linear skin defects (MLS): A clue to the pathogenesis of oncocytic cardiomyopathy? Am J Med Genet 1994;53:141.

14. Birnbaum SE, McGahan JP, Janos GG, et al. Fetal tachycardia and intramyocardial tumors. J Am Coll Cardiol 1985;6:1358.

15. Bjorkhem G, Lundstrom N-R, Lingman G. Intracardiac rhabdomyomas in neonates: Report of three cases. Acta Paediatr 1992;81:712.

16. Burke A, Johns JP, Virmani R. Hemangiomas of the heart. A clinicopathologic study of ten cases. Am J Cardiovasc Pathol 1990;3:283.

17. Burke AP, Virmani R. Cardiac myxoma. A clinicopathologic study. Am J Clin Pathol 1993;100:671.

18. Cartagena AM, Levin TL, Issenberg H, et al. Pericardial effusion and cardiac hemangioma in the neonate. Pediatr Radiol 1993;23:384.

19. Catton RW, Guntheroth WG, Reichenbach DD. A myxoma of the pulmonary valve causing severe stenosis in infancy. Am Heart J 1963;66:248, 1963.

20. Chan HSL, Sonley MJ, Moes CAF, et al. Primary and secondary tumors of childhood involving the heart, pericardium and great vessels: A report of 75 cases and review of the literature. Cancer 1985;56:825.

21. Chitayat D, McGillivray BC, Diamant S, et al. Role of prenatal detection of cardiac tumours in the diagnosis of tuberous sclerosis—Report of two cases. Prenatal Diagn 1988;8:577.

22. Coffin CM. Case 1. Congenital cardiac fibroma associated with Gorlin syndrome. Pediatr Pathol 1992;12:255.

23. Coffin CM, Dehner LP. Congenital tumors. *In* Stocker JT, Dehner LP (eds): Pediatric Pathology, Vol 1, p 325. Philadelphia: JB Lippincott, 1992.

24. Corno A, De Simone G, Catena G, et al. Cardiac rhabdomyoma: Surgical treatment in the neonate. J Thorac Cardiovasc Surg 1984;87:725.

25. Costas C, Williams RL, Fortune RL. Intracardiac teratoma in an infant. Pediatr Cardiol 1986;7:179.

26. Cyr DR, Guntheroth WG, Nyberg DA, et al. Prenatal diagnosis of an intrapericardial teratoma. A cause for nonimmune hydrops. J Ultrasound Med 1988;7:87.

27. Davy T, Helmer F, Horcher E, et al. Intrapericardial teratoma. Pediatr Cardiol 1982;3:243.

28. Deenadayalu RP, Tuuri D, Dewall RA, et al. Intrapericardial teratoma and brochogenic cyst. Review of the literature and report of successful surgery in an infant with intrapericardial teratoma. J Thorac Cardiovasc Surg 1974;67:945.

29. De Geeter B, Kretz JG, Nisand I, et al. Intrapericardial teratoma in a newborn infant: Use of fetal echocardiography. Ann Thorac Surg 1983;35:664.

30. Dehner LP: Pediatric Surgical Pathology, 2nd ed. Baltimore: Williams & Wilkins, 1987.

31. Dein JR, Frist WH, Stinson EB, et al. Primary cardiac neoplasms. J Thorac Cardiovasc Surg 1987;93:502.

32. DeVore GR, Hakim S, Kleinman CS, et al. The in utero diagnosis of an interventricular septal cardiac rhabdomyoma by means of real-time–directed, M-mode echocardiography. Am J Obst Gynecol 1982;143:97.

33. Dianzumba SB, Char G. Large calcified right atrial myxoma in a newborn. Rare cause of neonatal death. Br Heart J 1982;48:177.

34. DiLollo L, Castellani R, Maioran A. Ultrasonic patterns of a cardiac rhabdomyoma detected in utero. J Perinatal Med 1984;12:339.

35. Duncan WJ. Left ventricular rhabdomyoma. Pediatr Control 1983;4:170.

36. Engle MA, Ebert PA, Redo SF. Recurrent ventricular tachycardia due to resectable cardiac tumor. Circulation 1974;50:1052.

37. Engle MA, Glenn F. Primary tumor of the heart in infancy: Case report and review of the subject. Pediatrics 1955;15:562.

38. Farooki ZQ, Henry JG, Arciniegas E, et al. Ultrasonic pattern of ventricular rhabdomyoma in two infants. Am J Cardiol 1974;34:842.

39. Farooki ZQ, Ross RD, Paridon SM, et al. Spontaneous regression of cardiac rhabdomyomas. Am J Cardiol 1989;64:416.

40. Fenoglio JJ Jr, Diana DJ, Bowen TE, et al. Ultrastructure of a cardiac rhabdomyoma. Hum Pathol 1977;8:700.

41. Fenoglio JJ JR, McAllister HA, Ferrens VJ. Cardiac rhabdomyoma: A clinicopathologic and electron microscopic study. Am J Cardiol 1976;38:241.

42. Ferrans VJ, Roberts WC. Structural features of cardiac myxomas: Histology, histochemistry, and electron microscopy. Hum Pathol 1973;4:11.

43. Fischer DJ, Beerman LB, Park SC, et al. Diagnosis of intracardiac rhabdomyoma by two-dimensional echocardiography. Am J Cardiol 1984;53:978.

44. Freedom RM, Benson LN. Cardiac neoplasms. *In* Freedom RM, Benson LN, Smallhorn JF (eds): Neonatal Heart Disease, p 723. London: Springer-Verlag, 1992.

45. Fyke FE, Seward JB, Edwards WD, et al. Primary cardiac tumors: Experience with 30 consecutive patients since the introduction of two dimensional echocardiography. J Am Coll Cardiol 1985;5:1465.

46. Fyler DC. Report of the New England Regional Infant Cardiac Program. Pediatrics 1980;65(Suppl):376.

47. Geha AS, Wiedman WH, Soule EH, et al. Intramural ventricular cardiac fibroma. Circulation 1967;36:427.

48. Geva T, Santini F, Pear W, et al. Cardiac rhabdomyoma. Rare cause of fetal death. Chest 1991;99:139.

49. Giacoia GP. Fetal rhabdomyoma: A prenatal echocardiographic marker of tuberous sclerosis. Am J Perinatol 1992;9:111.

50. Golding R, Reed G. Rhabdomyoma of the heart. Two unusual clinical presentations. N Engl J Med 1967;276:597.

51. Gonzalez-Crussi F, Eberts TJ, Mirkin DL. Congenital fibrous hamartoma of the heart. Arch Pathol Lab Med 1978;102:491.

52. Gorlin RJ. Nevoid-basal cell carcinoma syndrome. Medicine 1987;66:98.

53. Gresser CD, Shime J, Rakowski H, et al. Fetal cardiac tumor: A prenatal echocardiographic marker for tuberous sclerosis. Am J Obstet Gynecol 1987;156:689.

54. Groves AMM, Fagg NLK, Cook AC, et al. Cardiac tumours in intrauterine life. Arch Dis Child 1992;67:1189.

55. Guereta LG, Burgueros M, Elorza MD, et al. Cardiac rhabdomyoma presenting as fetal hydrops. Pediatr Cardiol 1986;7:171.

56. Hals J, Ek J, Sandnes K. Cardiac myxoma as the cause of death in an infant. Acta Paediatr Scand 1990;79:999.

57. Harding CO, Pagon RA. Incidence of tuberous sclero-

sis in patients with cardiac rhabdomyomas. Am J Med Genet 1990;37:443.

58. Harrison MR, Goldbus MS, Phili RA. The Unborn Patient: Prenatal Diagnosis and Treatment. Orlando, FL: Grune & Stratton, 1984.

59. Houser S, Forbes N, Stewart S, et al. Rhabdomyoma of the heart: A diagnostic and therapeutic challenge. Ann Thorac Surg 1980;29:373.

60. Ilbawi M, DeLeon S, Riggs T. Primary vascular tumors of the heart in infancy. Report of a case with successful surgical management. Chest 1982;81:511.

61. Iliff PJ, Nicholls JM, Keeling JW, et al. Non-immunologic hydrops fetalis: A review of 27 cases. Arch Dis Child 1983;58:979.

62. Isaacs H Jr. Tumors of the Newborn and Infant. St. Louis: Mosby–Year Book, 1991.

63. Kauffman SL, Stout AP. Congenital mesenchymal tumors. Cancer 1965;18:460.

64. Kearney DL, Titus JL, Hawkins EP, et al. Pathologic features of myocardial hamartomas causing childhood tachyarrhythmias. Circulation 1987;75:705.

65. Kleinman CS, Donnerstein RL, DeVore GR, et al. Fetal electrocardiography for evaluation of in utero congestive heart failure. A technique for study of nonimmune fetal hydrops. N Engl J Med 1982;306:568.

66. Kuehl KS, Perry LW, Chandra R, et al. Left ventricular rhabdomyoma: A rare cause of subaortic stenosis in the newborn infant. Pediatrics 1970;46:464.

67. Lababidi Z, Wu JR, Walls J, et al. Neonatal cyanosis caused by cardiac rhabdomyomas. Am Heart J 1984; 108:624.

68. Lazarus KH, D'Orsogna DE, Bloom KR, et al. Primary pericardial sarcoma in a neonate. Am J Pediatr Hematol Oncol 1989;11:343.

69. Lintermans JP, Shoevaertds JC, Fiasse L, et al. Intrapericardial teratoma. A curable cause of cardiac tamponade in infancy. Clin Pediatr 1973;12:316.

70. Longino LA, Meeker IA Jr. Primary cardiac tumors in infancy. J Pediatr 1953;43:724.

71. Lubin BH, Friedman S, Miller WW. Intrapericardial teratoma associated with pericardial effusion: An acute surgical problem in infancy. J Pediatr Surg 1967;2:336.

72. Mair DD, Titus JL, Davis GD. Cardiac rhabdomyoma simulating mitral atresia. Chest 1977;71:102.

73. Marin-Garcia J, Fitch CW, Shenenfelt RE. Primary right ventricular tumor (fibroma) simulating cyanotic heart disease in a newborn. J Am Coll Cardiol 1984; 3:868.

74. Marx GR, Bierman FZ, Matthews E, et al. Two-dimensional echocardiographic diagnosis of intracardiac masses in infancy. J Am Coll Cardiol 1984;3:827.

75. McAllister HA Jr. Primary tumors of the cyst and the heart and pericardium. Curr Probl Cardiol 1979;4:2.

76. McAllister HA Jr, Fenoglio JJ Jr. Tumors of the Cardiovascular System, Fascicle 15, Second series. Washington, DC: Armed Forces Institute of Pathology, 1978.

77. McComb RD. Heterogeneous expression of factor VIII/von Willebrand factor by cardiac myxoma cells. Am J Surg Pathol 1984;8:539.

78. McCue CM, Henningar GR, Davis E, et al. Congenital subaortic stenosis caused by a fibroma of the left ventricle. Pediatrics 1955;16:372.

79. Nadas AS, Ellison RC. Cardiac tumors in infancy. Am J Cardiol 1968;21:363.

80. Neal WA, Knight L, Bleiden LC, et al. Clinical pathologic conference. Am Heart J 1975;89:514.

81. Patterson K, Donnelly WH, Dehner LP. The cardiovascular system. In Stocker JT, Dehner LP (eds): Pediatric Pathology, Vol 1, p 575. Philadelphia: JB Lippincott, 1992.

82. Potter EL, Craig JM. Pathology of the Fetus and Infant, 3rd ed, p 177. Chicago: Year Book Medical Publishers, 1975.

83. Rasmussen SL, Hwang WS, Harder J, et al. Intrapericardial teratoma. Ultrasonic and pathological features. J Ultrasound Med 1987;6:159.

84. Reddy DJ, Rao TS, Venkiaih KR, et al. Congenital myxoma of the heart. Indian J Pediatr 1956;23:210.

85. Reddy JK, Shinke RN, Chang CHJ, et al. Beckwith-Wiedemann syndrome, Wilms' tumor, cardiac hamartoma, persistent visceromegaly, and glomeruloneogenesis in a 2-year-old boy. Arch Pathol 1972;94: 523.

86. Reece EA. Fetal neoplasm. In Reece EA, Hobbins JC, Mahoney MJ, Petrie RH (eds): Medicine of the Fetus and Mother, p 617. Philadelphia: JB Lippincott, 1992.

87. Reece IJ, Cooley DA, Frazier OH, et al. Cardiac tumors: Clinical spectrum and prognosis of lesions other than classical benign myxoma in 20 patients. J Thorac Cardiovasc Surg 1984;88:439.

88. Reece IJ, Houston AB, Pollock JCS. Interventricular fibroma: Echocardiographic diagnosis and successful surgical removal in infancy. Br Heart J 1983;50:590.

89. Rees AH, Elbl FE, Minhas KV, et al. Echocardiographic evidence of left ventricular tumor in a neonate. Chest 1978;73:433.

90. Reynolds JL, Donahue JK, Pearce CW. Intrapericardial teratoma: A cause of acute pericardial effusion in infancy. Pediatrics 1969;43:71.

91. Riggs T, Sholl JS, Ilbawi M, et al. Neonatal diagnosis of pericardial tumor with successful surgical repair. Pediatr Cardiol 5:23, 1984.

91a. Rosenberg HS, Stenback WA, Spjut HJ. The fibromatoses of infancy and childhood. In Rosenberg HS, Bolande RP (eds): Perspectives in Pediatric Pathology, Vol 4, p 269. Chicago: Year Book Medical Publishers, 1978.

92. Russell GA, Dhasmana JP, Berry PJ, et al. Coexistent cardiac tumors and malformations of the heart. Int J Cardiol 1989;22:89.

93. Schaffer RM, Cabbad M, Minkoff H, et al. Sonographic diagnosis of fetal cardiac rhabdomyoma. J Ultrasound Med 1986;5:531.

94. Schmaltz AA, Apitz J. Primary heart tumors in infancy and childhood. Cardiology 1981;67:12.

95. Schmaltz AA, Apitz J. Primary rhabdomyosarcoma of the heart. Pediatr Cardiol 1982;2:73.

96. Schwartz J, Saldivar V, Tio F, et al. Interventricular fibroma and cystic renal dysplasia in a newborn. Pediatr Pathol 1984;2:187.

97. Selzer A, Sakai FJ, Popper RW. Protean clinical manifestations of primary tumors of the heart. Am J Med 1972;52:9.

98. Shaher RM, Farina M, Alley R, et al. Congenital subaortic stenosis in infancy caused by rhabdomyoma of the left ventricle. J Thorac Cardiovasc Surg 1972;63: 157.

99. Shaher RM, Mintzer J, Farina M, et al. Clinical presentation of rhabdomyoma of the heart in infancy and childhood. Am J Cardiol 1972;30:95.

100. Sharratt GP, Lacson AG, Cornel G, et al. Echocardiography of intracardiac filling defects in infants and children. Pediatr Cardiol 1986;7:189.

101. Shiraishi H, Yanagisawa M, Kuramatsu T, et al. Car-

diac tumour in a neonate with tuberous sclerosis: Echocardiographic demonstration and magnetic resonance imaging. Eur J Pediatr 1988;148:50.

102. Sholler GF, Hawker RE, Nunn GR, et al. Primary left ventricular rhabdomyosarcoma in a child: Noninvasive assessment and successful resection of a rare tumor. J Thorac Cardiovasc Surg 1987;93:465.

103. Shrivastava S, Jacks JJ, White RS, et al. Diffuse rhabdomyomatosis of the heart. Arch Pathol Lab Med 1977; 101:78.

104. Silverman JF, Kay S, McCue CM, et al. Rhabdomyoma of the heart. Ultrastructural study of three cases. Lab Invest 1976;35:596.

105. Simcha A, Wells BG, Tynan MJ, et al. Primary cardiac tumors in childhood. Arch Dis Child 1971;46:508.

106. Small EJ, Gordon GJ, Dahms BB. Malignant rhabdoid tumor of the heart in an infant. Cancer 1985;55:2850.

107. Smythe JF, Dyck JD, Smallhorn JF, et al. Natural history of cardiac rhabdomyoma in infancy and childhood. Am J Cardiol 1990;66:1247.

108. Spooner EW, Farina MA, Shaher RM, et al. Left ventricular rhabdomyoma causing subaortic stenosis—the two-dimensional echocardiographic appearance. Pediatr Cardiol 1982;2:67.

109. Sterns LP, Eliot RS, Varco RL, et al. Intracavitary cardiac neoplasms. Br Heart J 1966;28:75.

110. Sumner TE, Crowe JE, Klein A, et al. Intrapericardial teratoma in infancy. Pediatr Radiol 1980;10:51.

111. Van der Hauwaert LG. Cardiac tumors in infancy and childhood. Br Heart J 1971;33:125.

112. Van der Hauwaert LG, Corbeel L, Maldague P. Fibroma of the right ventricle producing severe tricuspid stenosis. Circulation 1965;32:451.

113. Vidaillet HJ. Cardiac tumors associated with hereditary syndromes. Am J Cardiol 1988;61:1355.

114. Webb DW, Thomas RD, Osborne JP. Cardiac rhabdomyomas and their association with tuberous sclerosis. Arch Dis Child 1993;68:367.

115. Weber HS, Kleinman CS, Hellenbrand WE, et al. Development of a benign intrapericardial tumor between 20 and 40 weeks of gestation. Pediatr Cardiol 1988;9:153.

116. Williams GEG. Teratoma of the heart. J Pathol Bacteriol 1961;82:281.

117. Williams WG, Trusler GA, Fowler RS, et al. Left ventricular myocardial fibroma: A case report and review of cardiac tumors in children. J Pediatr Surg 1972;7: 324.

118. Yabek SM, Isabel-Jones J, Gyepes MT, et al. Cardiac fibroma in a neonate presenting with severe congestive heart failure. J Pediatr 1977;91:310.

119. Zerella JT, Halpe DCE. Intrapericardial teratoma—Neonatal cardiorespiratory distress amenable to surgery. J Pediatr Surg 1980;15:961.

TUMORS OF THE LUNG

17

Although primary lung tumors are unusual in the newborn, benign and malignant neoplasms have been described in this age group.[17,23,27,29,30,47,97] Hemangioma, myofibromatosis, bronchopulmonary fibrosarcoma, and pulmonary blastoma are examples (Tables 17–1 and 17–2).[1,4,23,40,46,58,97,103] Metastatic neoplasms occur more often than do primary ones. Non-neoplastic diseases of the lung are far more prevalent than neoplastic lesions and may, in some instances, mimic a tumor as, for example, with an abscess, organizing bacterial pneumonia, or the congenital anomalies bronchogenic cyst and adenomatoid malformation (see Figs. 17–2 and 17–3).[29,60,76,85]

EMBRYOLOGY

The lower respiratory tract develops from a midline laryngotracheal groove in the floor of the primitive pharynx during the fourth week of gestation.[78] By the fifth week, an outgrowth arises from the caudal end of this groove, forming the laryngotracheal or respiratory diverticulum, which becomes separated from the foregut by a condensation of mesenchyme, the tracheoesophageal septum. Following this event, the laryngotracheal tube and esophagus are formed. The epithelium of the lower respiratory tract, including that of the bronchi and alveoli, and the tracheobronchial glands develop from the endoderm of the laryngotracheal tube. The surrounding mesenchyme is the source of the connective tissue, cartilage, muscle, and blood and lymphatic vessels of the respiratory tract.[78]

During the fourth week, the distal end of the laryngotracheal tube forms a lung bud that divides into two bronchial buds. The two bronchial buds become the secondary (stem) bronchi and precede the formation of the two lobes of the left lung and the three lobes of the right lung. Subsequently, each bronchial bud undergoes multiple, dichotomous branchings, invading the adjacent splanchnic mesenchyme of the developing lung, until 17 successive bronchial branchings are completed by the 17th week. Development of the lung continues after birth until 24 or more orders of branches are attained.[78]

Fetal lung development occurs in several stages. The earliest—the pseudoglandular stage, which lasts 5 to 17 weeks—is characterized by the formation of the bronchi and terminal bronchioles. The glycogen-rich, epithelial-lined branching channels are surrounded by abundant, pale-staining, loose-appearing mesenchyme (Fig. 17–1). The respiratory bronchioles and alveolar ducts develop and the lung becomes highly vascular during the canalicular period (16 to 25 weeks). During the terminal sac stage (24 weeks to birth), the terminal sacs (alveoli) bud off the alveolar ducts. The cuboidal epithelium of the alveoli begins to differentiate into the squamous alveolar type I and type II epithelial lining cells. The alveolar stage begins in the late fetal period after the 36th week and extends into mid-childhood as the lungs mature.[78]

BENIGN TUMORS AND TUMOR-LIKE CONDITIONS

Inflammatory Pseudotumor

Because so many different names have been applied to this lesion (e.g., plasma cell gran-

Table 17–1. Tumors and Tumor-Like Conditions of the Lung in the Fetus and Newborn

---

Inflammatory pseudotumor
Cystic mesenchymal hamartoma*
Rhabdomyomatous dysplasia (rhabdomyomatosis)
Cystic adenomatoid malformation
Congenital pulmonary lymphangiectasis
Lymphangioma
Hemangioma
Myofibromatosis (fibromatosis)
Bronchopulmonary myofibrosarcoma
Pleuropulmonary blastoma
Primitive neuroectodermal tumor (Askin tumor)*
Langerhans cell histiocytosis (Letterer-Siwe disease)
Tumors metastatic to the lung
    Leukemia
    Hepatoblastoma
    Rhabdomyosarcoma
    Neuroblastoma
    Wilms' tumor
    Rhabdoid tumor
    Yolk sac tumor

---

*Usually occurs in older children.

uloma, "round pneumonia" [nonspecific inflammatory reactions], inflammatory myofibroblastic tumor, and sclerosing hemangioma), "inflammatory pseudotumor" is a rather confusing entity.[30,60,97] Nevertheless, it is the leading tumor or tumor-like condition of the lung in children, accounting for more than 80% of cases.[5,9,29,47,77,82,97] Inflammatory pseudotumor rarely occurs in infants. Of 34 cases reviewed at the Armed Forces Institute of Pathology, only 1 (3%) was noted in a child younger than 1 year of age,[97] likewise, only 1 of 40 patients included in Bahadori and Liebow's review was an infant.[5] However, the condition has been described in the newborn (Fig. 17–2). It should be kept in mind that this benign condition, which most likely represents a reactive inflammatory process, can mimic a malignant tumor.[77] Inflammatory pseudotumor is characterized by slow growth, instances of spontaneous resolution, and a favorable prognosis. It is conceivable that many such lesions, some of which are discovered incidentally on imaging studies, represent organizing pneumonias and simply are not operated upon. Inflammatory pseudotumor can also occur in extrapulmonary sites, such as the soft tissues, orbit, heart, and spleen.[24,29,83,94,97,108] Again, this is a rare event in the newborn.

The gross appearance of inflammatory pseudotumor is a firm, circumscribed, grayish-white to yellow nodule that is usually situated in the periphery of the lung. Three different histologic patterns are described: organizing pneumonia, fibrous histiocytoma, and lymphoplasmacytic pattern.[72,97] Immunohistochemical and ultrastructural studies show that the spindle cells are fibroblasts and myofibroblasts; hence, the ominous term myofibroblastic tumor has been applied to some.[14]

Essentially all pediatric inflammatory pseudotumors have been resected surgically without evidence of recurrence or metastases.[82] Because of their benign behavior, the treatment of choice, if surgery is required to establish the diagnosis, is the most minimal lung resection possible.[9,82]

Congenital Pulmonary Cystic Diseases

Congenital cystic diseases of the lung, cystic mesenchymal hamartoma, and cystic adenomatoid malformation may mimic a neoplasm clinically, and occasionally, they are a source of malignancy within the cyst(s).[8,23,38,50,66,70,93,104]

Congenital cystic adenomatoid malformation is an uncommon developmental anomaly involving the entire lung or a portion of it.[76,98] Bronchial absence or atresia, according to Moerman et al., is believed to play a role in its etiology.[76] According to Langston, a segmental obstructive lesion can produce this anomaly, particularly type II (Claire Langston, MD, personal communication). The lesion presents clinically in a stillborn or newborn with hydrops fetalis or in a neonate with progressive respiratory distress secondary to an expanding mass in one hemithorax.[60,76,98] The malformation is detected antenatally by sonography.[60,74,90]

On the basis of gross and histologic findings, cystic adenomatoid malformation is divided into three main types, designated as types I, II, and III. Type I contains one or more large cysts with fibrous septa lined by columnar or cuboidal epithelial cells. Type II consists of many smaller cysts lined by ciliated columnar epithelial cells, and resembles ectatic terminal bronchioles (Fig. 17–3). Skeletal muscle may be found in the septa or adjacent to the cysts. The solid type III is composed of a firm, bulky mass that occupies much of a lung lobe. Histologically, type III is characterized by dilated, irregularly branching structures resembling bronchioles and separated by alveolar-like spaces lined by low cuboidal epithelium.[60,76,98] In particular, the solid type (type III) can mimic a tumor on

Table 17–2. 17 Newborn Tumors and Tumor-Like Conditions of the Lung*

Case No.	Sex	Histologic Diagnosis	Presenting Findings	Status	Reference
1	M	Lymphangioma	Respiratory distress	L	Milovic and Oluic[75]
2	M	Lymphangioma	Respiratory distress	L	Zimmerman and Habenicht[109]
3	M	Cavernous hemangioma	Signs of upper respiratory infection; RLL mass on chest x-ray films	L	Galliani et al.[40]
4	M	Papillomatosis	Hoarseness, progressive respiratory distress	L	Kramer et al.[65]
5	F	Inflammatory pseudotumor "plasma cell granuloma"	Mass, LUL	L	Walker (see Fig. 17–2)
6	M	Pulmonary blastoma†	Respiratory distress	D	Ashworth[4]
7	F	Pulmonary blastoma	Oligohydramnios, dyspnea, cyanosis, pneumothorax	L	Jetley et al.[56]
8	F	Pulmonary blastoma	Polyhydramnios, respiratory distress	D	Cappuccino et al.[18]
9	M	Bronchopulmonary fibrosarcoma	Respiratory distress, pleural effusions	L	Pettinato et al.[84]
10	M	Bronchopulmonary fibrosarcoma	Respiratory distress, pleural effusions	L	Pettinato et al.[84]
11	M	Bronchopulmonary fibrosarcoma [myofibroblastic tumor]‡	Hydrops, hydramnios, respiratory distress	D	McGinnis et al.[73]
12	F	Bronchopulmonary fibrosarcoma [mesenchymal malformation]‡	Hydramnios, cyanosis respiratory distress	D	Warren et al.[103]
13	M	Bronchopulmonary fibrosarcoma [leiomyosarcoma]‡	Hydrops, hydramnios, respiratory distress	L	Jimenez et al.[58]
14	M	Bronchopulmonary fibrosarcoma [leiomyosarcoma]‡	?Respiratory distress	D	Guccion and Rosen[43]
15	F	Bronchopulmonary fibrosarcoma [mesenchymal tumour]‡	Hydrops, respiratory distress	D	Haller et al.[45]
16	F	Bronchopulmonary fibrosarcoma [hamartoma]‡	Respiratory distress	D	Jones[59]
17	M	Bronchopulmonary fibrosarcoma [neonatal fibrosarcoma]‡	Respiratory distress	L	Robb[87]

*Selected from the literature.
†Diagnosed at necropsy.
‡The diagnosis within the brackets is the original histologic diagnosis cited in the publication.
RLL = right lower lobe of lung; LUL = left upper lobe; L = living; D = dead.

imaging studies, as well as on gross and microscopic examination.

Rhabdomyosarcoma and pulmonary blastoma are two examples of malignant lesions developing from lung cysts.[23,38,50,66,70,100,104] Although the cysts may be evident at birth, the neoplasms are not discovered until after the first year of life.

Vascular Conditions

Vascular lesions seldom occur in the lungs of infants and newborns. Whether they represent true neoplasms, hamartomas, or congenital malformations has been the subject of some debate.[30] The author believes that most of these lesions represent malformations and hamartomas.

Hemangiomas of the lung are uncommon.[40] Some occur together with multiple lesions in other organs (e.g., the skin, liver, central nervous system) in an invariably fatal syndrome termed diffuse neonatal hemangiomatosis.[16,49,107] Some lesions that are reported as hemangiomas in infants and children are congenital malformations of the pulmonary vasculature and have been variously called pulmonary arteriovenous fistula or aneurysms, congenital arteriovenous varix, and pulmonary angiomatosis.[27]

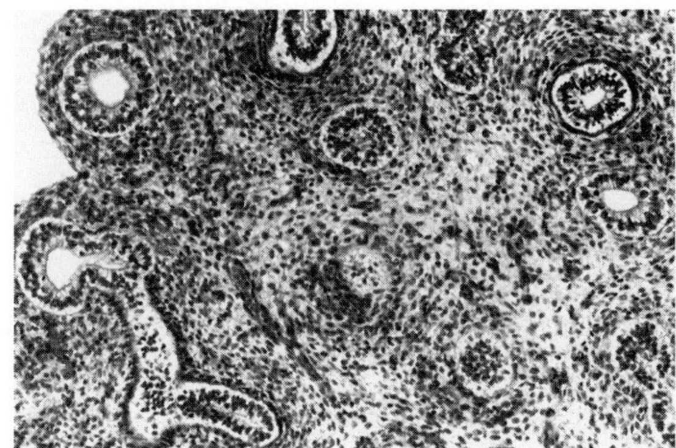

Figure 17–1. Developing lung. Branches of the pulmonary tree are uniformly lined by tall columnar cells and widely separated by primitive mesenchyme (hematoxylin-eosin, ×120). This specimen was obtained from a fetus of an estimated 10 to 12 weeks' gestation.

Patients with these conditions may have associated vascular malformations in other organs, such as in the mucous membranes, skin, and brain, forming part of a more generalized syndrome of hereditary telangiectasia, such as the Rendu-Osler-Weber disease. Familial occurrence has been documented.[27]

Vascular lesions tend to occur in the periphery of the lung or in the subpleural space. They are situated more often in the lower lobes, occurring as localized lesions that may be single, multiple, diffuse, or bilateral.[27,102] Multiple hemangiomas (hemangiomatosis) involving the pleura are a rare cause of bloody pleural effusion in the newborn. When congestive heart failure and consumptive coagulopathy accompany this disorder, the prognosis is generally poor.[53]

Like soft tissue hemangiomas, these hemangiomas are composed of either capillary or cavernous components, or both. They have prominent "feeding" arterial and venous blood vessels, which sometimes form large arteriovenous malformations. Capillary and cavernous hemangiomas are lined by regular plump or flattened, endothelial cells, respectively (see Chapter 4 "Soft Tissue Tumors").

Lymphangioma

Lymphangioma may occur as a localized or as a diffuse congenital malformation (lymphangiomatosis) of the lung.[30] Cervical cystic lymphangiomas (hygromas) are common, but primary isolated intrathoracic lesions are exceedingly rare. Two newborns with pulmonary lymphangiomas who presented with respiratory distress—one a 2-day-old-male infant and another a 2-week-old infant—were described by Milovic and Oluic[75] and by Zimmermann and Habenicht,[109] respectively. Congenital diaphragmatic hernia and lung cyst were considered in the imaging differential diagnosis. In this disease, the involved lung is partially or totally replaced by a mass of thin-walled, dilated, vascular channels of variable size filled with pink proteinaceous fluid and lined by rows of regular endothelial cells.[30,75]

Congenital Pulmonary Lymphangiectasis

Pulmonary lymphangiectasis is a congenital malformation characterized by cystic dilatation of the lymphatics. In this disease, the septal and subpleural lymphatic channels are primarily in-

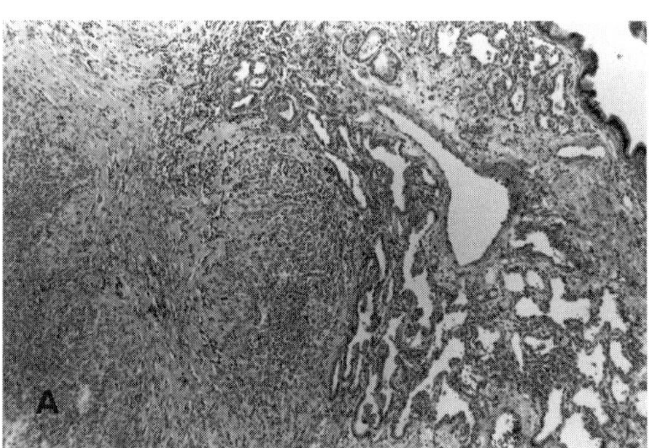

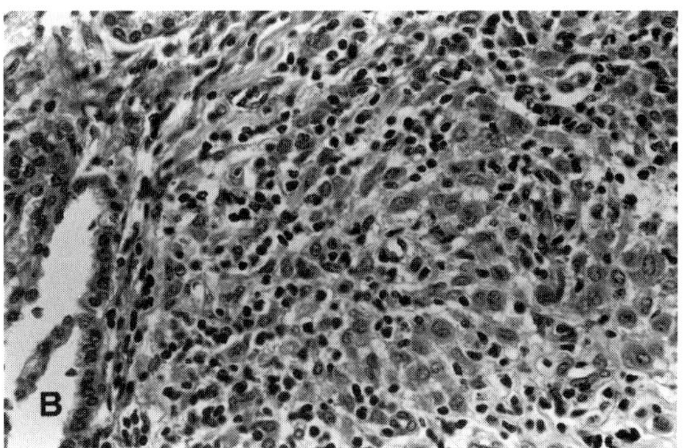

Figure 17–2. Inflammatory pseudotumor. *A*, The microscopic appearance of a 3.5 × 2.5 cm, subpleural mass from the left upper lung lobe, which was removed from a 1-week-old female infant. Within the lung, there is an inflammatory cell infiltrate accompanied by fibrosis (hematoxylin-eosin, ×48). *B*, The infiltrate is composed mostly of lymphocytes and histiocytes with a rare plasma cell (hematoxylin-eosin, ×300). (Courtesy of Frederick Walker, MD, Department of Pathology, Kaiser Permanente, San Diego, CA.)

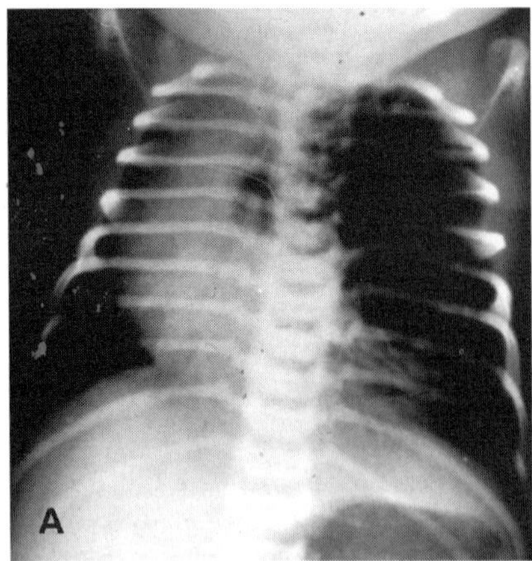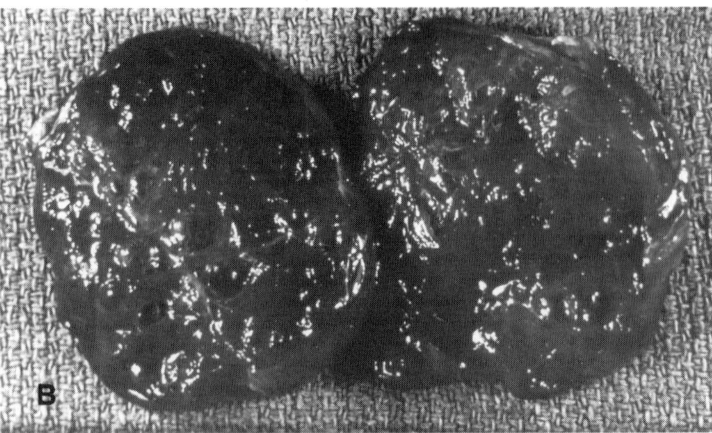

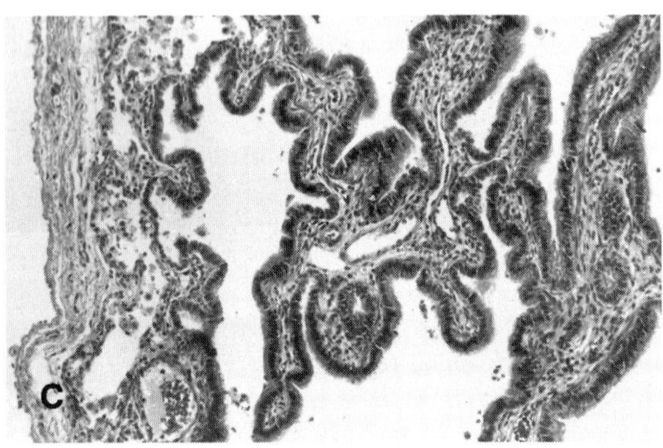

Figure 17–3. Cystic adenomatoid malformation. *A,* A chest x-ray film of a newborn with respiratory distress demonstrates a cystic lesion in the left lung, upper lobe, which has produced a mediastinal shift to the right. *B,* The excised specimen consists of cysts that blend with the pulmonary parenchyma. *C,* The cysts are lined by cuboidal to columnar epithelium. The wall contains only a few, scattered, smooth muscle fibers (hematoxylin-eosin, ×120).

volved.[35,37,39,41,52,60,67] Therefore, the lesion has essentially the same histologic features as a diffuse lymphangioma. Few cases have been reported in siblings.[92] Fronstin et al. reviewed 32 cases, including one of their own.[39] Three of the patients were stillborn and almost half had cardiac or other significant anomalies. Prenatal pleural effusion has been described in association with lymphangiectasis.[106] In contrast to lymphangioma, the outcome of this disease is invariably fatal.

Congenital pulmonary lymphangiectasis is further classified into three main types: primary, secondary, and generalized.[60] The gross and microscopic features of all three types are essentially the same in that the involved lung is firm and bosselated and the microscopic features consist of cystically dilated lymphatics. Factor VIII–related antigen and CD31 can be used to demonstrate lymphatic endothelium if this is considered necessary to establish the diagnosis.[86]

Primary pulmonary lymphangiectasis is most likely the result of failure of the pulmonary lymphatics to establish connection with systemic lymph channels, particularly the thoracic duct.

In practically all instances, this rare condition is fatal, and affected newborns die of respiratory distress shortly after birth. Secondary lymphangiectasis is associated with certain cardiac defects in which there is obstruction to pulmonary venous return, such as in total anomalous pulmonary venous drainage.[37] Generalized lymphangiectasis affects the lung as part of a systemic abnormality (lymphangiomatosis), with lymphangiomas and, occasionally, hemangiomas in the bones, viscera, and soft tissues; sometimes, it is impossible to distinguish between the two vascular components by microscopic study.[10,37,60,86] Interstitial emphysema in the newborn following vigorous resuscitative measures is common and can be mistaken for lymphangiectasis on the basis of histologic features.

Mesenchymal Cystic Hamartoma of the Lung

Pulmonary mesenchymal cystic hamartomas are nodules or cysts composed of both mesenchymal and epithelial elements.[71] Initially, the hamartoma consists of a nodule that grows slowly in size, becoming cystic when reaching approximately 1 cm in diameter. The cysts are lined by respiratory epithelium forming papillary projections. Beneath the epithelium, there is a cambium layer composed of mesenchymal cells resembling somewhat botryoid, embryonal rhabdomyosarcoma.[30,71] However, the main difference is that the mesenchymal cells of the hamartoma do not display the immaturity, the mitotic activity, or the cellular atypia found in rhabdomyosarcoma. The hamartomas usually occur as solitary lesions in the young, but they may be multifocal or bilateral in older individuals. Clinically, the cysts and nodules cause hemoptysis, pneumothorax, hemothorax, chest pain, or mild dyspnea.[71] The youngest patient in Mark's series of 5 patients was a 1½-year-old boy who presented with dyspnea and who was alive and well 4 years after surgical excision.[71] Although the possibility exists that these lesions may be congenital, they have not been documented in newborns. Probably the most important aspect of this lesion is that infants and children with pulmonary cysts, particularly mesenchyml cystic hamartomas, are at risk for developing malignant disease within these cysts.[105] Becroft and Jagusch described three 2-year-old boys with pleuropulmonary blastomas arising from mesenchymal cystic hamartomas.[7] Bove reported two similar cases, one with rhabdomyosarcoma and another with pulmonary blastoma.[12] Ueda et al. and Domizio et al. reported cases in older children.[33,100] Because of their malignant potential, pulmonary cysts should definitely be removed. According to Holland-Moritz and Heyn, 31% (5/16) of the children with pulmonary blastoma in their review had cystic lesions.[50]

Fibromatosis (Myofibromatosis)

Fibromatosis of the lung(s) occurs as part of a congenital disseminated disease called generalized or visceral fibromatosis.[1,13,30,88,89] This condition is characterized by multiple fibrovascular nodules found in the skin, musculoskeletal system, and viscera. The tumors are composed of myofibroblasts and fibroblasts displaying storiform, vascular, and hemangiopericytomatous growth patterns on microscopic examination.

Rosenberg et al.[89] classified congenital generalized fibromatosis into two main types. Type I included cases involving the skin, subcutaneous tissue, muscle, and bone, whereas type II described cases with visceral involvement. Brill and associates collected 63 examples of congenital generalized fibromatosis and added one of their own.[13] Adickes et al. culled 28 cases, plus one of their own, noting that 18 patients (64%) had lesions involving the lung.[1] Pulmonary involvement in generalized fibromatosis usually portends a poor prognosis (see also Chapter 4, "Soft Tissue Tumors").[13,88]

Laryngotracheal Papilloma

Laryngotracheal papillomas (juvenile papillomas, squamous papillomas) are relatively common, benign tumors arising most often in the larynx; in 5% to 10% of individuals, they extend distally into the trachea, and in less than 1%, the adjacent lung is involved.[29,97] Their stated incidence is 1500 to 2000 infants and children in the United States per year. Human papilloma virus is considered to be the etiologic agent.[25,26,29,48,79,97] The tumor is found most often during the first 3 years of life.[55]

Laryngeal papillomas are responsible for hoarseness and inspiratory stridor and, eventually, to severe respiratory distress.[55,65,97] These symptoms can occur in the newborn.[65] Typically, the clinical course is characterized by multiple recurrences requiring numerous resections and a tracheostomy as a safeguard. Laser therapy has been used with some success.[28,55,61] Spontaneous regression often occurs by late adolescence, and sometimes, there is extension of the papillomas distally into the peripheral airway and lungs, along with cavity formations and subpleural involvement.[62,65,97] Progression to squamous cell carcinoma in the second decade of life has been documented.[3,48,95] Laryngeotracheal papillomatosis is a cause of sudden, unexpected death in young children due to obstruction and suffocation caused by these lesions.

The papillomas are manifested as one or more tiny, papillary or sessile, wart-like excrescences projecting from the laryngeal mucosa and, less often, the tracheal mucosa. Occasionally, the mucosa is covered by numerous lesions obstructing the airway. On microscopic examination, they are seen to consist of papillary formations composed of nonkeratinized, stratified, squamous epithelium displaying maturation toward the surface and varying degrees of poikilocytosis (Fig. 17–4).[54] Focal atypia and increased mitotic activity are common. The epi-

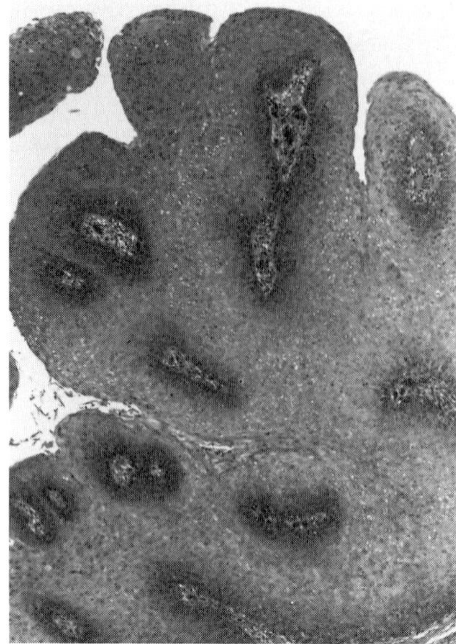

Figure 17–4. Laryngeal papilloma. Papillary formations composed of nonkeratinized, stratified, squamous epithelium are resting on a fibrovascular core. Minimal poikilocytotic atypia is present (hematoxylin-eosin, ×60).

thelium rests on a delicate fibrovascular core. A variable amount of nonspecific, chronic inflammation is present.

When the disease begins during childhood, it is usually self-limiting if properly treated, but sometimes in adults, the disease runs a more protracted course and carries an increased risk for developing squamous cell carcinoma.[3,25,95]

Langerhans Cell Histiocytosis

Although Langerhans cell histiocytosis is currently regarded as a reactive process, rather than a neoplastic one, when disseminated, the disease is treated by the pediatric oncologist.[30,55a] The pulmonary lesions of disseminated Langerhans cell histiocytosis (Letterer-Siwe disease) are characteristically diffuse and bilateral.[19,27] On gross inspection, the lungs show consolidated areas with foci of necrosis and abscess formation. Pneumothorax is a complication. The granuloma-like infiltrates are composed of Langerhans-type histiocytes, giant cells with similar, infolded nuclei, and variable numbers of eosinophils and neutrophils (see Fig. 8–2). The histiocytes are reactive with S-100 protein and display characteristic racket-shaped Birbeck granules on electron microscopy.[30,36] Older lesions are composed of granu-

lation tissue, extensive fibrosis, and histiocytic foam cells, a histologic picture similar to that of fibroxanthoma. Pulmonary involvement is one of the main causes of death from this disease in the newborn and infant.[55a]

MALIGNANT TUMORS

In patients of all ages, the most frequent malignant tumors in the lung are metastatic.[27,29,30,70,97] Rhabdomyosarcoma, Wilms' tumor, hepatoblastoma, and yolk sac tumor are the main malignant neoplasms metastasizing to the lungs during the first year of life. In leukemia, the pulmonary vessels may contain leukemic cells that may infiltrate the alveolar wall. Perivascular collections are found in severe cases.[27] Primary malignant tumors are uncommon in the perinatal period, and only a few examples of bronchopulmonary fibrosarcoma (myofibrosarcoma) and pleuropulmonary blastoma have been described. (see Table 17–2).[4,18,23,43,45,46,56,58,59,84,87,97]

Pleuropulmonary Blastoma

Pleuropulmonary blastoma (pulmonary blastoma of childhood, malignant mesenchymoma of the lung) is a highly aggressive, malignant tumor of childhood that is distinct from pulmonary blastoma (carcinosarcoma) affecting adults.[31,44,70] The entity was first described by Barnard in 1952, who called it "embryoma" based on its histologic similarity to the developing fetal lung (see Figs. 17–1 and 17–5).[6] Ten years later, Spencer described three examples and coined the term pulmonary blastoma, suggesting that the tumor originated from pluripotential mesoderm (pulmonary blastema) analagous to Wilms' tumor being derived from renal metanephric blastema.[96] Since then, more cases have been reported.[31,38,44,50,64,70,81,93] Less than 14% of these tumors affect children, and only 4% to 7% of those with the tumor are infants and newborns (see Table 17–2).[4,11,18,38,56,70] There is a male predominance approaching 3:1 in older children. Of 29 pediatric patients reviewed by Manivel et al., 2 were younger than 12 months of age.[70] Three newborns with pleuropulmonary blastoma are listed in Table 17–2. One was a male newborn with respiratory distress and a diffuse opacity of the right lung noted at birth. At 32 days of age, he died suddenly and the tumor was diagnosed at post-

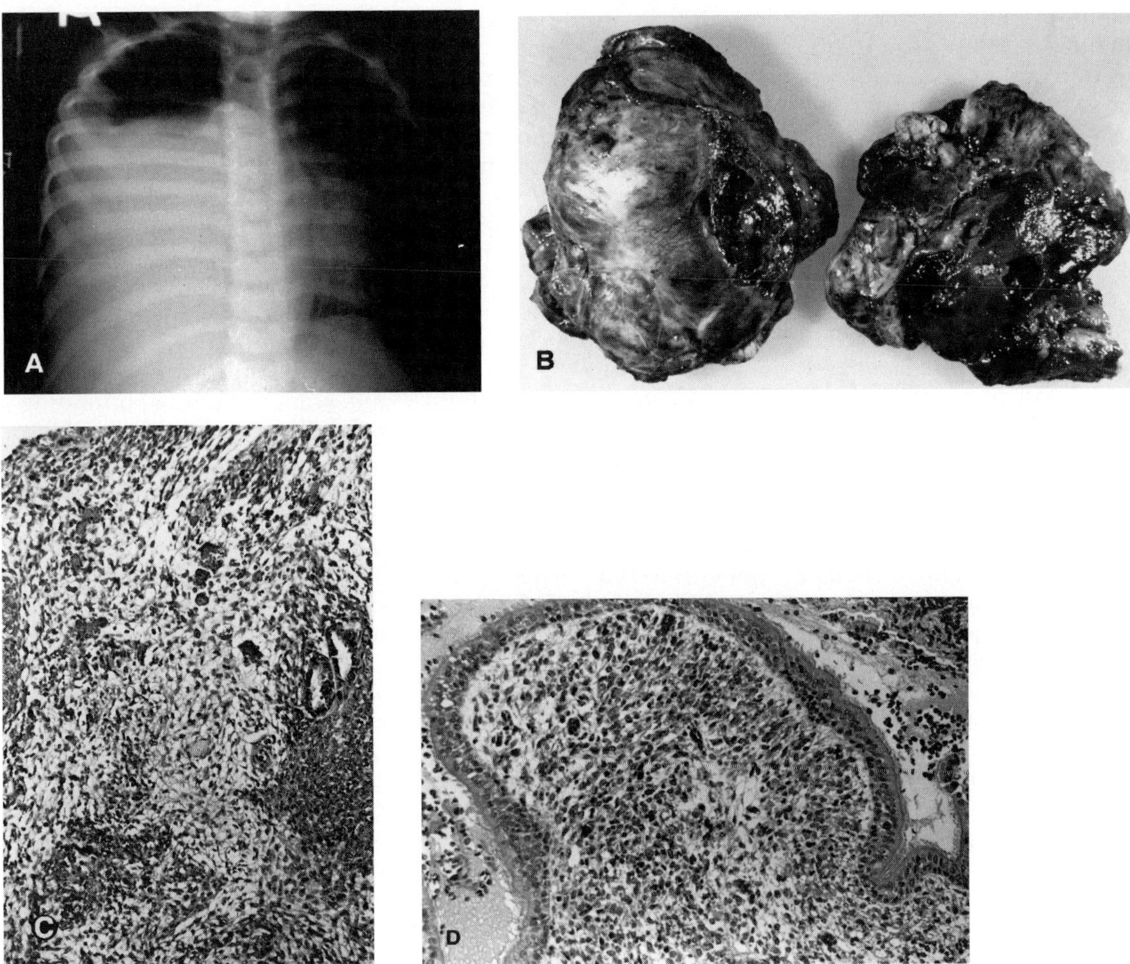

Figure 17–5. Pulmonary blastoma. *A*, A chest x-ray film of a 2-year-old girl with progressive respiratory distress and a low-grade fever shows opacification of the right hemithorax (''white-out''). *B*, The tumor is light tan-gray and friable, with extensive necrosis and hemorrhage. *C*, Blastemal (darkly cellular) areas alternate with pale, myxoid areas composed of tiny stellate and spindle-shaped cells. Small, primitive-appearing, bronchial-like structures are present at the right side of the photomicrograph (hematoxylin-eosin, ×120). *D*, When the tumor grows beneath the respiratory mucosa, it assumes a polypoid or botryoid appearance similar to that of embryonal rhabdomyosarcoma (hematoxylin-eosin, ×150).

mortem examination.[4] Another case involved a 3.2-kg female of 37 weeks' gestation with a maternal history of polyhydramnios.[18] After delivery, the baby had severe respiratory distress with Apgar scores of 0 and 2 at 1 and 5 minutes, respectively. Shortly after birth, an unsuccessful attempt was made to resect a 7 × 7 cm tumor that occupied the right upper and middle lobes. The third neonate, a 2.8-kg female infant, presented with a maternal history of oligohydramnios and respiratory distress, cyanosis, and pneumothorax.[56] The lesion occupied the right middle and lower lung lobes. She recovered uneventfully following a right middle and right lower lobectomy. No metastases, either lo-

cal or distant, were noted in these three newborns.

Pleuropulmonary blastoma is associated with pulmonary cysts, particularly cystic mesenchymal hamartoma and cystic adenomatoid malformation.[50] Multilocular cyst of the kidney has been described in patients with this neoplasm.[32] In a study by Dehner and associates, 10 (26%) of 38 children with this malignant disease had a family history of childhood tumors, including pleuropulmonary blastomas in siblings.[31]

In the older child, the clinical findings are a nonproductive cough, fever, and chest pain suggestive of a respiratory infection.[38,44,70] By contrast, respiratory distress, cyanosis, and pneumothorax are the presenting findings in the newborn.[4,18,56] Imaging studies reveal opacification of part of an entire lung and a mediastinal shift to the opposite side.[18,70] Tumors are located beneath the pleura or in the mediastinum. However, in the Children's Hospital, Los Angeles study, all but one of seven tumors originated from within the lung.[44]

The gross, histologic, immunohistochemical, and ultrastructural features of pleuropulmonary blastoma have been well documented (see Fig. 17–5).[33,44,63,64,70] Nevertheless, the histogenesis of this neoplasm remains unclear. The tumors tend to be large, some weighing more than 1 kg, and they have a multilobulated appearance. They are located at the periphery of the lung, occupying a part of or the entire lobe. Portions of visceral pleura may be attached to the specimen. The appearance of the cut surfaces varies, ranging from firm, light gray to red regions to pale tan, gelatinous areas, with or without necrosis, hemorrhage, and cyst formations.[29] On the basis of their gross appearance, pleuropulmonary blastomas are divided into three categories (types 1, 2, and 3) depending on whether they are purely cystic (type 1), predominantly solid (type 3), or intermediate between the 2 (type 2).[31]

Microscopically, the tumor has a distinctive appearance that varies from one field to the next. There are nests of small, undifferentiated, blastemal cells with round or oval, dark-staining nuclei, inconspicuous nucleoli, and scant cytoplasm. The nests of blastemal cells are surrounded by pale areas of loosely arranged spindle-shaped and stellate cells and, occasionally, bizarre, multinucleated giant cells (Fig. 17–5*C* and *D*). Both intracytoplasmic and extracytoplasmic globules (which are periodic acid-Schiff [PAS]–positive and diastase-resistant) are present. Characteristically, two or more different kinds of malignant mesenchymal components constitute the tumor. Cells displaying myoblastic, fibroblastic, chondroblastic, lipoblastic, and fibrohistiocytic differentiation have been described.[44,70] Epithelial and mesothelial structures are present and are histologically benign, probably representing reactive, entrapped elements rather than neoplastic ones.[31,44,70] There is a histologic spectrum, with the predominantly cystic lesion (type 1) with its rhabdomyosarcomatous component on one end and the solid type 2 tumor with its mixed mesenchymal elements on the other.[31] It may be difficult to distinguish between a pleuropulmonary blastoma without a cartilaginous component and a cystic rhabdomyosarcoma, especially with a small biopsy specimen.[29] Perhaps because of this, some pleuropulmonary blastomas have been mistakenly diagnosed as rhabdomyosarcoma.

Immunohistochemical studies show that these tumor cells stain positively for vimentin, desmin, alpha$_1$-antitrypsin, and alpha$_1$-chymotrypsin, and stain focally positive for S-100 protein. The entrapped epithelial elements show positivity for epithelial membrane antigen and cytokeratin.[31,44,70] Ultrastructurally, the blastemal cells are primitive-appearing, with round to oval nuclei and scant cytoplasm containing a few organelles. Spindle-shaped myofibroblastic cells with a well-formed endoplasmic reticulum, actin-like filaments with focal condensations beneath the cytoplasmic membrane, and rhabdomyoblasts showing thick and thin filaments and Z-band formations are present. In addition, fibrohistiocytoid and histiocytoid cells with numerous lysosomes have been described.[44,70]

The prognosis for patients with pleuropulmonary blastoma is dismal. Seven of the 11 patients in the series of Manivel et al. died of progressive disease with metastases to the brain, liver, lungs, spinal cord, and bones.[70] Five of the seven children included in the Children's Hospital, Los Angeles study died within 26 months after diagnosis.[44] Only two patients whose tumors were totally resected were alive after 2 years of follow-up evaluation. The newborn described by Jetley et al. survived following a right middle and lower lobectomy.[56] Two others with this disease, listed in Table 17–2, died. Thus, a cure is only possible if total en bloc resection is performed before metastasis has occurred.[31] Chemotherapy and/or radiotherapy may not be indicated in the absence of metastases or residual tumor.[56]

Bronchopulmonary Fibrosarcoma

Primary bronchopulmonary fibrosarcoma (congenital leiomyosarcoma, congenital peribronchial myofibroblastic tumor) is a relatively uncommon entity, although it is the most prevalent neonatal lung tumor (see Table 17–2).[43,45,46,58,59,73,84,87,103] Some tumors that were reported previously were classified as leiomyosarcomas, but recent immunohistochemical and ultrastructural studies do not support this diagnosis.[84] In 1993, McGinnis et al. concluded that the tumor was of myofibroblastic origin and suggested the term "congenital peribronchial myofibroblastic tumor."[73] They theorized that the neoplasm actually developed from splanchnic mesenchyme surrounding developing bronchi (Fig. 17–1).[73] Moreover, they believed it to be histologically analogous to the congenital mesoblastic nephroma (cellular variant) and the spindle cell tumor of the intestine.[73]

Typically, young patients with this neoplasm present with severe respiratory distress occurring soon after birth.[58,73,84] Of the nine patients reviewed by McGinnis et al. (of which 6 were males and 3 were females), four were born prematurely and six had evidence of in utero cardiac failure.[73] Nonimmune fetal hydrops and hydramnios occur in association with this neoplasm and may be the initial perinatal findings.[45,58,73,103] For example, both of the newborns described by Jimenez et al.[58] and by McGinnis et al.[73] had the combination of hydramnios, hydrops fetalis, a right lung mass noted on imaging studies, and increasing respiratory distress.

Bronchopulmonary fibrosarcomas arise from either the bronchus or from the adjacent lung parenchyma. There is no predilection for right versus left lung, nor for upper versus lower lobes.[73] The neoplasms range in size from 3.5 cm to 6 cm. Grossly, they are firm, gray, and yellow or light tan, with foci of hemorrhage and cyst formation. Histologic examination reveals a cellular tumor composed of spindle-shaped cells forming interdigitating fascicles similar to those observed in the soft tissue congenital fibrosarcoma. There is a moderately high mitotic rate. Foci of extramedullary hematopoiesis are found in the tumor. Immunohistochemical findings, such as positive vimentin staining, suggest a myofibroblastic origin, the muscle markers desmin and actin may be focally positive. The tumor cells are nonreactive for neuron-specific enolase (NSE), S-100 protein, leu-7, and alpha$_1$-antichymotrypsin.[84] The cartilaginous areas are reactive with S-100 protein.[73] Ultrastructurally, the spindle-shaped tumor cells display indented nuclei and infrequent nucleoli. The cytoplasm contains a prominent rough endoplasmic reticulum and intermediate filaments. Primitve cell junctions and extracellular deposits of collagen are noted.[58,84,103] In addition, there are spindle-shaped cells with cytoplasmic actin filaments, dense bodies, and attachment plaques, interpreted as myofibroblasts.[73] Cytometric DNA analysis performed by McGinnis et al. revealed a diploid pattern.[73]

Bronchopulmonary fibrosarcoma should probably be regarded as a low-grade malignant lesion that has a favorable prognosis following complete resection, despite its worrisome histologic appearance.[23,58,84,97] Because of the age and immaturity of the patients involved, the prognosis is guarded. About 50% of the neonates with this tumor survive (see Table 17–2). In the review of nine patients by McGinnis et al., there were four survivors; three patients died of complications attributed to prematurity and hydrops, and two died intraoperatively.[73]

Skeletal Muscle Tumors

There are several well-documented examples of striated muscle occurring in the lungs of fetuses and newborns[20–22,34,85] and in lungs with cystic and solid adenomatoid malformation,[15,22,30,98] as well as extralobar sequestration.[34] To the author's knowledge, however, primary pulmonary rhabdomyosarcoma has not been documented in the perinatal period. The presence of striated muscle in the lungs—termed rhabdomyomatous dysplasia, striated muscle heteroplasia, or rhabdomyomatosis—is associated with significant cardiac and pulmonary malformations.[22,34,101] The left or right lung may be equally involved, and both lungs may be affected.[22,34] The skeletal muscle fibers demonstrated by hematoxylin-eosin staining and by actin and myoglobin immunoperoxidase methods are widely distributed throughout the pulmonary interstitium, including the alveolar septa and the bronchial and bronchiolar walls.[20,21,34] Ultrastructurally, the striated muscle cells are composed of well-developed sarcomeric structures.[21]

Primary pulmonary rhabdomyosarcoma in childhood is rare.[2,47,80] Hartman and Schochat[47] reported 10 cases in children, Murphy et al. described 3 cases,[80] and Allan and associates[2] added two additional cases. None of these patients were infants or newborns. Rhabdomyosarcoma of the lung in children originates most frequently from bronchi, and less often, from congenital pulmonary cysts.[80] Cystic mesenchymal hamartoma, peripheral bronchogenic cyst, and cystic adenomatoid malformation are the types of cysts that have been described.[71,80] Because of the significant risk for the development of rhabdomyosarcoma within congenital pulmonary cysts, the latter should be resected as early as possible in an attempt to prevent this complication.

Primitive Neuroectodermal Tumor (PNET) of Thoracopulmonary Origin

The small cell malignant tumor of thoraco-pulmonary origin (Askin's tumor, PNET of the chest wall and lung) is one of the small blue cell tumors of childhood associated with a rapidly progressive, downhill clinical course and a poor outcome. The current view, based on immuno-histochemical, ultrastructural, and cytogenetic studies, is that this tumor is probably the same as the extraskeletal Ewing's sarcoma and PNET involving the soft tissues.[51,69,91,99] A neural crest origin has been proposed for these malignant lesions.

The PNET of thoracopulmonary origin occurs with two age peaks, one in late infancy and another in adolescence.[29] Clinically, the malignant tumor produces symptoms of fever, chest pain, a palpable mass in the chest wall, and pleural effusion.[29,51] The tumor probably arises from the soft tissues of the chest wall, but because of its proximity, the lung and pleura become involved during the course of the disease.

On gross examination, the chest wall and adjacent lung are effaced by one or more pale gray tumor nodules measuring up to 10 cm in greatest diameter. The cut surfaces show foci of necrosis, hemorrhage, and cyst formation.[29] Histologically, the tumor is highly cellular, consisting of small, round, darkly staining cells with scant cytoplasm that is sometimes arranged in lobules. Occasionally, pseudorosettes are noted. In contrast to light microscopic studies, which are often nonspecific, the electron microscopic findings are usually diagnostic. The neoplasm exhibits neural differentiation manifested by the presence of neuritic processes, dense core granules, and neurotubules. Glycogen deposits are seen in some tumors. NSE and, more specifically, the cell surface antigen HBA71, are positive immunohistochemical markers; these are unreactive in neuroblastoma, leukemic cells, and rhabdomyosarcoma (see Table 4–5). Chromosomal analysis of tissue culture material reveals a t(11;22) translocation, which also confirms the diagnosis.[51,91,99] To the author's knowledge, thoracopulmonary PNET has not been described in the newborn.

REFERENCES

1. Adickes ED, Goodrich P, AuchMoedy J, et al. Central nervous system involvement in congenital visceral fibromatosis. Pediatr Pathol 1985;3:329.
2. Allan BT, Day DL, Dehner LP. Primary pulmonary rhabdomyosarcoma of the lung in children. Report of two cases presenting with spontaneous pneumothorax. Cancer 1987;59:1005.
3. Al-Saleem T, Peale AR, Norris CM. Multiple papillomatosis of the lower respiratory tract. Clinical and pathology study of eleven cases. Cancer 1968;22:1173.
4. Ashworth TG. Pulmonary blastoma, a true congenital neoplasm. Histopathology 1983;7:585.
5. Bahadori M, Liebow AA. Plasma cell granuloma of the lung. Cancer 1973;31:191.
6. Barnard WG. Embryoma of the lung. Thorax 1952;7:299.
7. Becroft DMO, Jagusch MF. Pulmonary sarcomas arising in mesenchymal hamartomas. Pediatr Pathol 1987;7:478.
8. Benjamin DR, Cahill JL. Bronchoalveolar carcinoma of the lung and congenital cystic adenomatoid malformation. Am J Clin Pathol 1991;95:889.
9. Berardi RS, Lee SS, Chen HP. Inflammatory pseudotumors of the lung. Surg Gynecol Obstet 1983;156:89.
10. Bhatti MHK, Ferrante JW, Gielchinsky I, et al. Pleuropulmonary and skeletal lymphangiomatosis with chylothorax and chylopericardium. Ann Thor Surg 1985;40:398.
11. Blair JD, Al-Doroubi QI. Pulmonary blastoma in an infant. Am J Pathol 1976;82:90a.
12. Bove KE. Sarcoma arising in pulmonary mesenchymal cystic hamartoma. Pediatr Pathol 1989;9:785.
13. Brill PW, Yandow DR, Langer LO. Congenital generalized fibromatosis. Case report and literature review. Pediatr Radiol 1982;12:269.
14. Buell R, Wang N, Seemayer TA, et al. Endobronchial plasma cell granuloma (xanthomatous pseudotumor). A light and electron microscopy study. Hum Pathol 1976;7:411.
15. Buntain WL, Isaacs H, Payne VC Jr, et al. Lobar emphysema, cystic adenomatoid malformation and pulmonary sequestration: A clinical group. J Pediatr Surg 1974;9:85.
16. Byard RW, Burrows PE, Izakawa T, et al. Diffuse infantile haemangiomatosis: Clinicopathologic features and management problems in five fatal cases. Eur J Pediatr 1991;150:224.
17. Cangir A. Miscellaneous childhood tumors. *In* Fernbach DJ, Vietti TJ (eds): Clinical Pediatric Oncology, 4th ed, p 627. St. Louis: Mosby–Year Book, 1991.
18. Cappuccino H, Heleotis T, Krumerman M. Pulmonary blastoma as a unique cause of fatal respiratory distress in a newborn. J Pediatr Surg 1995;30:886.
19. Carlson RA, Hattery RR, O'Connell EJ, et al. Pulmonary involvement by histiocytosis X in the pediatric age group. Mayo Clin Proc 1976;51:542.
20. Chellam VG. Rhabdomyomatour dysplasia of the lung: A case report and review of the literature. Pediatr Pathol 1988;8:391.
21. Chen MF, Onerheim R, Wang NS, et al. Rhabdomyomatosis of newborn lung: A case report with immuno-histochemical and electron microscopic characterization of striated muscle cells in the lung. Pediatr Pathol 1991;11:123.
22. Chi JG, Shong Y-K. Diffuse striated muscle heteroplasia of the lung: An autopsy case. Arch Pathol Lab Med 1982;106:641.
23. Coffin CM, Dehner LP: Congenital tumors. *In* Stocker JT, Dehner LP (eds): Pediatric Pathology, Vol 1, p 325. Philadelphia: JB Lippincott, 1992.
24. Coffin CM, Watterston J, Priest JR, et al. Extrapulmo-

nary myofibroblastic tumor (inflammatory pseudotumor): A clinicopathologic and immunohistochemical study of 84 cases. Am J Surg Pathol 1975;19:859.

25. Cohen SR, Geller KA, Selzer S, et al. Papilloma of the larynx and tracheobronchial tree in children. A retrospective study. Ann Otol Rhinol Laryngol 1980;89:497.

26. Costa J, Howley MP. Presence of human papilloma viral antigens in juvenile multiple laryngeal papilloma. Am J Clin Pathol 1981;75:194.

27. Cox JN. Respiratory system. *In* Berry CL (ed): Paediatric Pathology, 2nd ed, p 293. London: Springer-Verlag, 1989.

28. Crockett DM, McCabe BF, Shive CJ. Complication of laser surgery for recurrent respiratory papillomatosis. Ann Otol Rhinol Laryngol 1987;96:639.

29. Dehner LP. Pediatric Surgical Pathology, 2nd ed. Baltimore: Williams & Wilkins, 1987.

30. Dehner LP. Tumors and tumor-like lesions of the lung and chest wall in childhood: Clinical and pathologic review. *In* Stocker JT (ed): Pediatric Pulmonary Disease, p 207. Washington, DC: Hemisphere, 1989.

31. Dehner LP, Watterston J, Priest J. Pleuropulmonary blastoma: A unique intrathoracic-pulmonary neoplasm of childhood. *In* Askin FB, Langston C, Rosenberg HS, Bernstein J (eds): Pulmonary Disease, Perspectives in Pediatric Pathology, Vol 18, p 214. Basel: Karger, 1995.

32. Delahunt B, Thomson KJ, Ferguson AF, et al. Familial cystic nephroma and pleuropulmonary blastoma. Cancer 1993;71:1338.

33. Domizio P, Liesner RJ, Dicks-Mireaux C, et al. Malignant mesenchymoma associated with a congenital lung cyst in a child: Case report and review of the literature. Pediatr Pathol 1990;10:785.

34. Drut RM, Quijano G, Drut R, et al. Rhabdomyomatous dysplasia of the lung. Pediatr Pathol 1988;8:385.

35. Esterly JR, Oppenheimer EH. Lymphangiectasis and other pulmonary lesions in the asplenia syndrome. Arch Pathol 1970;90:553.

36. Flint A, Lloyd RV, Colby TV, et al. Pulmonary histiocytosis. Immunoperoxidase staining for HLA-DR antigen and S-100 protein. Arch Pathol Lab Med 1986;110:930.

37. France NE, Brown RJK. Congenital pulmonary lymphangiectasis. Arch Dis Child 1971;46:528.

38. Francis D, Jacobsen M. Pulmonary blastoma. Curr Top Pathol 1983;73:265.

39. Fronstin MH, Hooper GS, Beese BE, et al. Congenital pulmonary cystic lymphangiectasis. Am J Dis Child 1967;114:330.

40. Galliani CA, Beatty JF, Grosfeld JL. Cavernous hemangioma of the lung in an infant. Pediatr Pathol 1992;12:105.

41. Gau GS. The respiratory system. *In* Keeling JW (ed): Fetal and Neonatal Pathology, p 363. London: Springer-Verlag, 1987.

42. Gibbons JRP, McKeown F, Field TW. Pulmonary blastoma with hilar lymph node metastases. Cancer 1981;47:152.

43. Guccion JG, Rosen SH. Bronchopulmonary leiomyosarcoma and fibrosarcoma. A study of 32 cases and review of the literature. Cancer 1972;30:386.

44. Hachitanda Y, Aoyama C, Sato JK, et al. Pleuropulmonary blastoma in childhood: A tumor of divergent differentiation. Am J Surg Pathol 1993;17:382.

45. Haller JO, Kaufman SL, Kassner EG. Congenital mesenchymal tumour of the lung. Br J Radiol 1977;50:217.

46. Hancock BJ, Di Lorenzo M, Youssef S, et al. Childhood primary pulmonary neoplasms. J Pediatr Surg 1993;28:1133.

47. Hartman GE, Schochat SJ. Primary pulmonary neoplasms of childhood: A review. Ann Thorac Surg 1983;36:108.

48. Helmuth RA, Strate RW. Squamous carcinoma of the lung in a nonirradiated, nonsmoking patient with juvenile laryngotracheal papillomatosis. Am J Surg Pathol 1987;11:643.

49. Holden KR, Alexander F. Diffuse neonatal hemangiomatosis. Pediatrics 1970;46:411.

50. Holland-Moritz RM, Heyn RM. Pulmonary blastoma associated with cystic lesions in children. Med Pediatr Oncol 1984;12:85.

51. Horowitz ME, DeLaney TF, Malawer MM, et al. Ewing's sarcoma family of tumors: Ewing's sarcoma of bone and soft tissue and the peripheral primitive neuroectodermal tumors. *In* Pizzo PA, Poplack DG (eds): Principles and Practice of Pediatric Oncology, 2nd ed, p 795. Philadelphia: JB Lippincott, 1993.

52. Hunter WS, Becroft DMO. Congenital pulmonary lymphangiectasis associated with pleural effusions. Arch Dis Child 1984;59:278.

53. Hurvitz CH, Greenberg SH, Song CH, et al. Hemangiomatosis of the pleura with hemorrhage and disseminated intravascular coagulation. J Pediatr Surg 1982;17:73.

54. Incze JS, Lui PS, et al. The morphology of human papillomas of the upper respiratory tract. Cancer 1977;39:1634.

55. Irwin BC, Hendrickse WR, Pincott CM, et al. Juvenile laryngeal papillomatosis. J Laryngol Otol 1986;100:435.

55a. Isaacs H Jr. Perinatal (congenital and neonatal) neoplasms: A report of 110 cases. Pediatr Pathol 1985;3:165.

56. Jetley NK, Bhatnagar V, Krishna A, et al. Pulmonary blastoma in a neonate. J Pediatr Surg 1988;23:1009.

57. Jimenez JF. Pulmonary blastoma in childhood. J Surg Oncol 1987;34:87.

58. Jimenez JF, Uthman EO, Townsend JW, et al. Primary bronchopulmonary leiomyosarcoma in childhood. Arch Pathol Lab Med 1986;110:348.

59. Jones CJ. Unusual hamartoma of the lung in a newborn infant. Arch Pathol 1949;48:150.

60. Katzenstein A-LA, Askin FB. Surgical pathology of non-neoplastic lung disease. *In* Bennington JL (ed): Major Problems in Pathology, 2nd ed, Vol 13. Philadelphia: WB Saunders, 1990.

61. Kavuru MS, Mehta AC, Eliachar I. Effect of photodynamic therapy and external beam radiation therapy on juvenile laryngotracheobronchial papillomatosis. Annu Rev Resp Dis 1990;141:509.

62. Kawanami T, Bowen A. Juvenile laryngeal papillomatosis with pulmonary parenchymal spread. Case report and review of the literature. Pediatr Radiol 1985;15:102.

63. Korbi S, M'Boyo A, Dusmet M, et al. Pulmonary blastoma. Immunohistochemical and ultrastructural studies of a case. Histopathology 1987;11:753.

64. Koss MN, Hochholzer L, O'Leary T. Pulmonary blastomas. Cancer 1991;67:2368.

65. Kramer SS, Wehunt WD, Stocker JT, et al. Pulmonary manifestations of juvenile laryngotracheal papillomatosis. AJR 1985;144:687.

66. Krous HF, Sexauer CL. Embryonal rhabdomyosarcoma arising within a congenital bronchogenic cyst in a child. J Pediatr Surg 1981;16:506.

67. Laurence KM. Congenital pulmonary lymphangiectasis. J Clin Pathol 1959;12:62.

68. Lin JJ, Svoboda DJ. Multiple congenital mesenchymal tumors. Multiple vascular leiomyomas in several organs of a newborn. Cancer 1971;28:1046.

69. Linnoila RI, Tsokos M, Triche TJ, et al. Evidence for neural origin and PAS-positive variants of the malignant small cell tumor of thoracopulmonary region ("Askin tumor"). Am J Surg Pathol 1986;10:124.

70. Manivel JC, Priest JR, Watterson J, et al. Pleuropulmonary blastoma: The so-called pulmonary blastoma of childhood. Cancer 1988;62:1516.

71. Mark EJ. Mesenchymal cystic hamartoma of the lung. N Engl J Med 1986;315:1255.

72. Matsubara O, Tan Liu NS, Kenney RM, et al. Inflammatory pseudotumor of the lung: Progression from organizing pneumonia to fibrous histiocytoma or to plasma cell granuloma in 32 cases. Hum Pathol 1988; 19:807.

73. McGinnis M, Jacobs G, El-Naggar A, et al. Congenital peribronchial myofibroblastic tumor (so-called "congenital leiomyosarcoma"). A distinct neonatal lung lesion associated with nonimmune hydrops fetalis. Mod Pathol 1993;6:487.

74. Mendoza A, Wolf P, Edwards DK, et al. Prenatal ultrasonographic diagnosis of congenital adenomatoid malformation of the lung. Correlation with pathology and implication for pregnancy management. Arch Pathol Lab Med 1986;110:402.

75. Milovic I, Oluic D. Lymphangioma of the lung associated with respiratory distress in a neonate. Pediatr Radiol 1992;22:156.

76. Moerman P, Fryns JP, Vanden Berghe K, et al. Pathogenesis of congenital cystic adenomatoid malformation of the lung. Histopathology 1992;21:315.

77. Monzon CM, Gilchrist GS, Burget EO Jr, et al. Plasma cell granuloma of the lung in children. Pediatrics 1982;70:268.

78. Moore KL. The Developing Human—Clinically Oriented Embryology, 5th ed. Philadelphia: WB Saunders, 1993.

79. Mounts P, Kashima H. Association of human papilloma virus subtype and clinical course in respiratory papillomatosis. Laryngoscope 1984;94:28.

80. Murphy JJ, Blair GK, Fraser GC, et al. Rhabdomyosarcoma arising within congenital pulmonary cysts: Report of three cases. J Pediatr Surg 1992;27:1364.

81. Ozkaynak MF, Ortega JA, Laug W, et al. Role of chemotherapy in pediatric pulmonary blastoma. Med Pediatr Oncol 1990;18:53.

82. Pearl M, Woolley MM. Pulmonary xanthomatous postinflammatory pseudotumors in children. J Pediatr Surg 1973;8:255.

83. Pearson PJ, Smithson WA, et al. Inoperable plasma cell granuloma of the heart: Spontaneous decrease in size during an 11-month period. Mayo Clin Proc 1988; 63:1022.

84. Pettinato G, Manivel C, Saldana MJ, et al. Primary bronchopulmonary fibrosarcoma of childhood and adolescence. Reassessment of a low grade malignancy—Clinicopathologic study of five cases and a review of the literature. Hum Pathol 1989;20:463.

85. Potter EL, Craig JM. Pathology of the Fetus and Infant, 3rd ed, p 344. Chicago: Year Book Medical Publishers, 1975.

86. Ramani P, Shah A. Lymphangiomatosis: Histologic and immunohistochemical analysis of four cases. Am J Surg Pathol 1993;17:329.

87. Robb D. A case of neonatal fibrosarcoma of lung. Br J Surg 1958;46:173.

88. Roggli VL, Hawkins E. Congenital generalized fibromatosis with visceral involvement: A report of a case. Cancer 1980;45:954.

89. Rosenberg HS, Stenback WA, Spjut HJ. The fibromatoses of infancy and childhood. *In* Rosenberg HS, Bolande RP (eds): Perspectives in Pediatric Pathology, Vol 4, p 269. Chicago: Year Book Medical Publishers, 1978.

90. Saltzman DH, Adzick NS, Benacerraf BR. Fetal cystic adenomatoid malformation of the lung: Apparent improvement in utero. Obstet Gynecol 1989;71:1000.

91. Schmidt D, Harms D, Burdach S. Malignant peripheral neuroectodermal tumours of childhood and adolescence. Virchows Arch [A] 1985;406:351.

92. Scott-Emuakpor AB, Warren ST, Kapur S, et al. Familial occurrence of congenital pulmonary lymphangiectasis: Genetic implications. Am J Dis Child 1981;135: 532.

93. Senac MO, Wood BP, Isaacs H, Weller M. Pulmonary blastoma—A rare childhood malignancy. Radiology 1991;179:743.

94. Shehan K, Wolf G, Nieman RS. Inflammatory pseudotumor of the spleen: A clinicopathologic study of three cases. Hum Pathol 1988;19:1024.

95. Siegel SE, Cohen SR, Isaacs H Jr, et al. Malignant transformation of tracheobronchial juvenile papillomatosis without prior radiotherapy. Ann Otol Rhinol Laryngol 1979;88:192.

96. Spencer H. Pulmonary blastomas. J Pathol 1961;82: 161.

97. Stocker JT. The respiratory tract. *In* Stocker JT, Dehner LP (eds): Pediatric Pathology, Vol 1, p 505. Philadelphia: JB Lippincott, 1992.

98. Stocker JT, Madewell JE, Drake RM. Congenital cystic adenomatoid malformation of the lung. Classification and morphologic spectrum. Hum Pathol 1977;8:155.

99. Tsokos M. Peripheral primitive neuroectodermal tumors: Diagnosis, classification and prognosis. Perspect Pediatr Pathol 1992;16:27.

100. Ueda K, Gruppo R, Unger F, et al. Rhabdomyosarcoma of the lung arising in a congenital cystic adenomatoid malformation. Cancer 1977;40:383.

101. Vilanova JR, Burgos-Bretones J, Aguirre JM, et al. Rhabdomyomatous dysplasia of lung and congenital diaphragmatic hernia. J Pediatr Surg 1983;18:201.

102. Wagenvoort CA, Beetstra A, Spijker J. Capillary haemangiomatosis of the lungs. Histopathology 1978;2: 401.

103. Warren JS, Seo IS, Mirkin LD. Massive congenital mesenchymal malformation of the lung. A case report with ultrastructural study. Pediatr Pathol 1985;3:321.

104. Weinberg AG, Currarino G, Moore GC, et al. Mesenchymal neoplasia and congenital pulmonary cysts. Pediatr Radiol 1980;9:179.

105. Weinblatt ME, Siegel SE, Isaacs H. Pulmonary blastoma associated with cystic lung disease. Cancer 1982; 49:669.

106. Wilson RH, Duncan A, Hume R, et al. Prenatal pleural effusion associated with congenital lymphangiectasis. Prenatal Diag 1985;5:73.

107. Wu T-J, Teng R-J. Diffuse neonatal haemangiomatosis with intra-uterine haemorrhage and hydrops fetalis: A case report. Eur J Pediatr 1994;153:759.

108. Zapatero J, Logo J, Madrigal L, et al. Subglottic inflammatory pseudotumor in a 6-year-old child. Pediatr Pulmonol 1989;6:268.

109. Zimmermann H, Habenicht R. Kongenitales lymphangiom der lunge. Z Kinderchir 1989;44:111.

BONE TUMORS

18

Primary tumors and tumor-like conditions of bone (Table 18–1) are uncommon in the fetus and newborn. Langerhans cell histiocytosis, congenital myofibromatosis, and fibrous dysplasia can produce single or multiple bone lesions. In one series, vascular lesions were reported as the dominant condition.[25a] A Children's Hospital, Los Angeles study reported that, of 249 patients with bone tumors who were younger than 10 years of age, 16 were infants.[34] Langerhans cell histiocytosis was the leading neoplasm with 10 cases (3 newborns), followed, in order of frequency, by 2 congenital chest wall hamartomas, and 1 each of fibrous dysplasia of the turbinate and myofibromatosis of the mandible.

Symptoms of bone tumors tend to be nonspecific, occasionally leading to an erroneous diagnosis. Because skeletal neoplasms can mimic benign conditions, such as osteomyelitis or trauma, the possibility that a lesion may be a tumor should always be kept in mind.[34]

CHEST WALL HAMARTOMA

Chest wall hamartoma has been variously referred to as benign mesenchymoma, aneurysmal bone cyst, and cartilaginous hamartoma.[1a,5,10,12,15,22,27,28,30,31] It is a tumor-like condition of newborns and infants that involves one or more adjacent ribs and produces a bulging mass and deformity of the chest wall (Figs. 18–1 and 18–2).[10,15,20,25a] Occasionally, the hamartoma is extensive; when it impinges upon the lungs, it causes neonatal respiratory distress and occasionally, death.[23,28,31] The lesion has been detected by prenatal ultrasonography, presenting as a large mass within the hemithorax and chest wall.[23] In one neonate described by Jung et al., sonography was performed because the mother was large for dates and polyhydramnios was noted.[23]

On gross examination, the involved rib is expanded, and is partially or totally replaced by a cystic lesion composed of cartilaginous, osseous, fibrous, and vascular elements. Microscopically, the hamartoma resembles an aneurysmal bone cyst with striking proliferation of hyaline cartilage plus bone and fibrous connective tissue formation (see Figs. 18–1 and 18–2).[21,27,28] Because of their proliferative appearance, hamartomas have been misdiagnosed as sarcomas. However, malignant change has been known to occur several years after the initial surgery.[15]

McLeod and Dahlin[28] and McCarthy and Dorfman[27] have suggested that the lesion probably represents a hamartoma or malformation, rather than a true neoplasm. The typical presentation at birth or in infancy, and the benign behavior of the lesion further support this idea.[27]

Conservative surgical excision is the treatment of choice. Nevertheless, several staged procedures may be required because of the extensive nature of these lesions and the disfiguration produced by some chest wall hamartomas.[15,20,31,32] Although spontaneous regression can occur, the usual outcome is progressive growth and deformity.[5,15,30,31] Scoliosis is a serious sequela in about 25% of the patients with chest wall hamartoma (see Fig. 18–2).[15]

CONGENITAL FIBROMATOSIS (INFANTILE MYOFIBROMATOSIS)

Congenital fibromatosis (discussed also in Chapter 4, "Soft Tissue Tumors") is character-

Table 18–1. Fetal and Newborn Tumors and Tumor-Like Conditions of Bone

Chest wall hamartoma
Langerhans cell histiocytosis
Congenital myofibromatosis
Congenital fibrosarcoma
Fibrous dysplasia*
Osteofibrous dysplasia
Melanotic neuroectodermal tumor of infancy
Ewing's sarcoma*
Enchondroma (Ollier's disease)*

*Generally seen in older infants and children.

ized by multiple nodular lesions of the skin, subcutaneous tissue, soft tissues, bone, and viscera.[7,33,35] The disease may be familial, as evidenced by the four cases occurring in one family described by Bartlett and colleagues.[2] Based on a study of 33 cases, Rosenberg and co-workers classified congenital generalized fibromatosis into two main types: I and II.[33] Infants with type I disease have multiple lesions involving the skin, subcutaneous tissue, muscle, and bone, whereas those with type II have, in addition, visceral tumors. This classification has prognostic significance in that, of 16 infants with type I disease, 15 survived, whereas 14 of 17 patients with type II disease subsequently died.[33]

Bone lesions can occur in either type I (63%) or type II (47%) congenital generalized fibromatosis.[33] A newborn with generalized fibromatosis involving the kidney and skeleton (the skull, pelvis, and long bones) has been reported by Teng and associates.[36] The bone lesions completely regresssed by 2 years of age, resulting in no bone deformity. Rarely, the disease may be manifested predominantly by bone lesions or may even be limited entirely to the bones.[6,17,19,25] Chan and colleagues described a male newborn who had multiple osteolytic metaphyseal bone lesions and a single soft tissue lesion at the knee.[6] A lytic lesion in the femur was associated with a pathologic fracture. Several years after the lesions spontaneously regressed, the child was left with left knee flexion contracture and bilateral ankle equinus deformities.

Less than 10% of the cases of the solitary form of congenital myofibromatosis involve bone alone.[6,17,19,37] Kindblom and Angervall depicted a 3-month-old male infant with a solitary lesion in the right ulna presenting as a swollen wrist since birth.[25] Radiographs showed shortening of the ulna and an osteolytic lesion in the distal metaphysis extending to the epiphysis.

The tumor was curetted on three occasions and was filled with bone transplants before it finally healed when the patient was 2½ years of age.

The radiologic features of osseous myofibromatosis consist of a lytic lesion with a sclerotic rim involving, in particular, the craniofacial bones, femur, tibia, vertebra, and rib.[6,17,19] Periosteal new bone formation and pathologic fracture are additional findings.

Osseous myofibromatosis has essentially the same histologic appearance as that involving the skin, soft tissue, and viscera. It consists of bundles of spindle-shaped fibroblasts, myofibroblasts, and cells intermediate between the two, arranged in bundles or whorls (Fig. 18–3). Central, cleft-like, vascular spaces are present. The immunohistochemical and ultrastructural features also are identical, and are discussed by Hasegawa et al.[17]

Myofibromatosis involving primarily bone, as well as those arising from the skin and soft tissues, should be treated conservatively, as most regress spontaneously.[6,19]

LANGERHANS CELL HISTIOCYTOSIS

Typically, the newborn with disseminated Langerhans cell histiocytosis (Letterer-Siwe disease) presents with a salmon-colored maculopapular rash, hepatosplenomegaly, lymphadenopathy, thrombocytopenia, and generally, "failure to thrive."[21] Lytic bone lesions eventually develop, although they may not always be present at the time of diagnosis. Osseous lesions characteristically involve the skull (most common site), the sinuses, ribs, pelvis, and scapula, but also may occur in the long bones and vertebra[21,34] (see Chapter 8, "Histiocytoses") (Fig. 18–4).

The exceedingly rare Hand-Schüller-Christian disease, characterized by exophthalmos, diabetes insipidus, and membrane bone infiltrates, occurs in the 2- to 4-year-old age group. Solitary bone lesions ("eosinophilic granuloma") typically are found in older children. In Dehner's study, the youngest patient with this lesion was 2 years of age.[14]

In a Children's Hospital, Los Angeles study of 249 primary bone lesions in infants and children younger than 10 years of age, there were 54 (22%) cases of Langerhans cell histiocytosis.[34] Three newborns had the disseminated form (Letterer-Siwe disease), with either bone

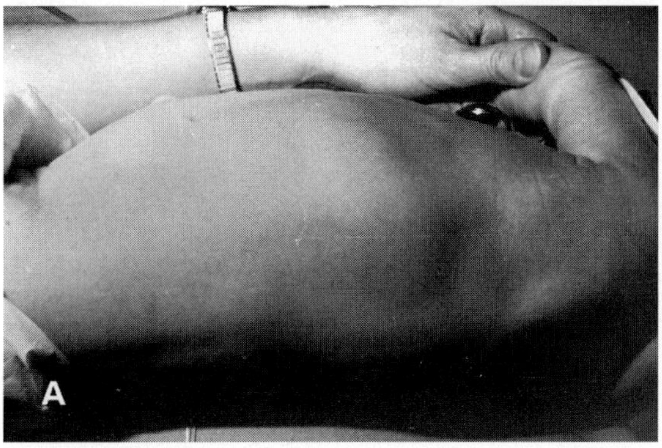

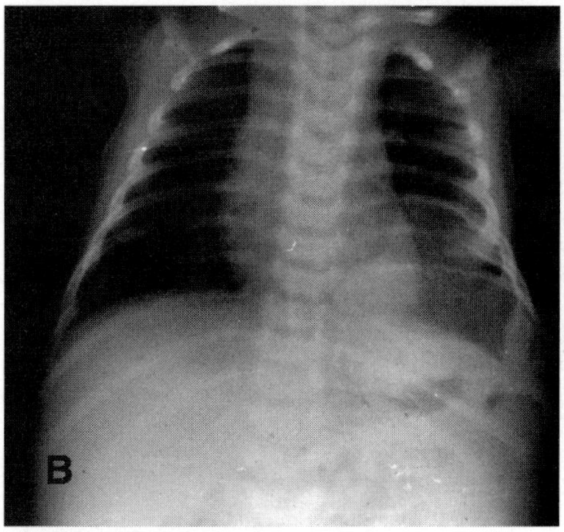

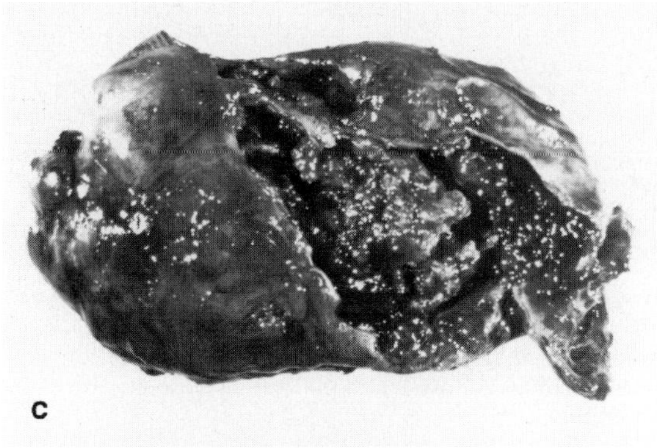

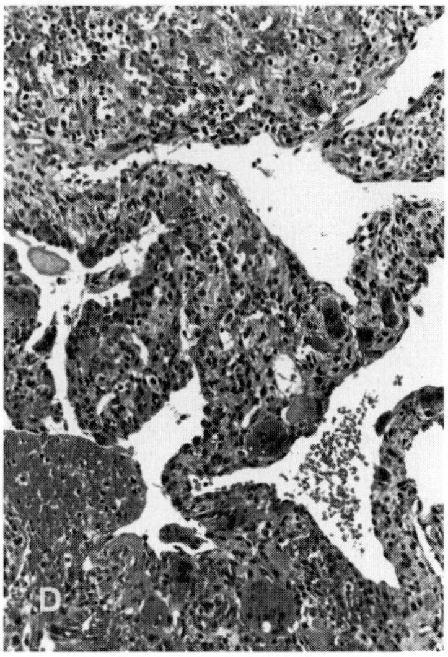

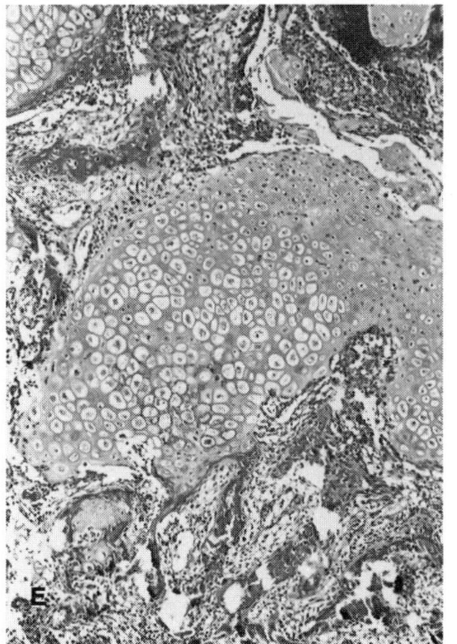

Figure 18–1. Chest wall hamartoma. *A,* A 1-month-old male infant presented with a history of a bulge over the chest wall since birth. *B,* A cystic, expansile lesion involving the left eighth rib is evident on radiographic examination. *C,* The soft, hemorrhagic contents of the rib are covered by a thin, "eggshell" layer of bone. *D,* The vascular component consists of spaces filled with blood and separated by fibrovascular tissue containing osteoclasts (hematoxylin-eosin, ×150). *E,* Proliferating cartilage and spicules of partially decalcified bone are surrounded by vascular connective tissue (hematoxylin-eosin, ×48). (*D* and *E:* From Isaacs H Jr. Neoplasms in infants: A report of 265 cases. Pathol Annu 1983;18(2):165. Used by permission of Appleton & Lange.)

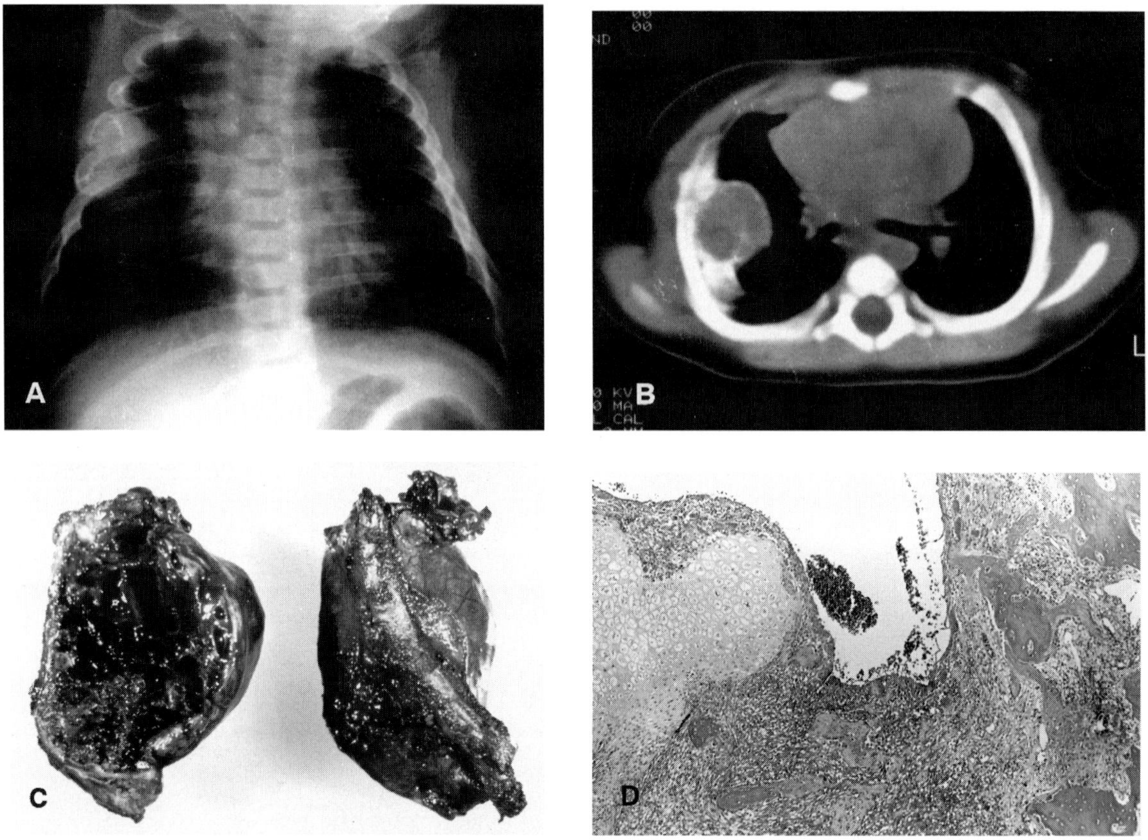

Figure 18–2. Chest wall hamartoma. *A,* A cystic, expansile lesion is seen to involve the right fourth rib of a 5-month-old male infant. Scoliosis and chest deformity, which are complications of this entity, are evident. *B,* A CT scan reveals a defect in the right chest wall and a cystic lesion bulging into the thoracic cavity. *C,* The involved rib was bisected, revealing an expansile, sponge-like mass occupying the rib; the mass was reminiscent of an aneurysmal bone cyst. *D,* Vascular, cartilaginous, and osseous components are illustrated (hematoxylin-eosin, ×48).

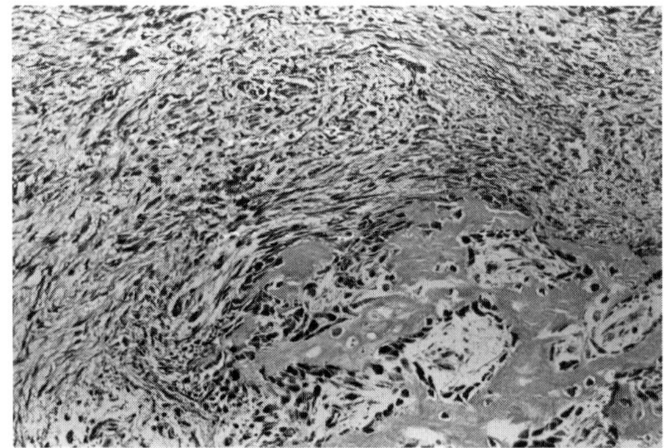

Figure 18–3. Myofibromatosis. A 3-week-old male infant presented with multiple subcutaneous nodules in the face, chest, arms, and bones. The jaw lesion shows an island of reactive bone surrounded by spindle-shaped myofibroblastic cells (hematoxylin-eosin, ×150).

lesions in the skull (n = 2) or in the mastoid (n = 1).

FIBROUS DYSPLASIA

Fibrous dysplasia has many variations, presents clinically in different ways, and involves one or more bones. Although it is considered to be a congenital developmental defect of unknown etiology, in some instances, because of its extensive growth, it mimics a neoplasm. Fibrous dysplasia may be apparent at birth, but most often, it does not become manifest until later in childhood.[16a,32]

The monostotic form usually affects children or young adults, occurring only rarely in infants. The bones most often involved are the ribs, tibia, femur, mandible, and maxilla. The first sign may be a fracture, or there may be

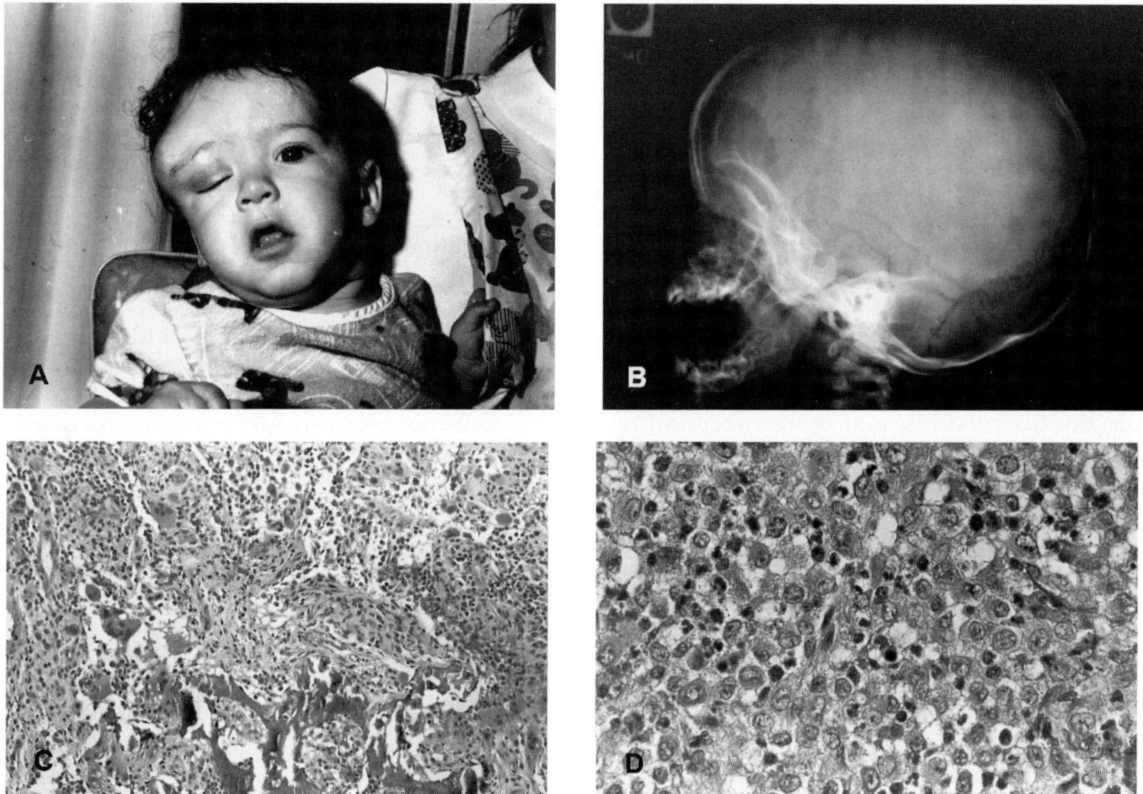

Figure 18–4. Langerhans cell histiocytosis. *A,* A 7-month-old male infant had painful swelling in a 3 × 3 cm area over the right orbital ridge noted 1 month prior to biopsy. The skull is the bone most commonly affected by this disease. *B,* A skull film, lateral view, reveals a lytic defect in the right frontal bone. Characteristically, no reaction is present along the advancing margins of the lesion. *C,* Bone is seen to have been replaced by a cellular infiltrate. The multinucleated giant cells are osteoclasts (hematoxylin-eosin, ×48). *D,* The infiltrate consists of histiocytes with eosinophilic cytoplasms, which occasionally are vacuolated, infolded nuclei, and one or two small nucleoli. A few lymphocytes and neutrophils are also present. S-100 protein is strongly positive in the histiocytes (hematoxylin-eosin, ×150). (From Isaacs H Jr. Neoplasms in infants: A report of 265 cases. Pathol Annu 1983;18(2):165. Used by permission of Appleton & Lange.)

local swelling and tenderness that eventually result in deformity. The child is usually otherwise normal. Histologically, the marrow and osseous structures in sharply delineated areas are replaced by fibrous connective tissue and poorly formed, immature bone that is deficient in osteoblasts.

Children with paranasal sinus involvement manifest the disease at an earlier age than those with lesions in the long bones.[34] Indeed, one female newborn in the Children's Hospital, Los Angeles study who had sinus involvement was 17 days old at the time of biopsy. The craniofacial lesions produce swelling, deformity, and/or exophthalmos.[34]

Polyostotic fibrous dysplasia is characterized by lesions in many bones, café au lait spots in the skin, and occasionally, mental retardation. Portions of the flat bones may be expanded into tumor-like masses, whereas the long bones may be curved, shortened, and thickened.[11,32] Serum calcium and phosphorus levels are normal, but serum phosphatase levels are elevated. When the disease affects female patients, the endocrine system may be involved, and may be associated with precocious puberty. This condition is known as the McCune-Albright syndrome.

OSTEOFIBROUS DYSPLASIA

Osteofibrous dysplasia, a tumor or tumor-like condition affecting young children, is characterized by a cystic, expansile lesion associated with a mass and bowing deformity.[1,17a] The mass may be present at birth; if there is a pathologic fracture, it may cause pain.[17a] The tibia is the bone most often involved, and the ipsilateral fibula is affected in 20% of cases.[17a]

The radiologic features of osteofibrous dysplasia include a cystic, lytic lesion in the mid-diaphysis of the tibia, with expansion of the cortex and curvature (bowing). A pathologic fracture may be present. Irregular trabeculae of bone, bordered by prominent osteoblasts and surrounded by a bland-appearing fibrous stroma composed of small numbers of fibroblasts and loose fibrous connective tissue, are among the histologic findings.[1,17a]

In the newborn, the differential diagnosis of osteofibrous dysplasia includes fibrous dysplasia, myofibromatosis, and congenital fibrosarcoma. Osteofibrous dysplasia differs from fibrous dysplasia in that the latter occurs more often in older children and involves almost any bone. Moreover, microscopically, the immature bone spicules show little or no osteoblastic activity, and the surrounding stroma is more cellular in fibrous dysplasia. Patients with fibrous dysplasia have a more progressive and disfiguring bone disease. Myofibromatosis occurs in one or several different bones. On x-ray study, it is seen to consist of lytic lesions with a sclerotic rim that typically regress completely by the age of 2 years, resulting in no bone deformity. Myofibroblastic cells and a central vascular pattern with hemorrhage and necrosis are the salient histologic findings. Congenital fibrosarcoma can arise from almost any bone, forming a destructive, expansile lesion with soft tissue extension. It is a highly cellular neoplasm displaying mitotically active, atypical, spindle-shaped cells surrounded by a myxoid stroma and foci of necrosis. The tumor frequently recurs but seldom metastasizes. Amputation may be required for cure.

The clinical course of osteofibrous dysplasia is characterized by slow progression of disease and eventually, by spontaneous regression during adolescence. Following a biopsy-proven diagnosis, the recommended treatment is careful observation without surgical intervention unless the child becomes symptomatic.[1,17a]

ENCHONDROMATOSIS (OLLIER'S DISEASE)

Endochondromatosis, although rarely recognized at birth, may be identified in patients as young as 6 months of age.[11,32] It consists of multiple, cartilaginous tumors originating in the enchondral growth zone; the tumors grow within the remainder of the shaft and extend in a triangular fashion toward the diaphysis. Radiologically, these tumors appear as rarefactions in the metaphysis and the end of the diaphysis, with expansion of the cortex around the tumor.[11,34] The process is accompanied by shortening and bowing of the tumor-containing long bones and by distortion of the nearby joints. The tumors are usually unilateral and are irregularly distributed. Histologically, enchondromas are lobulated and are composed of chondrocytes displaying marked variations in cellularity, organization, calcification, and degeneration. In about one third of the adult cases, the enchondromas undergo malignant change into chondrosarcomas.[11,16a]

Unless sarcomas develop, the prognosis for affected patients is favorable. However, fractures or joint disability may be a handicap in later life.

Some cases are complicated by vascular anomalies, particularly angiomas, phlebectasia, or hemangiomas.[3,11,16a] When these vascular lesions are present, the condition is known as the Maffucci syndrome.

EWING'S SARCOMA

Ewing's sarcoma seldom occurs in infancy. It is primarily a tumor of older children and adolescents. Of the 734 patients enrolled in the Intergroup Ewing's Sarcoma Study, 3 (0.4%) were younger than 1 year of age.[26] Kim et al. reported a case of a 5½-month-old female infant with a left femoral lesion,[24] and Kozlowski et al. described a 4-month-old female infant with a rib primary.[25a] The youngest patient with this sarcoma in the Children's Hospital, Los Angeles study of 18 children in the first decade of life was a 10-month-old girl with a scapular primary.[34] This tumor occurs much more often in girls than in boys during the first 3 years of life.[25a,26]

The clinical findings in young patients with Ewing's sarcoma include pain and swelling of the affected part of several weeks' duration, occasionally accompanied by fever and leukocytosis, suggesting the diagnosis of osteomyelitis. Additionally, pathologic fracture may be a presenting sign.[25a,26,34]

On plain films or computed tomography (CT) scans, the tumor has a lytic, destructive appearance, frequently affecting a rib or flat bone. The diaphysis is the site of involvement in the long bones, such as the humerus, tibia, or femur. A soft tissue mass and layers of periosteal new bone formation ("onion skin" appearance) may or may not be present about the periphery.[25a,34] The radiographic differential diagnosis of Ewing's sarcoma in the infant includes osteomyelitis, Langerhans cell histiocytosis, and metastatic neuroblastoma. Consultation with a pediatric radiologist is requisite before rendering a final diagnosis on a biopsy of a bone lesion in this age group.

Tumor curettage or biopsy specimens are soft, mushy, and light gray, with extensive necrosis. Some are almost liquid in consistency. Ewing's sarcoma is an outstanding example of one of the small blue cell malignant tumors of infancy and childhood. Typically, the neoplasm consists of sheets or nests of small cells containing round or oval nuclei with a fine, diffuse chromatin pattern and tiny nucleoli. Periodic acid-Schiff (PAS) staining for glycogen yields positive results in about 50% of these tumors. Immunoperoxidase studies show that the cells test positive for vimentin and for cell surface antigen HBA71, and occasionally, focally express neuron-specific enolase (NSE) and S-100 protein (see Table 4–5).[18,29] The skeletal muscle markers desmin and actin are unreactive. Ultrastructural studies reveal primitive-appearing, small cells with a high nuclear:cytoplasmic ratio, sparse organelles, variable glycogen deposits, and rudimentary cell junctions. Occasionally, dense core granules and neurofilaments are noted.[18,29]

The current thinking is that Ewing's sarcoma and primitive neuroectodermal tumor (PNET) are histogenetically related, both arising from the neural crest. The two highly malignant tumors have a consistent cytogenetic abnormality, a translocation t(11;22)(q24;Q12), and a similar histologic appearance.[14,18,26,29]

According to the results of the Intergroup Ewing's Sarcoma Study, the overall survival rate for affected patients younger than 3 years of age is 56%, which is almost identical to the survival rates of the older children included in this study.[26] The treatment of patients with this malignant disease is beyond the scope of this chapter, but is discussed elsewhere.[18,26]

CONGENITAL FIBROSARCOMA

Congenital fibrosarcoma of the soft tissues is relatively common, but primary osseous fibrosarcoma in the newborn is unusual.[4,11a,32] Distinguishing between congenital fibrosarcoma and fibromatosis of bone may be difficult.[16] Dahlin maintains that the latter is less cellular and more fibrogenic in its histologic appearance than the former.[11a] Congenital fibrosarcoma is a highly cellular neoplasm composed of small spindle cells arranged in a whorling pattern with relatively little collagen. Nuclei are uniform, displaying many mitotic figures.[11a]

Bernado et al.[4] and Dahlin[11a] described rapidly growing fibrosarcomas of the femur in a 3-month-old male infant and a 9-day-old female infant, respectively; both patients eventually required amputation. Another case of congenital fibrosarcoma, this time involving the humerus, was described by Faure and colleagues.[16] This patient underwent biopsy at the age of 2 months, followed by tumor excision at 11 months, disarticulation at the shoulder at 20 months of age, and finally, 6 years later, a scapulothoracic disarticulation. The three patients just described survived following surgical resection as the main treatment, and none of them developed metastases.

MISCELLANEOUS CONDITIONS

A chordoma arising from the clivus and manifesting as a cervical and paravertebral mass in a 1-month-old male infant was reported by Coffin et al.[8] The tumor was partially resected, and the patient expired 3 weeks later with metastases to the adrenal and kidney. These pathologists concluded from their study that childhood chordomas are more variable histologically and they pursue a more aggressive clinical course than their adult counterpart.[8]

Melanotic neuroectodermal tumor should be considered in the differential diagnosis of a maxillary mass in the young.[14] (This entity is discussed in greater detail in Chapter 4, "Soft Tissue Tumors.") An unusual example of a reparative giant cell granuloma involving the base of the skull in a 4-month-old female infant was described by Cohen and Granda-Ricart.[9] The tumor eroded the squamous and petrous portions of the temporal bone, displaced the adjacent brain, and formed a mass in the retroauricular area. Cranial fasciitis has been discussed in Chapter 4, "Soft Tissue Tumors." Pedunculated odontogenic tumors, which have been treated successfully by simple excision, have also been observed in the newborn.[14]

REFERENCES

1. Anderson MJ, Townsend DR, Johnston JO, et al. Osteofibrous dysplasia in the newborn: Report of a case. J Bone Joint Surg 1993;75-A:265.

1a. Baretton G, Stehr M, Nerlich A, et al. Chest wall hamartoma in infancy: A case report with immunohistochemical analysis of various interstitial collagen types. Pediatr Pathol 1994;14:3.

2. Bartlett RC, Otis RD, Laakso AO. Multiple congenital neoplasms of soft tissues. Report of 4 cases in 1 family. Cancer 1961;14:914.

3. Bean WB. Dyschondroplasia and hemangiomata (Maffucci's syndrome). Arch Intern Med 1955;95:757.

4. Bernado L, Admella C, Lucaya J, et al. Infantile fibrosarcoma of the femur. Pediatr Pathol 1987;7:201.

5. Blumenthal BI, Capitanio MA, Queloz JM, et al. Intrathoracic mesenchymoma: Observations in two infants. Radiology 1972;104:107.

6. Chan Y-F, Lau JHK, Tong CY. Congenital generalized fibromatosis with predominant osseous involvement in a Chinese newborn. J Pediatr Orthopaed 1989;9:64.

7. Chung EB, Enzinger FM. Infantile myofibromatosis. Cancer 1981;48:1807.

8. Coffin CM, Swanson PE, Wick MR, et al. Chordoma in childhood and adolescence. A clinicopathologic analysis of 12 cases. Arch Pathol Lab Med 1993;117:927.

9. Cohen D, Granda-Ricart MC. Giant cell reparative granuloma of the base of the skull in a 4-month-old infant—CT findings. Pediatr Radiol 1993;23:319.

10. Cohen MC, Drut R, Garcia C, et al. Mesenchymal hamartoma of the chest wall: A cooperative study with review of the literature. Pediatr Pathol 1992;12:525.

11. Dahlin DC. Bone Tumors, 3rd ed. Springfield, IL: CC Thomas, 1978.

11a. Dahlin DC. Case report 189. Skeletal Radiol 1982;8:77.

12. Dehner LP. Neoplasms of the fetus and neonate. In Naeye RL, Kissane JM, Kaufman N. (eds): Perinatal Diseases, International Academy of Pathology, Monograph No. 22, p 286. Baltimore: Williams and Wilkins, 1981.

13. Dehner LP. Neuroepithelioma (primitive neuroectodermal tumor) and Ewing's sarcoma. At least a partial consensus. Arch Pathol Lab Med 1994;118:606.

14. Dehner LP. Tumors of the mandible and maxilla in children. I. Clinicopathologic study of 46 histologically benign lesions. Cancer 1973;31:364.

15. Dounies R, Chwals WJ, Lally KP, et al. Hamartomas of the chest wall in infants. Ann Thorac Surg 1994;57:868.

16. Faure C, Gruner M, Boccon-Gibod L. Case report 149. Skeletal Radiol 1981;6:208.

16a. Fechner RE, Mills SE. Tumors of the Bones and Joints, Atlas of Tumor Pathology, Third Series, Fascicle 8. Washington, DC: Armed Forces Institute of Pathology, 1991.

17. Hasegawa T, Hirose T, Seki K, et al. Solitary infantile myofibromatosis of bone: An immunohistochemical and ultrastructural study. Am J Surg Pathol 1993;17:308.

17a. Hindman BW, Bell S, Russo T, et al. Neonatal osteofibrous dysplasia: Report of two cases. Pediatr Radiol 1996;26:203.

18. Horowitz ME, DeLaney TF, Malawer MM, et al. Ewing's sarcoma family of tumors: Ewing's sarcoma of bone and soft tissue and the peripheral primitive neuroectodermal tumors. In Pizzo PA, Poplack DG (eds): Principles and Practice of Pediatric Oncology, 2nd ed, p 795. Philadelphia: JB Lippincott, 1993.

19. Inwards CY, Unni KK, Beabout JW, et al. Solitary congenital fibromatosis (infantile myofibromatosis) of bone. Am J Surg Pathol 1991;15:935.

20. Isaacs H Jr. Neoplasms in infants: A report of 265 cases. Pathol Annu 1983;18(2):165.

21. Isaacs H Jr. Perinatal (congenital and neonatal) neoplasms: A report of 110 cases. Pediatr Pathol 1985;3:165.

22. Ishiguro Y, Murahashi O, Esaki M, et al. Mesenchymal hamartoma of the chest wall in infancy: 7-year follow-up. Pediatr Surg Int 1993;8:521.

23. Jung AL, Johnson DG, Condon VR, et al. Congenital chest wall mesenchymal hamartoma. J Perinatol 1994;14:487.

24. Kim TH, Zaatari G, Atkinson GO, et al. Ewing's sarcoma of a lower extremity in an infant: A therapeutic dilemma. Cancer 1986;58:187.

25. Kindblom L-G, Angervall L. Congenital solitary fibromatosis of the skeleton: Case report of a variant of congenital generalized fibromatosis. Cancer 1978;41:636.

25a. Kozlowski K, Beluffi G, Cohen DH, et al. Primary bone tumours in infants: Short literature review and report of 10 cases. Pediatr Radiol 1985;15:359.

26. Maygarden SJ, Askin FB, Siegel GP, et al. Ewing's sarcoma of bone in infants and toddlers: A clinicopathologic report from the Intergroup Ewing's Study. Cancer 1993;71:2109.

27. McCarthy EF, Dorfman HD. Vascular and cartilaginous hamartoma of the ribs in infancy with secondary aneurysmal bone cyst formation. Am J Surg Pathol 1980;4:247.

28. McLeod RA, Dahlin DC. Hamartoma (mesenchymoma) of the chest wall in infancy. Radiology 1979;131:657.

29. Navarro S, Cavazzana AO, Llombart-Bosch A, et al. Comparison of Ewing's sarcoma of bone and peripheral neuroepithelioma. An immunocytochemical and ultrastructural analysis of two primitive neuroectodermal neoplasms. Arch Pathol Lab Med 1994;118:608.

30. Oakley RH, Carty H, Cudmore RE. Multiple benign mesenchymomata of the chest wall. Pediatr Radiol 1985;15:58.

31. Odell M, Benjamin DR. Mesenchymal hamartoma of chest wall in infancy: Natural history of two cases. Pediatr Pathol 1986;5:135.

32. Potter EL, Craig JM. Pathology of the Fetus and Infant, 3rd ed, p 177. Chicago: Year Book Medical Publishers, 1975.

33. Rosenberg HS, Stenback WA, Spjut HJ. The fibromatoses of infancy and childhood. In Rosenberg HS, Bolande RP (eds): Perspectives in Pediatric Pathology, Vol 4, p 269. Chicago: Year Book Medical Publishers, 1978.

34. Senac MO Jr, Isaacs H, Gwinn JL. Primary lesions of bone in the 1st decade of life: Retrospective survey of biopsy results. Radiology 1986;160:491.

35. Stout AP. Juvenile fibromatosis. Cancer 1954;7:953.

36. Teng P, Warden J, Cohn WL. Congenital generalized fibromatosis (renal and skeletal) with complete spontaneous remission. J Pediatr 1963;62:748.

37. Wiswell TE, Davis J, Cunningham BE, et al. Infantile myofibromatosis: The most common fibrous tumor of infancy. J Pediatr Surg 1988;23:314.

19

SALIVARY GLAND TUMORS

Primary neoplasms of the salivary glands seldom occur in infants and children. Including all age groups, less than 5% of these neoplasms are reported to occur in childhood.[4,9,11,16,21,22,27] Their incidence is even lower in the newborn, as they account for 8% or less of the total number of childhood cases.[4,11,17,23] Overall, the parotid gland is the most common primary site, being involved more frequently (10:1) than the submandibular or sublingual glands (Table 19–1).[4]

Vascular tumor-like conditions (e.g., hemangioma and lymphangioma) are more prevalent in the young than are epithelial salivary gland tumors. For example, in the Boston Children's Medical Center review, the ratio of vascular conditions to epithelial tumors was 2:1.[23] Moreover, capillary hemangioma is recognized as the leading parotid tumor in infancy, and may present as a facial mass in the neonate.[7,20,21,23,26] Kauffman and Stout reviewed 11 cases of salivary gland hemangiomas in children, all occurring in newborns.[21] These lesions were treated by excision, resulting in facial palsy in three patients. The recommended therapeutic course is a biopsy-proven diagnosis followed by careful observation, as many of these lesions regress spontaneously.[20,23] Surgery should be postponed in light of the natural history of hemangiomas.

Plexiform neurofibroma involving the major salivary glands and producing gland enlargement is sometimes found in newborns with neurofibromatosis. Even at an early age, this lesion can cause considerable disfigurement.[23]

Although sialoblastoma ("embryoma") is probably the most common epithelial salivary gland tumor,[1–3,14,23,33] pleomorphic adenoma,[8,12,13,19,24] mucoepidermoid carcinoma,[15,22] and un-

differentiated carcinoma[17,18,21] also are known to occur in the perinatal period (Fig. 19–1).

EMBRYOLOGY

The salivary glands begin as localized proliferations of cells or buds from either the ectodermal epithelium of the stomodeum (primitive mouth)—the parotid glands—or from the endoderm of the floor of the mouth—the submandibular glands—during the sixth to eighth weeks of development.[25] These buds ramify, forming solid cords that develop lumina, forming ducts. The rounded ends of the cords develop into acini (undifferentiated pluripotential cells), which differentiate into ductal cells, acinar secretory cells, and myoepithelial cells.[9] The capsule and interstitial connective tissue are derived from the surrounding mesenchyme, which is penetrated by the branching buds. The sublingual glands are seen during the eighth week as multiple buds of the endoderm in the groove between the lower jaw and tongue.[25]

SIALOBLASTOMA

The congenital salivary gland tumor initially described and termed "embryoma" by Vawter and Tefft in 1966,[33] as well as the monomorphic adenoma, congenital basal cell adenoma, basaloid adenocarcinoma, congenital hybrid basal cell adenoma, adenoid cystic carcinoma, and congenital carcinoma all share certain histologic features, namely, the presence of epithelial and myoepithelial cell components.[1–3,5,6,14,]

Table 19–1. 16 Cases of Sialoblastoma of the Newborn*

Case No.	Diagnosis	Location	Size (cm)	Associated Findings and Treatment	Status	Reference
1	Sialoblastoma	RPG	5	Excision, RT; 2 recurrences, NED	NED	Lack and Upton[23]
2	Sialoblastoma	LPG	7	Excision, RT, CT	NED	Lack and Upton[23]
3	Sialoblastoma	?	5	Excision	NED	Krolls et al.[22]
4	Sialoblastoma	LPG	9	Dystocia; excision; recurrence	DOD	Fonseca et al.[11]
5	Sialoblastoma	RSG	2	Excision	NED	Harris et al.[14]
6	Sialoblastoma	RSG	3	Excision	NED	Canalis et al.[5]
7	Sialoblastoma	PG	?	Excision	NED	Bianchi and Cudmore[4]
8	Sialoblastoma	RPG	1.5	Facial palsy; excision, CT; regional lymph node metastases	NED	Simpson et al.[28]
9	Sialoblastoma	LPG	2.5	Excision	NED	Adkins[1]
10	Sialoblastoma	LPG	15	Dystocia; excision, RT; 3 recurrences	NED	Taylor[31]
11	Sialoblastoma	RPG	2.2	Excision; recurrence	NED	Hsueh and Gonzalez-Crussi[16]
12	Sialoblastoma	LPG	5	Excision, CT, RT	NED	Vawter and Tefft[33]
13	Sialoblastoma	RPG	7	Excision, RT; 2 recurrences	NED	Vawter and Tefft[33]
14	Sialoblastoma	LPG	5	Excision	NED	Roth and Micheau[26]
15	Sialoblastoma	RPG	8	Excision	NED	Roth and Micheau[26]
16	Sialoblastoma	LPG	4.5	Excision	NED	Batsakis et al.[3]

*Selected from the literature.

RPG = right parotid gland; LPG = left parotid gland; RSG = right submandibular gland; PG = parotid gland; RT = radiotherapy; CT = chemotherapy; NED = no evidence of disease; DOD = died of disease.

[16,22,23,26,28,30–32] Currently, the preferred term for this confusing group of neoplasms is "sialoblastoma," which seems appropriate because the histologic appearance of the tumor does, in some respects, resemble the developing salivary gland.[31] Moreover, Taylor[31] and Harris and colleagues[14] argue that congenital salivary gland neoplasms arise from cells of a primitive blastema and are comparable to blastomas, originating in other organs, that have the ability to differentiate along more than one cell line (e.g., nephroblastoma or hepatoblastoma). To

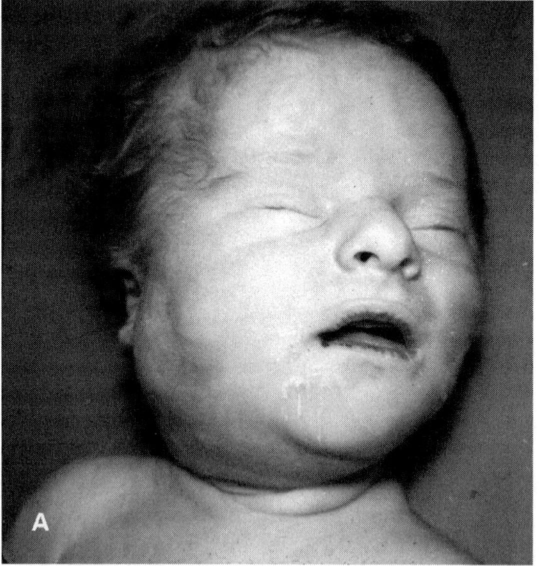
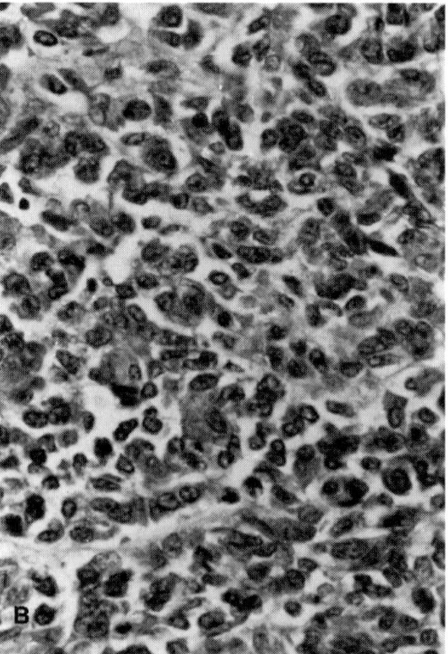

Figure 19–1. Adenocarcinoma of the submaxillary gland. *A*, A 1-day-old, 2300-g male infant presented with a large cervicofacial mass, respiratory distress, and a maternal history of polyhydramnios. *B*, The tumor consists of cells with pleomorphic, atypical nuclei and vacuolated cytoplasms. Mitoses are present. In the lower left hand corner, the tumor is forming a ductlike structure (hematoxylin-eosin, ×380). (From Pediatr Pathol 1985;3:165, Isaacs H Jr, Taylor & Francis, Inc., Washington, DC. Reproduced with permission. All rights reserved.)

date, only a few cases have been reported (see Table 19–1).

Clinically, sialoblastoma presents as an obvious facial or submandibular mass that may be noted at birth. When the parotid gland is involved, a seventh nerve facial palsy may be present. Because of its size, the tumor may be responsible for dystocia.[11,31] Of the 16 cases reviewed (see Table 19–1), 13 originated from the parotid gland and 2 from the submandibular gland; 1 site was not identified.

On gross examination, sialoblastoma varies in size, ranging from 1 cm to 15 cm in diameter, and has a tan-grey to yellow, lobulated, sometimes cystic, and focally necrotic cut surface. The tumors tend to be well circumscribed.[14,16,23,31,33] The characteristic histologic features include nodular, solid nests of epithelial cells containing small, duct-like structures surrounded by narrow bands of fibrous connective tissue.[11,14,16,33] The tumor cells are composed of round to oval nuclei with a fine chromatin pattern, one or more large nucleoli, and a pale- to amphophilic-staining cytoplasm. Small to moderate numbers of mitoses are found. Periodic acid-Schiff (PAS) staining before and after diastase digestion confirms the presence of intracytoplasmic glycogen deposits.[23]

Immunohistochemical studies show that only the ductal cells stain positively for cytokeratin, whereas both ductal cells and epithelial cells express vimentin.[11,14,16,31] The spindle-shaped myoepithelial cells situated peripherally about the epithelial cell nests stain positively with smooth muscle actin, myosin, and S-100 protein. Electron microscopy confims the immunohistochemical findings.[3,16] The cells comprising the epithelial nests contain smooth, oval nuclei, abundant endoplasmic reticulum, numerous ribosomes, and few primitive cell junctions. The ductal epithelial cells are larger, with irregular nuclei and less prominent cytoplasms containing many lysosomes and free ribosomes. Tight junctions and microvilli are present in these cells. The ductal epithelium is partially surrounded by slender myoepithelial cells with elongated nuclei, intracytoplasmic thin filaments, and replicated basement membranes.[3,16]

Lack and Upton reported two full-term newborns with parotid gland sialoblastomas ("congenital carcinomas") presenting at birth as large facial masses.[23] Both patients underwent biopsy studies, followed by an attempt at total resection. In addition, one received radiotherapy; this patient had two recurrences, at the ages of 6 and 10 months, followed by a curative resection. The other infant received irradiation and chemotherapy after a wide local excision. Both patients survived with a residual facial nerve palsy. In another case, a large congenital tumor recurred and invaded the patient's skull, but was eventually cured following additional surgery and radiotherapy.[31] In contrast, Roth and Micheau described two newborns with parotid sialoblastomas, one measuring 8 cm in diameter, who were cured by surgical resection alone without recurrence.[26]

Local recurrence (sometimes occurring three times) was noted in one third (5/16) of the patients listed in Table 19–1; regional lymph node metastases occurred in 1 patient. There was a single death from local extension by tumor. Nine of 16 newborns underwent surgical resection as the sole treatment, and 8 of these patients survived.

The findings indicate that sialoblastoma is locally aggressive, slow to metastasize, and will recur if inadequately excised. For these reasons, it should be considered and treated as a low-grade malignant disease. Surgery is the treatment of choice, with complete excision, if at all possible, undertaken at the first operative procedure. Radiation therapy and chemotherapy are probably contraindicated.[16] The long-term prognosis is favorable.

CONGENITAL PLEOMORPHIC ADENOMA (SALIVARY GLAND ANLAGE TUMOR)

The congenital pleomorphic adenoma of the nasopharynx, described initially by Har-El et al.[13] and later by Dehner and co-workers,[8,9] presents in the first 3 months of life with airway obstruction, progressive respiratory distress, and feeding problems. The manifestations of larger lesions may mimic choanal atresia because of the obstructive symptoms.

The midline, pedunculated, polypoid tumors of the nasopharynx measure 1 to 3 cm in diameter. On histologic examination, these lesions show an outer surface epithelium composed of nonkeratinized, stratified, squamous, epithelial cells; a hypocellular submucosa with duct-like structures and nests of squamous epithelium communicating with the surface mucosa; and central (mesenchymal), stroma-like nodules blending with ductules.[9]

Immunohistochemical studies performed on 9 patients in the series of Dehner et al. reveal diffuse reactivity for salivary gland amylase, cytokeratin, and epithelial membrane antigen positivity in epithelial structures, as well as reactivity with vimentin, cytokeratin, and muscle-specific actin in the stroma-like nodules.[9] According to these authors, myoepithelial cells characteristically express cytokeratin and actin. Electron microscopic findings confirm the immunohistochemical studies. Myoepithelial cells with basal lamina, desmosomes, and bundles of microfilaments are noted in the nodules, in addition to cells with epithelial features.[9]

Salivary gland anlage tumor should be distinguished from sialoblastoma, which occurs predominantly within the parotid, has a different histologic appearance, and probably represents a different stage of development of the salivary gland.[9]

Dehner et al. argue that the tumor represents a hamartoma of minor salivary gland origin and histologically recapitulates the development of the salivary gland because of the presence of the myxoid stroma with ductules and squamous nests.[9] Although potentially fatal in the neonate if left untreated, surgical excision results in cure.[8,9,13] All but one of the 9 patients reviewed by Dehner et al. survived; one patient died 6 months later from sepsis without evidence of residual tumor.[9]

MISCELLANEOUS SALIVARY GLAND TUMORS

Salivary gland neoplasms other than sialoblastoma and salivary gland anlage tumor have been recorded in the newborn.[17,21,22] Of the 34 major salivary gland tumors reviewed by Kauffman and Stout, 2 occurred in newborns, both of which were diagnosed as undifferentiated carcinoma.[21] The carcinomas were depicted as rapidly growing, inoperable tumors that were fixed to adjacent structures; the clinical course was characterized by local and distant metastases and a short survival.[21] This malignant lesion was described also in a 2300-g male newborn with a maternal history of polyhydramnios who had a large submandibular gland primary tumor that metastasized to the bones of the face and skull, as well as to the larynx, palate, regional lymph nodes, and adrenal (see Fig. 19–1).[17] Krolls et al. reported a parotid mucoepidermoid carcinoma in a 6-month-old male infant that had metastasized to the maxilla and regional lymph nodes.[22]

Unusual congenital anomalies, such as cystic choristomas of the submandibular gland composed of gut and respiratory epithelium, have been described.[29,30] Kauffman and Stout have reported a case of gastric heterotopia occurring in a cyst of the submandibular gland in an 8-month-old male infant.[21] In addition, a glial heterotopia has been reported in a submandibular salivary gland of a 2-month-old male infant.[23]

REFERENCES

1. Adkins GF. Low grade basaloid adenocarcinoma of salivary gland in childhood—The so-called hybrid basal cell adenoma–adenoid cystic carcinoma. Pathology 1990;22:187.
2. Batsakis JG, Frankenthaler R. Embryoma (sialoblastoma) of salivary glands. Ann Otol Rhinol Laryngol 1992;101:958.
3. Batsakis JG, Mackay B, Ryka AF, et al. Perinatal salivary gland tumours (embryomas). J Laryngol Otol 1988; 102:1007.
4. Bianchi A, Cudmore RE. Salivary gland tumors in children. J Pediatr Surg 1978;13:519.
5. Canalis RF, Mok MW, Fishman SM, et al. Congenital basal cell adenoma of the submandibular gland. Arch Otolaryngol 1980;106:284.
6. Coffin CM, Dehner LP. Congenital tumors. *In* Stocker JT, Dehner LP (eds): Pediatric Pathology, Vol 1, p 325. Philadelphia: JB Lippincott, 1992.
7. Dehner LP. Neoplasms of the fetus and neonate. *In* Naeye RL, Kissane JM, Kaufman N (eds): Perinatal Diseases, International Academy of Pathology, Monograph No. 22, p 286. Baltimore: Williams and Wilkins, 1981.
8. Dehner LP. Salivary gland anlage tumor (congenital pleomorphic adenoma): A clinicopathologic and immunohistochemical study (abstract). Society of Pediatric Pathology, Atlanta, GA, March, 1992.
9. Dehner LP, Valbuena L, Perez-Atayde A, et al. Salivary gland anlage tumor ("congenital pleomorphic adenoma"). A clinicopathologic, immunohistochemical and ultrastructural study of nine cases. Am J Surg Pathol 1994;18:25.
10. Donath K, Seifert G, Lentrodt J. The embryonal carcinoma of the parotid gland: A rare example of an embryonal tumor. Virchows Arch [A] 1984;403:425.
11. Fonseca I, Martins AG, Soares J. Epithelial salivary gland tumors of children and adolescents in southern Portugal. Oral Surg 1991;72:696.
12. Galich R. Salivary gland neoplasms in childhood. Arch Otolaryngol 1969;89:878.
13. Har-EL G, Zirkin HY, Tovi F, et al. Congenital pleomorphic adenoma of the nasopharynx (report of a case). J Laryngol Otol 1985;99:1281.
14. Harris MD, McKeever P, Robertson JM. Congenital tumours of the salivary gland: A case report and review. Histopathology 1990;17:155.
15. Hendrick JW. Mucoepidermoid cancer[?] in the parotid gland in a one-year-old child. Am J Surg 1964; 108:907.
16. Hsueh C, Gonzalez-Crussi F. Sialoblastoma: A case report and review of the literature on congenital epithelial tumors of salivary gland origin. Pediatr Pathol 1992;12:205.
17. Isaacs H Jr. Perinatal (congenital and neonatal) neoplasms: A report of 110 cases. Pediatr Pathol 1985;3: 165.

18. Ito M, Nakagawa A, Nakayama A, et al. Undifferentiated carcinoma of the parotid gland in a 10-month-old child. Acta Pathol Jpn 1990;40:149.
19. Jaques DA, Krolls SO, Chambers RG. Parotid tumors in children. Am J Surg 1976;132:469.
20. Karlan MS, Snyder WH. Salivary gland tumors and sialadenitis in children: Experience at Children's Hospital of Los Angeles. Calif Med 1968;108:423.
21. Kauffman SL, Stout AP. Tumors of the major salivary glands in children. Cancer 1963;16:1317.
22. Krolls SO, Trodahl JN, Boyers RC: Salivary gland lesions in children: A survey of 430 cases. Cancer 1972;30:459.
23. Lack EE, Upton MP. Histopathologic review of salivary gland tumors in childhood. Arch Otolaryngol Head Neck Surg 1988;114:898.
24. Lucas RB. Pathology of Tumours of the Oral Tissues, 4th ed, p 297. Edinburgh: Churchill Livingstone, 1984.
25. Moore, KL. The Developing Human: Clinically Oriented Embryology, 5th ed. Philadelphia: WB Saunders, 1993.
26. Roth A, Micheau C. Embryoma (or embryonal tumor) of the parotid gland: Report of two cases. Pediatr Pathol 1986;5:9.
27. Schuller DE, McCabe BF. Salivary gland neoplasms in children. Otolaryngol Clin North Am 1977;10:399.
28. Simpson PR, Rutledge JC, Schaefer SD, et al. Congenital hybrid basal cell adenoma—Adenoid cystic carcinoma of the salivary gland. Pediatr Pathol 1986;6:199.
29. Smart PJ, Lendon M. Choristoma of the submandibular gland: A rare cause of cervical swelling. J Pediatr Surg 1992;27:1498.
30. Tang TT, Glicklich M, Siegesmund KA, et al. Neonatal cystic choristoma in submandibular salivary gland simulating cystic hygroma. Arch Pathol Lab Med 1979;103:537.
31. Taylor GP. Case 6. Congenital epithelial tumor of the parotid—Sialoblastoma. Pediatr Pathol 1988;8:447.
32. Thackray AC, Lucas RB. Tumors of the major salivary glands. In Atlas of Tumor Pathology, 2nd Series, Fascicle 10, p 125. Washington, DC: Armed Forces Institute of Pathology, 1974.
33. Vawter GF, Tefft M. Congenital tumors of the parotid gland. Arch Pathol 1966;82:242.

Index

Note: Pages in *italics* indicate illustrations; those followed by t refer to tables.

ISBN 0-7216-3813-9

MAJOR PROBLEMS IN PATHOLOGY

MAJOR PROBLEMS IN PATHOLOGY (MPP) series provides current, accurate, and detailed information on specific areas of diagnostic pathology.

The volumes reflect the distilled wisdom of their authors, providing a scholarly review of the topic and practical guidance for the reader. Excellence of text, illustration, and reference are hallmarks of the series.

Now—you can preview the **MPP** volumes of your choice **FREE for 30 days!** Simply indicate your selections on the postage-paid order card…**call toll-free 1-800-545-2522** (8:30–7:00 Eastern Time)… or **FAX us FREE at 1-800-874-6418.** Be sure to mention **DM#39971.**

Become an MPP series subscriber! You'll receive each new volume in the **MPP series** as soon as it's published—1 to 3 titles per year—and save shipping costs!

If you're not completely satisfied with any volume you order through the mail or the toll-free numbers, just return the book(s) with the invoice within 30 days at no further obligation. You keep only the volumes you want. *Your satisfaction is guaranteed!*

VALUABLE ADDITIONS TO YOUR WORKING LIBRARY!

Available from your bookstore or the publisher.

Complete and mail today for a FREE 30-day preview!

☑ **YES!** Please send me the **MAJOR PROBLEMS IN PATHOLOGY** titles I've indicated below. If not completely satisfied with any volume, I may return the book(s) with the invoice within 30 days at no further obligation.

☐ W3813-9 **Tumors of the Fetus and Newborn** (*Isaacs*)

☐ W4252-7 **Perinatal Pathology, 2nd Edition** (*Wigglesworth*)

☐ W4337-X **Pathology of the Thymus and Mediastinum** (*Kornstein*)

☐ B1594-6 **Liver Biopsy Interpretation, 5th Edition** (*Scheuer & Lefkowitch*)

☐ W3298-X **Pathology of the Peripheral Nerve** (*Richardson & De Girolami*)

☐ W5136-4 **Surgical Pathology of the Lymph Nodes and Related Organs, 2nd Edition** (*Jaffe*)

☐ W4482-1 **Solid Organ Transplantation Pathology** (*Hammond*)

☐ W5263-8 **Pathology of Adrenal and Extra-Adrenal Paraganglia** (*Lack*)

☐ W6457-1 **Pathology of Incipient Neoplasia, 2nd Edition** (*Henson & Albores-Saavedra*)

☐ W6459-8 **Surgical Pathology of the Pituitary Gland** (*Lloyd*)

☐ W6462-8 **Immunomicroscopy: A Diagnostic Tool for the Surgical Pathologist, 2nd Edition** (*Taylor & Cote*)

☐ W5755-9 **Katzenstein and Askin's Surgical Pathology of Non-Neoplastic Lung Disease, 3rd Edition** (*Katzenstein*)

☐ W3232-7 **Cardiovascular Pathology** (*Virmani, Atkinson & Fenoglio*)

☐ W6192-0 **Mucosal Biopsy of the Gastrointestinal Tract, 5th Edition** (*Whitehead*)

☐ W6412-1 **The Renal Biopsy, 3rd Edition** (*Striker, Striker & D'Agati*)

☐ **SXMPP** Enroll me in the **MPP Subscriber Plan** so that I may receive future titles immediately upon publication and save shipping costs! I may preview each new volume FREE for 30 days—and keep only the volumes I want.

Name____

Address ____

City ______________________________State _____Zip________Telephone (______)____________

Staple this to your purchase order to expedite delivery. © W.B. SAUNDERS COMPANY 1997. Printed in USA. Shipping additional outside the USA.

C#14862   DM#39971